Advances in Internal Medicine®
Volume 39

Advances in Internal Medicine®

Volumes 1 through 36 (Out of Print)

Volume 37

The Current Management of the Patient With Uncomplicated Myocardial Infarction, *by Robert C. Schlant*
Cocaine Abuse, *by Scott A. Mackler and Charles P. O'Brien*
Systolic Hypertension in Older Persons, *by William B. Applegate*
Controversies in the Diagnosis and Management of Benign Prostatic Hypertrophy, *by Catherine E. DuBeau and Neil M. Resnick*
Progressive Renal Insufficiency: The Role of Angiotensin Converting Enzyme Inhibitors, *by Susan Savage and Robert W. Schrier*
Diabetic Foot Ulcers: Etiology, Treatment, and Prevention, *by Carl Grunfeld*
Management of the Complications of Human Immunodeficiency Virus Infection, *by Sharon Safrin and Paul Volberding*
The Molecular Genetics of Lung Cancer, *by David P. Carbone and John D. Minna*
Hemorrhagic Colitis Associated With *Escherichia Coli* 0157:H7, *by Mitchell B. Cohen and Ralph A. Giannella*
Non-A, Non-B Hepatitis: Impact of the Emergence of the Hepatitis C Virus, *by Patricia C. Hsia and Leonard B. Seeff*
Thyroid Dysfunction in Older Persons, *by Clark T. Sawin*
Chylomicronemia Syndrome, *by Alan Chait and John D. Brunzell*
Primary Hyperparathyroidism: Recent Advances in Pathogenesis, Diagnosis, and Management, *by Hunter Heath, III*
Autoimmunity to hsp65 and the Immunologic Paradigm, *by Irun R. Cohen*
C-Reactive Protein and the Acute Phase Response, *by Stanley P. Ballou and Irving Kushner*
Lung Biopsy, *by James P. Utz, Mark A. Perrella, and Edward C. Rosenow, III*
Balloon Valvuloplasty, *by David R. Holmes, Jr. and Rick A. Nishimura*
Diagnostic Paracentesis, *by John C. Hoefs and Gavin M. Jonas*
Coxsackievirus Myocarditis, *by Noel R. Rose, David A. Neumann, and Ahvie Herskowitz*
Parvovirus B19 and Human Disease, *by Thomas J. Török*

Volume 38

HDL and Coronary Artery Disease, *by Diane L. Tribble and Ronald M. Krauss*
Left Ventricular Mass, Diastolic Dysfunction, and Hypertension, *by John S. Gottdiener*

Advances in Internal Medicine®

Editor

Robert W. Schrier, M.D.

Professor and Chairman, Department of Medicine, University of Colorado School of Medicine; Attending Physician, Renal Division, University Hospital, University of Colorado Health Sciences Center, Denver, Colorado

Associate Editors

François M. Abboud, M.D.

Edith King Pearson Professor of Medicine, Head, Department of Internal Medicine, University of Iowa College of Medicine; Director of Cardiovascular Research Center, University of Iowa Hospitals and Clinics, Iowa City, Iowa

John D. Baxter, M.D.

Professor of Medicine, University of California; Director, Metabolic Research Unit and Chief, Division of Endocrinology, Moffitt Hospital, San Francisco, California

Anthony S. Fauci, M.D.*

Chief, Laboratory of Immunoregulation, Director, National Institute of Allergy and Infectious Diseases, National Institutes of Health, Bethesda, Maryland

*Dr. Fauci edited this book in his private capacity and no official endorsement or support by the National Institutes of Health is intended or should be inferred.

Mosby

Volume 39 • 1994

St. Louis Baltimore Boston Chicago London Madrid Philadelphia Sydney Toronto

Mosby
Dedicated to Publishing Excellence

Vice President, Continuity Publishing: Kenneth H. Killion
Sponsoring Editor: Kelly Poirier
Project Manager: Denise Dungey
Project Supervisor: Maria Nevinger
Production Editor: Laura Pelehach
Staff Support Administrator: Barbara M. Kelly

Printed in the United States of America
Composition by The Clarinda Company
Printing/binding by The Maple-Vail Book Manufacturing Group

Mosby–Year Book, Inc.
11830 Westline Industrial Drive
St. Louis, Missouri 63146

Editorial Office:
Mosby–Year Book, Inc.
200 North LaSalle Street
Chicago, Illinois 60601

International Standard Serial Number: 0065–2822
International Standard Book Number: 0–8151–83127

Contributors

William T. Abraham, M.D.

Instructor of Medicine, University of Colorado, School of Medicine, Denver, Colorado

Pamela W. Anderson, M.D.

Assistant Professor of Medicine, University of Southern California School of Medicine, Los Angeles

John H. Bloor, M.D., Ph.D.

Instructor, University of Colorado School of Medicine, Department of Medicine, Division of Gastroenterology and Hepatobiliary Research Center, Staff Physician, Denver Veterans Administration Medical Center, Department of Medicine, Division of Gastroenterology, Denver, Colorado

Vreny A. Briner, M.D.

Department of Medicine, University Hospital Bern, Bern, Switzerland

Jay N. Cohn, M.D.

Professor of Medicine, Head, Cardiovascular Division, Department of Medicine, University of Minnesota Medical School, Minneapolis, Minnesota

Pamela S. Douglas, M.D.

Charles A. Dana Research Institute, Harvard-Thorndike Laboratory of the Department of Medicine (Cardiovascular Division), Associate Professor of Medicine, Harvard Medical School, Director, Non-Invasive Cardiology, Beth Israel Hospital, Boston, Massachusetts

David P. Faxon, M.D.

Professor of Medicine, University of Southern California School of Medicine, Chief, Division of Cardiology, University of Southern California Medical Center, Los Angeles, California

Eric R. Fearon, M.D., Ph.D.

Assistant Professor of Pathology and Biology, Boyer Center for Molecular Medicine, Yale University School of Medicine, New Haven, Connecticut

Gary S. Hoffman, M.D.

Head, Vasculitis and Related Diseases Section, Laboratory of Immunoregulation, National Institute of Allergy and Infectious Diseases, National Institutes of Health, Bethesda, Maryland; Chairman, Department of Rheumatic and Immunologic Diseases, Cleveland Clinic Foundation, Cleveland, Ohio

Jay H. Hoffnagle, M.D.

Director, Division of Digestive Diseases and Nutrition, National Institute of Diabetes and Digestive and Kidney Diseases, National Institutes of Health, Bethesda, Maryland

Willa A. Hsueh, M.D.
Professor of Medicine, University of Southern California School of Medicine, Los Angeles, California

Bruce E. Johnson, M.D.
Chief, Lung Cancer Biology Section, Navy Medical Oncology Branch, National Cancer Institute, National Naval Medical Center, Bethesda, Maryland

John P. Kane, M.D., Ph.D.
Professor of Medicine, Professor of Biochemistry and Biophysics, Cardiovascular Research Institute, University of California, San Francisco, School of Medicine, San Francisco, California

Paul Katz, M.D.
Professor and Vice Chairman, Department of Medicine, Chief, Division of Rheumatology, Immunology and Allergy, Georgetown University Medical Center, Washington, D.C.

Michael J. Kelley, M.D.
Medical Staff Fellow, Navy Medical Oncology Branch, National Cancer Institute, National Naval Medical Center, Bethesda, Maryland

Spencer H. Kubo, M.D.
Associate Professor of Medicine, Director, Heart Failure—Heart Transplantation Program, Cardiovascular Division, Department of Medicine, University of Minnesota Medical School, Minneapolis, Minnesota

T.F. Lüscher, M.D.
Professor, Clinical Pharmacology, University Hospital Basel, Basel, Switzerland

Mary J. Malloy, M.D.
Clinical Professor of Medicine and Pediatrics, Cardiovascular Research Institute, University of California, San Francisco, School of Medicine, San Francisco, California

John E. Mapoles, Ph.D.
Assistant Professor, University of Colorado School of Medicine, Department of Microbiology, Hepatobiliary Research Center; Research Biologist, Denver Veterans Administration Medical Center, Denver, Colorado

Adolph Mares, Jr., M.D.
Fellow, Section of Cardiology, Baylor College of Medicine, Houston, Texas

E.R. McFadden, Jr., M.D.
Argyl J. Beams Professor of Medicine, Director, Airway Disease Center, Department of Medicine, Case Western Reserve University School of Medicine, Cleveland, Ohio

Peter Oettgen, M.D.

Charles A. Dana Research Institute, Harvard-Thorndike Laboratory of the Department of Medicine (Cardiovascular Division), Instructor of Medicine, Harvard Medical School, Codirector, Cardiovascular Health and Lipid Center, Beth Israel Hospital, Boston, Massachusetts

Allan I. Pack, M.D., Ch.B., Ph.D.

Professor of Medicine, Pulmonary and Critical Care Division, Director, Center for Sleep and Respiratory Neurobiology, University of Pennsylvania Medical Center, Philadelphia, Pennsylvania

Thomas C. Quinn, M.D.

Laboratory of Immunoregulation, National Institute of Allergy and Infectious Diseases, National Institutes of Health, Bethesda, Maryland; Division of Infectious Diseases, Johns Hopkins University School of Medicine, Baltimore, Maryland

Robert Roberts, M.D.

Professor of Medicine and Cell Biology, Chief of Cardiology, Baylor College of Medicine; Director, Bugher Foundation Center for Molecular Cardiology, Houston, Texas

Anne Rompalo, M.D.

Division of Infectious Diseases, Johns Hopkins University School of Medicine, Baltimore City Health Department, Sexually Transmitted Diseases Clinics, Baltimore, Maryland

Thomas J. Ryan, M.D.

Professor of Medicine, Evans Department of Clinical Research and Department of Medicine, Chief of Cardiology, Section of Cardiology, University Hospital, Boston University Medical Center, Boston, Massachusetts

Peter N. Schlegel, M.D.

Assistant Professor of Urology, James Buchanan Brady Foundation, Department of Urology, The New York Hospital-Cornell Medical Center, New York; Staff Scientist, The Population Council, Center for Biomedical Research, New York, New York

Steven M. Schnittman, M.D.

Chief, Medical Branch, Division of AIDS, National Institute of Allergy and Infectious Diseases, National Institutes of Health, Bethesda, Maryland

Francis R. Simon, M.D.

Professor, University of Colorado School of Medicine, Department of Medicine, Division of Gastroenterology, Director, Hepatobiliary Research Center; Staff Physician, Department of Medicine, Division of Gastroenterology, Denver Veterans Administration Medical Center, Denver, Colorado

Andrea T. Slotkoff, M.D.

Post Doctoral Fellow, Division of Rheumatology, Immunology and Allergy, Department of Medicine, Georgetown University Medical Center, Washington, D.C.

J. Blake Tyrrell, M.D.

Metabolic Research Unit, Department of Medicine, University of California, San Francisco School of Medicine, San Francisco, California

Jonathan Zenilman, M.D.

Division of Infectious Diseases, Johns Hopkins University School of Medicine, Baltimore City Health Department, Sexually Transmitted Diseases Clinics, Baltimore, Maryland

Publisher's Preface

Advances in Internal Medicine®, volume 39, marks the beginning of a new era of editorship for this publication. We at Mosby hope you will join us in welcoming Robert W. Schrier, M.D., Professor and Chairman of the Department of Medicine at the University of Colorado School of Medicine, to his new role as Editor-in-Chief along with Associate Editors, Francois Abboud, M.D., Edith King Pearson Professor of Medicine and Head of the Department of Internal Medicine at the University of Iowa College of Medicine; John D. Baxter, M.D., Professor of Medicine at the University of California; and Anthony S. Fauci, M.D., Chief of the Laboratory of Immunoregulation and Director of the National Institute of Allergy and Infectious Diseases at the National Institutes of Health.

Under the stellar leadership of Drs. Schrier, Abboud, Baxter, and Fauci, we are certain that *Advances in Internal Medicine*® will continue to provide readers with insightful, important, thought-provoking, and clinically relevant information. Again, welcome.

Mosby–Year Book, Inc.

Contents

Role of Vascular Endothelial Abnormalities in Clinical Medicine: Atherosclerosis, Hypertension, Diabetes, and Endotoxemia

Vreny A. Briner, M.D.

Department of Medicine, University Hospital Bern, Bern, Switzerland

T. F. Lüscher, M.D.

Professor, Clinical Pharmacology, University Hospital Basel, Basel, Switzerland

Vascular tone and glomerular filtration rate are highly dependent on the balance between endothelium-derived vasoactive factors to modulate contraction and relaxation in the vascular smooth muscle cell (VSMC) and the smooth muscle–like glomerular mesangial cell (GMC). In addition to their constricting and dilating properties, these substances may also modify extracellular matrix and VSMC and GMC proliferation and thus induce both functional as well as structural changes in the vessel wall and glomeruli.

Endothelium-Derived Relaxing Factors

Endothelium-dependent relaxation occurs in response to hormones, platelet-derived factors, and shear stress and is mediated, at least in part, by nitric oxide (NO) produced within endothelial cells.[1] Nitric oxide stimulates the production of cyclic 3′5′-guanosine monophosphate (cGMP) in VSMCs and GMCs (Fig 1). The constitutive NO synthase requires a rise in cytosolic-free Ca^{2+} concentration for activation.[2] In contrast, the function of the inducible NO synthase is Ca^{2+} independent. This latter enzyme is expressed in a great number of cells other than the endothelial cell (EC) after exposure to endotoxin and several cytokines.[3, 4] Stimulation of the constitutive NO synthase generates NO of pmol/L concentration, while the

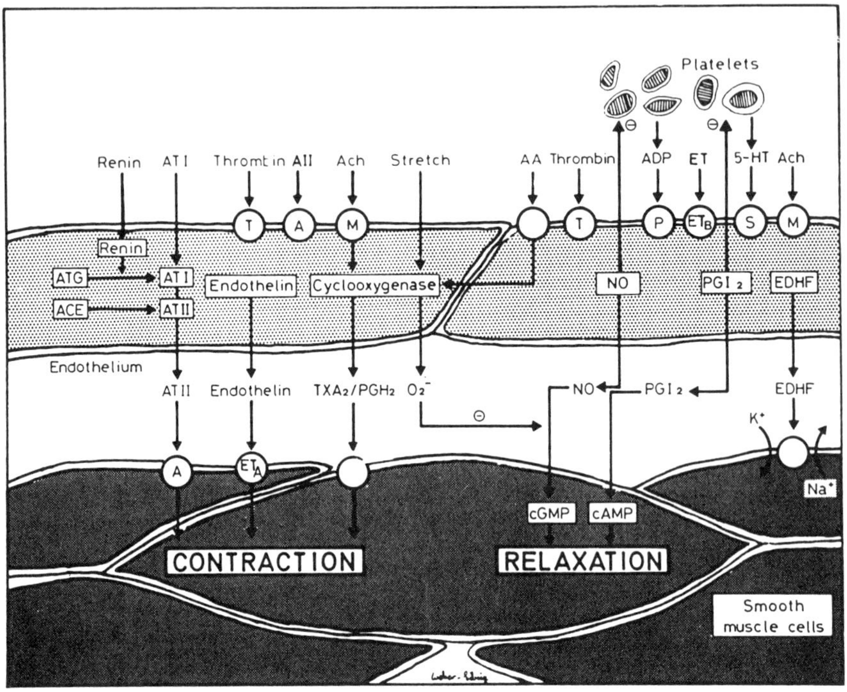

FIG 1.

Endothelium as a source of vasoactive substances. *AA* = arachidonic acid; *ACE* = angiotensin-converting enzyme; *Ach* = acetylcholine; *ADP* = adenosine diphosphate; *AT I* = angiotensin I; *AT II* =angiotensin II; *ATG* =angiotensinogen; *cGMP* = cyclic 3′5′-guanosine monophosphate; *EDCF* = endothelium-derived contracting factor; *EDRF* = endothelium-derived relaxing factor; *5-HT* = 5-hydroxytryptamine (serotonin); *PGI_2* = prostacyclin. *Round circles* represent receptors: *A* = angiotensin; H_1/H_2 = histamine; *M* = muscarinic; P_1 = purinergic; S_1 = serotonin; *T* = thrombin; *V* = vasopressin receptor. (Adapted from Lüscher TF, Bock HA, Yang Z, et al: *Kidney Int* 1991; 39:575–590. Used by permission.)

amount of NO produced after exposure to endotoxin or cytokines is much greater, i.e., in the range of nmol/L. Under physiologic conditions there is basal NO production in ECs to regulate blood flow. Indeed, the infusion of L-N^G-monomethyl arginine (L-NMMA), an inhibitor of NO synthesis, causes a rise in blood pressure, demonstrating that the circulation normally is in a continuous state of vasodilation. Nitric oxide elicits antithrombotic effects by inhibiting platelet aggregation and through local vasodilation and is released by platelet products (e.g., serotonin, adenosine diphosphate, and adenosine triphosphate).

Another endothelium-derived vasodilator is prostacyclin, a product of the cyclooxygenase pathway.[5] Its generation is induced by mechanisms similar to those that stimulate NO synthesis. Prostacyclin triggers the production of cyclic 3′5′-adenosine monophosphate (cAMP) in VSMCs and

GMCs.[5] However, the potency of cAMP to induce vascular relaxation is negligible compared to the effect of cGMP, the second messenger of NO stimulation.

Endothelium-derived hyperpolarizing factor, products of the lipoxygenase or cytochrome 450 pathway, may also contribute to VSMC and GMC relaxation; however, the significance of these effectors is less well known.

Endothelium-Derived Contracting Factors

Endothelial cells produce the peptide hormone endothelin-1 (ET-1) in response to mediators such as thrombin, transforming growth factor-β_1, angiotensin II, arginine vasopressin, cytokines, and Ca^{2+} ionophores.[1, 6] The hormone is produced as preproendothelin and cleaved into big endothelin and finally converted to the active hormone ET-1 by the endothelin-converting enzyme. At low concentrations, ET-1 exposure causes vasodilation via generation of prostacyclin and NO, and at high concentrations ET-1 induces prolonged and strong vasoconstriction via hydrolysis of membranous phospholipids and generation of second messengers, such as inositol 1,4,5-trisphosphate and diacylglycerol.[7] Circulating levels of ET-1 are low, suggesting that the release of the hormone occurs preferentially toward the contraluminal side. A number of inhibitory mechanisms exist to regulate ET-1 production and its effects, such as cGMP-dependent[8] and cAMP-dependent inhibition[9] and a yet unknown mediator produced in VSMC.[10] Activation of the cyclooxygenase pathway in ECs induces the generation of thromboxane A_2 (TxA_2), endoperoxides (prostaglandin H_2), and superoxide anions that may stimulate VSMC and GMC contraction. Superoxide anions attenuate the NO effect by accelerating its breakdown.[11] The cyclooxygenase pathway is the important source for endothelium-derived contracting factors in veins and cerebral vasculature.[1]

Taken together, the ECs play a key role in the production of vasoactive substances to maintain and regulate vascular tone and glomerular filtration rate. Endothelial cell dysfunction, therefore, is likely to alter the balance of mediators necessary to maintain homeostasis. Physical and chemical stress may affect EC function and contribute to the pathogenesis of atherosclerosis, hypertension, diabetic angiopathy, and impaired vascular function in endotoxemia. This chapter reviews the role of vascular endothelial abnormalities in these diseases.

Atherosclerosis

Morbidity and mortality in Western countries are highest from atherosclerosis and coronary artery diseases. The development of atherosclerosis is enhanced in patients with hyperlipidemia, hypercholesterolemia, hypertension, smoking habits, and diabetes mellitus. This indicates the importance of cumulative effects in the development of the disease.

The pathogenesis of atherosclerosis may be divided into three types: (1)

functional alterations of EC; (2) proliferation and migration of VSMCs in arterial intima; and (3) endothelial denudation and plaque rupture with damage to both intima and media and in turn massive platelet aggregation. All these changes result in impairment of vascular responses to vasoactive substances. Endothelial damage favors the interaction of ECs monocyte-macrophages, VSMCs, and T lymphocytes,[12] resulting in the synthesis and release of lipases, elastases, growth factors, and cytokines, which act in co-operation or antagonistically to modulate vascular tone, to stimulate intimal VSMC migration and proliferation, and to stimulate changes in matrix composition and vessel wall structure. These events result in further endothelial damage and fatty streaks and subsequently plaque formation.[13] Although functional changes of the endothelial layer may be very prominent in atherosclerosis, morphologic changes in the endothelial layer occur only in the late stage of the disease. In the central region of atherosclerotic lesions, oxidized low-density lipoprotein accumulates. Low-density lipoprotein may attract monocyte-macrophages to invade the tissue to become foam cells, which incorporate low-density lipoprotein. The significance of lipids in the development and progression of atherosclerosis is supported by the fact that in rabbits hypercholesterolemia induces functional alterations of EC and reduces endothelium-dependent relaxation in the absence of macroscopic lesions.[14] Epidemiologic studies indicate that estrogen reduces the risk of cardiovascular events through its effects to increase the high-density lipoprotein cholesterol–to–low-density protein cholesterol ratio, which may explain why premenopausal women are at lower risk of atherosclerosis and coronary heart disease than men of similar age.[15]

In established atherosclerosis in human coronary arteries, basal NO production is reduced.[16] Furthermore, endothelium-dependent relaxation to substance P, serotonin, bradykinin, and aggregating platelets is attenuated[16–19]; however, the receptor-independent (i.e., calcium ionophore A23187–induced) relaxation remains preserved until late stages of atherosclerosis.[17]

The mechanism responsible for the severe impairment of endothelium-dependent relaxation in atherosclerosis is a matter of debate. Release of biologically active NO in coronary arteries of hypercholesterolemic pigs is markedly reduced.[19] In the aorta of rabbits treated with a high cholesterol chow, the release of NO as measured by chemiluminescence, which also measures inactive products (NO_2^-, NO_3^-), is increased.[20] This latter observation suggests an increased formation of products that inactivate NO (i.e., superoxide radicals) and/or a decreased activity of superoxide dismutase. Endothelium-independent relaxation in response to nitroglycerin is decreased only in late stages of atherosclerosis[21]; the response remains preserved in morphologically normal coronaries.[22] These findings may suggest that impaired endothelium-dependent relaxation in atherosclerotic arteries is the result of impaired hormone binding or signal transmission in ECs and not an inability of VSMCs to respond to NO.

In addition to the decrease in the dilatory response of atherosclerotic

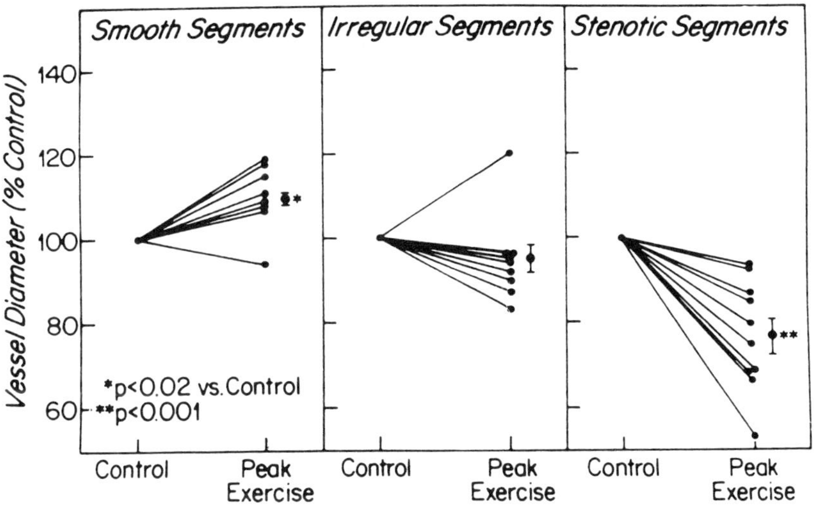

FIG 2.
Vasomotor response of smooth, irregular, and stenotic coronary arteries during exercise. All of the stenosed and all of the irregular coronary segments constricted during exercise. In contrast, all but one of the smooth segments dilated during exercise. (From Gordon JB, Ganz P, Nabel EG, et al: *J Clin Invest* 1989; 83:1946–1952. Used by permission.)

vessels, augmented responses to vasoconstrictors that may predispose to vasospasm have been observed.[23] These findings may be the result of decreased NO formation, increased ET production, and alteration in VSMC reactivity. The adhesion of platelets with subsequent increase in the concentration of vasoconstrictors such as TxA_2 and serotonin may be particularly important at the site of severe and unstable coronary artery lesions.[24] Coronary spasm provoked by the administration of histamine occurs in miniature swines only at sites of previous endothelial denudation and atherosclerosis.[25] Furthermore, acetylcholine and serotonin[26] and exercise[21] (Fig 2) may cause paradoxical constriction[125] of epicardial coronary arteries in the presence of atherosclerosis while disease-free segments dilate.

Vascular Smooth Muscle Cell Growth in the Blood Vessel

Endothelial cells may both stimulate and inhibit VSMC proliferation. Endothelial denudation leads to intimal hyperplasia, while NO and NO-generating vasodilators, prostacyclin, heparin, and transforming growth factor β_1 inhibit mitogenesis and proliferation of cultured VSMCs.[27] However, endothelial cells may also produce growth factors, such as platelet-derived growth factor and fibroblast growth factor. These contrasting endothelial effects are balanced under normal conditions. The mechanisms that disrupt the regulating cascade of growth in disease is less well known. The migratory activity of VSMCs derived from atherosclerotic plaques of human coronaries is reduced in vitro by the addition of SIN-1, a NO-generating vasodilator substance.[28] This finding may suggest that levels of NO are insufficient in the area of plaque formation, resulting in VSMC proliferation and perpetuation of the atherosclerotic process.

Hypoxia, Ischemia, and Reperfusion

In areas of stenotic coronary sclerosis, blood supply may be insufficient and result in hypoxia. Hypoxia-induced impairment of endothelium function primarily mediates the impairment of VSMC function in the canine vasculature, resulting in decreased NO production and rise in vascular tone.[29] After experimental coronary ligation and reperfusion in canine coronary arteries, thrombin-induced endothelium-dependent relaxation is impaired.[30] Similar observations of impaired arterial function in a state of deficient blood supply are found in afferent arterioles of the kidney after ischemia-induced renal failure.[31] Under these experimental conditions, bradykinin- and acetylcholine-stimulated endothelium-dependent relaxation is attenuated[31] and autoregulation of the vessel to dilate during decreases in perfusion pressor is lost.[32] Nitric oxide production is reduced. In addition, the inhibitory effect of NO on renin[33] and natriuretic peptide[34] production may decrease, thus resulting in further increase of renal vascular resistance. The NO deficiency may explain the increased sensitivity of VSMC to contracting substances and increased basal tone of the microvasculature. Hypoxia triggers the production of ET-1 by the damaged endothelium and further augments the contractile response.[35]

Severe hypoxia resulting in myocardial infarction or acute renal failure is associated with increased concentrations of circulating levels of ET-1.[36] The significance of ET in hypoxia- or anoxia-induced vascular damage is supported in experimental models. The administration of ET antibodies reduces the size of myocardial infarction and enhances glomerular filtration rate in the setting of ischemia-induced damage.[37] Hypoxia also stimulates the generation of free radicals, TxA_2, and angiotensin II.[11] All these vasoactive substances may augment ischemia-induced damage. Furthermore, in chronic renal failure an endogenous inhibitor of NO synthesis is insufficiently excreted in the urine and therefore may accumulate.[38]

Coronary Bypass Function

In patients with coronary artery disease, bypass grafts derived from the arteries demonstrate a better patency rate than do those derived from the veins.[39] In vitro pulsatile stretch stimulates proliferation of VSMCs derived from the saphenous vein, but has no effect on VSMCs derived from internal mammary artery.[40] In addition, the internal mammary artery demonstrates much more pronounced endothelium-dependent relaxation than does the saphenous vein in response to adenosine diphosphate and aggregating platelets[41, 42] (Fig 3). These differences in endothelium and VSMC function may play an important role in graft function and patency and thus in the survival of patients after coronary bypass surgery.

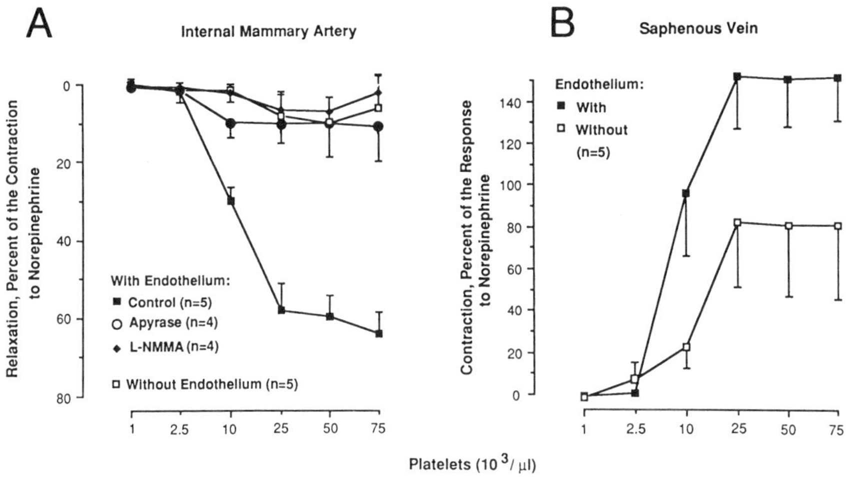

FIG 3.
Effect of aggregating platelets to induce endothelium-dependent relaxation in internal mammary artery **(A)** and saphenous vein **(B).** Aggregating platelets induced endothelium-dependent relaxation in the mammary artery. This effect was blocked by L-N^G-monomethyl arginine (L-NMMA), an inhibitor of NO production. In contrast, aggregating platelets evoked potent contraction in the saphenous vein. (Modified from Yang Z, Stultz P, von Segesser L, et al: *Lancet* 1991; 337:939–943. Used by permission.)

Hypertension

In the regulation of systemic blood pressure, endothelium-derived substances are important. The inhibition of NO generation by infusion of L-NMMA increases peripheral vascular resistance and blood pressure.[43, 44] Essential hypertension is characterized by increased vascular resistance, which results at least in part from functional and morphologic alterations of the endothelium.[45] In the forearm of patients with essential hypertension[46] and in the microcirculation and aorta of hypertensive rats,[47] endothelium-dependent relaxation to acetylcholine is blunted. In spontaneously hypertensive rats, the reduced response results from the production of a cyclooxygenase-dependent, endothelium-derived constricting factor (i.e., prostaglandin H_2),[48] while in most other forms of experimental hypertension a reduced production of endothelium-derived NO is suggested.[46,47] The inhibitory effect of NO on renin production may decrease, thereby contributing to increasing vascular resistance.[32, 33] Endothelial cells may mediate vasoconstriction not only by releasing prostaglandin H_2 but also ET-1, angiotensin II, TxA_2, and prostaglandin F_1. The concentration of ET-1 in hypertension has been reported to be increased,[49] but others have found it to be normal[50] except in the presence of arteriosclerosis and/or impairment of renal function. The circulating level, however, may not reflect the local concentration of ET-1. In addition, threshold concentrations

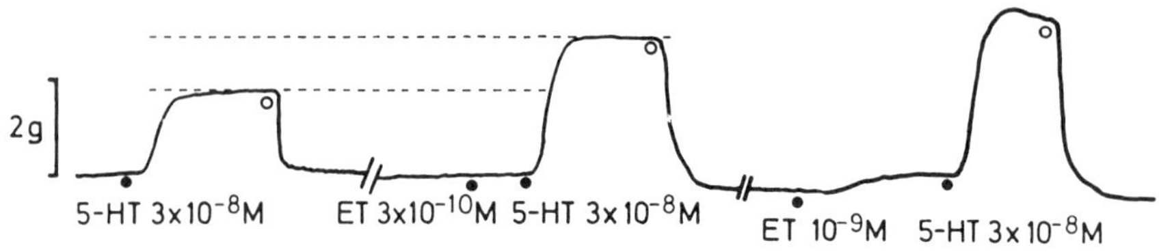

FIG 4.
Endothelin-1 potentiation of vasoconstrictor responses in human coronary arteries. In isolated rings of the left anterior descending coronary artery 5-hydroxytryptamine *(5-HT)* (serotonin)-induced contraction was potentiated by subthreshold concentrations of ET-1. (From Yang Z, Richard V, von Segesser L, et al: *Circulation* 1990; 82:188–195. Used by permission.)

of ET-1 can augment the action of other vasoconstrictors[51] (Fig 4). In addition to the impaired function of the endothelium in the presence of hypertension, the sensitivity of VSMCs to epinephrine and angiotensin II is enhanced, possibly in part due to a decreased basal NO formation.[47] Multiple abnormalities of membrane phospholipid composition and transporter systems in VSMCs may be responsible for the increased contractile response to vasoconstrictor hormones, BayK 8644, a calcium channel activator, or ouabain, a blocker of sodium-potassium exchange.[52]

Hypertension and aging result in similar morphologic changes in the arterial wall. These include intimal and medial thickening, accumulation of VSMC and macrophages within the intima, and an increase in arterial connective tissue content.[53] Both conditions stimulate focal endothelial replication, as estimated by ^{3}H-thymidine incorporation in the rat aorta,[54] and have an increased proliferative response of VSMCs to balloon-catheter injury.[55] Angiotensin II, serotonin, and norepinephrine may enhance VSMC migration and proliferation. Hypercholesterolemia may accentuate these proliferative processes further. A progressive increase in receptor number for growth factors such as platelet-derived growth factor and transforming growth factor-β_1 in the aortic tissue is also observed.[56] The coronary arteries of spontaneous hypertensive rats suggest less vulnerability to hypertensive endothelial dysfunction and aging.[57] However, interspecies and anatomic differences might exist. Taken together, these findings still provide support for the concept that hypertension may accelerate the arterial changes associated with aging.

Under physiologic conditions, endogenous vasodilators that activate adenylate cyclase, such as prostacyclin, prostaglandin E_2, and adenosine, or vasodilators that activate guanylate cyclase, such as NO and atrial natriuretic peptide, inhibit VSMC growth.[27, 28, 58, 59] Thus, ECs may regulate vascular function in the short term by controlling vascular tone and in the long term by influencing vascular structure. Impaired function of the endothelium, as may occur in hypertension, may result in enhanced VSMC growth and vascular remodeling and result in medial hypertrophy of resistance vessels. The increased muscle mass may amplify the constrictive response to vasoconstrictor hormones and thus amplify hypertension by accentuating systemic vascular resistance.

Diabetes

Early diabetes is characterized by hyperperfusion of many tissues and an increase in glomerular filtration rate.[60] These changes are the result of a diminished responsiveness of contractile cells, such as VSMCs and GMCs, to vasoconstrictor hormones[61] and loss of vascular autoregulation.[62] These changes correlate with the degree of glucose control. Vascular autoregulation in cerebral[63] and renal vasculature[64] is dependent on Ca^{2+} uptake. In diabetic patients, Ca^{2+} uptake by several tissues (e.g., cultured VSMCs and myocardial muscle) is reduced and is the result of impaired function of voltage gated Ca^{2+} channels.[65, 66] Aortas from diabetic rabbits and rats and those from normal rabbits exposed to elevated concentrations of glucose in vitro demonstrate impaired endothelium-dependent relaxation in response to acetylcholine, enhanced contractile response to norepinephrine, and augmented generation of vasoconstrictor prostanoids.[67] Impaired vasodilation in part is mediated by free radicals that are generated through the increased cyclooxygenase activity occurring in the endothelium.[68] Thus, in diabetic patients with hypertension, administration of antioxidants may cause an acute antihypertensive effect[69] (Fig 5). Although high glucose levels may stimulate ET-1 release from vascular endothelial cells in vitro, circulating ET-1 is not elevated in most diabetic patients with or without vascular complications.[70] However, high glucose or insulin exposure of cultured EC inhibits[71] and stimulates ET-1 gene expression,[72] respectively. Acute hyperinsulinemia in streptozotocin rats results in vasoconstriction, an event which may relate to the triggering of a variety of vasoactive mechanisms,[73] because it is unlikely that insulin is acting alone as a vasoactive hormone. In vitro, high glucose supplementation of culture medium results in a decrease in receptor number for vasoconstrictor hormones such as arginine vasopressin, angiotensin II in VSMCs and GMCs,[74] and ET-1 in VSMCs,[75] to diminish the contractile response to these hormones. This effect of diminishing receptor number is mediated by sustained activation of protein kinase C and reversed by inhibiting its activation or down-regulation.[74] These divergent in vivo and in vitro effects on contraction may in part result from differences in time exposure to hyperglycemia. Not only glucose but also insulin modulates contraction in VSMCs. In human coronary arteries, insulin stimulates endothelium-dependent relaxation.[76] Increased blood flow and leakage of proteins are largely prevented by inhibitors of NO.[77] However, enhanced NO synthesis is not the sole trigger mechanism of diabetic vascular complications. In vivo studies suggest that factors other than hyperglycemia and hyperinsulinemia are important for the development of diabetic nephropathy.[78]

Structural Changes in the Vessel Wall and Kidney

In cultured bovine ECs, high-glucose concentration in the culture medium increases the permeability of the monolayer by activation of protein kinase C. (For review see Mandarino LI, Schrier RW: *Diabetes Care* 1992;

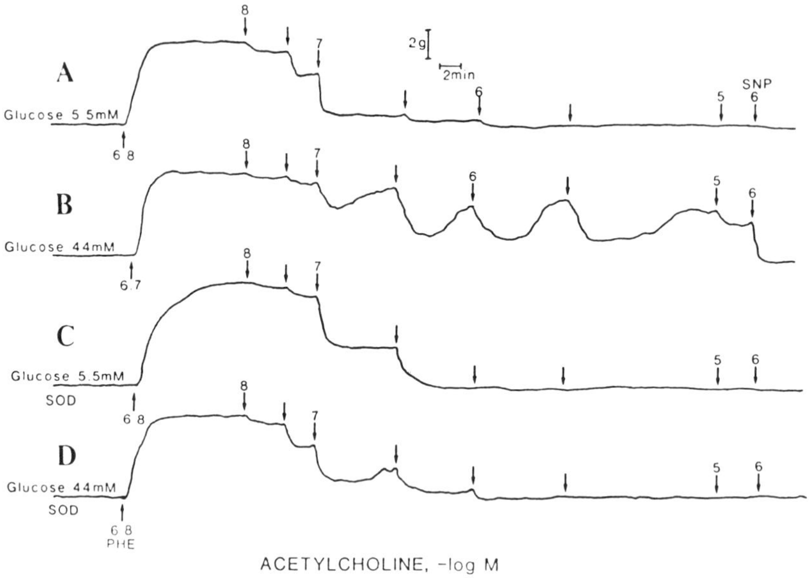

FIG 5.
Effect of high glucose exposure to impair acetylcholine-induced relaxation. Aortas incubated for 6 hours in 5.5 mM glucose showed normal relaxation in response to acetylcholine *(Ach)* **(A),** but those exposed to 44 mM glucose demonstrated impaired dilation **(B).** Nitroprusside-mediated relaxation *(SNP)* (10^{-6}M) was not altered **(B).** Treatment of aortic rings with superoxide dismutase *(SOD)* (150 U/mL) did not alter Ach effects **(C),** but prevented impaired relaxation caused by high glucose **(D).** (From Tesfamariam B, Cohen RA: *Am J Physiol* 1992; 263:H321–H326. Used by permission.)

15:1892–1901.) Protein kinase C activation may result from enhanced de novo synthesis of diacylglycerol formation from glucose, which subsequently may stimulate sustained activation of protein kinase C, a key enzyme in regulating cell function. Biochemical alteration of the basement membrane by nonenzymatic glycosylation of type IV collagen may lead to unphysiologic cross-linking. This in turn may contribute to the alteration of the barrier function of the endothelium and initiation and progression of diabetic angiopathy. In proximal tubular cells, elevated glucose stimulates transforming growth factor β_1 gene expression,[79] which stimulates extracellular matrix formation, e.g., collagen and fibronectin synthesis,[80] which may contribute to the progression of diabetic angiopathy and nephropathy. In vivo and in vitro prostaglandin production is also altered.[81] An increased production of vasodilatory prostaglandins occurs in acute exposure of cultured VSMCs and GMCs to high concentrations of glucose. Acetylcholine causes endothelium-dependent contraction in the isolated diabetic aorta.[68] This contractile response is prevented by cyclooxygenase inhibitors and the prostaglandin H_2/TxA_2 receptor antagonist SQ 29548.

Inhibition of TxA_2 synthesis has also been shown to diminish glomerular permeability to proteins and proteinuria in streptozotocin-induced diabetic rats. The relationship between enhanced glomerular TxA_2 formation and development and progression of renal disease has been shown in other experimental models of nephropathy, e.g., toxic nephritis and progressive glomerulosclerosis.[82] Inhibition of TxA_2 synthase ameliorates progressive diabetic nephropathy and prevents the increase in type IV collagen mRNA levels in diabetic mice. Once microalbuminuria has occurred, diabetic angiopathy is very likely to be present, especially in tissues demonstrating end-organ damage. Thus, the predictive mortality from cardiovascular events in diabetic patients with proteinuria is nearly 40 times, and that of diabetics without proteinuria four times, that of an age-matched population.[83]

The inhibition of angiotensin-converting enzyme slows down the progression of diabetic nephropathy, not only by affecting the angiotensin system but also by reducing blood pressure.[84] The importance of blood pressure in the development of diabetic complications is demonstrated in patients with one-sided renal or carotid artery stenosis. Unilateral renal artery stenosis prevents the development of diabetic complications, while the kidney, without arterial stenosis and therefore higher perfusion pressure, develops nephropathy. Cross-sectional studies demonstrate the presence of rising blood pressure with the development of nephropathy,[85] diabetic retinopathy,[86] and diabetic neuropathy.[87] This finding may suggest that in diabetic patients, hemodynamic- and pressure-induced damage of the microvasculature may occur despite systemic blood pressure levels within the accepted normal range.[88]

Endotoxemia

Endotoxins are lipopolysaccharides that are present in the outer membrane of gram-negative bacteria and play a pivotal role in the development of gram-negative septicemia. Despite increased activity of the adrenergic nervous system, systemic vascular resistance is decreased. Endotoxin effects are time dependent. They may be mediated by (1) the release of cytokines and other mediators, particularly from blood cells and the endothelium, to modulate vascular tone and blood clotting; (2) toxic effects resulting in morphologic alterations and changes in permeability of the endothelial layer; and (3) the induction of NO synthase in almost all cells tested so far, in particular the contractile cells such as VSMCs and GMCs.

Release of Vasoactive Substances

In septicemia, endotoxin may activate coagulation, fibrinolysis, the kallikrein-kinin system and the complement cascade.[89] The interaction of endotoxin with humoral and cellular targets, e.g., monocytes and ECs,[90] causes synthesis of a number of mediators,[91] such as metabolites of O_2,[92] interleukin (IL-1),[93] IL-4, IL-6, IL-8, tissue necrosis factor, and also tissue necrosis factor–1 and IL-1 receptors[91, 94] prostaglandins,[95] platelet-activating factor,[96] thrombin, leukotrienes, and ET-1.[97] These mediators are released and initiate and maintain functional changes in many tissues, including the cardiovasculature. However, cytokines are likely not to work individually but form a network of interacting signals with overlapping activity. These mediators may be protective of the host in one setting but may be injurious in another.

Endotoxin-Induced Cytotoxicity

In cultured ECs, endotoxin causes a time- and concentration-dependent reduction in the viability of ECs.[98] Tissue necrosis factor α and IL-1 enhance endotoxin-mediated EC injury.[92, 99] Endothelial cells of the renal medulla, glomeruli, and pulmonary microvasculature seem especially vulnerable.[100] The cytotoxic effect reaches a maximum at 24 hours and is inhibited by (1) L-NMMA, an inhibitor of NO synthesis, (2) simultaneous incubation with glucocorticoids,[101] and (3) platelet-derived growth factor.[4] The down-regulation and negative feedback of mediators and generation of natural inflammatory inhibitors, such as IL-4 and IL-8 may no longer occur in damaged endothelium. Furthermore, in the presence of endothelial damage, e.g., in the lung and kidney, endothelium-dependent vasodilators such as bradykinin or platelet-activating factor, which have increased production in endotoxemia, have the potential to become vasoconstrictors rather than vasodilators by exerting direct effects on VSMCs and GMCs (Fig 6). Endotoxin, tissue necrosis factor, platelet-activating factor, thrombin, and leukotrienes may also contribute to increase endothelial permeability, resulting in a capillary leak syndrome.[91] In sepsis and adult respiratory distress syndrome, circulating ET-1 elimination is impaired, thereby resulting in severe pulmonary vasoconstriction while peripheral vascular resistance is decreased.[102] Endothelial damage may allow new organisms to enter the bloodstream; thus, sepsis can become self-perpetuating. In an autocrine manner, IL-1 may enhance EC procoagulant activity[103] and enhance the expression of intercellular adhesion molecules (ICAM-1), thus leading to adherence of leucocytes[104] and the neutralization of cytokines. Tissue necrosis factor has multiple actions on ECs that, like those of IL-1, serve to promote coagulation and inflammation.[105] Platelet-activating factor exhibits a variety of biologic activities, including contraction of VSMCs and GMCs, increase in vascular permeability, platelet aggregation, decrease in cardiac output, and hypotension. In addition, platelet-activating factor may also cause cross desensitization and blunting of receptor-mediated effects.[106] Platelet-activating factor, IL-1, tissue necrosis factor, and endotoxin induce similar metabolic responses.[91] In the microenvironment, the beneficial effects of these mediators probably outweigh the negative effects. However, if the infection is not brought under control, endotoxin and these mediators may leak into the circulation and trigger systemic responses.

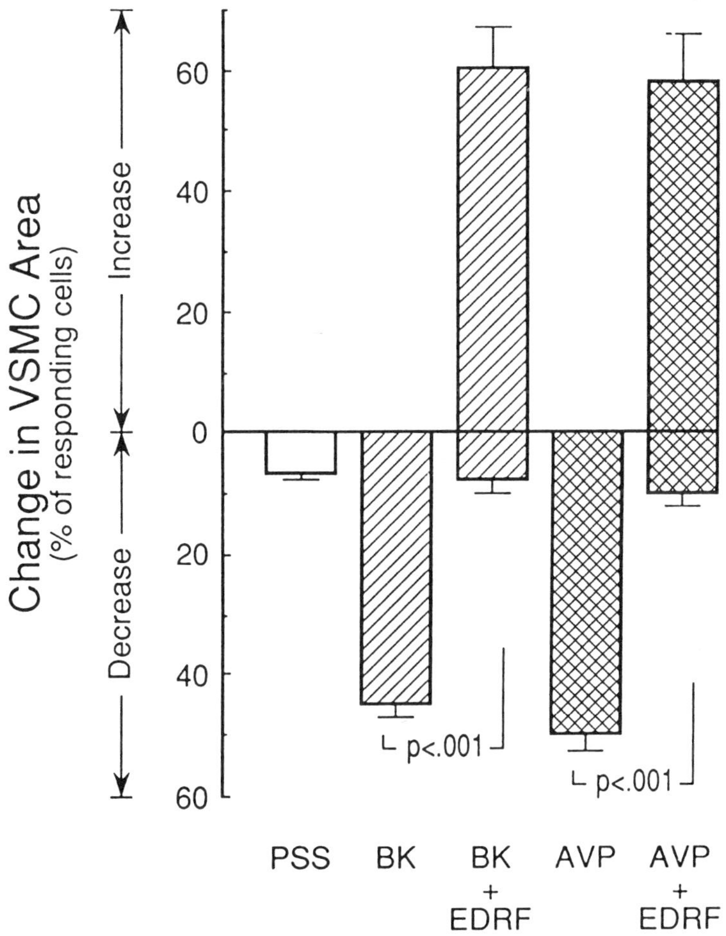

FIG 6.
Effect of endothelium-derived supernatant *(EDRF)* after bradykinin *(BK)* stimulation to reverse BK- and arginine vasopressin *(AVP)*–induced contractile response in vascular smooth muscle cells *(VSMC)*. Exposure of VSMC to BK or AVP induced a significant decrease in their area by more than 10%. In the presence of BK-stimulated endothelial-derived supernatant, VSMC area increased with BK, AVP, and physiologic saline solution. (From Briner VA, Tsai P, Schrier RW: *Am J Physiol* 1993; 264:F322–F327. Used by permission.)

Effects of Endotoxin Exposure via Different NO Synthases

Volunteers treated with a single injection of endotoxin demonstrate hyporeactivity to vasoconstrictors such as norepinephrine and angiotensin II.[107] In the rat, vascular responsiveness to norepinephrine is restored by inhibitors of the L-arginine–NO pathway and cyclooxygenase inhibition[108, 109] or B4148, a bradykinin receptor blocker.[95] These observations suggest that NO derived from stimulation of the constitutive NO synthase, prostaglandin E_2 formation, and activation of the kallikrein-kinin system are important in hypotension occurring immediately after endotoxin injection. The administration of L-arginine, the precursor of NO, exacerbates endotoxin-induced hypotension.[109] The acute endotoxin effect to cause vasodilation is endothelium-dependent[110, 113]; however, endothelium-denuded vessels demonstrate unaltered contractile response. In another experimental setting, endotoxin infusion impairs flow-, bradykinin-, and acetylcholine-induced vasodilation. This endotoxin effect is antagonized by L-arginine, suggesting that this form of arteriolar dysfunction is the result of diminished release of endothelium-derived relaxing factor.[111] These findings of acute endotoxin exposure suggest direct toxic effects on endothelium-dependent vasodilation and thus endotoxin-induced impairment of EC function.

Prolonged more than 1- or 2-hour exposure to endotoxin impairs both vasodilation and contractile response[95, 112, 113] (Fig 7). The endothelium-dependent action of endotoxin is expressed earlier than the effect on smooth muscle.[113, 114] In vitro studies suggest diminished activity of Ca^{2+} channels, and thus reduced Ca^{2+} uptake, on exposure to vasoconstrictors or depolarization and impaired contractile response.[110] Furthermore, α_1-adrenergic receptor number is down-regulated in septicemia, which results in diminished vasoconstriction on exposure to an agonist.[115] In addition, prolonged exposure to endotoxin and cytokines such as IL-1 and tissue necrosis factor, initiates the transcription of the gene for the inducible NO synthase, which in turn results in the appearance of this distinct enzyme in the blood vessel, myocardium, and glomeruli.[4, 114]

The activity of the inducible NO synthase does not depend on Ca^{2+} and is also independent of endothelial function. Once the enzyme has been induced, it will produce NO continuously for the lifetime of the enzyme, resulting in a persistent stimulation of guanylate cyclase and increased production of cGMP. Characteristic features to induce this effect are the lag period of about 2 to 3 hours and the requirement of new protein synthesis.

The induction can be substantially inhibited by simultaneous administration of platelet-derived growth factor[4] and glucocorticoids.[101] The preventive effect of steroids requires early administration after endotoxin exposure; later applications are ineffective. Once the induction process of the enzyme has been triggered by endotoxin or cytokines, glucocorticoids are of no benefit.

In addition to enhanced vasodilation by increased cGMP, both IL-1 and tissue necrosis factor stimulate the production of vasodilatory prostaglandin E_2.[116]

Implications for Treatment

Treatment of septic shock with antibodies that block endotoxins is of limited benefit because of the antibodies' lack of effect on endotoxin-induced

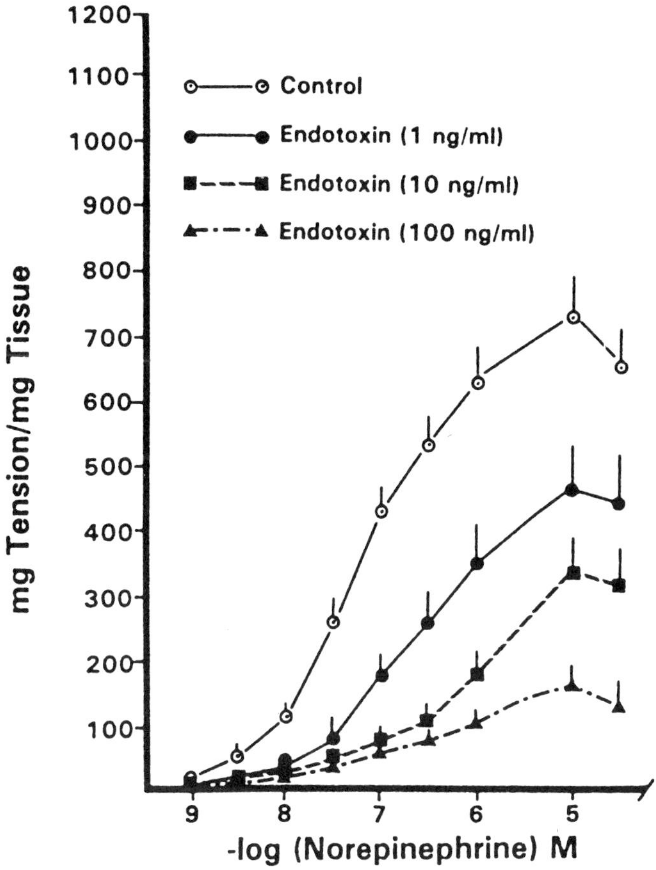

FIG 7.
Endotoxin inhibition of noradrenaline-stimulated contraction. Rat aortic rings incubated for 16 hours with control medium or medium supplemented with 1, 10, or 100 ng/mL of endotoxin demonstrated dose-dependent inhibition of maximal contraction in response to noradrenaline. (From McKenna TM: *J Clin Invest* 1990; 86:160–168. Used by permission.)

mediators and cytokines that, once produced, maintain the vascular effects. Other targets for treating septicemia include neutralizing antibodies to the complement C5a, leukotriene, platelet-activating factor,[117] ECAM-1, and IL-1. Anti–tissue necrosis factor antibodies prevent septic shock during lethal bacteremia.[118] The IL-1 receptor antagonist,[119, 120] a naturally occurring antagonist,[121] anti–IL-6 antibody,[122] and soluble IL-1 and tissue necrosis factor receptors, which bind their respective cytokine, may ameliorate the disease. The acute increase in renal vascular resistance and decrease in glomerular filtration rate are prevented by early inhibition of TxA_2 synthesis in a rat model of endotoxin-induced acute renal failure.[123, 124] Despite these favorable results in the treatment of experimental sepsis, results in humans seem less favorable. The diagnosis of sepsis and initiation of therapy is probably late and endotoxin has triggered the production of a great number of vasoactive substances. At that point it is not very likely that inhibition of one of the many mediators may stop the self-perpetuating process of septicemia.

References

1. Lüscher TF, Vanhoutte PM: *The Endothelium-Modulator of Cardiovascular Function.* Boca Raton, FL, CRC Press, 1990.
2. Bredt DS, Snyder SH: Isolation of nitric oxide synthase, a calmodulin-requiring enzyme. *Proc Natl Acad Sci USA* 1990; 87:682–685.
3. Rees DD, Cellek S, Palmer RMJ, et al: Dexamethasone prevents the induction by endotoxin of a nitric oxide synthase and the associated effects on vascular tone: An insight into endotoxin shock. *Biochem Biophys Res Commun* 1990; 173:541–547.
4. Pfeilschifter J: Platelet-derived growth factor inhibits cytokine induction of nitric oxide synthase in rat glomerular mesangial cells. *Eur J Pharmacol* 1991; 208:339–340.
5. Moncada S, Vane JR: Pharmacology and endogenous release of prostaglandin endoperoxides, thromboxane A_2 and prostacyclin. *Pharmacol Rev* 1979; 30:293–331.
6. Yanagisawa M, Kurihara H, Kimura S, et al: A novel potent vasoconstrictor peptide produced by vascular endothelial cells. *Nature* 1988; 332:411–415.
7. Lüscher TF, Yang Z, Tschudi M, et al: Interaction between endothelin-1 and endothelium-derived relaxing factor in human arteries and veins. *Circ Res* 1990; 66:1088–1094.
8. Boulanger C, Lüscher TF: Release of endothelin from the porcine aorta: Inhibition by endothelium-derived nitric oxide. *J Clin Invest* 1990; 85:587–590.
9. Yokokawa K, Kohno M, Yasunari K, et al: Endothelin-3 regulates endothelin-1 production in cultured human endothelial cells. *Hypertension* 1991; 18:304–315.
10. Stewart DJ, Langleben D, Cernacek P, et al: Endothelin release is inhibited by coculture of endothelial cells with cells of vascular media. *Am J Physiol* 1990; 259:H1928–H1932.
11. Katusic ZS, Vanhoutte PM: Superoxide anion is an endothelium-derived contracting factor. *Am J Physiol* 1989; 257:H33–H37.
12. Libby O, Hansson GK: Involvement of the immune system in human atherogenesis: Current knowledge and unanswered questions. *Lab Invest* 1991; 64:5–12.
13. Fagiotto A, Ross R: Studies of hypercholesterolemia in the non-human primate. II: Fatty streak conversion to fibrous plaques. *Arteriosclerosis* 1984; 4:341–356.
14. Jayakody L, Kappagoda T, Senaratne MPJ, et al: Impairment of endothelium-dependent relaxation: An early marker for atherosclerosis in the rabbit. *Br J Pharmacol* 1988; 94:335–346.
15. Godsland IF, Wynn V, Crook D, et al: Sex, plasma lipoproteins, and athero-

sclerosis: Prevailing assumptions and outstanding questions. *Am Heart J* 1987; 11:1467–1503.
16. Chester AH, O'Neil GS, Moncada S, et al: Low basal and stimulated release of nitric oxide in atherosclerotic epicardial coronary arteries. *Lancet* 1990; 336:897–900.
17. Bossaller C, Habib GB, Yamamoto H, et al: Impaired muscarinic endothelium-dependent relaxation and cyclic guanosine 5′-monophosphate formation in atherosclerotic human coronary artery and rabbit aorta. *J Clin Invest* 1987; 79:170–174.
18. Berkenboom G, Depierreux M, Fontaine J: The influence of atherosclerosis on the mechanical response of human isolated coronary arteries to substance P, isoprenaline and noradrenaline. *Br J Pharmacol* 1987; 92:113–120.
19. Shimokawa H, Vanhoutte PM: Impaired endothelium-dependent relaxation to aggregating platelets and related vasoactive substances in porcine coronary arteries in hypercholesterolemia and atherosclerosis. *Circ Res* 1989; 64:900–914.
20. Minor RL Jr, Myers PR, Guerra R Jr, et al: Diet-induced atherosclerosis increases the release of nitrogen oxides from rabbit aorta. *J Clin Invest* 1990; 86:2109–2116.
21. Gordon JB, Ganz P, Nabel EG, et al: Atherosclerosis influences the vasomotor response of epicardial coronary arteries to exercise. *J Clin Invest* 1989; 83:1946–1952.
22. Verbeuren TJ, Jordaens FH, Zonnekeyn LL, et al: Effects of hypercholesterolemia on vascular reactivity in the rabbit. *Circ Res* 1986; 58:552–564.
23. Heistadt DD, Armstrong ML, Marcus ML, et al: Augmented responses to vasoconstrictor stimuli in hypercholesterolemic and atherosclerotic monkeys. *Circ Res* 1984; 54:711–718.
24. Schmitz JM, Apprill PG, Buja LM, et al: Vascular prostaglandin and thromboxane production in a canine model of myocardial ischemia. *Circ Res* 1985; 57:223–231.
25. Shimokawa H, Tomoike H, Nabeyama S, et al: Coronary artery spasm induced in atherosclerotic miniature swine. *Science* 1983; 221:560–562.
26. Ludmer PL, Selwyn AP, Shook TL, et al: Paradoxical vasoconstriction induced by acetylcholine in atherosclerotic coronary arteries. *N Engl J Med* 1986; 315:1046–1051.
27. Garg UC, Hassid A: Nitric oxide-generating vasodilators and 8-bromo-cyclic guanosine monophosphate inhibit mitogenesis and proliferation of cultured vascular smooth muscle cells. *J Clin Invest* 1989; 83:1774–1777.
28. Bauriedel G, Windstetter U, Ganesh S, et al: SIN-1 decreases migratory activity of smooth muscle cells cultivated from human coronary plaques (abstract). *Eur J Clin Invest* 1991; 21:53.
29. Rubanyi GM, Vanhoutte PM: Hypoxia releases a vasoconstrictor substance from canine vascular endothelium. *Am J Physiol* 1985; 364:45–56.
30. Ku DD: Coronary vascular reactivity after acute myocardial infarction. *Science* 1982; 218:576–578.
31. Conger JD, Robinette JB, Schrier RW: Smooth muscle calcium and endothelium-derived relaxing factor in the abnormal vascular response of acute renal failure. *J Clin Invest* 1988; 82:532–537.
32. Kelleher SP, Robinette JB, Conger JD: Sympathetic nervous system in the loss of autoregulation in acute renal failure. *Am J Physiol* 1984; 246:379–386.

33. Vidal MJ, Romero JC, Vanhoutte PM: Endothelium-derived relaxing factor inhibits renin release. *Eur J Pharmacol* 1988; 149:401–402.
34. Sanchez-Ferrer CF, Burnett JC, Lorenz RR, et al: Possible modulation of release of atrial natriuretic factor by endothelium derived relaxing factor. *Am J Physiol* 1990; 259:H982–H986.
35. Rakugi H, Tabuchi Y, Nakamaru M, et al: Evidence for endothelin-1 release from resistance vessels of rats in response to hypoxia. *Biochem Biophys Res Commun* 1990; 169:973–977.
36. Miyuauchi T, Yanagisawa M, Tomizawa T, et al: Increased plasma concentrations of endothelin-1 and big endothelin-1 in acute myocardial infarction. *Lancet* 1989; 2:53–54.
37. Kon V, Yoshioka T, Fogo A, et al: Glomerular actions of endothelin in vivo. *J Clin Invest* 1989; 83:1762–1767.
38. Vallance P, Leone A, Calver A, et al: Accumulation of an endogenous inhibitor of nitric oxide synthesis in chronic renal failure. *Lancet* 1992; 339:572–575.
39. Loop FD, Lytle BW, Cosgrove DM, et al: Influence of the internal mammary-artery graft on 10-year survival and other cardiac events. *N Engl J Med* 1986; 314:1–6.
40. Predel HG, Yang Z, von Segesser L, et al: Implications of pulsatile stretch on growth of saphenous vein and mammary artery smooth muscle. *Lancet* 1992; 340:878–879.
41. Lüscher TF, Diederich D, Siebenmann R, et al: Difference between endothelium-dependent relaxations in arterial and in venous coronary bypass grafts. *N Engl J Med* 1988; 319:462–467.
42. Yang Z, Stulz P, von Segesser L, et al: Different interactions of platelets with arterial and venous coronary bypass vessels. *Lancet* 1991; 337:939–943.
43. Rees DD, Palmer RMJ, Moncada S: The role of endothelium-derived nitric oxide in the regulation of blood pressure. *Proc Natl Acad Sci USA* 1989; 86:3375–3378.
44. Romero JC, Lahera V, Salom MG, et al: Role of the endothelium-dependent relaxing factor nitric oxide on renal function. *J Am Soc Nephrol* 1991; 2:1371–1387.
45. Panza JA, Quyyumi AA, Brush JE, et al: Abnormal endothelium-dependent vascular relaxation in patients with essential hypertension. *N Engl J Med* 1990; 323:22–27.
46. Linder L, Kiowski W, Bühler FR, et al: Indirect evidence for release of endothelium-derived relaxing factor in human forearm circulation in vivo: Blunted response in essential hypertension. *Circulation* 1990; 81:1762–1767.
47. Dohi Y, Thiel MA, Bühler FR, et al: Activation of endothelial L-arginine pathway in resistance arteries. *Hypertension* 1990; 16:170–179.
48. Kato T, Iwana Y, Okumura K, et al: Prostaglandin H_2 may be the endothelium-derived contracting factor released by acetylcholine in the aorta of the rat. *Hypertension* 1990; 15:475–482.
49. Shichiri M, Hirata Y, Ando K, et al: Plasma endothelin levels in hypertension and chronic renal failure. *Hypertension* 1990; 15:493–496.
50. Davenport AP, Ashby MJ, Easton P, et al: A sensitive radioimmunoassay measuiring endothelin-like immunoreactivity in human plasma: Comparison of levels in patients with essential hypertension and normotensive control subjects. *Clin Sci* 1990; 78:261–264.

51. Yang Z, Richard V, von Segesser L, et al: Threshold concentrations of endothelin-1 potentiate contractions to norepinephrine and serotonin in human arteries: A new mechanism of vasospasm? *Circulation* 1990; 82:188–195.
52. Storm DS, Turla MB, Todd KM, et al: Calcium and contractile response to phorbol ester and the calcium channel agonist Bay K 8644, in arteries from hypertensive rats. *Am J Hypertens* 1990; 3:245S–248S.
53. Wolinsky H: Long-term effects of hypertension on the rat aortic wall and their relation to concurrent aging changes: Morphologic and chemical studies. *Circ Res* 1972; 30:301–309.
54. Haudenschild CC, Prescott MF, Chobanian AV: Aortic endothelial and subendothelial cells in experimental hypertension and aging. *Hypertension* 1981; 3(suppl):I148–I153.
55. Berkenboom G, Depierreux M, Fontaine J: The influence of atherosclerosis on the mechanical response of human isolated coronary arteries to substance P, isoprenaline and noradrenaline. *Br J Pharmacol* 1987; 92:113–120.
56. Sarzani R, Arnaldi G, Takasaki I, et al: Effects of hypertension and aging on platelet-derived growth factor and platelet-derived growth factor receptor expression in rat aorta and heart. *Hypertension* 1991; 18(suppl):III93–III99.
57. Tschudi MR, Criscione L, Lüscher TF: Effect of age and hypertension on endothelial function of rat coronary arteries. *J Hypertens* (suppl.) 1991; 9:5164–5165.
58. Bell L, Madri JA: Effect of platelet factors on migration of cultured bovine aortic endothelial and smooth muscle cells. *Circ Res* 1989; 65:1057–1065.
59. Jonzon B, Nilsson J, Fredholm BB: Adenosine receptor-mediated changes in cyclic AMP production and DNA synthesis in cultured arterial smooth muscle cells. *J Cell Physiol* 1985; 124:451–456.
60. Fajans SS, Lernmark A, Nerup J, et al: Diabetes mellitus, in DeGroot LJ (ed): *Endocrinology,* Philadelphia, WB Saunders, 1989, pp 1346–1542.
61. Ballerman BJ, Skorecki KL, Brenner BM: Reduced glomerular angiotensin II receptor density in early diabetes mellitus in the rat. *Am J Physiol* 1984; 247:F110–F116.
62. Sullivan Sparkes HV: Diminished contractile response of aorta from diabetic rat. *Am J Physiol* 1980; 239:E412–E421.
63. Bentsen N, Larsen B, Lassen NA: Chronically impaired autoregulation of cerebral blood flow in long-term diabetics. *Stroke* 1975; 6:497–502.
64. Mauer MS, Brown DM, Steffes MW, et al: Studies of renal autoregulation in pancreatectomized and streptozotocin diabetic rats. *Kidney Int* 1990; 37:909–917.
65. Lechuga E, Williams B, Schrier RW: Effect of elevated extracellular glucose concentrations on transmembrane calcium ion fluxes in cultured rat vascular smooth muscle cells. *J Am Soc Nephrol* 1990; 1:634.
66. Bielefeld DR, Pace CS, Boshell BR: Altered sensitivity of chronic diabetic hearts to calcium. *Am J Physiol* 1983; 245:E560–E567.
67. Abebe W, MacLeon KM: Protein kinase C-mediated contractile responses of arteries from diabetic rats. *Br J Pharmacol* 1990; 101:465–471.
68. Tesfamariam B, Cohen RA: Free radicals mediated endothelial cell dysfunction caused by glucose. *Am J Physiol* 1992; 263:H321–H326.
69. Ceriello A, Giugliano D, Quatraro A, et al: Anti-oxidants show an anti-hypertensive effect in diabetic and hypertensive subjects. *Clin Sci* 1991; 81:739–742.

70. Kanno K, Hirata Y, Shichiri M, et al: Plasma endothelin-1 levels in patients with diabetes mellitus with or without vascular complication. *J Cardiovasc Pharmacol* 1991; 17 (suppl 7):S475–S476.
71. Oliver FJ, de la Rubia G, Feener EP, et al: Stimulation of endothelin-1 gene expression by insulin in endothelial cells. *J Biol Chem* 1991; 266:23251–23256.
72. Hattori Y, Kasai K, Nakamura T, et al: Effect of glucose and insulin on immunoreactive endothelin-1 release from cultured porcine endothelial cells. *Metabolism* 1991; 40:165–169.
73. Tucker BJ, Anderson CM, Thies RS, et al: Glomerular hemodynamic alterations during acute hyperinsulinemia in normal and diabetic rats. *Kidney Int* 1992; 42:1160–1168.
74. Williams B, Tsai P, Schrier RW: Angiotension II and arginine vaopression receptor desensitization in rat vascular smooth muscle cell due to glucose activated protein kinase C. *J Am Soc Nephrol* 1990; 1:483.
75. Awazu M, Parker RE, Harvie BR, et al: Down-regulation of endothelin-1 receptors by protein kinase C in streptozotocin diabetic rats. *J Cardiovasc Pharmacol* 1991; (suppl 7):S500–S502.
76. Thom S, Hughs A, Sever PS: Endothelium dependent responses in human arteries, in Vanhoutte PM (ed): *Relaxing and Contracting Factors. Biological and Clinical Research.* Clifton, NJ, Humana Press, 1988, pp 511–528.
77. Corbett JA, Tilton RG, Chang K, et al: Aminoguanidine, a novel inhibitor of nitric oxide formation, prevents diabetic vascular dysfunction. *Diabetes* 1992; 41:552–556.
78. Zatz R, Dunn BR, Meyer TW, et al: Prevention of diabetic glomerulopathy by pharmacological amelioration of glomerular capillary hypertension. *J Clin Invest* 1986; 77:1925–1930.
79. Rocco MV, Chen Y, Goldfarb S, et al: Elevated glucose stimulates TGF-β gene expression and bioactivity in proximal tubule. *Kidney Int* 1992; 41:107–114.
80. Roberts AB, Sporn MB: Transforming growth factor β. *Adv Cancer Res* 1988; 51:107–145.
81. Gerrard JM, Stuart MJ, Rao GHR, et al: Alteration in the balance of prostaglandin and thromboxane synthesis in diabetic rats. *J Lab Clin Med* 1980; 95:950–954.
82. Remuzzi G, FitzGerald GA, Patrono C: Thromboxane synthesis and action within the kidney. *Kidney Int* 1992; 41:1483–1493.
83. Borch-Johnson K, Kreiner S: Proteinuria: Value as a predictor of cardiovascular mortality in insulin dependent diabetes mellitus. *Br Med J* 1987; 294:1651–1654.
84. Taguma Y, Kitamoto Y, Futaki G, et al: Effect of captopril on heavy proteinuria in azotemic diabetics. *N Engl J Med* 1985; 13:1617–1620.
85. Morgens CE: Long term antihypertensive treatment inhibiting the progression of diabetic nephropathy. *Br Med J* 1982; 285:685–688.
86. Parving HH, Hommel E, Mathiesen E, et al: Prevalence of microalbuminuria, arterial hypertension, retinopathy and neuropathy in patients with insulin dependent diabetes. *Br Med J* 1988; 296:156–160.
87. Epidemiological correlates of diabetic neuropathy. Report from the Pittsburgh Epidemiology of Diabetic Complication Study. *Diabetes* 1989; 38:1456–1461.

88. Zatz R, Meyer TW, Rennke HG, et al: Predominance of hemodynamic rather than metabolic factors in the pathogenesis of diabetic glomerulopathy. *Proc Natl Acad Sci USA* 1985; 82:5963–5967.
89. Badr KF, Kelley VE, Brenner BM: Selective antagonism of thromboxane A2 and sulfidopeptide leukotrienes ameliorates endotoxin-induced renal ischemia (abstract). *Kidney Int* 1985; 27:22.
90. Libby P, Ordovas JM, Auger KR, et al: Endotoxin and tumor necrosis factor induce interleukin 1 gene expression in adult human vascular endothelial cells. *Am J Pathol* 1986; 125:179–185.
91. Bone RC: The pathogenesis of sepsis. *Ann Intern Med* 1991; 115:457–469.
92. Brigham KL, Meyrick B, Berry LC, et al: Antioxidants protect cultured bovine lung endothelial cells from injury by endotoxin. *Am J Physiol* 1987; 63:840–850.
93. Miossec P, Cavender D, Ziff M: Production of interleukin 1 by human endothelial cells. *J Immunol* 1986; 136:2486–2491.
94. Spinas GA, Keller U, Brockhaus M: Release of soluble receptors for tumour necrosis factor (TNF) in relation to circulating TNF during experimental endotoxemia. *J Clin Invest* 1992; 90:533–536.
95. Suttorp N, Seeger W, Uhl J, et al: Pseudomonas aeruginosa cytotoxin stimulates prostacyclin production in cultured endothelial cells: Membrane attack and calcium influx. *J Cell Physiol* 1985; 123:64–72.
96. Camussi G, Aglietta M, Malavasi F, et al: The release of platelet activating-factor from human endothelial cells in culture. *J Immunol* 1983; 131:2397–2403.
97. Sugiura M, Inagami T, Kon V: Endotoxin stimulates endothelin-release in vivo and in vitro as determined by radioimmunoassay. *Biochem Biophys Res Commun* 1989; 161:1220–1227.
98. Salvemini D, Korbut R, Anggard E, et al: Immediate release of a nitric oxide-like factor from bovine aortic endothelial cells by *Escherichia coli* lipopolysaccharide. *Proc Natl Acad Sci USA* 1990; 87:2593–2597.
99. Sharma SA, Olchowy TW, Breider MA: Tumor necrosis factor alpha and interleukin 1 alpha enhances lipopolysaccharide-mediated bovine endothelial cell injury. *J Leukoc Biol* 1992; 51:579–585.
100. Kikeri D, Pennell JP, Hwantg KH, et al: Endotoxemia acute renal failure in awake rat. *Am J Physiol* 1986; 250:F1098–F1106.
101. Palmer RMJ, Bridge L, Foxwell NA, et al: The role of nitric oxide in endothelial cell damage and its inhibition by glucocorticoids. *Br J Pharmacol* 1992; 105:11–12.
102. Druml W, Wagner O, Gasic S, et al: Pulmonary endothelin-1 handling in lung failure (abstract 45P). *J Am Soc Nephrol* 1992; 3:435.
103. Bevilacqua MP, Pober JS, Majeau GR, et al: Interleukin-1 induces biosynthesis and cell surface expression of procoagulant activity on human vascular endothelial cells. *J Exp Med* 1984; 160:618–623.
104. Dejana E, Brevario F, Erroi A, et al: Modulation of endothelial cell function by different molecular species of interleukin-1. *Blood* 1987; 69:695–699.
105. Pober JS, Cotran RS: Cytokines and endothelial biology. *Physiol Rev* 1990; 70:427–451.
106. Schwertschlag US, Whorton AR: Platelet-activating factor–induced homologous and heterologous desensitization in cultured vascular smooth muscle cells. *J Biol Chem* 1988; 263:13791–13796.

107. Greisman SE, Hornick RB, Carozza FA, et al: The role of endotoxin during typhoid fever and tularemia in man. II. Altered cardiovascular response to catecholamines. *J Clin Invest* 1964; 43:986–999.
108. Gray GA, Schott C, Julou-Schaeffer G, et al: The effect of inhibitors of the L-arginine/nitric oxide pathway on endotoxin-induced loss of vascular responsiveness in anaesthetized rats. *Br J Pharmacol* 1991; 103:1218–1224.
109. Julou-Schaeffer G, Gray GA, Fleming I, et al: Loss of vascular responsiveness induced by endotoxin involves L-arginine pathway. *Am J Physiol* 1990; 259:H1038–H1043.
110. McKenna TM: Prolonged exposure of rat aorta to low levels of endotoxin in vitro results in impaired contractility. *J Clin Invest* 1990; 86:160–168.
111. Kuo L, Chilial WM, Davis MJ, et al: Endotoxin impairs flow-induced vasodilation of porcine coronary arterioles. *Am J Physiol* 1992; 262:H1838–H1845.
112. McKenna TM, Martin FM, Chernow B, et al: Vascular endothelium contributes to decreased aortic contractility in experimental sepsis. *Circ Shock* 1986; 19:267–273.
113. Beasley D, Cohen RA, Levinsky NG: Endotoxin inhibits contraction of vascular smooth muscle in vitro. *Am J Physiol* 1990; 258:H1178–H1192.
114. Beasley D: Interleukin-1 and endotoxin activate soluble guanylate cyclase in vascular smooth muscle. *Am J Physiol* 1990; 259:R38–R44.
115. Carcillo JA, Litten RZ, Suba EA, et al: Alterations in rat aortic $alpha_1$-adrenoreceptors and $alpha_1$-adrenergic stimulated phosphoinositide hydrolysis in intraperitoneal sepsis. *Shock* 1988; 26:331–339.
116. Pfeilschifter J, Mühl H: Interleukin 1 and tumor necrosis factor potentiate angiotensin II– and calcium ionophore–related prostaglandin E2 synthesis in rat renal mesangial cells. *Biochem Biophys Res Commun* 1990; 169:585–595.
117. Tolins JP, Vercellotti GM, Wilkowske M, et al: Role of platelet activating factor in endotoxemic acute renal failure in the male rat. *J Lab Clin Med* 1989; 113:316–324.
118. Tracey KJ, Fong Y, Hesse DG, et al: Anti-cachectin/TNF monoclonal antibodies prevent septic shock during lethal bacteremia. *Nature* 1987; 330:662–664.
119. Ohlsson K, Bjork P, Bergenfeldt M, et al: Interleukin-1 receptor antagonist reduces mortality from endotoxin shock. *Nature* 1990; 348:550–552.
120. Dinarello CA: The proinflammatory cytokines interleukin-1 and tumour necrosis factor and treatment of the septic shock syndrome. *J Infect Dis* 1991; 163:1177–1184.
121. Arend WP, Malyak M, Bigler CF, et al: The biological role of naturally-occurring cytokine inhibitors. *Br J Rheumatol* 1991; 30(suppl 2):49–52.
122. Starnes HF Jr, Pearce MK, Tewari A, et al: Anti-IL-6 monoclonal antibodies protect against lethal *Escherichia coli* infection and lethal tumor necrosis factor-alpha challenge in mice. *J Immunol* 1990; 145:4185–4191.
123. Remuzzi A, Viberti G, Ruggenenti P, et al: Glomerular response to hyperglycemia in human diabetic nephropathy. *Am J Physiol* 1990; 259:F545–F552.
124. Lüscher TF, Bock HA, Yang Z, et al: Endothelium-derived relaxing and contracting factors: Perspectives in nephrology. *Kidney Int* 1991; 39:575–590.
125. Briner VA, Tsai P, Schrier RW: Bradykinin: Potential for vascular constriction in the presence of endothelial injury. *Am J Physiol* 1993; 264:F322–F327.

Body Fluid Volume Regulation in Health and Disease

William T. Abraham, M.D.

Instructor of Medicine, University of Colorado School of Medicine, Denver, Colorado

Robert W. Schrier, M.D.

Professor and Chairman, Department of Medicine, University of Colorado School of Medicine, Attending Physician, Renal Division, University Hospital, University of Colorado Health Sciences Center, Denver, Colorado

An understanding of body fluid volume regulation, as modulated by renal sodium and water excretion, has considerable implications for the practice of clinical medicine. In particular, a unifying hypothesis of body fluid volume regulation permits a rational approach to comprehending the pathogenesis of the sodium and water retention that characterizes certain edematous states, including cardiac failure, cirrhosis, and pregnancy. In these clinical circumstances, it is clear that the integrity of the kidney as the ultimate effector organ of body fluid volume regulation is intact. For example, transplantation of the kidney from edematous cirrhotic patients to subjects with normal liver function totally reverses the renal sodium and water retention.[1] Moreover, transplantation of a normal liver into a cirrhotic patient with ascites and edema has been shown to abolish the renal sodium and water retention.[2] Thus, in such edematous states, the kidney must be responding to extrarenal signals from the afferent limb of a volume regulatory system. The study of these edematous states has led to our proposal of a unifying hypothesis of body fluid volume regulation that applies both to health and to disease.[3–8] The purpose of this chapter is to review the afferent and efferent mechanisms that constitute this body fluid volume regulatory system.

Afferent Mechanisms Involved in Body Fluid Volume Regulation

In humans, an increase in sodium and water intake is associated with an expansion of the extracellular fluid volume, including expansion of the interstitial fluid and plasma volumes. This enlargement of total body fluid

Advances in Internal Medicine®, vol 39

volume normally results in an increase in renal sodium and water excretion, followed by restoration of the normal extracellular fluid volume. However, in patients with edematous states, avid sodium and water retention persists despite expansion of these body fluid compartments. Thus, the afferent volume receptors participating in the body fluid volume regulatory system must not primarily sense total extracellular fluid or blood volume. Rather, in such patients, there must be some body fluid compartment that is still inadequately filled even in the presence of expansion of these body fluid compartments.

The Concept of Effective Blood Volume

In 1948, Peters[9] coined the term *effective blood volume* to refer to the component of blood volume to which the volume regulatory system responds by causing renal sodium and water retention in the setting of cardiac or hepatic failure even though total blood and plasma volumes may be increased. That is, in cardiac failure or cirrhosis, extrarenal signals that enhance tubular sodium and water reabsorption by the otherwise normal kidney are initiated by this decrease in effective blood volume. In this regard, it is clear that renal sodium and water retention can occur in patients with cardiac or liver failure before any decrease in glomerular filtration rate.

Borst and deVries[10] first suggested cardiac output as the primary regulator of renal sodium and water excretion. In this context, a diminished cardiac output would constitute effective blood volume, serving as the stimulus for renal sodium and water retention in patients with edematous disorders. Although this concept is attractive, there exist several states of sodium and water retention that are associated with an increased rather than a diminished cardiac output. For example, a significant elevation in cardiac output may occur in the presence of avid renal sodium and water retention and expansion of extracellular fluid volume in association with cirrhosis, high-output cardiac failure, pregnancy, and large arteriovenous (AV) fistulae. Thus, there must exist some other or additional determinant(s) of effective blood volume.

The Integrity of the Arterial Circulation as the Determinant of Effective Blood Volume

Our body fluid volume regulation hypothesis suggests that the relative integrity or fullness of the arterial circulation constitutes the primary afferent signal through which the kidneys either increase or decrease their excretion of sodium and water. This hypothesis explains why an increase in the volume of blood on the venous side of the circulation may cause a rise in total blood volume while a decrease in the relative volume of blood in the arterial circulation may promote continued renal sodium and water retention (Fig 1). A decrease in cardiac output is the most obvious means whereby a decrease in arterial circulatory integrity may occur. However, if this were the only afferent signal for underfilling of the arterial circulation, a unifying hypothesis of body fluid volume regulation would not be possible

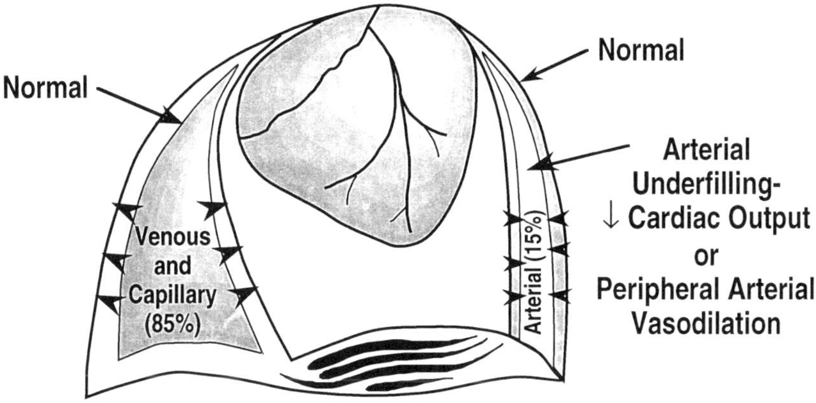

FIG 1.
Total blood volume may be expanded because of venous congestion while the arterial vascular compartment is underfilled either because of decreased cardiac output or peripheral arterial vasodilation. This may occur because ≥ 85% of total blood volume resides in the venous circulation while only about 15% of blood volume is in the arterial circulation. (From Schrier RW: *J R Coll Physicians Lond* 1992; 26:295–306. Used by permission.)

given the above-mentioned edematous disorders that are associated with increased cardiac outputs. Thus, we have proposed peripheral arterial vascular resistance and the compliance of the arterial vasculature as the second determinant of the fullness of the arterial circulation. Peripheral arterial vasodilation therefore provides another afferent signal for arterial underfilling, which causes renal sodium and water retention. Thus, with our unifying schema of body fluid volume regulation, either a decrease in cardiac output or peripheral arterial vasodilation may constitute the afferent signal for arterial underfilling, with its resultant renal sodium and water retention that lead to expansion of total blood volume (Fig 2).

Arterial blood pressure is not a sensitive index of the presence of arterial underfilling, because of the rapidity of the compensatory efferent responses. Rather, it is only with advanced disease states that the compensatory responses to arterial underfilling are insufficient to maintain mean arterial pressure. Even if sensitive methods for accurately measuring the volume of blood in the arterial circulation, which is generally less than 2% of total body fluid, were available, the absolute measured arterial blood volume could be greater than that of normal subjects despite relative arterial underfilling caused by peripheral arterial vasodilation.

Afferent Volume Receptors

The afferent volume receptors for this volume regulatory system must reside in the arterial vascular compartment and predominate over low-pressure receptors. Stimulation of the low-pressure volume receptors of the

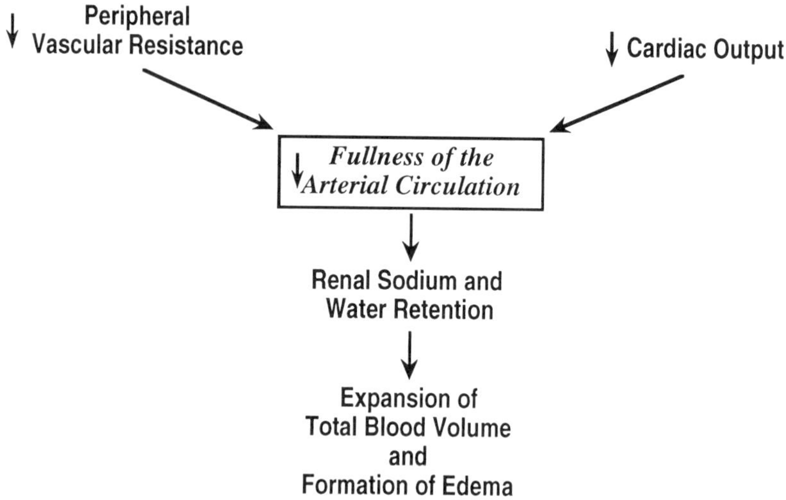

FIG 2.
A decrease in either cardiac output or peripheral vascular resistance, the determinants of the integrity of the arterial circulation, results in diminished fullness of the arterial vascular compartment; subsequent renal sodium and water retention lead to expansion of total blood volume and edema formation.

thorax, including the atria, right ventricle, and pulmonary vessels, does result in enhanced release of atrial natriuretic peptide (ANP)[11] and suppression of arginine vasopressin (AVP).[12] However, patients with advanced cardiac failure or cirrhosis exhibit avid sodium and water retention despite elevated atrial pressures and increased circulating concentrations of ANP. Thus, the high-pressure baroreceptors in the left ventricle, carotid sinus, aortic arch, and juxtaglomerular apparatus have been implicated as the primary afferent receptors involved in the regulation of renal sodium and water excretion.[13–21]

The presence of volume-sensitive receptors in the arterial circulation in humans was first suggested by observations made in patients with traumatic AV fistulas.[22] In such patients, closure of the AV fistulas is associated with a decrease in the rate of emptying of the arterial blood into the venous circulation, as demonstrated by closure-induced increases in diastolic arterial pressure and decreases in cardiac output, and results in an immediate increase in renal sodium excretion without changes in either glomerular filtration rate or renal blood flow[22] (Fig 3). Further data implicating high-pressure volume receptors, and thus the integrity of the arterial vascular tree, as sensors in modulating renal sodium excretion can be found in denervation experiments. In these studies, pharmacologic or surgical interruption of sympathetic afferent neural pathways emanating from high-pressure areas inhibited the natriuretic response to volume expansion.[23–29] Moreover, reduction of pressure or stretch at the carotid sinus has been shown to activate the sympathetic nervous system and to promote renal

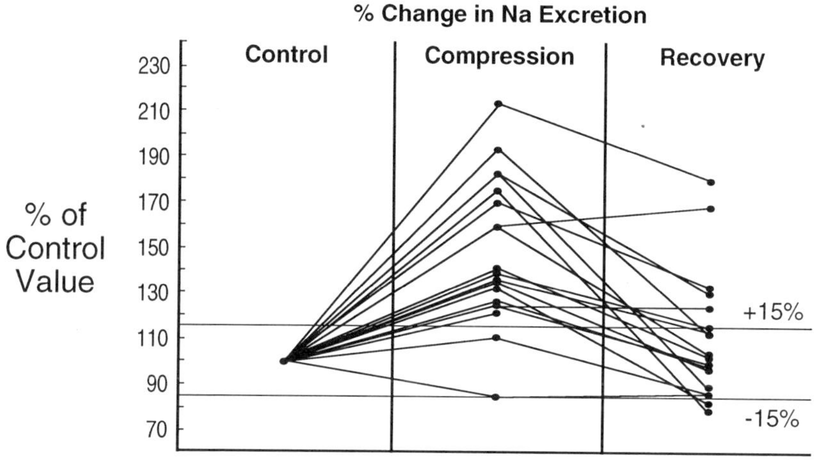

FIG 3.
Compression of arteriovenous fistulas is associated with an immediate increase in renal sodium excretion. The increase in renal sodium excretion occurs without changes in either glomerular filtration rate or renal blood flow and is likely mediated by an increase in the fullness of the arterial vascular compartment caused by the compression-induced decrease in the rate of emptying of the arterial blood into the venous circulation. (From Epstein FH, Post RS, McDowell M: *J Clin Invest* 1953; 32:233–241. Used by permission.)

sodium and water retention.[30, 31] High-pressure baroreceptors also appear to be important factors in regulating the nonosmotic release of vasopressin and thus renal water excretion.[32, 33] The juxtaglomerular apparatus, a high-pressure receptor located in the afferent arterioles within the kidney, responds to decreased stretch or increased renal sympathetic tone with enhanced secretion of renin.[30] Hence, this baroreceptor is an important factor in the control of angiotensin II formation and aldosterone secretion and ultimately in renal sodium retention.

Efferent Mechanisms Involved in Body Fluid Volume Regulation

Unloading of high-pressure ventricular and arterial volume receptors results in diminution of the tonic inhibitory effect of afferent vagal and glossopharyngeal neural traffic to the central nervous system and results in stimulation of the sympathetic nervous system, activation of the renin-angiotensin-aldosterone system, and the nonosmotic release of vasopressin. Baroreceptor stimulation of the sympathetic nervous system appears to be the primary integrator of this neurohormonal vasoconstrictor response to arterial underfilling, because activation of the renin-angiotensin-aldosterone system involves renal β-adrenergic stimulation[34] and the nonosmotic release of AVP involves sympathetic stimulation of the supraoptic and paraventricular nuclei in the hypothalamus[35] (Fig 4). Activation of these three neurohumoral vasoconstrictor systems, by altering renal hemodynamics and tubular function, mediates the avid renal sodium and water retention characteristic of patients with cardiac failure, cirrhosis, pregnancy, and other states associated with either a decrease in cardiac output or peripheral arterial vasodilation (Figs 5 and 6). In this regard, the natriuretic peptides, such as ANP and brain natriuretic peptide, and vasodilating prostaglandins may play important counter-regulatory roles. The pathogenesis of the sodium and water retention associated with cardiac failure, cirrhosis, and pregnancy will now be reviewed in the context of the unifying hypothesis of body fluid volume regulation.

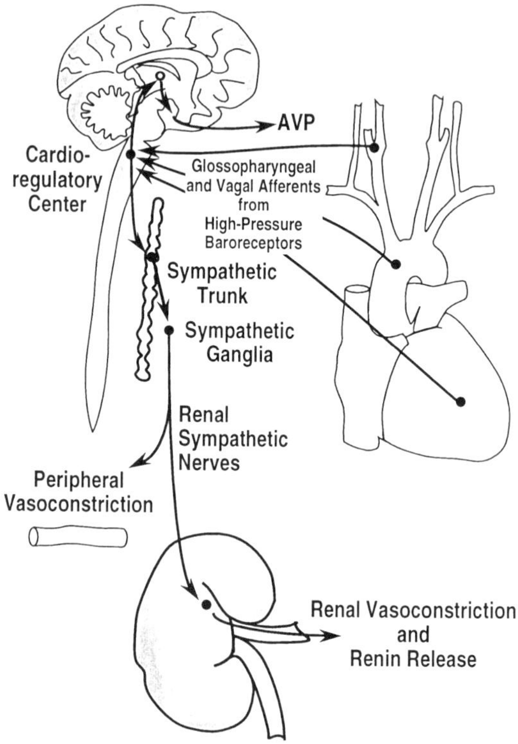

FIG 4.
Unloading of high-pressure baroreceptors in the ventricles, carotid sinus, and aortic arch stimulates cardioregulatory centers in the brain, resulting in activation of the sympathetic nervous system. Activation of the sympathetic nervous system appears to be the primary integrator of the neurohormonal vasoconstrictor response to arterial underfilling; activation of renal nerves stimulates the release of renin, thus activating the renin-angiotensin-aldosterone system, and sympathetic stimulation of the supraoptic and paraventricular nuclei in the hypothalamus results in the nonosmotic release of vasopressin. Sympathetic activation also causes peripheral vasoconstriction.

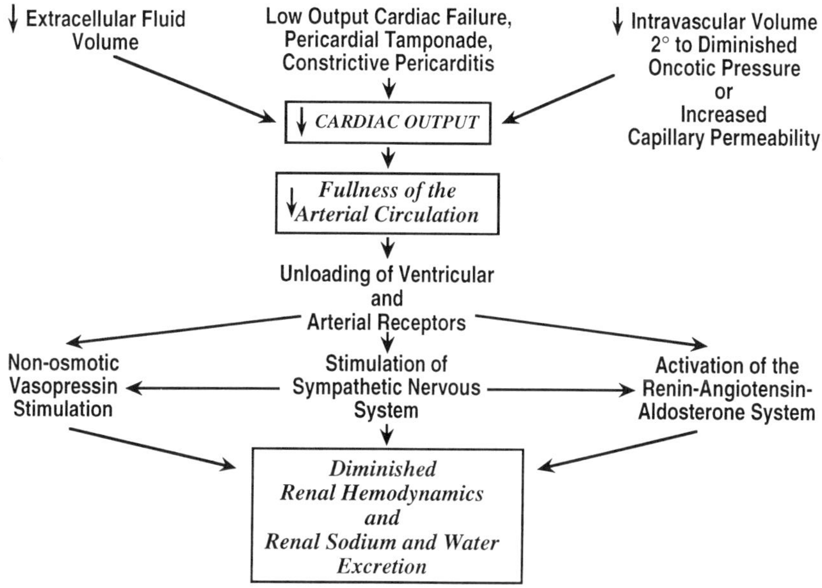

FIG 5.
Sequence of events by which a decrease in cardiac output initiates renal sodium and water retention.

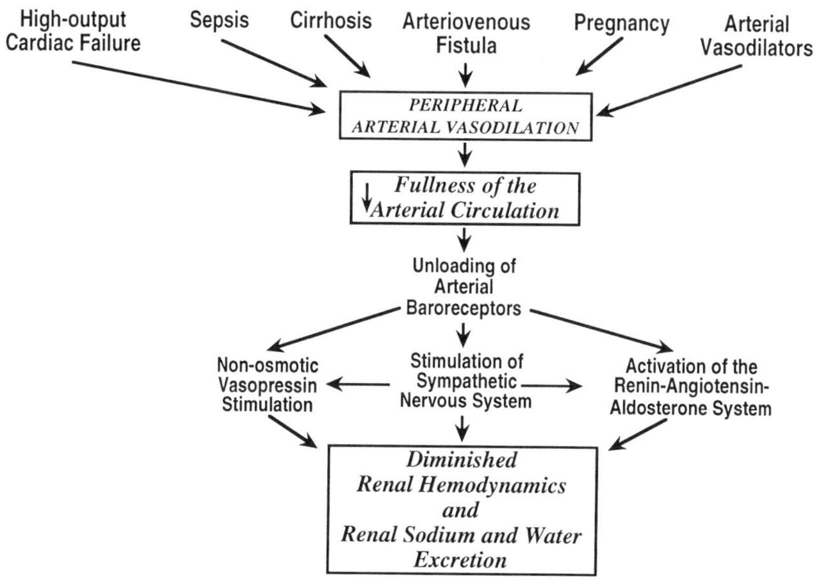

FIG 6.
Sequence of events by which peripheral arterial vasodilation initiates renal sodium and water retention.

Cardiac Failure

Numerous studies have documented elevated circulating plasma norepinephrine concentrations in patients with congestive heart failure.[36–40] The degree of plasma norepinephrine elevation in patients with heart failure correlates with the severity of the left ventricular dysfunction and with mortality.[36, 37, 41, 42] Tritiated norepinephrine kinetics studies in patients with cardiac dysfunction have shown that these elevated plasma norepinephrine concentrations are primarily due to increased norepinephrine release rather than to decreased norepinephrine clearance, suggesting activation of the adrenergic nervous system[38–40] (Fig 7). Studies employing the technique of peroneal nerve microneurography to directly assess sympathetic nerve activity to muscle have confirmed the presence of increased adrenergic activity in patients with congestive heart failure.[43] Through renal vasoconstriction and a direct effect on the proximal convoluted tubule, increased renal sympathetic activity may directly contribute to the avid sodium and water retention of congestive heart failure. In fact, intrarenal adrenergic blockade has been shown to cause a natriuresis in experimental animals and humans with heart failure.[44–46] Moreover, it has recently been shown that the intravenous administration of the α_2-receptor agonist clonidine to rats with heart failure results in a marked decrease in renal sympathetic nerve activity and a concomitant increase in urinary volume excretion.[47]

As previously noted, high-pressure baroreceptor-mediated activation of the sympathetic nervous system appears to be the primary integrator of the

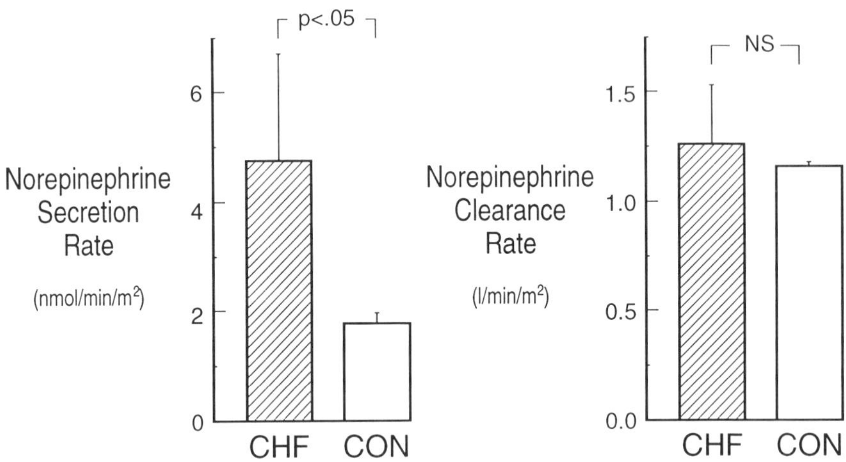

FIG 7.

The plasma norepinephrine secretion rate is greater in patients with mild-to-moderate congestive heart failure *(CHF)* than in normal controls *(CON)*, but the clearance rates of both groups are similar. These findings are consistent with early activation of the sympathetic nervous system in cardiac failure. (From Abraham WT, Hensen J, Schrier RW: *Clin Sci* 1990; 79:429–435. Used by permission.)

neurohormonal response to arterial underfilling; sympathetic activation of renal β-adrenergic receptors stimulates the renin-angiotensin-aldosterone system and central adrenergic stimulation increases the nonosmotic release of AVP. Thus plasma aldosterone and AVP, in addition to increased renal sympathetic activity, would be expected to be involved in the sodium and water retention of cardiac failure. In this regard, the specific receptor antagonist for aldosterone, spironolactone, has been shown to increase sodium excretion in sodium-retaining patients with chronic heart failure[48] (Fig 8). That aldosterone-mediated sodium retention is a compensatory response to arterial underfilling is supported by the finding that the spironolactone-induced natriuresis is associated with further stimulation of plasma renin activity and plasma norepinephrine and a decrease in plasma ANP concentration.[48]

A sensitive radioimmunoassay has been used to show that plasma AVP

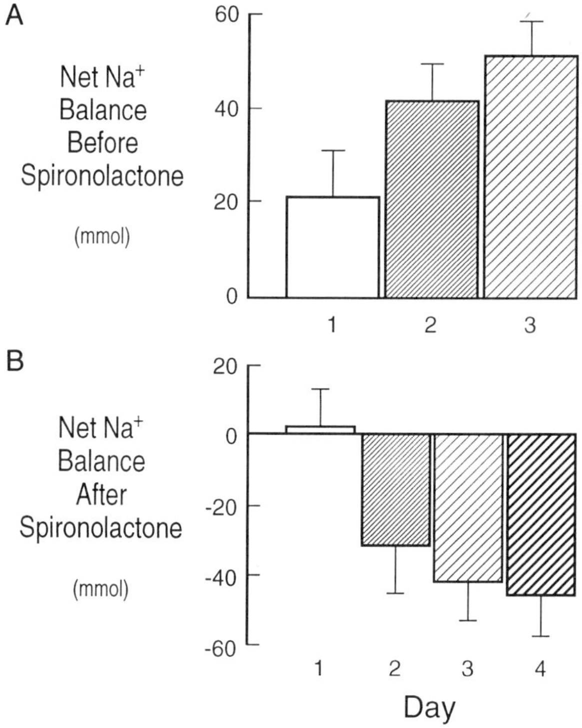

FIG 8.
Aldosterone antagonism reverses the sodium retention in patients with congestive heart failure. Net positive cumulative sodium balance, by day, for the period before spironolactone **(A)** and net negative cumulative sodium balance after the initiation of spironolactone, 400 mg/d **(B),** are shown. The increase in sodium excretion with aldosterone antagonism is significant ($P < .01$). (From Hensen J, Abraham WT, Durr JA, et al: *Am J Nephrol* 1991; 11:441–446. Used by permission.)

is increased relative to the decreased plasma osmolality in patients with cardiac failure, a finding that is consistent with the nonosmotic stimulation of AVP release in heart failure.[49] An antagonist of the antidiuretic or V_2 receptor for vasopressin has been shown to totally reverse the abnormal water excretion in rats with acutely diminished cardiac outputs, supporting a role for AVP in the water retention of congestive heart failure.[50]

An increase in plasma ANP has been found to be the earliest hormonal change in cardiac failure. However, the normal plasma concentrations of renin, norepinephrine, and aldosterone in patients with early cardiac dysfunction can be considered relatively high with respect to the observed plasma volume expansion, which in normal subjects would suppress these plasma hormone concentrations. Moreover, plasma ANP is also known to suppress plasma renin and aldosterone.[51] Thus, the increased plasma ANP may contribute to the normal plasma concentrations of these hormones in early cardiac failure.

The unifying hypothesis of body fluid volume regulation also provides a potential explanation for the failure of edematous patients to escape from the sodium-retaining effect of aldosterone and for the resistance to the natriuretic and diuretic effects of elevated endogenous and of exogenous ANP. Because arterial underfilling that occurs secondary to a decrease in cardiac output or peripheral arterial vasodilation activates mediators that decrease filtered sodium load and increase proximal tubular sodium reabsorption, the distal delivery of sodium to the collecting duct site of action of aldosterone and ANP is diminished. It is therefore proposed that diminished distal sodium delivery accounts for the ANP resistance[52] and impaired aldosterone escape that characterize cardiac failure[3, 4] (Fig 9). Atrial natriuretic peptide receptor down-regulation or ANP inactivation by increased neutral endopeptidase activity in the proximal tubule do not seem to account for ANP resistance in cardiac failure, because a linear correlation between plasma ANP and its secondary messenger, urinary cyclic guanosine monophosphate (cGMP), has been found in cardiac failure patients.[53] Studies in rats with experimental cardiac failure have also demonstrated that renal denervation reverses the resistance to ANP.[54] Because proximal sodium reabsorption is enhanced by adrenergic stimulation, this effect of renal denervation to enhance ANP sensitivity in cardiac failure is also compatible with a role of distal sodium delivery.

Compensatory response to arterial underfilling can become maladaptive in advanced cardiac failure. Evidence for this can be found in several angiotensin-converting enzyme (ACE) inhibitor heart failure trials demonstrating positive outcomes on morbidity and mortality.[55–58] For example, the Cooperative North Scandinavian Enalapril Survival Study, or CONSENSUS, has shown that in New York Heart Association Class IV cardiac failure patients with the highest plasma concentrations of angiotensin II, norepinephrine, aldosterone, and ANP, the ACE inhibitor enalapril improves 6-month survival in association with diminished circulating levels of angiotensin II, aldosterone, ANP, and norepinephrine.[55] It should be emphasized, however, that if the dose of ACE inhibitor is too large, then

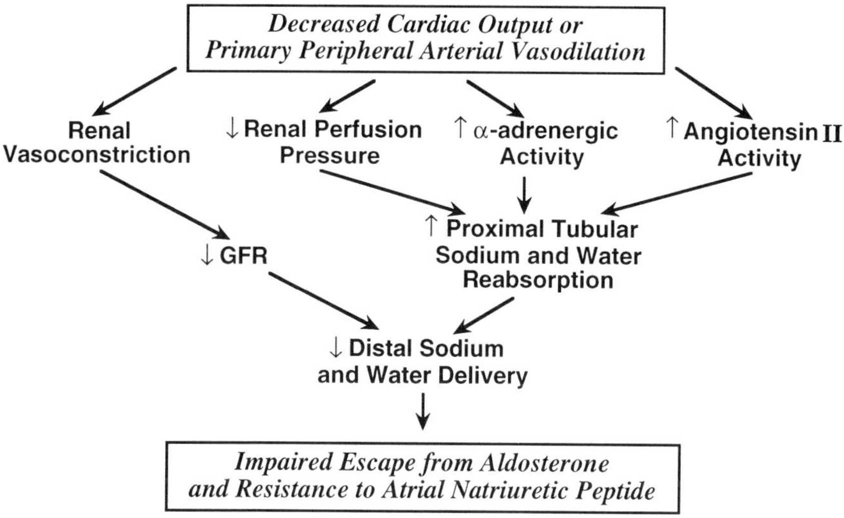

FIG 9.
A decrease in cardiac output or peripheral arterial vasodilation initiates events that diminish sodium delivery to the distal renal tubule, thereby impairing aldosterone escape and causing resistance to the natriuretic effect of atrial natriuretic peptide. (From Schrier RW, Better OS: *Eur J Gastroenterol Hepatol* 1991; 3:721–729. Used by permission.)

diminished vascular resistance may decrease blood pressure and obscure any improvement in cardiac function.

Cirrhosis

Prior to the unifying hypothesis of body fluid volume regulation, two theories explaining the pathogenesis of sodium and water retention in cirrhosis were proposed.[59, 60] With the classic Underfilling Hypothesis, ascites formation secondary to portal hypertension is proposed to decrease plasma volume and cause secondary renal sodium and water retention.[59] However, results of animal studies have shown that sodium and water retention precede ascites formation in cirrhotic animals, thus contradicting the hypothesis.[60] Thus, primary renal sodium and water retention, secondary to a hepatorenal reflex, has been proposed to lead to plasma volume expansion of both the venous and arterial compartments and cause overflow ascites.[60] This Overflow Hypothesis of ascites formation in cirrhotic patients, however, does not explain the progressive stimulation of the neurohumoral profile that is observed in cirrhotic patients and is characteristic of arterial underfilling.[3–7] Against this background, we have proposed the Peripheral Arterial Vasodilation Hypothesis for the initiation of renal sodium and water retention in cirrhosis.[7] This theory encompasses the entire range from compensated to decompensated cirrhosis to the hepatorenal syndrome (Fig 10), and is a part of the unifying hypothesis of body fluid volume regulation.

According to this hypothesis, splanchnic vasodilation occurs early in cirrhosis, and the resultant arterial underfilling stimulates sodium and water retention with plasma volume expansion prior to ascites formation. The normal plasma hormone concentrations in these compensated cirrhotic patients are relatively increased for the degree of plasma volume expansion. The mediators of the early splanchnic vasodilation in cirrhosis are unknown but may include the opening of existing shunts, activation of vasodilating hormones, and ultimately the development of collaterals. As cirrhosis progresses, vasodilation may occur at other sites, including the skin, muscles, and lungs. Increased synthesis and release of the potent vasodilator nitric oxide, perhaps caused by increased circulating levels of endotoxin in cirrhosis, has been proposed to account for the hemodynamic changes found in cirrhotic patients.[61] However, nitric oxide activity is difficult to assess in vivo, and to date only indirect evidence supports this hypothesis. For example, urinary cGMP, the second messenger of nitric oxide as well as of ANP,[62] is increased in cirrhotic patients prior to the development of ascites and in some patients prior to an increase in circulating ANP concentrations.[63] This observation is compatible with nitric oxide–mediated vasodilation early in cirrhosis. Endogenous opioids may also contribute to the peripheral vasodilation and to the renal sodium and water retention of cirrhosis as the administration of the opioid antagonist naloxone increases sodium and water excretion after water loading in patients with cirrhosis and

	COMPENSATED CIRRHOSIS (NO ASCITES)	DECOMPENSATED CIRRHOSIS (ASCITES)	HEPATORENAL SYNDROME
Peripheral Arterial Vasodilation	↑	↑↑	↑↑↑
Plasma Hormones (AVP, Renin, Aldosterone, NE)	Normal	↑	↑↑
Plasma Volume	↑	↑↑	↑↑↑

FIG 10.
The Peripheral Arterial Vasodilation Hypothesis of sodium and water retention in cirrhosis explains the entire range of pathophysiology from compensated and decompensated cirrhosis to the hepatorenal syndrome. In compensated cirrhosis, normal plasma hormone concentrations indicate relative stimulation in the presence of volume expansion. As cirrhosis becomes decompensated, progressive arterial vasodilation is associated with greater stimulation of neurohormonal vasoconstrictor systems, despite expansion of plasma volume. *AVP* = arginine vasopressin; *NE* = norepinephrine.

ascites.[64] Other factors that have been proposed to mediate this splanchnic and peripheral vasodilation in cirrhosis include vasodilating prostaglandins, glucagon, calcitonin gene–related peptide, platelet-activating factor, substance P, and vasoactive intestinal peptide; however, definitive proof is lacking for all of them.

As with cardiac failure, pretreatment hyponatremia and high plasma concentrations of renin, norepinephrine, and aldosterone portend a poor prognosis in the cirrhotic patient.[6] The highest plasma concentrations of these hormones and the lowest blood pressures occur as the decompensated cirrhotic patient with ascites progresses toward the hepatorenal syndrome.

The major detraction from the Peripheral Arterial Vasodilation Hypothesis in cirrhosis is the finding that some compensated cirrhotic patients exhibit lower plasma aldosterone and renin activity and greater natriuresis than do normal subjects in the supine position[65] and with head-out water immersion.[66] These findings can, however, be explained by centralization of excessive splanchnic venous blood volume in cirrhotic patients in the supine position or during head-out water immersion. In this regard, the compensated cirrhotic patients who exhibit an exaggerated natriuresis with head-out water immersion also exhibit the highest plasma ANP concentrations, suggesting an increase in cardiac preload caused by centralization of venous blood volume.[66] Moreover, compensated cirrhotic patients with low plasma renin activity in the supine position demonstrate normal or increased plasma renin activity in the upright position.[67]

As with other states of arterial underfilling, the neurohumoral responses to the peripheral arterial vasodilation of cirrhosis are associated with factors that diminish distal sodium delivery.[68] The impaired aldosterone escape[68] and resistance to ANP[69] that occur in cirrhosis are therefore most likely mediated by diminished distal sodium delivery. As with experimental cardiac failure, renal denervation has been shown to reverse the resistance to ANP in experimental cirrhosis[70] (Fig 11). This finding supports a role of diminished distal sodium delivery in the ANP resistance, particularly since Skorecki et al.[69] have demonstrated a normal increase in urinary cGMP but no natriuresis in some cirrhotic patients infused with ANP. Moreover, the addition of low-dose ACE inhibition (captopril 20 to 25 mg/d) to furosemide and spironolactone in patients with diuretic-resistant decompensated cirrhosis results in restoration of diuretic responsiveness, likely caused by a decrease in angiotensin II–mediated proximal tubular sodium reabsorption and renal vascular resistance.[71]

In a recent report from the Barcelona group, the presence of aldosterone escape was studied in compensated cirrhotic patients without ascites.[72] While there was no difference in liver enzymes, serum albumin, electrolytes, creatinine, and blood urea nitrogen between those cirrhotic patients who escaped vs. those who did not escape from the sodium-retaining effect of mineralocorticoid hormone, the lowest peripheral vascular resistances were present in those patients with impaired mineralocorticoid escape. There were no differences in the hepatic venous pressure gradients

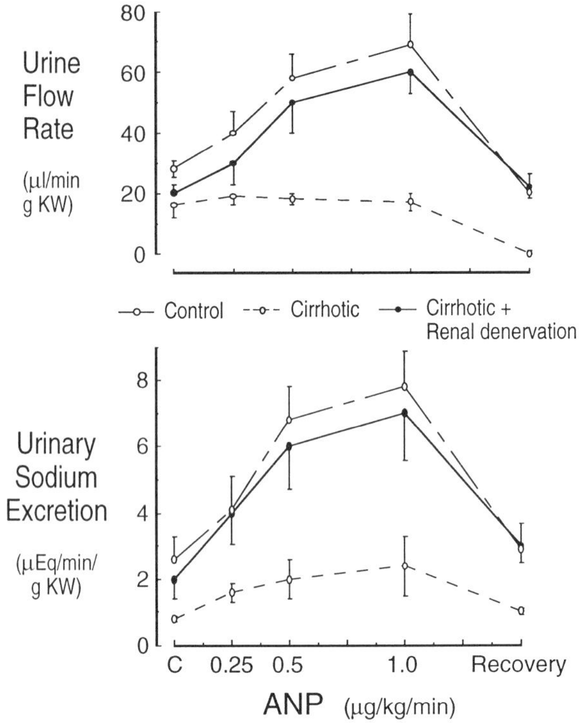

FIG 11.
Renal denervation reverses the resistance to the diuretic and natriuretic effects of atrial natriuretic peptide *(ANP)* in a rat model of cirrhosis. (From Koepke JP, Jones S, DiBona GF: *Am J Physiol* 1987; 252:R1019–R1023. Used by permission.)

between the two groups. Taken together, these findings do not support increased intrahepatic pressure as the primary determinant of sodium and water retention in cirrhosis,[73] but rather support the Peripheral Arterial Vasodilation Hypothesis.[7]

The role of peripheral arterial vasodilation has been studied in decompensated cirrhotic patients with and without exogenous norepinephrine and head-out water immersion.[74] This combined maneuver was found to acutely normalize renal sodium and water excretion in these ascitic patients. A statistically high correlation between the diuretic response and the increment in peripheral vascular resistance was observed in these studies (Fig 12). Moreover, peripheral vasoconstriction with infused norepinephrine has been shown to partly restore renal responsiveness to ANP in patients with cirrhosis and ascites.[75] However, any advantage to the kidney from peripheral vasoconstriction induced by norepinephrine infusion may be limited over time by norepinephrine-induced renal vasoconstriction.[76] The acute administration of ornipressin, an agonist of the vascular (V_1) receptor of AVP, has been shown to increase systemic vascular resistance

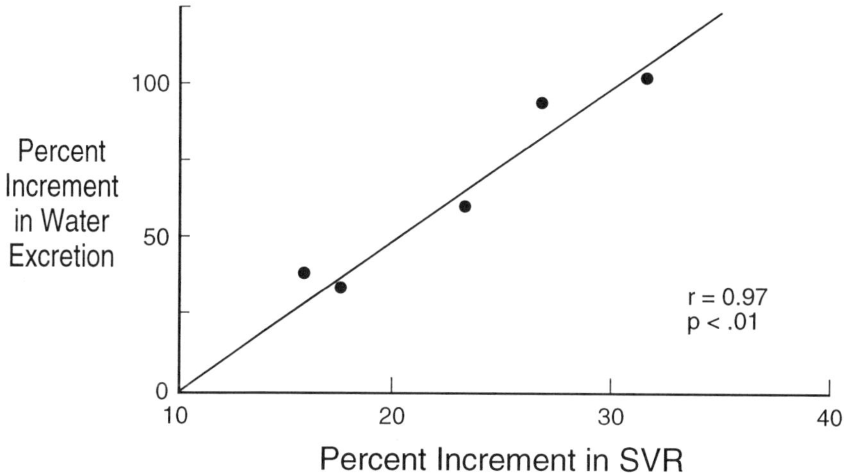

FIG 12.
The increase in systemic vascular resistance *(SVR)* with norepinephrine infusion during head-out water immersion correlates with the increase in water-load excretion from immersion alone to immersion with norepinephrine infusion, supporting a role for peripheral arterial resistance as a determinant of arterial circulatory integrity. (From Shapiro MD, Nicholls KM, Groves BM, et al: *Kidney Int* 1985; 28:206–211. Used by permission.)

and decrease renal vascular resistance, resulting in a marked increase in renal function and excretory capacity in patients with decompensated cirrhosis.[77] Moreover, chronic ornipressin treatment has been demonstrated to increase glomerular filtration rate, renal blood flow, diuresis, and natriuresis in hepatorenal syndrome patients, serving as a bridge to liver transplantation.[78] These observations provide further support for the Peripheral Arterial Vasodilation Hypothesis.

Pregnancy

Pregnancy is associated with a 30% to 50% increase in total plasma, blood, and extracellular fluid volume, which is accompanied by a similar increase in cardiac output, renal blood flow, and glomerular filtration rate. It has been suggested that the plasma volume expansion may account for the increase in renal hemodynamics. However, the rise in cardiac output, glomerular filtration rate, and renal blood flow precede the plasma volume expansion in pregnancy[79] (Fig 13). In addition, stimulation of the renin-angiotensin-aldosterone system, a hormonal index of arterial underfilling, is seen in pregnancy. In nonpregnant individuals, a 30% to 50% expansion of plasma volume would suppress the renin-angiotensin-aldosterone system. This observation, as well as other characteristics of pregnancy that will be discussed, are not compatible with primary renal sodium and water retention leading to expansion of plasma and extracellular fluid volume.

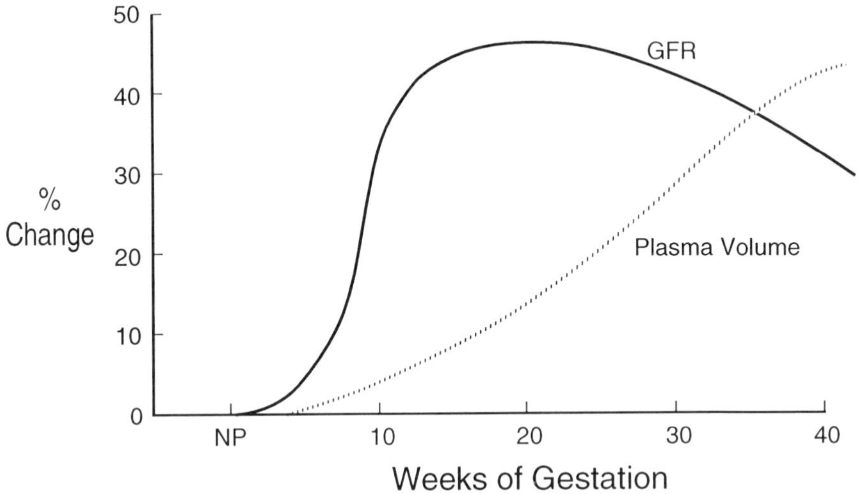

FIG 13.
Glomerular filtration rate *(GFR)* rises before plasma volume expansion occurs in pregnant women. (From Davison JM: *Scand J Clin Lab Invest [Suppl]* 1984; 169:15–21. Used by permission.)

According to our unifying hypothesis of body fluid volume regulation, primary peripheral arterial vasodilation is the major initiating factor in pregnancy that causes arterial underfilling and the resultant compensatory responses.[8] For example, in the first trimester of normal pregnancy, blood pressure falls as cardiac output rises in association with a primary decrease in peripheral vascular resistance. In contrast, primary volume expansion with an increase in cardiac output and a secondary peripheral vasodilation would not explain the decrease in blood pressure that occurs during the first trimester of pregnancy. Moreover, it is known that primary peripheral arterial vasodilation is associated with stimulation of the renin-angiotensin-aldosterone system, a normal occurrence in pregnancy.[3]

The decrease in plasma sodium and osmolality that occurs in pregnancy is likewise most compatible with peripheral vasodilation and arterial underfilling. An increase in thirst and water intake is also known to occur in the first trimester of pregnancy,[80] another effect most compatible with arterial underfilling caused by peripheral arterial vasodilation.

If the plasma volume expansion of pregnancy involves both the venous and arterial circulatory compartments, then the blood volume threshold (mL/kg body weight) for the nonosmotic release of vasopressin during volume depletion should approximate that of the nonpregnant state. It has, however, been shown in the rat that the nonosmotic stimulation of vasopressin in pregnancy occurs at a blood volume that is 40% greater than that found in the nonpregnancy state.[81] The expected blunting of the tubuloglomerular feedback with volume expansion in the nonpregnant rat also does not occur with pregnancy.[82] Moreover, either an angiotensin antagonist or an angiotensin-converting enzyme inhibitor lowers blood pressure more in the anesthetized pregnant rat than in the anesthetized nonpregnant rat.[83] Taken together, these findings are best explained by a mechanism in which primary peripheral arterial vasodilation causes arterial underfilling and secondary stimulation of the renin-angiotensin-aldosterone system.

Hormonal and hemodynamic measurements in the pregnant baboon support this arterial underfilling hypothesis.[84] This investigation demonstrated that early peripheral arterial vasodilation and an increase in cardiac output preceded the plasma volume expansion of pregnancy (Fig 14). In these pregnant baboons, the hemodynamic changes were associated with activation of vasoconstrictor and antinatriuretic hormones, suggesting that the increase in cardiac output did not totally compensate for the peripheral vasodilation. This observation explains the normal occurrence of a lower blood pressure during the first trimester of pregnancy and is consistent with the theory that predominant peripheral arterial vasodilation initiates the hemodynamic and neurohormonal changes of pregnancy.

In the absence of preeclampsia and eclampsia, the sodium and water retention in pregnancy are not of the degree observed with other states of arterial underfilling, such as cardiac failure and cirrhosis. There also is no good evidence of impaired mineralocorticoid escape with normal pregnancy. This capacity to handle salt and water normally in pregnancy in spite of arterial underfilling most likely relates to the 30% to 50% increase in glomerular filtration rate and thus filtered sodium and water. Support for this interpretation comes from the observation that more avid sodium and water retention occurs during preeclampsia and eclampsia, states associated with a fall in glomerular filtration rate to nonpregnant levels.

A major challenge is to identify the factors that mediate the hemodynamic changes, including enhanced renal blood flow and glomerular filtration rate, during pregnancy. Renal vasodilation not only antedates the blood volume expansion of pregnancy but also occurs in spite of peripheral arterial vasodilation, an event that generally is associated with reflex renal vasoconstriction. While a fall in vasodilating prostaglandins may be involved in preeclampsia and eclampsia, there is considerable experimental evidence that these hormones cannot be the sole mediator of the enhanced renal hemodynamics of normal pregnancy. Specifically, inhibition of prostaglandin synthesis has been shown not to reverse the increase in glomerular filtration rate and renal blood flow in the pregnant rat.[85] There is emerging evidence that the source of the potent systemic and renal vasodilation of pregnancy may be the endothelium. Several recent investigations of nitric oxide synthesis inhibition in pregnant rats suggest a role for nitric oxide in the vasodilation of pregnancy.[86–89] Moreover, the administration of L-arginine, a substrate for nitric oxide production, is associated with a greater fall in mean arterial pressure in pregnant versus nonpregnant rats.[89] In addition, urinary excretion of nitrate and cGMP are increased and strongly correlated with one another in pregnant rats.[88] Increased concentrations of circulating cGMP are also observed in the gravid rat.[90] Nitric

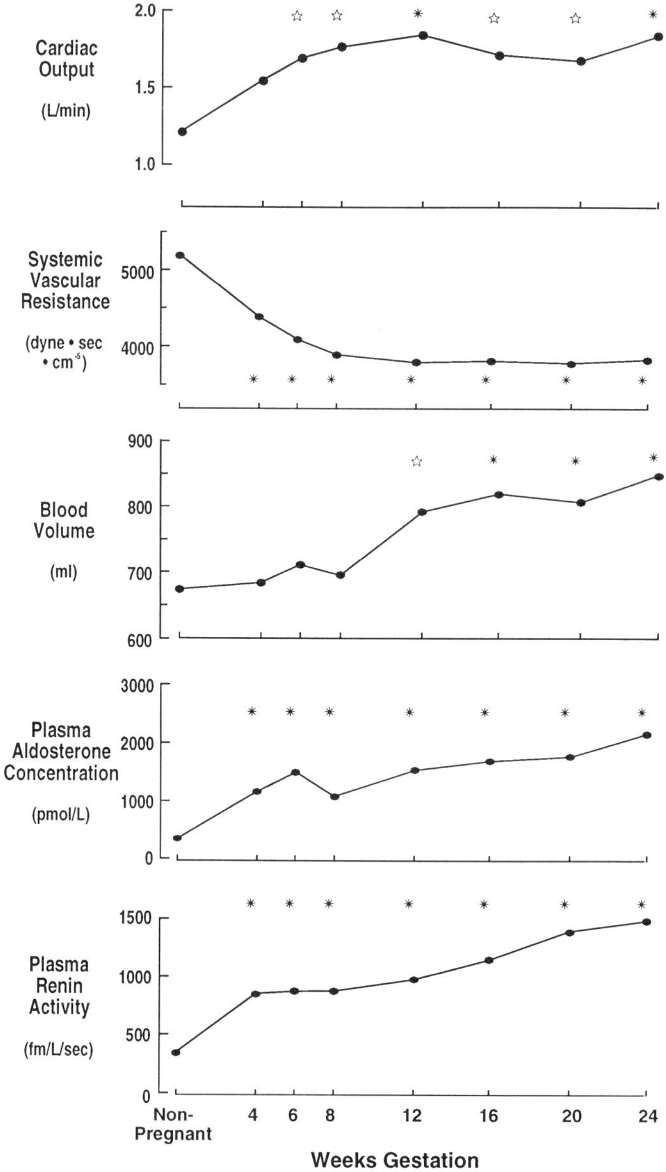

FIG 14.
Peripheral arterial vasodilation, an increase in cardiac output, and activation of the renin-angiotensin-aldosterone system precede blood volume expansion in pregnant baboons (*Open star* = $P < .05$; $^*P < .01$). (Adapted from Phippard AF, Horvath JS, Glynn EM: *J Hypertension* 1986; 4:773–779. Used by permission.)

oxide hemoglobin has been detected in the blood of pregnant, but not nonpregnant, rats.[88] Collectively, these observations suggest that endogenous nitric oxide production is increased in gravid rats and may be involved in the vasodilation of pregnancy. However, in another study, the acute administration of maximal doses of nitric oxide antagonists in the pregnant rat did not support a role for nitric oxide as the mediator of the systemic renal vasodilation of pregnancy.[91]

Recently relaxin, a peptide hormone produced predominantly by the corpus luteum of pregnancy, has been shown to have powerful chronotropic and inotropic effects on the rat heart with a potency that is greater than that of endothelin, angiotensin II, and isoprenaline.[92] Serum relaxin concentrations are undetectable in nonpregnant women; however, they can be detected in the peripheral sera of women within 10 days after conception.[93, 94] Moreover, the pattern of serial relaxin concentrations determined throughout pregnancy mirrors the hemodynamic changes: an early first-trimester increase, followed by a slight second-trimester decline and stable levels throughout the second and third trimesters.[92, 93] However, a definitive role for nitric oxide, relaxin, or some other vasodilating substance in the hemodynamic alterations of pregnancy requires further study. The discovery of the nature of the systemic and renal vasodilator(s) of pregnancy would have important potential implications for the treatment of not only preeclampsia and eclampsia but also states of acute and chronic renal failure.

The understanding of the physiology of normal pregnancy in the context of our unifying hypothesis of body fluid volume regulation provides potential insights for the preeclampsia and eclampsia states. Our pathogenetic proposal for the preeclampsia and eclampsia states is that they are initiated by endothelial damage with increased endothelin and result in increased vascular sensitivity to angiotensin II, norepinephrine, and vasopressin[8] (Fig 15). The hallmarks of preeclampsia and eclampsia, including the observed increased sensitivity to angiotensin, fall in glomerular filtration rate and renal blood flow, hypertension, edema, and proteinuria, can be explained by this hypothesis.

Summary

The unifying hypothesis of body fluid volume regulation explains the renal handling of sodium and water in health and in various disease states associated with edema formation and no intrinsic renal parenchymal disease. According to this hypothesis, underfilling of the arterial vascular compartment, resulting from either a decrease in cardiac output or peripheral arterial vasodilation, initiates a sequence of events that results in activation of the sympathetic nervous and renin-angiotensin-aldosterone systems and the nonosmotic release of AVP. Activation of these neurohormonal vasoconstrictor systems causes diminished renal hemodynamics and renal sodium and water retention that persist despite an increase in total extracel-

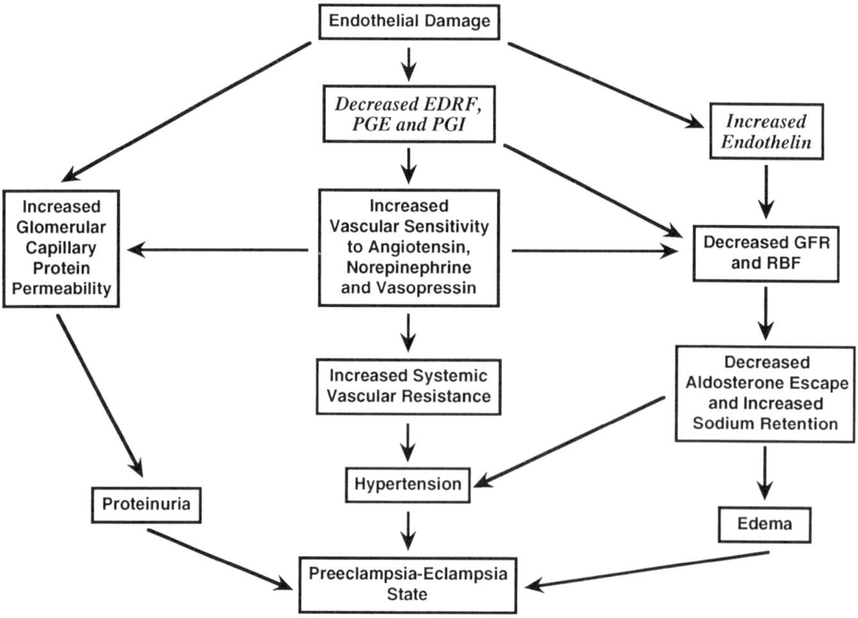

FIG 15.
Proposed pathophysiologic events for preeclampsia and eclampsia. (From Schrier RW, Briner VA: *Obstet Gynecol* 1991; 77:632–639. Used by permission.)

lular and blood volume. In edematous patients, a vasoconstrictor-mediated increase in proximal tubular sodium reabsorption results in diminished sodium delivery to the distal tubular sites of action of aldosterone and ANP; this explains the failure of such patients to escape from the sodium-retaining effects of aldosterone and the resistance to the natriuretic and diuretic effects of ANP. In pregnancy, an early decrease in systemic vascular resistance associated with activation of the neurohormonal vasoconstrictor systems precedes the normal expansion of blood and plasma volumes and is consistent with the arterial underfilling hypothesis. The loss of this peripheral vasodilatory response in some pregnancies may contribute to the development of preeclampsia and eclampsia.

References

1. Koppel MH, Coburn JW, Mims MM, et al: Transplantation of cadaveric kidneys from patients with hepatorenal syndrome: Evidence for the functional nature of renal failure in advanced liver disease. *N Engl J Med* 1969; 280:1367–1371.
2. Iwatsuki S, Popovtzer MM, Corman JL, et al: Recovery from hepatorenal syndrome after orthotopic liver transplantation. *N Engl J Med* 1973;289: 1155–1159.

3. Schrier RW: Pathogenesis of sodium and water retention in high-output and low-output cardiac failure, nephrotic syndrome, cirrhosis, and pregnancy. *N Engl J Med* 1988; 319:1065–1072 (Part 1); 1127–1134 (Part 2).
4. Schrier RW: Body fluid volume regulation in health and disease: A unifying hypothesis. *Ann Intern Med* 1990; 113:155–159.
5. Schrier RW: A unifying hypothesis of body fluid volume regulation: The Lilly Lecture 1992. *J R Coll Physicians Lond* 1992; 26:295–306.
6. Schrier RW: An odyssey into the milieu interieur: Pondering the enigmas. *J Am Soc Nephrol* 1992; 2:1549–1559.
7. Schrier RW, Arroyo V, Bernardi M, et al: Peripheral arterial vasodilation hypothesis: A proposal for the initiation of renal sodium and water retention in cirrhosis. *Hepatology* 1988; 8:1151–1157.
8. Schrier RW, Briner VA: Peripheral arterial vasodilation hypothesis of sodium and water retention in pregnancy: Implications for pathogenesis of preeclampsia-eclampsia. *Obstet Gynecol* 1991; 77:632–639.
9. Peters JP: The role of sodium in the production of edema. *N Engl J Med* 1948; 239:353–362.
10. Borst JG, deVries LA: Three types of "natural" diuresis. *Lancet* 1950; 2:1–6.
11. Bichet DG, Schrier RW: Cardiac failure, liver disease and nephrotic syndrome, in Schrier RW, Gottschalk CW (eds): *Diseases of the Kidney*, ed 4. Boston, Little, Brown, 1988, pp 2703–2742.
12. de Torrente A, Robertson GL, McDonald KM, et al: Mechanism of diuretic response to increased left atrial pressure in the anesthetized dog. *Kidney Int* 1975; 8:355–361.
13. Goetz KL, Bond GC, Bloxham DD: Atrial receptors and renal function. *Physiol Rev* 1975; 55:157–205.
14. Zucker IH, Earle AM, Gilmore JP: The mechanism of adaptation of left atrial stretch receptors in dogs with chronic congestive heart failure. *J Clin Invest* 1977; 60:323–331.
15. Schrier RW, Lieberman RA, Ufferman RC: Mechanism of antidiuretic effect of beta adrenergic stimulation. *J Clin Invest* 1972; 51:97–111.
16. Schrier RW, Berl T: Mechanism of effect of alpha-adrenergic stimulation with norepinephrine on renal water excretion. *J Clin Invest* 1973; 52:502–511.
17. Berl T, Cadnapaphornchai P, Harbottle JA, et al: Mechanism of suppression of vasopressin during alpha-adrenergic stimulation with norepinephrine. *J Clin Invest* 1974; 53:219–227.
18. Berl T, Cadnapaphornchai P, Harbottle JA, et al: Mechanism of stimulation of vasopressin release during beta adrenergic stimulation with isoproterenol. *J Clin Invest* 1974; 53:857–867.
19. Anderson RJ, Cadnapaphornchai P, Harbottle JA, et al: Mechanism of effect of thoracic inferior vena cava constriction on renal water excretion. *J Clin Invest* 1974; 54:1473–1479.
20. Anderson RJ, Pluss RG, Berns AS, et al: Mechanism of effect of hypoxia on renal water excretion. *J Clin Invest* 1978; 62:769–777.
21. Schrier RW, Berl T: Mechanism of antidiuretic effect of interruption of parasympathetic pathways. *J Clin Invest* 1972; 51:2613–2620.
22. Epstein FH, Post RS, McDowell M: Effects of an arteriovenous fistula on renal hemodynamics and electrolyte excretion. *J Clin Invest* 1953; 32:233–241.
23. Schrier RW, Humphreys MH: Factors involved in the antinatriuretic effects of acute constriction of the thoracic inferior and abdominal vena cava. *Circ Res* 1971; 29:479–489.

24. Schrier RW, Humphreys MH, Ufferman RC: Role of cardiac output and the autonomic nervous system in the antinatriuretic response to acute constriction of the thoracic superior vena cava. *Circ Res* 1971; 29:490–498.
25. Gilmore JP: Contribution of baroreceptors to the control of renal function. *Circ Res* 1964; 14:301–317.
26. Gilmore JP, Daggett WM: Response of chronic cardiac denervated dog to acute volume expansion. *Am J Physiol* 1966; 210:509–512.
27. Knox FG, Davis BB, Berliner RW: Effect of chronic cardiac denervation on renal response to saline infusion. *Am J Physiol* 1967; 213:174–178.
28. Pearce JW, Sonnenberg H: Effects of spinal section and renal denervation on the renal response to blood volume expansion. *Can J Physiol Pharmacol* 1965; 43:211–224.
29. Schedl HP, Bartter FC: An explanation for and experimental correction of the abnormal water diuresis in cirrhosis. *J Clin Invest* 1967; 46:1297–1308.
30. Davis JO: The control of renin release. *Am J Med* 1973; 55:333–350.
31. Guyton A, Scanlon CJ, Armstrong GG: Effects of pressoreceptor reflex and Cushing's reflex on urinary output. *Fed Proc* 1952; 11:61–62.
32. Schrier RW, Berl T, Anderson RJ: Osmotic and nonosmotic control of vasopressin release. *Am J Physiol* 1979; 236:F321–F332.
33. Schrier RW, Berl T, Anderson RJ, et al: Nonosmolar Control of Renal Water Excretion, in Andreoli T, Grantham J, Rector F (eds): *Disturbances in Body Fluid Osmolality*. Bethesda, MD, American Physiological Society, 1977, pp 149–178.
34. Berl T, Henrich WL, Erickson AL, et al: Prostaglandins in the beta adrenergic and baroreceptor-mediated secretion on renin. *Am J Physiol* 1979; 235:F472–F477.
35. Sklar AH, Schrier RW: Central nervous system mediators of vasopressin release. *Physiol Rev* 1983; 63:1243–1280.
36. Thomas JA, Marks BH: Plasma norepinephrine in congestive heart failure. *Am J Cardiol* 1978; 41:233–243.
37. Levine TB, Francis GS, Goldsmith SR, et al: Activity of the sympathetic nervous system and renin-angiotensin system as assessed by plasma hormone levels and their relation to hemodynamic abnormalities in congestive heart failure. *Am J Cardiol* 1982; 49:1659–1666.
38. Davis D, Bailey R, Zelis R: Abnormalities in systemic norepinephrine kinetics in human congestive heart failure. *Am J Physiol* 1988; 254:E760–E766.
39. Hasking JG, Esler MD, Jennings GL, et al: Norepinephrine spillover to plasma in patients with congestive heart failure: Evidence of increased overall and cardiorenal sympathetic nervous activity. *Circulation* 1986; 73:615–621.
40. Abraham WT, Hensen J, Schrier RW: Elevated plasma noradrenaline concentrations in patients with low-output cardiac failure: Dependence on increased noradrenaline secretion rates. *Clin Sci* 1990; 79:429–435.
41. Chidsey CA, Braunwald E, Morrow AG: Catecholamine excretion and cardiac stores of norepinephrine in congestive heart failure. *Am J Med* 1965; 39:442–451.
42. Cohn JN, Levine BT, Olivari MT: Plasma norepinephrine as a guide to prognosis in patients with chronic congestive heart failure. *N Engl J Med* 1984; 311:819–823.
43. Leimbach WN, Wallin BG, Victor RG, et al: Direct evidence from intraneural recordings for increased sympathetic outflow in patients with heart failure. *Circulation* 1986; 73:913–919.

44. Brod J, Fejfar Z, Fejfarová MH: The role of neuro-humoral factors in the genesis of renal haemodynamic changes in heart failure. *Acta Med Scand* 1954; 148:273–290.
45. Gill JR Jr, Mason DT, Bartter FC: Adrenergic nervous system in sodium metabolism: Effects of guanethidine and sodium-retaining steroids in normal man. *J Clin Invest* 1964; 43:177–184.
46. DiBona GF, Herman PJ, Swain LL: Neural control of renal function in edema-forming states. *Am J Physiol* 1988; 254:R1017–R1024.
47. Feng QP, Carlsson S, Thorén P, et al: Effects of clonidine on renal sympathetic nerve activity, natriuresis and diuresis in chronic congestive heart failure rats. *J Pharmacol Exp Ther* 1992; 261:1129–1135.
48. Hensen J, Abraham WT, Durr JA, et al: Aldosterone in congestive heart failure: Analysis of determinants and role in sodium retention. *Am J Nephrol* 1991; 11:441–446.
49. Szatalowicz VL, Arnold PE, Chaimovitz C, et al: Radioimmunoassay of plasma arginine vasopressin in hyponatremic patients with congestive heart failure. *N Engl J Med* 1981; 305:263–266.
50. Ishikawa S, Saito T, Okada K, et al: Effect of vasopressin antagonist on water excretion in inferior vena cava constriction. *Kidney Int* 1986; 30:49–55.
51. Lee ME, Miller WL, Edwards BS, et al: Role of endogenous atrial natriuretic factor in acute congestive heart failure. *J Clin Invest* 1990; 84:1962–1966.
52. Koepke JP, DiBona GF: Blunted natriuresis to atrial natriuretic peptide in chronic sodium-retaining disorders. *Am J Physiol* 1987; 252:F865–F871.
53. Abraham WT, Hensen J, Kim JK, et al: Atrial natriuretic peptide and urinary cyclic guanosine monophosphate in patients with chronic heart failure. *J Am Soc Nephrol* 1992; 2:1697–1703.
54. Pettersson A, Hedner J, Hedner T: Renal interaction between sympathetic activity and ANP in rats with chronic ischaemic heart failure. *Acta Physiol Scand* 1989; 135:487–492.
55. CONSENSUS Trial Study Group: Effects of enalapril on mortality in severe congestive heart failure: Results of the Cooperative North Scandinavian Enalapril Survival Study (CONSENSUS). *N Engl J Med* 1987; 316:1429–1435.
56. SOLVD Investigators: Effect of enalapril on survival in patients with reduced left ventricular ejection fractions and congestive heart failure. *N Engl J Med* 1991; 325:293–302.
57. SOLVD Investigators: Effect of enalapril on mortality and the development of heart failure in asymptomatic patients with reduced left ventricular ejection fractions. *N Engl J Med* 1992; 327:685–691.
58. Captopril-Digoxin Multicenter Research Group: Comparative effects of captopril and digoxin in patients with mild to moderate heart failure. *JAMA* 1988; 259:539–544.
59. Papper S: The role of the kidney in Laennec's cirrhosis of the liver. *Medicine* 1958; 37:299–316.
60. Lieberman FL, Denison EK, Reynolds TB: The relationship of plasma volume, portal hypertension, ascites, and renal sodium and water retention in cirrhosis: The "overflow" theory of ascites formation. *Ann NY Acad Sci* 1970; 170:202–206.
61. Vallance P, Moncada S: Hyperdynamic circulation in cirrhosis: A role for nitric oxide? *Lancet* 1991; 337:776–778.
62. Burton GA, MacNeil S, de Jonge A, et al: Cyclic GMP release and vasodilation induced by EDRF and atrial natriuretic factor in the isolated perfused kidney of the rat. *Br J Pharmacol* 1990; 99:364–368.

63. Miyase S, Fujiyama S, Chikazawa H, et al: Atrial natriuretic peptide in liver cirrhosis with mild ascites. *Gastroenterol Jpn* 1990; 25:356–362.
64. Leehey DJ, Gollapudi P, Deakin A, et al: Naloxone increases water and electrolyte excretion after water loading in patients with cirrhosis and ascites. *J Lab Clin Med* 1991; 118:484–491.
65. Trevisani F, Bernardi M, Gasbarrini A, et al: Bed rest-induced hypernatriuresis in cirrhotic patients without ascites: Does it contribute to maintain "compensation"? *J Hepatol* 1992; 16:190–196.
66. Campbell PJ, Leung WM, Logan AG, et al: Hyperresponsiveness to water immersion in sodium retaining cirrhotics: The role of atrial natriuretic factor. *Clin Invest Med* 1988; 11:392–395.
67. Bernardi M, DiMarco C, Trevisani F, et al: The hemodynamic status of preascitic cirrhosis: An evaluation under steady state condition and after postural change. *Hepatology* 1992; 16:341–346.
68. Schrier RW, Better OS: Pathogenesis of ascites formation: Mechanism of impaired aldosterone escape in cirrhosis. *Eur J Gastroenterol Hepatol* 1991; 3:721–729.
69. Skorecki KL, Leung WM, Campbell P, et al: Role of atrial natriuretic peptide in the natriuretic response to central volume expansion induced by head-out water immersion in sodium-retaining cirrhotic subjects. *Am J Med* 1988; 85:375–382.
70. Koepke JP, Jones S, DiBona GF: Renal nerves mediate blunted natriuresis to atrial natriuretic peptide in cirrhotic rats. *Am J Physiol* 1987; 252:R1019–1023.
71. van Vliet AA, Hackeng WH, Donker AJM, et al: Efficacy of low-dose captopril in addition to furosemide and spironolactone in patients with decompensated liver disease during blunted diuresis. *J Hepatol* 1992; 15:40–47.
72. La Villa G, Salmeron JM, Arroyo V, et al: Mineralocorticoid escape in patients with compensated cirrhosis and portal hypertension. *Gastroenterology* 1992; 102:2114–2119.
73. Unikowsky B, Wexler MJ, Levy M: Dogs with experimental cirrhosis of the liver but without intrahepatic hypertension do not retain sodium or form ascites. *J Clin Invest* 1983; 72:1594–1604.
74. Shapiro MD, Nicholls KM, Groves BM, et al: Interrelationship between cardiac output and vascular resistance as determinants of effective arterial blood volume in cirrhotic patients. *Kidney Int* 1985; 28:206–211.
75. Badalamenti S, Borroni G, Lorenzano E, et al: Renal effects in cirrhotic patients with avid sodium retention of atrial natriuretic factor injection during norepinephrine infusion. *Hepatology* 1992; 15:824–829.
76. Abraham WT, Schrier RW: The hepatorenal syndrome: Altered diuretic responsiveness with increased effective arterial blood volume. *Cardiovasc Rev Rep* 1988; 9:63–65.
77. Lenz K, Hörtnagl H, Druml W, et al: Ornipressin in the treatment of functional renal failure in decompensated liver cirrhosis. *Gastroenterology* 1991; 101:1060–1067.
78. Ruedin P, Giostra E, Cunningham M, et al: Sustained effect of chronic ornipressin treatment in hepato-renal syndrome. *J Am Soc Nephrol* 1992; 3:348.
79. Davison JM: Renal hemodynamics and volume homeostasis in pregnancy. *Scand J Clin Lab Invest [Suppl]* 1984; 169:15–21.
80. Davison JM, Gilmore EA, Durr J, et al: Altered osmotic thresholds for vasopressin and thirst in human pregnancy. *Am J Physiol* 1984; 246:F105–F109.

81. Barron WM, Stamoutsos B, Lindheimer MD: Osmoregulation during pregnancy in the rat: Evidence for resetting of the threshold for vasopressin secretion during gestation. *J Clin Invest* 1981; 68:337–346.
82. Baylis C, Blantz RC: Tubuloglomerular feedback activity in virgin and 12-day-pregnant rats. *Am J Physiol* 1985; 249:F169–F173.
83. Baylis C, Collins RC: Angiotensin II inhibition on blood pressure and renal hemodynamics in pregnant rats. *Am J Physiol* 1986; 250:F308–F314.
84. Phippard AF, Horvath JS, Glynn EM: Circulatory adaptation to pregnancy—Serial studies of haemodynamics, blood volume, renin and aldosterone in the baboon (Papio hamadryas). *J Hypertension* 1986; 4:773–779.
85. Conrad JP, Colpoys MC: Evidence against the hypothesis that prostaglandins are the vasodepressor agents of pregnancy: Serial studies in chronically instrumented, conscious rat. *J Clin Invest* 1986; 77:236–245.
86. Molnar M, Hertelendy F: N omega-nitro-L-arginine, an inhibitor of nitric oxide synthesis, increases blood pressure in rats and reverses the pregnancy-induced refractoriness to vasopressor agents. *Am J Obstet Gynecol* 1992; 166:1560–1567.
87. Ahokas RA, Mercer BM, Sibai BM: Enhanced endothelium-derived relaxing factor activity in pregnant, spontaneously hypertensive rats. *Am J Obstet Gynecol* 1991; 165:801–807.
88. Conrad KP, Joffe GM, Kruszyna H, et al: Identification of increased nitric oxide biosynthesis during pregnancy in rats. *J Am Soc Nephrol* 1992; 3:542.
89. Niederberger M, Schrier RW: Evidence for a physiological role of nitric oxide in pregnancy. *J Am Soc Nephrol* 1992; 3:549.
90. Conrad KP: Possible mechanisms for changes in renal hemodynamics during pregnancy: Studies from animal models. *Am J Kidney Dis* 1987; 9:253–259.
91. Umans JG, Lindheimer MD, Barron WM: Pressor effect of endothelium-derived relaxing factor inhibition in conscious virgin and gravid rats. *Am J Physiol* 1990; 259:F293–F296.
92. Kakouris H, Eddie LW, Summers RJ: Cardiac effects of relaxin in rats. *Lancet* 1992; 339:1076–1078.
93. Quagliarello J, Szlachter N, Steinetz BG, et al: Serial relaxin concentrations in human pregnancy. *Am J Obstet Gynecol* 1979; 135:43–44.
94. Eddie LW, Martinez F, Healy DL, et al: Relaxin in sera during the luteal phase of in-vitro fertilization cycles. *Br J Obstet Gynaecol* 1990; 97:215–220.

Alcoholic Liver Disease: New Concepts of Pathogenesis and Treatment*

John H. Bloor, M.D., Ph.D.

Instructor, University of Colorado School of Medicine, Department of Medicine, Division of Gastroenterology and Hepatobiliary Research Center, Staff Physician, The Denver Veterans Administration Medical Center, Department of Medicine, Division of Gastroenterology, Denver, Colorado

John E. Mapoles, Ph.D.

Assistant Professor, University of Colorado School of Medicine, Department of Microbiology, Hepatobiliary Research Center; Research Biologist, Denver Veterans Administration Medical Center, Denver, Colorado

Francis R. Simon, M.D.

Professor, University of Colorado School of Medicine, Department of Medicine, Division of Gastroenterology, Director, Hepatobiliary Research Center; Staff Physician, Denver Veterans Administration Medical Center, Department of Medicine, Division of Gastroenterology, Denver, Colorado

Ethanol is the most widely used drug in our society. Serious social and medical problems caused by abuse of and dependence on ethanol affect about 10% of the adults in the United States. At least 3% of deaths in this country are causally related to alcohol. Physiological and pathological effects of ethanol have been documented in most organ systems. This review will concentrate on the pathophysiology of ethanol in the liver and on recent developments in the treatment of alcoholic liver disease (ALD). This topic was last reviewed in this series 25 years ago.[1] To fully summarize the literature on alcoholic liver disease published since that time would require most of this volume. For information beyond what is discussed in the present article, the reader is referred to several excellent reviews on this subject published in the last several years.[2–5]

*This work was supported in part by NIH grants DK-42588 and P30-DK34914 (Dr. Simon); Veterans Administration Merit Review Grant entitled "Mechanism(s) of Ethanol Induced Injury" (Dr. Simon); the Denver Veterans Administration Research Center for Basic and Clinical Studies of Alcoholism; A Veterans Administration Associate Investigator Award entitled "Alcohol Metabolism and Hepatic Fibrosis" (Dr. Bloor); and a Basic Research Award from the Glaxo Institute for Digestive Health (Dr. Bloor).

Absorption, Distribution and Elimination of Ethanol

Alcohol is transferred across biological membranes by simple diffusion.[6,7] It appears to obey Fick's law in that the rate of diffusion is proportional to the concentration gradient.[6] Absorption can take place throughout the GI tract, but the rate of absorption in any region depends on the local concentration. This varies with the amount and type of beverage taken and whether it is consumed with a meal. Up to 75% of ethanol given with a meal can be absorbed through the stomach.[8] Under other circumstances the concentration of ethanol in the small bowel can reach 5%,[9,10] leading to significant intestinal absorption. Uptake from the gastrointestinal tract is rapid, and peak blood ethanol levels are generally reached within 30 minutes to 1 hour after intake.[7] Following absorption, alcohol is rapidly distributed throughout the total body water by simple diffusion.

The site of ethanol absorption from the GI tract is of clinical importance. The amount of alcohol that appears in the circulation as well as the peak level attained are generally lower when alcohol is taken with a meal. This is partly because ethanol can be metabolized by alcohol dehydrogenase (ADH) present in the gastric mucosa.[11,12,13] This "first pass" gastric metabolism of ethanol is abolished by gastrectomy.[14] Gastric ADH activity is reported to be higher in men than in women, which may account for higher peak blood alcohol concentrations in women after oral administration of ethanol.[15,16] It has been suggested that this difference may partially explain the greater susceptibility of women to alcoholic liver disease.[16,17] Gastric alcohol metabolism is lower in both male and female alcoholics, thus increasing the bioavailability of ethanol absorbed from the stomach in these populations.

The whole-body rate of ethanol elimination is approximately 0.1 gm/kg/hr,[7] but there is a twofold to threefold individual variation in this rate.[18,19] Twin studies have suggested that the origin of this variation is equally divided between genetic and environmental factors.[20] Although the rate of decrease in blood ethanol is linear at moderate concentrations, at high and low concentrations ethanol clearance rates can best be described by Michaelis-Menton kinetics.[7] This is explained to some extent by the existence of ethanol-metabolizing enzymes with high and low Michaelis constants (K_m) for ethanol.[21]

Metabolism of Ethanol

Although unmetabolized ethanol is eliminated through the kidneys, lungs, and skin, these processes contribute 5% or less to the overall rate of ethanol clearance.[7] Most ethanol is oxidatively metabolized to acetaldehyde and then to acetate, 80% to 90% of which takes place in the liver.[7] The enzymes catalyzing these reactions and their importance in vivo are discussed in this section.

Alcohol and Aldehyde Dehydrogenases

Within the liver, ethanol oxidation is predominantly catalyzed by ADH, which converts ethanol to acetaldehyde and by aldehyde dehydrogenase (ALDH) which oxidizes acetaldehyde to acetate. ADH is normally rate-limiting in this pathway.[22]

Alcohol Dehydrogenase

Alcohol dehydrogenases (EC 1.1.1.1) are broadly distributed throughout nature, and a wide variety of endogenous and exogenous substrates have been documented. The human enzymes were originally divided into three classes on the basis of their activity toward ethanol, their electrophoretic mobilities, and their sensitivity to 4-methylpyrazole inhibition.[23, 24] Recently this has been expanded to five classes.[25] All of these enzymes are dimers, each subunit having a molecular weight of approximately 40,000 daltons. ADH is responsible for 80% to 90% of ethanol oxidation in the body.[26] ADH isoforms have been detected in many tissues, although most ADH activity is in the liver with smaller amounts found in stomach, intestine, and kidney.[26, 27]

The class I enzymes correspond to what is usually regarded as the common liver ADH. They have a high affinity for ethanol, with K_ms of approximately 0.1 to 1.0mM (4.6 mg/dL), and they are very sensitive to inhibition by pyrazole. Based on starch gel analysis of liver enzyme activities, Smith et al.[27] proposed that humans have three class I ADH genes. Subsequent molecular biological analysis confirmed this hypothesis. These genes are referred to as ADH_1, ADH_2, and ADH_3 and are located close together on human chromosome 4. The encoded protein subunits designated α, β, and γ, respectively, have a 93% to 95% amino acid homology. This similarity allows the formation of heterodimers ($\alpha\beta$, $\alpha\gamma$, and $\beta\gamma$), in addition to homodimers ($\alpha\alpha$, $\beta\beta$, and $\gamma\gamma$). All of these combinations are active, although their specific activities differ.

Humans express one class II enzyme, π-ADH. It is detected principally in the liver[28] with minor activity in the intestine.[29] The subunit for π-ADH is encoded by the ADH_4 gene. The amino acid sequence is about 60% homologous with class I subunits and can only form π-homodimers.[24] The π-ADH has a K_m for ethanol of about 34mM (156 mg/dL), and the enzyme is less sensitive to 4-methylpyrazol inhibition than the class I enzymes. The liver enzyme activity is less than 10% of that of the class I ADH at low ethanol concentrations, but may become more important at higher ethanol concentrations.[28]

Class III ADH is of little interest in the context of ethanol oxidation, because of its very low affinity for ethanol ($K_m > 1M$). This is not surprising, since it was recently discovered that this enzyme normally functions in vivo as glutathione-dependent formaldehyde dehydrogenase (EC 1.2.1.1).[30]

An ADH with unique characteristics has recently been characterized from the human stomach.[11, 12] This enzyme, designated σ-ADH,[11] or μ-ADH,[12] appears to have enzymatic characteristics similar to class II enzymes with a high K_m for ethanol (41mM)[11] and inhibition of the enzyme by 4-methylpyrazole at concentrations similar to the class II enzymes. However, other properties clearly distinguish it from the class II enzymes. A new grouping, designated class IV, has been defined to encompass this and similar ADHs. The enzyme appears to be expressed predominantly in the stomach. At the high gastric ethanol concentrations that occur immediately following ingestion of alcoholic beverages, the contribution of this isoform to gastric ethanol metabolism is probably greater than that of the class I enzymes expressed there. However, the overall ADH activity in gastric mucosa is only about 1% of the hepatic activity,[11] and the quantitative significance of gastric ethanol oxidation remains unclear.

Class V ADHs consist of a single recently cloned gene, ADH_6.[31, 32] This gene encodes an ADH subunit with about 60% homology to the other ADHs. It is expressed in the liver and stomach and has a K_m for ethanol of about 28 mM (129 mg/dL). The role of this enzyme in the oxidation of ethanol is presently uncertain.

ADH Polymorphisms.—Class I ADH genes show polymorphism which may be important in explaining individual heterogeneity in the rates of ethanol elimination and the heritability of alcoholism and alcoholic liver disease.[33] Allelic variants at the ADH_2 and ADH_3 loci are known, but no polymorphisms have been reported at the ADH_1 locus. This probably reflects the lack of a careful search using modern molecular methods rather than a true absence of mutations. The three known polymorphic alleles at the ADH_2 locus have been designated ADH_2^1, ADH_2^2, and ADH_2^3. These encode the ADH β_1, β_2, and β_3 subunits, respectively.[24] ADH_2^1 has an allelic frequency of at least 95% in white Americans and Europeans. The ADH_2^2 allele is common throughout Asia with an allelic frequency of 85% in Japanese populations. The $\beta_2\beta_2$ enzyme is enzymatically distinct from $\beta_1\beta_1$ with an eighteenfold greater K_m for ethanol, a lower pH optimum, and a substantially higher V_{max}. The greater V_{max} leads to an increased rate of ethanol oxidation at high ethanol concentrations compared to the $\beta_1\beta_1$ form. ADH_2^3 has not been studied widely and has been found only in certain black American populations. There are two polymorphic alleles at the ADH_3 locus: ADH_3^1 which encodes γ_1 and ADH_3^2, which encodes γ_2. White American and European populations express these alleles at roughly equal frequencies, while Japanese and black American populations express the γ_1 subunit at much higher rates. The K_ms for ethanol of the $\gamma_1\gamma_1$ and $\gamma_2\gamma_2$ homodimers are approximately equal.

Because ADH is an important rate-limiting factor in ethanol metabolism, there have been attempts to correlate ethanol elimination rates and predisposition to alcoholism and alcoholic liver disease with ADH genotype. Although Orientals reportedly have a higher rate of ethanol clearance[34] and the allelic frequency of ADH_2^2 is high in these populations, there have been no studies seeking a correlation between ethanol elimination rate and this allele.

Several groups have looked for correlations between ADH_3 alleles and alcohol-elimination rate and between ADH_2 and ADH_3 variants and alcoholism or alcoholic cirrhosis. A French study found no significant difference in the rate of ethanol elimination in individuals homozygous for ADH_3^1 as compared to those homozygous for the ADH_3^2 allele.[35] A recent study correlating alcoholism and ADH genotype suggests that alcoholics have a significantly lower frequency of the ADH_2^2 and ADH_3^1 alleles.[36] Pupon et al.[37] showed no significant correlation between alleles at the ADH_3 locus and the occurrence of cirrhosis in alcoholics, while Day et al.[38] suggested that the frequency of ADH_3^1 may be higher in cirrhosis. However, both studies were small, and any single locus is expected to contribute only a little to the hereditability of alcoholic liver disease. It is possible that allelic variation at one or more of these loci does alter the risk of an alcoholic developing liver disease, but that the effect was missed due to inadequate statistical power (a type II error). Further studies with larger numbers of subjects and investigations of vertical transmission of linkage between allelic variants and alcoholic liver disease will be needed to resolve this question.

Some of the results just discussed suggest that variation in the rate of ethanol elimination is at least partly caused by specific ADH genotypes leading to differences in expression of hepatic ADH activity. In ethnic groups having a high frequency of an allele coding for an ADH isoform with a high enzymatic activity, aldehyde dehydrogenase may become rate-limiting for ethanol metabolism. In this situation acetaldehyde will accumulate, causing a mild disulfiram-like response (discussed later) with the consequent development of an aversion to alcohol. Such genotypes may be used in the future as negative markers for alcoholism or ALD. There is particular need for studies correlating ADH genotype (easily determined from lymphocyte DNA) and ethanol elimination rates measured using well-established methods. Such data will indicate which variants produce biologically significant changes in hepatic ethanol and acetaldehyde levels. These are more likely to be related to differences in relative risk for alcoholism and ALD.

Aldehyde Dehydrogenase

Acetaldehyde generated from ethanol is further oxidized to acetate by aldehyde dehydrogenase (EC 1.2.1.3, ALDH).[39] As with the ADHs, these enzymes display a broad substrate specificity. ALDHs are present in most cells of the body, but the highest activity is in the liver. Mammalian ALDHs are divided into three broad classes based on their cellular distribution and their inducibility.[40] ALDHs isolated from the cytosol belong to class I, while those isolated from the mitochondria are class II. Class III enzymes are associated with liver tumors and are of little interest in the present context.

$ALDH_1$ and $ALDH_2$ were first isolated from hepatic cytosol and mitochondria, respectively. They have a 68% amino acid sequence homology.[39] The active enzymes are homotetramers with a subunit molecular weight of approximately 54 kd. Although both have relatively low K_ms for acetaldehyde, the greater activity of $ALDH_2$ at low acetaldehyde concentrations suggests that it is in the major pathway for acetaldehyde oxidation.[41] $ALDH_3$ (cytosolic) and $ALDH_4$ (mitochondrial) can also be isolated from the liver but have K_ms greater than 1mM (4.6 mg/dL) for acetaldehyde. A recently described enzyme, γ-aminobutyraldehyde dehydrogenase, has a low K_m for acetaldehyde, but its importance in ethanol metabolism is unclear.

Hepatic ALDHs can be inhibited by a number of compounds, including disulfiram, cyanamide, pargyline, and reserpine. Disulfiram reacts with a critical sulfhydryl group, irreversibly inhibiting the enzyme. Marketed as Antabuse, it has been used since the 1950s to help maintain sobriety by aversion therapy in patients being treated for alcoholism.[42] In someone who has taken disulfiram, ethanol is oxidized to acetaldehyde, but further metabolism to acetate is impaired. This causes accumulation of acetaldehyde resulting in flushing, palpitation, hypotension, nausea, and vomiting.[43] This response can be fatal if a large amount of alcohol is consumed, making it potentially dangerous to use in alcoholics who cannot consciously control their drinking. Disulfiram is also reported to occasionally cause an acute hepatitis similar to that due to hepatotropic viruses.[44] Calcium carbimide (calcium cyanamide, marketed as Temposil or Abstem) and nitrefazole, neither of which is currently available in the United States, are also ALDH inhibitors that may be useful in maintaining abstinence in alcoholics by the same mechanism as disulfiram.[42]

ALDH Polymorphisms.—Polymorphism has been reported in the $ALDH_1$ and $ALDH_2$ genes.[33, 39] The most important clinically is $ALDH_2^2$,[45] expressed in approximately 50% of Orientals.[46] This allele encodes an inactive form of ALDH that can be detected immunologically in liver extracts. Sequence analysis indicates that the lack of activity is due to substitution of glutamine for a lysine residue in the polypeptide. $ALDH_2^2$ is dominant over $ALDH_2^1$ (both heterozygous and homozygous individuals lack $ALDH_2$ activity), because tetramers containing one or more $ALDH_2^1$ subunits are catalytically inactive. Presence of this mutation is closely associated with flushing in Oriental populations. The response to ethanol in affected individuals is similar to that caused by disulfiram and is presumably due to accumulation of acetaldehyde in the circulation.[47] Probably because of aversion to the symptoms induced by acetaldehyde, $ALDH_2^2$ is a negative marker for alcoholism.[48] Variation in the flushing reaction and in the blood levels of acetaldehyde among persons having the $ALDH_2^2$ allele may be due to an ADH variant (e.g., $ADH\beta_2\beta_2$) or another mutation in ALDH. This is an area that deserves further investigation.

Other Routes for Ethanol Metabolism

Lesser amounts of alcohol are oxidized to acetaldehyde by microsomal enzymes, by catalase, and by nonenzymatic reactions. A small amount of ethanol may also be sequestered by esterification, a nonoxidative pathway.

Ethanol Oxidation Associated With the Microsomes

Oxidation of ethanol by rat liver microsomes was originally described in the 1960s.[49, 50] Similar activities have subsequently been detected in many species, including humans.[3, 51] There appear to be a number of microsomal cytochromes which can oxidize ethanol. This activity collectively is referred to as the microsomal ethanol-oxidizing system or MEOS. One P450 isoform, now designated P450IIEI, appears to be the most important, accounting for 30% of the MEOS activity in normal rabbit liver. In rabbits fed ethanol this fraction increases to 70% to 80%,[52] illustrating the characteristic inducibility of this system. Levels of induction of MEOS activity in response to ethanol feeding are generally about threefold.[53] In addition to ethanol, P450IIEI is induced by other substrates such as pyrazole and acetone.[3, 51]

Whether P450IIEI contributes significantly to ethanol metabolism in vivo continues to be debated. The enzyme has a K_m for ethanol of 8 to 10mM (46 mg/dL), suggesting that it is most important at higher concentrations of ethanol.[3] In the baboon, MEOS activity is normally about one tenth that of ADH activity.[54] When the animals were fed a diet having 50% of the calories derived for ethanol for 2 to 7 years, the increased rate of ethanol elimination observed could be accounted for by the increase in MEOS activity. The importance of the MEOS in the elimination of ethanol in humans is less clear. Holtzman et al.[55] observed that treatment with cimetidine did not decrease the rate of ethanol elimination. Because cimetidine has been shown to inhibit P450-catalyzed reactions, they concluded that MEOS contributes little to the metabolism of ethanol in humans. However, the specificity of cimetidine for P450IIEI has not been completely established,[56] making this interpretation somewhat premature.

Despite the uncertainty concerning the activity of MEOS and its contribution to ethanol elimination, the induction of MEOS has important clinical implications. The induced activity of the MEOS system can increase metabolism of xenobiotics including carbon tetrachloride, isoniazid, and acetaminophen.[3] Many of these compounds have low toxicity if unmodified, but their metabolites are extremely hepatotoxic. For example, there are reports that normally therapeutic doses of acetaminophen can cause acute hepatic failure in alcoholics.[57, 58] The mechanism is not completely understood, but it is thought to be similar to that involved in the acute hepatitis caused by an acetaminophen overdose. In the alcoholic, an increased rate of oxidation of the analgesic to toxic metabolites by the ethanol-induced P450IIEI presumably overwhelms the normal detoxification mechanisms, leading to liver injury.

Minor Oxidative Pathways for Ethanol Elimination

Catalase (EC 1.11.1.6) can mediate the oxidation of ethanol by hydrogen peroxide (H_2O_2).[59] Nonenzymatic oxidation of ethanol by hydroxide radical has also been reported.[51, 60] Neither of these pathways appears to be important in terms of the bulk elimination of ethanol. Whether they are clinically important in other ways in the human is unknown.[51]

Nonoxidative Ethanol Metabolism

Ethanol can be metabolized via a nonoxidative pathway to form fatty acid ethyl esters.[61, 62] Although this pathway is present in the liver, heart, and pancreas, the greatest activities are found in the liver and pancreas. It is of particular interest in the heart and pancreas, which have little ethanol oxidative capacity, yet are major targets of alcohol-induced injury. The enzyme that catalyzes these reactions has been isolated from the heart. It has a K_m for ethanol of 1M. A blood alcohol level of 100 mg/dL—a level at which a person is considered legally impaired in many states—corresponds to an ethanol concentration of only 0.022M. Consequently, the enzyme is virtually never saturated, and the reaction is quantitatively of minor importance in ethanol metabolism. Although fatty acid ethyl esters have been detected in the cadavers of heavy drinkers,[63] a link between these compounds and injury to pancreas, liver, or any other tissue has not been demonstrated.

Pathological Effects of Ethanol and Ethanol Metabolism

It is now accepted that the etiology of ALD is multifactorial.[64] Its occurrence in well-nourished alcoholics has discredited the hypothesis that it is primarily caused by inadequate nutrition. Furthermore, malnourishment in humans who do not drink does not increase the risk of developing cirrhosis. As the toxic effects of ethanol and acetaldehyde have been documented, attention has turned to mechanisms whereby these substances can cause the hepatic injuries that are so familiar to those caring for these patients. Dietary deficiencies and other mechanisms may worsen the course of ALD and slow recovery in abstinent patients, but it is becoming obvious that both the presence and metabolism of ethanol are necessary for the development of the characteristic liver damage. As more and more effects of ethanol and acetaldehyde on the liver are documented, the problem becomes one of distinguishing primary effects of these toxins from epiphenomena that do not contribute to or that result from the injury.

A large number of model systems have been used to study the effects of ethanol and acetaldehyde.[65–69] These extend from cultured cells to a variety of animal models in species ranging from mice to baboons. None of these models truly reproduces human ALD, and many of them are difficult to use routinely in the laboratory. The baboon appears to be the model which most closely mimics the progression of the disease, but it is difficult and expensive to use. Lack of an adequate model has considerably slowed progress in understanding the pathogenesis of ALD. On the other hand, it has not inhibited the development of theories relating to the problem. Some of these will be discussed.

Ethanol

Ethanol is only weakly toxic to cells at concentrations normally achieved in the circulation. Nevertheless, it can affect properties of biological membranes,[70, 71] potentially leading to pathological changes in cell function. Changes in membrane fluidity have been observed in animals following chronic ethanol ingestion. This may alter the function of membrane-associated enzymes. Changes in the fatty acid composition of cell membranes have been documented, most of which produce a decrease in membrane fluidity. The direct fluidizing effect of ethanol on membranes can be offset in vitro by cholesterol,[72] phosphatidyl inositol,[73] and by members of all classes of phospholipids.[74] In contrast, several studies have demonstrated increased hepatocyte plasma membrane fluidity following chronic ethanol intake and exposure.[75] Thus, the importance of altered membrane fluidity in the pathogenesis of hepatic dysfunction remains uncertain.

Acetaldehyde

Acetaldehyde is the first metabolite of ethanol oxidation and is produced by all ethanol oxidative pathways. It has been suggested that acetaldehyde is a key factor in hepatic injury caused by alcohol.[3, 76–79] Acetaldehyde reacts readily with nucleophiles to form stable and unstable (reversible) adducts. Although the target is most often an amino group, some hydroxyl and sulfhydryl groups will also react with acetaldehyde. These adducts may directly damage a key function of the cell or may act as "neoantigens," stimulating an immune response and leading to immune-mediated cell injury. Acetaldehyde can also deplete cellular glutathione by reacting with it or by oxidizing other molecules which, in turn, oxidize glutathione. This can cause cellular injury through oxidative stress.[77]

Formation of Acetaldehyde Adducts

Although acetaldehyde can form adducts with proteins,[80] lipids,[81] and DNA,[82] most studies have concentrated on the interaction between acetaldehyde and proteins. Acetaldehyde is known to bind covalently to hemoglobin,[83, 84] albumin,[85] plasma and microsomal membranes,[86–88] enzymes,[89, 90] cytoskeletal proteins,[91, 92] and calmodulin.[93] These adducts appear to be reversible Schiff's bases between the carbonyl carbon of acetaldehyde and the ϵ-amino group of lysine or the α-amino group of the N-terminal amino acid residue. The tyrosine hydroxyl group can also react with acetaldehyde under some circumstances.[83] These Schiff's bases may be stabilized by reducing agents.[94, 95] Jennett et al.[80] have suggested that these stable adducts are the more important factors in causing cell injury.

Acetaldehyde adducts have been identified in a number of model systems including rat liver slices incubated with ethanol in vitro[96, 97] and in rats fed ethanol for up to 10 months.[88] Adducts of specific proteins, including hemoglobin,[83, 98] P450IIEI,[99] cytosolic proteins,[100, 101] and serum proteins,[86] have also been identified. Monoclonal or polyclonal antibodies specific for acetaldehyde-modified proteins[102] have been used to detect acetaldehyde adducts in the sera of ethanol-treated mice[102] and humans,[86, 103] as well as in rat liver.[100, 101]

The functional consequences of these adducts in vivo are poorly understood. It has been suggested but not rigorously proven that adducts may alter drug binding, oxygen affinity (of hemoglobin), enzyme activity, secretion of proteins, biogenesis of plasma membrane components, and tubulin depolymerization.[80] As mentioned earlier, whether these adducts actually cause hepatic injury and dysfunction or are of no pathological significance is unknown.

Acetaldehyde and the Cytoskeleton

All cells contain a complex filamentous cytoskeleton which lends structure to the cell and provides "roadways" for the intracellular movement of vesicles.[104–106] Components of this structure include microtubules (polymers of tubulin), actin filaments, and intermediate filaments. In hepatocytes, intermediate filaments contain cytokeratins, while those in fibroblasts are composed of vimentin. The cytokeratins are interesting because they are a major constituent of Mallory bodies (Mallory's hyaline), hepatocytic inclusions characteristically found in alcoholic hepatitis.[107, 108]

Considerable work in vitro has concentrated on the interaction of acetaldehyde with cytoskeletal elements.[92] The work with tubulin represents the best model of how acetaldehyde may interact with proteins and disrupt their function. α-Tubulin contains a lysine residue that is essential for polymerization and which is also highly reactive toward aldehydes. It has been termed the "highly reactive lysine" or HRL.[109] When acetaldehyde reacts with tubulin, it forms specific adducts with the HRL, as well as adducts with other free amino groups. Adducts formed with the HRL strongly inhibited polymerization, whereas the other adducts have no apparent effect on this process.[110, 111] This suggests that, in vivo, most adducts have only small effects on most proteins, but that modification of key residues can disrupt function.

Acute and chronic ethanol administration in several model systems impairs protein secretion,[80] causing proteins to accumulate in the Golgi apparatus. This effect appears to be mediated by acetaldehyde, since it can be blocked by ADH inhibitors[112] or increased by ALDH inhibitors.[113] The disruption may be due to the interaction of acetaldehyde with tubulin, preventing proper assembly of microtubules which are needed for normal membrane vesicle trafficking. This hypothesis is supported by reports of improper assembly of microtubules in rats chronically treated with ethanol[114] and by data discussed previously,[92] which demonstrate that acetaldehyde inhibits tubulin polymerization in vitro. If, in fact, this disruption of intracellular trafficking is related to the pathogenesis of liver disease, it is ironic that colchicine, which also disrupts microtubules, has been used in an attempt to block collagen secretion and prevent neutrophil degranulation for the purpose of treating alcoholic liver disease (discussed later).

Acetaldehyde and the Immune Response

The effect of ethanol on the function of the immune system is a large area which has been reviewed in detail elsewhere.[4, 115] There are many documented changes in the immune system associated with ALD. The majority of these are probably related to liver damage and are not a specific result of chronic ethanol exposure.

Some aspects of alcoholic hepatitis may result from the response of the immune system to acetaldehyde adducts.[115] A number of researchers have detected an increase in acetaldehyde-specific antibodies[116–118] or hemoglobin-acetaldehyde adducts[119, 120] in the serum of alcoholics or heavy drinkers. These antibodies have been used to detect acetaldehyde adducts in livers of heavy drinkers.[121] The formation of these or other adducts, perhaps on the plasma membrane, could be the source of neoantigens. A reaction to such antigens by the immune system could stimulate immune-mediated injury in the liver or in other tissues. Although the effect of adduct formation in vivo in humans is not clear, presence of the adducts has been used to evaluate alcohol consumption. Recently, Sillanaukee et al.[103, 122] demonstrated that a modified form of hemoglobin (HbA_{1ach}) is significantly increased in heavy drinkers and alcoholics. Measurement of HbA_{1ach} was as sensitive as other tests for alcohol abuse, but still detected only 50% of those judged to be alcoholics by other criteria.

Acetaldehyde and Oxidative Injury

Although the effects of ethanol and acetaldehyde on the oxidation state of the liver and the potential for oxidative or ischemic injury have received considerable attention, whether these phenomena are of clinical importance is still unknown. Glutathione[123, 124] and other thiols are the primary cellular defense against reactive metabolites. Glutathione can spontaneously form a reversible adduct with acetaldehyde,[125, 126] and chronic ethanol ingestion causes a modest decrease in total hepatic glutathione.[127, 128] Mitochondrial glutathione decreases independently of cytosolic glutathione, apparently due to a defect in the uptake from the cytosolic pool. Whether the reduction of glutathione in ethanol-exposed hepatocytes is directly due to ethanol or to acetaldehyde is not known. Changes in the concentration of reduced glutathione could also be secondary to variation in the reduction-oxidation ratio or in the activities needed to synthesize glutathione or reoxidize reduced glutathione.

Genetics of Alcoholic Liver Disease

In the mid-1970s, Lelbach[129] published data indicating that 40% to 50% of those drinking 200 g or more of ethanol per day for 20 years or more developed cirrhosis. This is approximately the maximum amount of ethanol that can be metabolized in 24 hours by a person weighing 70 kg. Lelbach's data have been criticized because, compared to other series, an unusually large fraction of his patients developed cirrhosis. Of great importance, however, is the fact that half of the drinkers did not develop cirrhosis, even at this almost inconceivably high level of consumption. Whether they would have eventually developed liver disease at higher doses consumed for longer periods is not known. From the data, no distinction can be made between a relative and an absolute resistance to alcohol-induced liver injury. Lelbach's data also provide no evidence that there is a threshold for either quantity or duration of consumption below which alcoholic liver disease does not occur. Together, these results emphasize the large and apparently continuous variability in the sensitivity to the hepatotoxic effects of alcohol that exists in the population.

Other epidemiologic data suggest that 85% to 100% of alcohol abusers develop fatty liver, about 40% to 50% eventually have alcoholic hepatitis, and only 10% to 20% go on to develop alcoholic cirrhosis. These results strongly indicate that there must be other factors, such as genetics, nutrition, environment, and perhaps the presence of other hepatotoxins, that have an important cofunction in causing liver disease in alcoholics. The presence of varying numbers of these factors in any individual alcoholic determines the point at which liver disease may or may not develop. A role for genetics in the development of liver disease is further supported by the 1981 report by Hrubec and Omenn.[130] Among male twin pairs concordant for alcoholism, 14.6% of monozygotic twins but only 5.4% of dizygotic twins were also concordant for alcoholic liver disease.[130]

Women are less likely to abuse alcohol than are men and to do so at a later age.[131] However, among women who do drink heavily, alcoholic hepatitis and cirrhosis develop sooner and at a lower amount of alcohol consumed,[132] and they progress more rapidly than in men.[133] The peak blood alcohol level is higher in women than in men after a given oral dose of ethanol. Factors contributing to this include a smaller volume of distribution, less lean body mass, and a lower level of gastric alcohol dehydrogenase (discussed earlier). The lower gastric enzyme level may increase the portal blood ethanol concentration, resulting in a greater exposure of the liver to ethanol and its metabolites. Hormonal differences may also contribute to this differential susceptibility to liver disease, as well as other factors yet to be defined.

Although this is an example of the role of genetics in determining susceptibility to ALD, it does not address the source of individual variability in the occurrence of liver disease among both men and women. Several genes other than those on the X and Y chromosomes must be involved, each one contributing a small amount to the individual risk for developing ALD. Likely candidate genes include those coding for proteins and enzymes involved in ethanol metabolism or those which contribute to alcohol-mediated hepatic injury. Individual variation in the quantities of specific proteins or the presence of abnormal proteins in the liver may affect whether alcoholic hepatitis or cirrhosis develops in response to alcohol or acetaldehyde.

As discussed previously, correlation between ADH and ALDH isoforms and alcoholic liver disease have been looked for but so far none have been found. The gene for P450IIEI is another candidate gene, particularly since it is inducible by ethanol, although its quantitative importance in ethanol metabolism in human liver is not known. In alcoholic hepatitis, which involves hepatic inflammation, genes encoding mediators of inflammation including transforming growth factor β1,[134] tumor necrosis factor α,[135–137] interleukins 1, 6, and 8,[138] and receptors for these molecules could contribute to differences in sensitivity to alcohol. All of these cytokines have been implicated in the development or progression of alcoholic hepatitis.

Hepatic fibrosis and cirrhosis due to alcohol or other causes is characterized by the accumulation of excess extracellular matrix (ECM) containing disproportionate amounts of type I collagen, fibronectin, laminin, and other normal ECM components. The increase in the amount of type I collagen is particularly dramatic and is the target of several molecular approaches to the prevention of hepatic fibrosis (discussed later, under Treatment). This collagen is composed of two chains encoded respectively by the $\alpha1(I)$ and $\alpha2(I)$ genes. Weiner et al.[139] examined the frequency of two polymorphisms in the $\alpha2(I)$ gene in alcoholics with and without cirrhosis and in nonalcoholics. They found that one combination of these polymorphisms occurred with greater frequency in alcoholics with cirrhosis than in alcoholics without cirrhosis or in nonalcoholics. Christa et al.[140] reported a similar finding in patients with alcoholic hepatitis. Both studies were small and the particular polymorphisms used have no known functional significance (i.e., they are not known to alter the rates of synthesis or degradation or the function of the collagen molecules). Nevertheless, this may be one marker for a predisposition to alcoholic liver disease in some individuals. Genes encoding other ECM proteins as well as enzymes involved in ECM remodeling (e.g., collagenases) are also likely candidate genes for studies of this type.

Another reason to be interested in ECM genes in this context is the observation that synthesis of $\alpha1(I)$ collagen protein is increased by acetaldehyde, at least partly due to increased transcription. Increased synthesis has been observed in human diploid fibroblasts (HDF),[141, 142] baboon myofibroblasts,[143] freshly isolated rat Ito cells,[144] and cultured rat Ito cells.[145, 146] The increase in collagen production in these cells appears to be due primarily to increased synthesis rather than decreased degradation, with control being at least partly transcriptional. Treatment of AF_2 cells, a human diploid fibroblast cell line that does not express ADH, with ascorbic acid, which can generate aldehydes by lipid peroxidation, also stimulated type I collagen gene transcription and the accumulation of collagen mRNA with no effect on collagenase gene transcription.[147] This suggests that the underlying mechanism may be important for process other than acetaldehyde-induced hepatic fibrogenesis.

Similar experiments have been carried out with rat Ito cells.[145, 146] After a 6-hour exposure to acetaldehyde, collagen and fibronectin mRNAs increased about threefold, while TGF-β mRNA was unaffected. This is of interest because TGF-β is reported to increase collagen $\alpha1(I)$ gene transcription by five- to tenfold. After 24 hrs of exposure, the response had fallen to 1.5-fold. These workers also showed that acetaldehyde affects collagen gene transcriptional activity.

The induction of gene transcription by acetaldehyde may be mediated by a variety of mechanisms. However, work with reductive methylation and the fd gene 5 protein[148] suggests that alkylation of lysine residues (for example, by acetaldehyde) may affect transcription factor binding and hence gene transcription. Lysine residues are critical for the binding of this single-stranded DNA-binding protein,[149] but do not affect overall protein conformation. Whether this factor is involved in collagen gene regulation is not known, but it indicates a mechanism whereby aldehydes could alter gene transcription.

Treatment of Alcoholic Liver Disease

Medicine is a scientific discipline in which application of the scientific method to observations of disease provides the basis for diagnosis and therapy. However, when applying this principle to patients with alcoholic liver disease, our poor understanding of its pathogenesis makes the development of rational therapy difficult at best. Thus there is, of necessity, a significant gap between the preceding discussion and that which follows. For each of the therapies to be discussed in this section, the theoretical basis for its trial is outlined. This should not be taken to mean that the relationship of the proposed mechanism to the effect of alcohol on the liver is understood. It is hoped that, as our grasp of the mechanisms underlying ethanol hepatotoxicity improve, so will the available therapy. A glimmer of hope may be contained under "Future Prospects."

It is important to distinguish three degrees of alcoholic liver injury. All may occur together or individually. *Fatty liver* is the mildest form of alcoholic liver disease. It is frequently asymptomatic and can be caused by drinking relatively small amounts of ethanol. As little as 10 ounces of pure ethanol (approximately 10 to 14 mixed drinks, three bottles of wine, or three 6-packs of beer) consumed over a weekend will cause fatty infiltration. Although it is considered to be benign, nonprogressive, and reversible with abstinence, there are no long-term studies of morbidity or mortality in patients with alcoholic steatosis who continue to drink. *Alcoholic hepatitis* is a much more serious inflammatory lesion characterized by polymorphonuclear leukocyte infiltration and pericentral hepatocellular necrosis. Mallory's hyalin is often present, and early fibrosis may be found. Mortality within 1 month of initial hospitalization with alcoholic hepatitis is as high as 50% to 60% in some series.[150] Factors associated with increased short-term mortality include age, markedly increased prothrombin time, presence of encephalopathy, serum bilirubin level greater than 25 mg/dL, decreased serum albumin, and serum creatinine level greater than 2.0 mg/dL. Alcoholic hepatitis is also a precursor lesion for cirrhosis. Which cases will progress cannot be predicted at present although continued ethanol abuse greatly increases the risk. *Alcoholic cirrhosis* is the end stage of alcoholic liver disease with fibrosis and micronodular or macronodular cirrhosis present on biopsy. In the absence of a concurrent alcoholic hepatitis, advanced alcoholic cirrhosis can be indistinguishable from endstage cirrhosis of other etiologies. If abstinence is established prior to the occurrence of serious complications (jaundice, ascites, hematemesis), 5-year survival can be 80% to 90%.[151] A history of complications reduces this to about 60%. Elevation of the portal-hepatic vein gradient causes esophageal varices and confers a poor prognosis.[151] For gradients < 15 torr, 4-year survival is 90%, decreasing to 40% when the gradient is ≥ 15 torr.

Abstinence remains the best monotherapy for these disorders and a necessary adjunct to all other forms of treatment. Patients with clinical or histologic evidence of liver disease who stop drinking have greatly improved survival compared to those who continue to drink.[152, 153] The goals of additional intervention are to shorten the period required for resolution, to reduce morbidity and mortality, and to prevent progression to fibrosis and cirrhosis. Towards these ends many approaches have been tried with little objective success. At the present time, orthotopic liver transplant is the only effective therapy for end-stage alcoholic liver disease. The theoretical basis and clinical results of some of these modalities will be summarized following. Progress in three promising new areas of research will also be discussed.

Nutritional Factors

The prevalence of malnutrition in alcoholics with alcoholic hepatitis or cirrhosis approaches 100%.[154] In contrast, nutritional status is relatively well maintained in alcoholics without liver disease.[154] Consequently, although an adequate diet is an important component of treatment for any alcoholic, it is of critical importance in alcoholics with liver disease. A recent issue of *Seminars in Liver Disease* is devoted to "Nutrition and the Liver".[155] It includes much information about the role of nutrition in the etiology and management of alcoholic liver disease.

This malnutrition is partly due to ingestion of alcohol as a large fraction of the caloric intake (i.e., consumption of "empty" or nonnutritive calories). Anorexia is also common in alcoholics and contributes to poor nutritional intake even in hospitalized patients. In reviewing eight studies totalling 362 patients, Achord[156] found that 87% of the patients were anorectic and 55% had nausea and vomiting. Ethanol, in excess, also drastically alters digestion, absorption, and metabolism (particularly when there is liver damage), producing specific deficiencies despite an apparently adequate diet. Protein-calorie malnutrition (marasmus) and deficiencies of zinc, selenium, iron, S-adenosylmethionine, lecithin, essential fatty acids, and vitamins A, D, E, K, thiamine, folate, pyridoxine, and B12 have all been reported to occur in alcoholic liver disease. While the importance of supplementation with thiamine and folate is well recognized, the significance of the deficiencies of most of the other compounds is less clear (but see *Future Prospects* later in this chapter). Most interest has focused on protein-calorie replacement, and several studies have examined the effect of this on morbidity and mortality in alcoholic liver disease. There has also been interest in abnormalities in the plasma amino acid profile. There is usually an overall decrease in total plasma amino acid concentration with a disproportionate reduction in the branched-chain amino acids (BCAA; valine, leucine, and isoleucine).[157] It has been suggested that these changes may be etiologically related to hepatic encephalopathy. Specific problems related to malnutrition in the context of orthotopic liver transplantation are reviewed by Porayko et al.[158]

Nutritional Supplementation

As has been noted, alcoholics with liver disease are usually malnourished. It has been hoped that improved nutritional status would accelerate healing of the liver and reduce complications (especially infections) during recuperation. In the past 15 years, a number of trials have been reported comparing a normal diet alone to the same diet supplemented with standard protein or amino acid formulas in the management of patients with acute and chronic alcoholic hepatitis and cirrhosis. Because anorexia is a major factor in determining food intake in these patients, the supplement was given parenterally or by enteral tube feeding. (It should be noted that the presence of esophageal varices is not a contraindication to placement of a soft, small-diameter esophageal feeding tube.) In many cases this led to considerable differences in the intake of both calories and protein between the treatment and control groups since their oral intake was usually similar. The studies also differed in the composition of the supplements used, the amounts given, patient selection, and duration of follow-up, making comparisons between studies difficult.

The principle conclusion from all of the studies was that nutritional status improved in both treatment and control groups. Although the improvement tended to be greater and more rapid in the supplemented patients, whether this was due to the greater intake of calories or protein or both could not be ascertained. Many studies also showed improved hepatic function as indicated by a decrease in bilirubin or serum transaminases. Decreased mortality was only evident in some studies, but the number of patients was usually small, increasing the likelihood of a type II error. The consensus is that supplementation in excess of a diet that is nutritionally adequate does not further improve morbidity or short-term mortality in this group of patients. However, in all of these studies it was clear that *provision* of an adequate diet did not mean that *intake of food* by the patient was satisfactory. Enteral or parenteral supplementation may be of value in situations where the patient cannot or will not eat an adequate amount on his or her own. Consultation with a dietitian having experience in the management of patients with alcoholic liver disease can be very valuable in achieving an adequate, palatable diet for individual patients.

Branched Chain Amino Acids

Branched chain amino acid (BCAA) supplementation in malnourished patients with hepatic encephalopathy was originally proposed in 1975 by Fischer et al.[159] Since that time many trials have investigated the benefit of BCAA in the management of patients with liver disease. The nutritional aspects of these studies have been critically reviewed by Muñoz.[160] From these studies it appears that BCAA supplementation is not nutritionally superior to standard—and much less expensive—protein and amino acid products. BCAA supplements may possibly be of use in management of alcoholics with liver disease who have proven intolerant to standard protein supplements, either by inability to maintain adequate protein intake or because of the development of hepatic encephalopathy.

Naylor et al.[161] performed a meta-analysis of five studies that had looked at the effect of BCAA on encephalopathy and mortality. Meta-analysis is ". . . a quantitative literature review technique . . . used to evaluate evidence from randomized controlled trials. . . when controversy persists after a number of trials have addressed the same issue. In essence, meta-analysis facilitates exploration of the reasons why trials differ in their conclusions, and permits aggregation of their results into a single best estimate or set of estimates of treatment effect size."[161] In this case the comparison was difficult due to the considerable heterogeneity in the study protocols and patient samples.[161, 162] Follow-up times were also all very brief and inadequate for accurate assessment of mortality. Although their analysis suggested that short-term mortality and recovery from encephalopathy were improved by BCAA supplementation, the authors conclude with the statement: ". . . it would seem premature to recommend general adoption of a controversial therapeutic modality that entails greater exposure and uncertain benefits relative to conventional management strategies."[161]

An interesting variant to the use of BCAA is supplementation with alpha-keto analogues of branched chain-amino acids.[160] These compounds are chemically identical to BCAA except that they have been oxidatively deaminated, leaving a carbonyl group on the alpha carbon in place of the alpha amino group. The purpose is to eliminate the addition of exogenous nitrogen, forcing the body to utilize toxic nitrogen compounds that have accumulated to convert the alpha-keto acids to alpha amino acids that can serve as protein precursors. Although results of several trials appear promising, larger studies with longer follow-up times will be needed before a conclusion concerning benefit of these expensive compounds can be reached.

Insulin and Glucagon Infusion

Because these hormones promote liver regeneration following partial hepatectomy and hasten recovery in a murine model of fulminant viral hepatitis,[163] several trials have examined their effect on morbidity and mortality in patients with acute alcoholic hepatitis. Using mortality as an endpoint, one study reported a significant effect after 3 weeks of treatment,[164] whereas three others showed no difference between treatment and control groups.[165–167] Results are summarized in Table 1. In addition, Bird et al.[166] found no difference in survival between the groups even 6 months after completion of treatment. Fehér et al.[164] reported an improvement in biochemical indices in their treatment group, an effect also described by Baker et al.,[165] but not by the other two groups. All of the studies appear sound and the reason for the different outcomes is unclear. Nevertheless, it appears reasonable to conclude that infusion of insulin and glucagon at the doses used here does not alter the course or outcome of acute alcoholic hepatitis. *There is no indication for this therapy in the treatment of liver disease at the present time.*

TABLE 1.
Summary of Published Trials of Insulin and Glucagon Infusion for the Treatment of Acute Alcoholic Hepatitis

	Length of Treatment	Dose Infused Over 24 Hours		Number of Deaths/Number in Group		
		Insulin	Glucagon	Treated	Control	
Baker, 1981[165]	3 weeks	24 U	2.4 mg	3/25	6/25	NS
Feher, 1987[164]	3 weeks	30 U	3.0 mg	5/33	14/33	$p < 0.05$
Bird, 1991[166]	3 weeks	30 U	3.0 mg	15/43	14/43	NS
Trinchet, 1992[167]	3 weeks	30 U	3.0 mg	10/35	5/37	NS

Pharmacologic Agents

Glucocorticoids

As discussed earlier in this review, the mechanism of injury in alcoholic hepatitis is not known. Because of the inflammatory component in the lesion and the evidence that immunological factors may be involved in its pathogenesis, many attempts have been made to treat acute alcoholic hepatitis with glucocorticoids due to their immunosuppressive properties. Since prednisone is hepatically metabolized to prednisolone, its active form, prednisolone itself or 6α-methylprednisolone have often been used, rather than prednisone. This is probably unnecessary since even severe liver disease appears to only minimally reduce this conversion.[168]

At least ten prospective clinical trials testing the efficacy of glucocorticoids in alcoholic hepatitis have been published since the first two appeared in 1971.[169, 170] Despite this mass of data, major authors remain sharply divided on whether these compounds should[151] or should not[171] be used in clinical practice. The problem lies in the inconsistent results of the studies. In addition, the small number of patients in each study and differences in patient selection, diagnostic criteria, and severity of illness make comparisons among the studies difficult. To circumvent these problems, Imperiale and McCullough[172] applied meta-analysis to the 11 studies that satisfied their inclusion criteria. The weight given to the results from each study depended on the quality of the study, judged according to specific criteria, and a quantitative analysis of the data. The pooled results were analyzed statistically for homogeneity. In addition to a pooled analysis of all trials, subgroups of subjects without active gastrointestinal bleeding and those with hepatic encephalopathy were also analyzed. The authors hypothesized that those without bleeding and with encephalopathy might benefit most from corticosteroids. Major results are summarized in Table 2. The authors conclude that corticosteroids reduce short-term mortality in patients with acute alcoholic hepatitis who are also encephalopathic. If those with gastrointestinal bleeding are excluded, the benefit seen is greater. Corticosteroids are of no value in reducing mortality in patients who are not encephalopathic. They also found no deleterious effect of treatment, suggesting that concerns about increased rates of infection and other side effects of corticosteroids may be unwarranted in this setting.

Two additional meta-analyses[173, 174] of these clinical trials reached similar conclusions regarding the benefit of corticosteroids in patients with severe alcoholic hepatitis. However, because of uncertainty in how best to define the subgroup that would benefit from treatment and the disagreement among the individual trials, both felt that additional studies were necessary before general clinical use could be recommended. Subsequently, Ramond et al.[175] randomized 61 patients with severe acute alcoholic hepatitis to prednisolone (40 mg/day for 28 days; 32 patients) or placebo (29 patients). All had biopsy-proven alcoholic hepatitis and either cirrhosis or fibrosis. Severe disease was defined as the presence of spontaneous he-

TABLE 2.
Summary of Selected Results of a Meta-analysis of Eleven Controlled Trials of Corticosteroids for the Treatment of Acute Alcoholic Hepatitis*

Subgroup Analyzed	Number of Trials (Max = 11)	Risk Ratio (Reduction in Risk)	95% Confidence Interval
All Trials	11	0.63 (37%)	0.50–0.80
Patients With Encephalopathy	11	0.66 (34%)	0.52–0.85
Patients With Encephalopathy and Without Bleeding	7	0.41 (59%)	0.28–0.60
Patients Without Encephalopathy	9	1.07 (−7%)	0.68–1.71
Patients Without Encephalopathy and Without Bleeding	5	1.01 (−1%)	0.36–2.81

*The risk ratio is the risk of short-term mortality in patients treated with corticosteroids compared to those who were not treated with corticosteroids. $P < 0.05$ that the actual risk ratio falls outside the 95% confidence interval. None of the analyses showed a statistically significant harmful effect of corticosteroids.

patic encephalopathy (4 patients), a discriminant function greater than 32 (42 patients), or both (15 patients). The discriminant function used[176] was:

$$4.6 \times (\text{prothrombin time} - \text{control time}) + (\text{serum bilirubin})/17$$

The prothrombin and control times are measured in seconds and serum bilirubin is expressed as micromoles per liter. At the start of treatment, nine of the experimental and ten of the placebo patients were encephalopathic. Survival at 2 months was 88 ± 5% (28/32) in the treatment group compared to 45 ± 8% (13/29) in the placebo group ($P = 0.001$). This survival difference was maintained when the patients were evaluated at 6 months. The only significant prognostic factor for survival was prednisolone treatment ($P = 0.02$). Of interest is that there was no difference in survival between treatment and placebo in patients with encephalopathy, in contrast to the data from the three meta-analyses. This led the authors to suggest that the discriminant function rather than the presence of encephalopathy should be used to select patients who would benefit from prednisolone therapy.

In summary, the consensus of these 12 controlled trials and three meta-analyses of the majority of the trials is that *short-term survival of patients with severe acute alcoholic hepatitis is improved by treatment with corticosteroids.* Whether long-term survival is also improved is not known. Treatment is discussed further under Recommendations.

Colchicine

Colchicine is thought to exert its antiinflammatory effects by disrupting microtubules needed for neutrophil chemotaxis, phagocytosis, and degranulation, thereby reducing the inflammatory infiltrate and preventing the release of proinflammatory substances. Part of this effect may also be a reduction in interleukin-1 by colchicine.[177] By thus treating alcoholic hepatitis, it has been hoped that progression to fibrosis and cirrhosis could be prevented. In animal models and in vitro, colchicine is also antifibrogenic. It is reported to prevent secretion of procollagen (probably by disruption of microtubular assembly),[178] increase collagenase synthesis,[179] and prevent $CC1_4$-induced cirrhosis in rats.[180]

Four controlled trials of colchicine for the treatment of alcoholic liver disease have been published. Kershenobich et al.[181] randomized 54 patients to colchicine and 46 to placebo. Of these, 73% were Child-Pugh class A, 26% class B, and 1% class C. A total of 45% had alcoholic cirrhosis, but the distribution of etiologies between treatment and control groups was not given. 92% of the patients had liver biopsies. The colchicine was given at a dose of 1 mg/day, 5 days/week, for the duration of the study (mean follow-up was 4.7 years). Although the proportion of the patients receiving colchicine who died of liver disease (37%) was comparable to that in controls (40%), the authors state that the median survival of the colchicine group was 11.0 years while that of the control group was 3.5 years. They also describe histologic improvement in 9/30 (30%) treated patients and 0/14 (0%) placebo patients. Significant problems with this study include poor compliance with medication, apparently poorer follow-up of placebo patients, and lack of information about interim characteristics of the patients during the trial. At most, the data suggest that chronic treatment of early liver disease does not affect the ultimate cause of death, but may prolong survival. How this applies to patients with alcoholic liver disease cannot be gleaned from the published data. A recent abstract[182] gives preliminary data from a small study testing the therapeutic effect of colchicine (1 mg/day, 5 days/wk) on patients with biopsy-proven alcoholic cirrhosis. A total of 23 patients received colchicine and an additional 20 were given placebo. From the abstract it appears that all subjects were Child-Pugh class A or B and that they were followed for 1 to 2 years. No significant effect of colchicine was seen on Child-Pugh class or on several laboratory parameters, including serum concentration of tumor necrosis factor. No posttreatment histologic data are given. Comparison of this report with that of Kershenobich et al.[181] is difficult because of different outcome criteria, but there is at least the suggestion that they may not agree. The study by Pinto et al.[182] cannot be fully evaluated until a detailed report, including data on survival and posttreatment histology, is published.

The other two studies both looked at the effect of colchicine in alcoholic hepatitis. Trinchet et al.[183] randomized 33 patients with alcoholic hepatitis to colchicine (1 mg/day for 6 months) and 34 to placebo. Cirrhosis was also present in 52% of the treatment group and 47% of the placebo group. All were actively drinking at the time of enrollment. Patients were fully evaluated (usually including liver biopsy) at 3 and 6 months from entry. Compliance with medication was reported to be "good" by pill counting and questioning. The dropout rate was quite high (48%), and the proportions of males and cirrhotics had increased in the colchicine group by 6 months. No significant changes were seen over the 6-month course of the study in biochemical parameters or histologic scores for alcoholic hepatitis or fibrosis for within either the treatment or the placebo groups or between the two groups. Akriviadis et al.[184] randomized 36 patients to colchicine (1 mg/day for 30 days) and 36 to placebo. All had alcoholic hepatitis by clinical criteria; patients with clinical evidence of advanced cirrhosis were excluded. Patients were all initially hospitalized and most completed the treatment before discharge. Colchicine had no significant effect on in-hospital deaths, serum bilirubin, aspartate aminotransferase level, prothrombin time, or leukocyte count. There was also no effect on mortality rates at follow-up evaluation 4 months after enrollment. Liver biopsies on 9 treated and 10 control patients at a mean of 19 days into the study showed no difference in any histologic parameters between the groups. These studies lead to the conclusion that there is no major effect of colchicine on acute alcoholic hepatitis. Both groups point out that much larger studies would be needed to identify more minor treatment responses.

In summary, although there are theoretical reasons to believe that colchicine may be helpful for treating alcoholic hepatitis, the somewhat limited study data do not support this hypothesis. Whether there is a beneficial effect of colchicine on long-term survival of cirrhotics (alcoholic or otherwise) would require a more carefully executed study than is so far available. It is unclear whether such a study is warranted. *At the present time colchicine should not be used in the routine management of alcoholic liver disease.*

Propylthiouracil

Propylthiouracil (PTU), used to treat hyperthyroidism, inhibits both thyroid hormone synthesis in the thyroid gland and peripheral conversion of thyroxine to triiodothyronine. Its use in the treatment of alcoholic hepatitis is based on the similarity to hyperthyroidism of the hypermetabolic state induced in rat liver by ethanol feeding.[185] Furthermore, in rat liver made hypermetabolic by ethanol feeding, hypoxemic insult causes centrilobular (zone 3) necrosis similar to that seen in alcoholic liver disease.[186] Large doses of PTU can partially prevent this injury.[186] Although early data were equivocal,[185] several recent studies suggest that a similar hypermetabolic state appears to exist in human alcoholics with either hepatitis or cirrhosis.[187–189] In these studies, resting energy expenditure was compared in controls and patients with alcoholic liver disease. No difference was seen until the values were corrected for lean body mass (i.e., muscle mass), based on urinary creatinine excretion. After correction, patients with alcoholic liver disease had increased energy expenditure, consistent with a hypermetabolic state. This correction is plausible since muscle metabolism is responsible for much of the resting energy expenditure.[190]

There are three published clinical trials of the efficacy of PTU in treating alcoholic hepatitis. The first[191] randomized 133 patients with both histological and clinical evidence (78 patients) or clinical evidence alone of alcoholic hepatitis. Those who had milder disease and received PTU showed more rapid improvement in a clinical index composed of 11 clinical and 6 laboratory parameters than did those on PTU with more severe hepatitis or those receiving placebo. Short-term mortality was not affected by PTU. In the second study,[192] 31 patients received PTU and 36 received placebo. All had severe alcoholic hepatitis based on clinical and laboratory data, making the patients fairly similar to the more severe subgroup in the previous study.[191] No difference in mortality or in changes in biochemical parameters was seen when the PTU and placebo groups were compared. This confirms the previous observation[191] that PTU has no affect on the course of severe alcoholic hepatitis but provides no information about its effect on milder disease. Furthermore, because of the relatively small numbers of patients, the likelihood of a type II error (failing to detect an effect of therapy when an effect actually exists) was high in both studies. To reduce the probability of a type II error to 10% would require enrollment of 200 to 300 patients.[192]

The most recent study examined the effect of long-term PTU therapy on survival of patients with alcoholic liver disease. Patients were followed for up to 2 years. Most continued to drink throughout the study, based on daily morning urinary alcohol concentrations.[193] Severity of liver disease was judged by a combined clinical and laboratory index (CCLI).[194, 195] This is similar to the index used by this group in earlier studies,[191] but several factors shown not to be related to mortality had been removed. This index should be useful in future studies of alcoholic liver disease as a complement to the Child-Pugh classification[196] and Maddrey's discriminant function.[176] The results of the study showed three things:

1. PTU reduced mortality overall by 48%, from 0.25 in the placebo group to 0.13 in the treatment group.
2. Mortality in the subgroup with a CCLI > 5 was reduced by 55%, from 0.55 in the placebo group to 0.25 in the treatment group. The number of deaths in the subgroup with CCLI ≤ 5 was too small for a similar analysis.
3. There was no reduction in mortality in the subgroup with mean morning urinary alcohol concentrations >8mM (37 mg/dL).

There was a very high dropout rate—68% in the PTU and 60% in the placebo group. Analysis showed that the dropouts from the PTU and placebo groups had similar characteristics (including mean CCLIs of <4) and that they withdrew for similar reasons, minimizing their effect on the composition of the study groups. Dropouts were followed for up to 2 years after withdrawal and had low cumulative mortality rates, consistent with the low CCLIs at withdrawal. Because the high attrition rate reduced the number of patients followed to the end of the study, weakening any conclusions regarding long-term effects, it is interesting that a beneficial effect of PTU was observed, nevertheless, in specific subgroups of the patients.

There has been little subsequent interest in the use of PTU for treatment of alcoholic hepatitis despite the apparently consistent results of the short-term studies and the encouraging effect on long-term mortality in some patients with severe disease. Potential difficulties with PTU include its apparent ineffectiveness in patients who continue to drink heavily[193] and the questionable compliance of alcoholics with a medication to be taken twice a day for many years. Now that there is more convincing evidence for the occurrence of hypermetabolism in alcoholics with liver disease, further studies of the clinical usefulness of PTU seem justified. *At the present time we cannot recommend the use of PTU for treating patients with alcoholic hepatitis outside of controlled trials.*

Surgery

In the past 10 years orthotopic liver transplantation has emerged as a successful treatment for end-stage liver disease of many etiologies.[197] Its use in treating alcoholic liver disease remains somewhat controversial, however. There is no question that alcoholic liver disease can be fatal or that it can be "cured" by liver transplantation. The controversy centers around whether there are social and moral reasons to refuse transplantation to alcoholics or, if alcoholics are to be transplanted, how to select optimal candidates for transplant. It should be noted that all of the available data are for transplantation of alcoholics with end-stage cirrhotic liver disease and not with acute alcoholic hepatitis alone. This is partly due to the highly variable course and potential reversibility of the acute lesion with abstinence from alcohol. Furthermore, data to be discussed later in this section suggest that prolonged abstinence prior to transplant predicts posttransplant abstinence. Since the presence of alcoholic hepatitis is usually associated with active alcohol consumption, this is likely to be a group at increased risk for recidivism and perhaps, as a consequence, poor transplant outcomes. The number of patients awaiting transplant and the number dying from liver disease while waiting are both increasing. It seems inadvisable to create additional transplant candidates who are likely to have a poor prognosis posttransplant. Until data are available that demonstrate a favorable outcome in this group of patients, acute alcoholic hepatitis should not be a general indication for orthotopic liver transplantation.

The nonmedical issues relevant to hepatic transplantation for alcoholic cirrhosis have been reviewed recently[198–200] and further discussion of them is beyond the scope of this article. Instead, we will focus on three medical questions which, at least potentially, can be answered with some objectivity.

1. Is there any difference in the posttransplant course of patients with alcoholic liver disease compared to those with liver disease of other etiologies?—In an early compilation of hepatic transplantation statistics, survival of patients transplanted for alcoholic cirrhosis was poor compared to those transplanted for other causes.[201] However, patients with alcoholic cirrhosis comprised only 5% of the number transplanted, and 80% of the transplants for alcoholic cirrhosis were performed prior to the introduction of cyclosporine. No information was given regarding comparability of the alcoholic and nonalcoholic patients with respect to comorbidities, age, severity of illness at transplant, and other factors that could have affected a successful outcome. Nevertheless, this report led to the perception that alcoholics were a poor risk for orthotopic liver transplant. In three subsequent reports of patients transplanted since 1980, actuarial 1-year survivals were 66%,[136, 202] 74%,[203] and 73%,[204] comparable to those for patients transplanted for other liver diseases in the same transplant programs. These studies are important because they demonstrate that the survival rate of liver transplantation for alcoholic cirrhosis can be comparable to that for other indications, using current surgical and immunosuppressive techniques. Two recent abstracts give additional support to this conclusion.[205, 206] There is no medical reason at the present time to categorically reject patients with alcoholic cirrhosis as candidates for orthotopic liver transplantation.

2. How can selection criteria be defined that maximize the likelihood of a satisfactory outcome for orthotopic liver transplantation in patients with alcoholic cirrhosis?—General medical and surgical selection criteria for liver transplant candidates have not changed much in some time.[207] Additional considerations in transplantation for alcoholic cirrhosis are the presence of extrahepatic alcohol-related disease, including malignancy,[208] and the likelihood of abstinence and compliance with treatment posttransplant.

Two studies have attempted to define criteria for selection of transplant candidates from amongst applicants with alcoholic liver disease. Beresford et al.[209] worked from the premise that the principal difference in outcome between patients with alcoholic and nonalcoholic liver disease was the presence of alcoholism. Using known prognostic indicators for short- and long-term abstinence from alcohol, they developed a flexible set of psychosocial criteria (the University of Michigan Alcoholism Prognosis Scale for Major Organ Transplant Candidates)[204] that they expected would predict transplant candidates who would have satisfactory posttransplant courses. This scale, together with usual medical and surgical criteria, was used to evaluate 99 alcoholics with liver disease who applied to the University of Michigan for orthotopic liver transplantation between 1985 and 1989.[204] Of these, 45 patients were selected as suitable candidates and received transplants. Actuarial survival in this group was 78% at 1 year and 73% at 2 years, similar to their nonalcoholic patients and to the results reported by other transplant centers.[136, 202–206] The rate of recidivism was 11%, also similar to rates from other programs. As the authors themselves point out, because their analysis was retrospective, it could not differentiate a positive effect of the selection process on survival and recidivism from effects of the transplant itself and postoperative medical and psychological management. Thus we are left with a plausible but unvalidated selection instrument that had no greater effect on short-term outcome than did the selection procedures used by other transplant programs.[136, 202–206]

In the second study, available only as an abstract, Gish et al.[210] prospectively categorized patients with respect to risk (high, medium, or low) for recidivism and noncompliance before and after transplant. No specific period of abstinence was required, but actual criteria for classification were not given. The authors concluded that they could accurately predict subsequent recidivism and noncompliance and that only low-risk patients are good transplant candidates. Additional details must await full publication of their results. The possibility that acceptance or rejection for transplant, the transplant itself, or the posttransplant care may contribute to a patient's subsequent behavior was not directly addressed in the abstract. This has been discussed by Lucey et al.[204] and is an important consideration in evaluating the outcome of studies such as this one.

Additional data are available from follow-up studies of patients transplanted for alcoholic cirrhosis. Bird et al.[136, 202] reported a recidivism rate for ethanol consumption of only 12.5% (3/24). However, the three patients that resumed alcohol consumption were the only ones who had not stopped drinking prior to transplant. In the series reported by Kumar et al.,[203] 15% (11/73) of the patients had been abstinent for less than six months pretransplant. Although overall posttransplant recidivism was 11.5%, it was 6.7% among patients abstinent 6 months or more compared to 43% among those with less than 6 months of abstinence. A similar pattern is described in a recent abstract.[205] Although the rate of recidivism posttransplant is consistently greater in patients who were abstinent for the shortest time pretransplant, the value of a fixed period of abstinence has been disputed.[203, 204] Long waiting periods for transplantation of alcoholics have been considered punitive and tantamount to a death sentence.[211] Whether longer abstinence truly decreases recidivism urgently needs to be tested in a controlled trial. If this observation is true, then the minimum duration of abstinence necessary for maximum benefit must be defined. The previous suggestion that at least 6 months of abstinence should be a requirement for candidacy[212] appears to have been made arbitrarily. In addition, although the recidivism rates previously cited seem fairly low, they are based on small numbers of patients and, more importantly, on short periods of follow-up. In the Pittsburgh cohort, at a mean follow-up of 4.5 years, actuarial 5-year survival was 55% and recidivism had risen to 23%.[206] It will be important to continue to collect long-term follow-up data on alcoholics posttransplant.

Also lacking (with the exception of the abstract by Gish et al.[210]) is information about the effect of posttransplant alcohol abuse on the outcome of orthotopic liver transplantation. Although it is intuitive to believe that it must be deleterious and much of the work described has focused on recidivism as being synonymous with poor outcome, few actual data are available. The effect of ethanol on the transplanted liver is addressed in the next section. Other potential consequences of alcohol abuse posttransplant include decreased compliance with medical care (particularly immunosuppressive medications), malnutrition, occurrence of alcohol-related extrahepatic diseases, and accidental death while intoxicated. These seem to be problems that are at least as serious as direct damage of the transplanted liver by alcohol. All of these concerns need to be evaluated in prospective studies.

3. If an alcoholic patient does not remain abstinent posttransplant, will alcoholic liver disease develop in the transplanted liver?—Since liver transplantation is a relatively new procedure and alcoholic cirrhosis usually requires 15 to 20 years or more to manifest itself, patience may be required to see an effect, if it is there. The apparently low recidivism rate cited previously may also make recurrence of alcoholic liver disease unlikely. Moreover, as discussed earlier, it is probable that genetic factors—presumably involving genes expressed in the liver—play a role in individual sensitivity to alcoholic liver disease. There is at least some hope that the transplanted liver, being genetically distinct from the injured liver, will not carry the same risk for an adverse response to ethanol.

To address the question of recurrence, the Pittsburgh group retrospectively analyzed 154 liver biopsies from 23 patients (mean of 7 ± 2 biopsies per patient) who had been transplanted for alcoholic cirrhosis between January 1981 and December 1991 and who were known to have abused alcohol again after transplantation. Their findings, published as an abstract[213] and summarized in Table 3, suggest a high rate of ethanol-related damage in the transplanted livers over a remarkably short time span. This seems surprising, and it is important to note that none of the changes seen are specific for alcoholic liver disease. Data bearing on other potential causes of injury to the transplanted livers (before or after transplant) are not included in the abstract.

If the reported changes do appear to be a consequence of alcohol consumption, why did they occur so rapidly? One possibility is the existence in alcoholics of circulating antibodies or committed B or T lymphocytes that recognize acetaldehyde adducts ("neo-antigens"; see earlier). Although the donor liver presumably has few or none of these antigens initially, after the recipient resumes alcohol consumption, acetaldehyde is available to create adducts in the new liver. The response of the immune system to these antigens could rapidly lead to hepatic injury. While this is an interesting and testable hypothesis, it is also possible that transplantation, immunosuppression, or some other variable may alter the effect of ethanol on the transplanted liver. If so, then it is an important consideration for all patients receiving a liver transplant, not just those who presented initially with alcoholic cirrhosis. Alternatively, are these lesions simply hitherto unrecognized (early?) effects of ethanol on the liver that are being detected here because of the close surveillance which these patients receive? In either case, is the

TABLE 3.
Histologic Effects of Ethanol Consumption on Transplanted Livers.*

Histologic Finding	Fraction of Patients With One or More Abnormal Biopsies	Days After Transplant That the Abnormal Biopsy was Obtained	Total Number of Biopsies (out of 154) With the Abnormality
Steatosis	22/23	3–752	72
Central Sclerosis	20/23	11–309	49
Pericellular Fibrosis	12/23	28–579	35
Mallory's Hyaline Cirrhosis	23/23	77–579	23
Cirrhosis	4/23	177–711	9
Individual Cell Necrosis	17/23	As early as 3–28	57
Piecemeal Necrosis	—	207–912	—

*Data from Baddour N, Demetris AJ, Shah G, et al: *Gastroenterology* 1992; 102(part 2):A777.

injury clinically relevant in the short- or long-term? If it is, is complete abstinence necessary to prevent it, or is "social" drinking possible without adverse effects? Answers to these intriguing questions must await publication of additional details from this and other groups. The value of such data for the understanding of alcoholic liver disease cannot be overestimated.

Recommendations

From the studies discussed previously, we believe that three recommendations can be made regarding treatment of alcoholic liver disease. The limitations inherent in these recommendations emphasize the areas in which further basic and clinical research is needed.

1. **Total abstinence from alcohol, together with good nutrition, are the most important prescriptions for recovery.**—The diet should supply 2500 to 3000 calories per day. If hepatic encephalopathy is not present, amounts of enteral protein sufficient to establish a positive nitrogen balance (80 to 120 g of protein/day) do not seem to precipitate encephalopathy. However, in starting a patient with unknown protein tolerance on enteral feedings, the amount of protein given should start at 20 to 30 g/day. It can be increased at 20 to 30 g/day until the desired amount is attained, provided encephalopathy does not occur. Branched chain amino acid supplements are expensive and, if used at all, they should be reserved for patients who do not tolerate adequate amounts of conventional protein or amino acid solutions. The diet should provide recommended daily allowances of all vitamins and minerals. Supplementation with thiamine and folate is generally indicated. Parenteral administration of vitamins K and B12 should be used as indicated by laboratory testing. Supranormal amounts of other trace elements should be used only if specific deficiencies are documented.
2. **Corticosteroids are useful for decreasing the short-term mortality of severe acute alcoholic hepatitis.**—Although there are slight differences in dosing, a reasonable regimen appears to be 40 mg of prednisolone per day for 4 weeks. Adjustment for its greater potency and molecular weight gives an equivalent daily dose of 33 mg of methylprednisolone. Only patients with a discriminant function greater than 32 or possibly those with encephalopathy, should be treated. Patients with gastrointestinal bleeding or intercurrent infections should not be treated. Beneficial effects of corticosteroids on morbidity, long-term mortality, or progression of alcoholic hepatitis to fibrosis and cirrhosis have not been documented.
3. **Patients with end-stage liver disease due to alcoholic cirrhosis are candidates for orthotopic liver transplantation.**—Selection criteria for alcoholics should be similar to those used for patients being evaluated for liver transplantation for other causes of liver failure. However, because of the psychosocial problems associated with alcohol abuse, particular care should be taken to establish that a stable, supportive environment exists to maintain abstinence from alcohol and to assure compli-

ance with posttransplant care. There are no data to support a specific period of abstinence as a criterion for transplantation. While pretransplant abstinence may predict posttransplant abstinence, the data are not strong enough to refuse transplantation to an alcoholic, who otherwise fulfills selection criteria, but who would not survive an extended waiting period. Moreover, although most people intuitively believe that resumption of alcohol abuse posttransplant is harmful, data to support this position are woefully lacking. Patients felt likely to eventually need hepatic transplant should be referred to a transplant center for evaluation as soon as possible. The rate of progression of liver disease—and the time needed for approval for transplantation—are both difficult to estimate accurately.

Future Prospects

Given the relatively poor results of "traditional" therapies for alcoholic liver disease, it is encouraging that there are several new approaches that appear promising. As often happens, these are the result of an improved understanding of the biologic mechanisms involved in the pathogenesis of the disease, again emphasizing the importance of basic research into disease processes. The agents to be discussed in this section are still in the early stages of investigation, although at least one of them—HOE 077—is undergoing phase I clinical trials.[214] Another area of great potential interest is cytokine antagonists. As mentioned earlier, a number of cytokines appear to be involved in the development of alcoholic liver disease.[134–138] Blocking the effects of these substances could ameliorate symptoms and prevent progression.

Prolyl-4-hydroxylase Inhibitors

Following synthesis, procollagen polypeptides undergo several posttranslational modifications. One of these is hydroxylation of proline residues, catalyzed by prolyl-4-hydroxylase (P4H[215]). 4-Hydroxyproline is needed for successful folding of the collagen monomers into the mature triple helical collagen molecule at body temperature. Under-hydroxylated (denatured) collagen may either leave the cell and disrupt extracellular collagen processing and deposition, or it can be rapidly degraded in the lysosomes.[216] HOE 077 is a pyridine-2,4-carboxylate diamide that can be activated only in the liver by deamidation to pyridine-2,4-dicarboxylic acid (2,4-PDCA), a competitive inhibitor of P4H.[217] The active compound, 2,4-PDCA, is hydrophilic and cannot readily cross biological membranes. Administration of HOE-077 to rats with $CC1_4$-induced hepatic fibrosis is reported to inhibit progression of the hepatic fibrosis. Doses five- to fifty-fold greater than those needed to block hepatic fibrogenesis reportedly do not alter the mechanical properties of skin, bones, or tendons, and do not impair wound healing,[217] consistent with its activation being confined to the liver. Such a drug could be useful for blocking progression of alcoholic hepatitis to fibrosis or preventing further deterioration in patients with hepatic fibrosis of varied etiologies. In preliminary studies, human metabolism of HOE 077 appears similar to that in animals, and no toxic effects in humans were noted following single doses of 250 to 1500 mg of the compound.[214] It will be of considerable interest to watch the progress of clinical trials of this and related compounds.

Anti-sense RNAs and DNAs

Complementary oligoribo- or deoxyribonucleotides which bind to specific sequences in mRNA or in genes (DNA), respectively, can prevent expression of the protein encoded by that gene.[218, 219] These molecules are short—20 to 30 base pairs—sequences of RNA or DNA that are complementary to coding regions of cellular polynucleotides. Their binding blocks transcription or translation, preventing expression of the gene product. Several such compounds show promise for treatment of specific viral illnesses, including AIDS, but they are still far from ready for clinical trials. Of interest to those caring for patients with liver disease is a recent report that an antisense oligodeoxyribonucleotide complementary to a sequence in the 5' region of the collagen $\alpha 1(I)$ gene decreased collagen synthesis in cultured fibroblasts by 60%.[220] Uptake of the antisense DNA by the fibroblasts was enhanced by coupling it to an asialoglycoprotein (ASG) which bound to and was taken up by ASG receptors expressed on the fibroblast plasma membrane. This same system can be used to target molecules to hepatocytes since only hepatocytes normally express ASG receptors in vivo.[221, 222] Since the myofibroblast seems to be the cell responsible for increased collagen synthesis in hepatic fibrosis, specific targeting to these cells will be needed for the collagen antisense DNAs to decrease collagen synthesis in hepatic fibrosis.[223] Other possible gene targets relevant to liver disease of many etiologies include prolyl 4-hydroxylase (discussed previously), other enzymes involved in the synthesis of collagen and other extracellular matrix proteins, and cytokines implicated in the pathogenesis of alcoholic hepatitis. The considerable potential of this approach to the treatment of alcoholic liver disease cannot be realized, however, until the mechanisms mediating the injurious effect of alcohol on the liver are identified. Without this, the most appropriate targets for antisense nucleotides cannot be selected. Introduction of antisense DNAs can also be used to define the role of specific genes and gene products in the pathogenesis of liver disease, thereby contributing to delineation of the pathways involved.

Lecithin (phosphatidyl choline) and SAMe (S-adenosylmethionine; SAM)

Over 40 years ago studies in rats suggested that deficiencies of choline and methionine might contribute to the hepatotoxicity of alcohol. However, in clinical trials, choline failed to ameliorate alcoholic liver injury when ethanol consumption continued[224] and did not inhibit the ability of ethanol to produce fatty liver in human volunteers[225] or fatty liver and fibrosis in baboons.[226] Methionine was similarly ineffective at preventing alcoholic liver injury.

Choline is a precursor for the synthesis of phosphatidyl choline (a membrane phospholipid) and methionine can be converted into S-adenosylmethionine (SAMe), needed for synthesis of phospholipids, glutathione, and for a number of other biological methylations. Both of these compounds are critical for maintenance of membranes and mitochondria and for other cellular functions. In 1988, activities of enzymes needed for utilization of these precursors were found to be decreased in cirrhotics.[227] Whether these enzymes are rate-limiting and hence are actually able to affect net flow through these pathways was not shown. In a recently published study, Lieber et al.[228] bypassed these enzymes by feeding baboons a liquid diet containing ethanol, with or without polyunsaturated lecithin (PUL), for up to 8 years. While PUL did not prevent fat accumulation, it was associated with a decrease in hepatic fibrosis. In seven baboons fed ethanol without PUL for 6 years or more, six developed septal fibrosis and one of these six progressed to cirrhosis. Two animals fed ethanol and PUL for more than 6 years developed only perivenular or interstitial fibrosis. When these two animals and a third who had received ethanol plus PUL for only 3 years were changed to a diet of ethanol without PUL, all progressed to cirrhosis within 18 months. Whether the antifibrotic effect was due to the PUL or to one of its components (unsaturated fatty acids or choline) is not known. Given the results of other studies, it seems unlikely that choline had a significant protective effect, but unsaturated fatty acids do protect against oxidative tissue injury in some systems. The number of animals used in this study was small but the use of primates would seem to make it more likely that these results may apply to humans.

SAMe is the source of methyl groups needed to convert phosphatidyl ethanolamine to lecithin. In liver this is a minor but significant pathway for the synthesis of membrane phospholipids. A decrease in phospholipid methylation can alter fluidity, thereby changing activities of membrane enzymes and having other effects on cellular function. SAMe is also essential for the synthesis of glutathione, a compound needed to protect cells against oxidative injury,[229] and serves as a methyl donor in a number of other reactions.[229] In clinical trials it is reported to relieve symptoms and improve liver function indices in patients with intrahepatic cholestasis.[230] In baboons fed a liquid diet containing ethanol with or without orally administered SAMe for 18 to 36 months, several liver-related measures were relatively better in animals receiving SAMe, although the same proportion of animals in each group (40%) developed significant fibrosis.[231] Patients with alcoholic or non-alcoholic liver disease have decreased serum levels of glutathione.[232] These are partially restored by oral administration of SAMe, although the clinical significance of this observation is not known.[232]

The data suggesting a beneficial effect of PUL and SAMe on alcoholic liver disease are encouraging but very preliminary. Whether the results can be transferred to humans must await clinical trials. The time has not arrived for supplementation of alcoholic beverages with lecithin or SAMe as has been suggested for thiamine.

References

1. Lieber CS: Metabolic effects produced by alcohol in the liver and other tissues. *Adv Intern Med* 1968; 14:151–199.
2. Zetterman RK: Modern approach to alcoholic liver disease. *Scand J Gastroenterol* 1992; 192 (Suppl 27):55–62.
3. Lieber CS: Hepatic, metabolic and toxic effects of ethanol: 1991 update. *Alcohol Clin Exp Res* 1991; 15:573–592.
4. Kennedy NP, Tipton KF: Ethanol metabolism and alcoholic liver disease. *Essays Biochem* 1990; 25:137–195.
5. Johnson RD, Williams R: Immune responses in alcoholic liver disease. *Alcohol* 1986; 10:471–486.
6. Kalant H: Absorption, diffusion, distribution, and elimination of ethanol: Effect on biological membranes, in Kissin B, Begleiter H (eds): *The Biology of Alcoholism:* Biochemistry, vol. I. New York, Plenum Press, 1971, pp 1–62.
7. Holford NHG: Clinical pharmacokinetics of ethanol. *Clinical Pharmacokinetics* 1987; 13:273–292.
8. Cortot A, Jobin G, Ducrot F, et al: Gastric emptying and gastrointestinal absorption of alcohol ingested with a meal. *Dig Dis Sci* 1986; 31:343–348.
9. Persson J: Alcohol and the small intestine. *Scand J Gastroenterol* 26:3–15, 1991.
10. Beck I, Dinda P: Acute exposure of small intestine to ethanol: effects on morphology and function. *Dig Dis Sci* 1981; 26:817–838.
11. Moreno A, Pares X: Purification and characterization of a new alcohol dehydrogenase from human stomach. *J Biol Chem* 1991; 266:1128–1133.
12. Yin A-J, Wang M-F, Liao C-S, et al: Identification of a human stomach alcohol dehydrogenase with distinctive kinetic properties. *Biochem Int* 1990; 22:829–835.
13. Seitz HK, Simanowski UA, Egerer G, et al: Human gastric alcohol dehydrogenase: in vitro characteristics and effect of cimetidine. *Digestion* 1992; 51:80–85.
14. Caballeria J, Frezza M, Hernandez-Munoz R, et al: The gastric origin of the first pass metabolism of ethanol in man: Effect of gastrectomy. *Gastroenterology* 1989; 97:1205–1209.
15. Julkunen RJK, DiPadova C, Lieber CS: First pass metabolism of ethanol-A gastrointestinal barrier against the systemic toxicity of ethanol. *Life Sci* 1985; 37:567–573.
16. Frezza M, DiPadova C, Pozzato G, et al: High blood alcohol levels in women: The role of gastric alcohol dehydrogenase activity and first-pass metabolism. *N Engl J Med* 1990; 322:95–99.
17. Saunders JB, Davis M, Williams R: Do women develop alcoholic liver disease more readily than men? *Br Med J* 1981; 282:1140–1143.
18. Keiding S, Christensen NJ, Damgaard SE, et al: Ethanol metabolism in heavy drinkers after massive and moderate alcohol intake. *Biochem Pharmacol* 1983; 22:337–344.
19. Bennion LJ, Li T-K: Alcohol metabolism in American Indians and whites. Lack of racial differences in metabolic rate and liver alcohol dehydrogenase. *N Engl J Med* 1976; 294:9–13.
20. Kopun M, Propping P: The kinetics of ethanol absorption and elimination in twins and supplementary repetitive experiments in singleton subjects. *Eur J Clin Pharmacol* 1977; 11:337–344.

21. Crabb D.W., Bosron WF, Li T-K: Ethanol metabolism. *Pharmacol Ther* 1987; 34:59–73.
22. Crow KE, Hardman MJ: Regulation of rates of ethanol metabolism, in Crow KE, Batt RD (eds): *Human Metabolism of Alcohol,* vol 2. Boca Raton, Fla, CRC Press, 1989, pp 3–16.
23. Vallee BL, Bazzone TJ: Isozymes of human liver alcohol dehydrogenase. *Isozymes Curr Top Biol Med Res* 1983; 8:219–244.
24. Burnell JC, Bosron WF: Genetic polymorphism of human liver alcohol dehydrogenase and kinetic properties of the isoenzymes, in Crow KE, Batt RD (eds): *Human Metabolism of Alcohol,* vol 2. Boca Raton, Fla, CRC Press, 1989, pp 65–75.
25. Pares X, Cederlund C, Moreno A, et al: Class IV alcohol dehydrogenase (the gastric enzyme): Structural analysis of human $\sigma\sigma$-ADH reveals class IV to be variable and confirms the presence of a fifth mammalian alcohol dehydrogenase class. *FEBS Lett* 1992; 303:69–72.
26. Li T-K: Enzymology of human alcohol metabolism. *Adv Enzymol* 1977; 45:427–483.
27. Smith ME, Hopkinson DA, Harris H: Developmental changes and polymorphism in human alcohol dehydrogenase. *Ann Hum Genet* 1971; 34:251–271.
28. Li T-K, Bosron WF, Dafeldecker WP, et al: Isolation of II-alcohol dehydrogenase of human liver: Is it a determinant of alcoholism? *Proc Natl Acad Sci USA* 1977; 74:4378–4381.
29. Smith ME, Hopkinson DA, Harris H: Alcohol dehydrogenase isozymes in adult human stomach and liver: evidence for activity of the ADH_3 locus. *Ann Hum Genet* 1972; 35:243–253.
30. Koivusalo M, Baumann M, Uotila L: Evidence for the identity of glutathione-dependent formaldehyde dehydrogenase and class III alcohol dehydrogenase. *FEBS Lett* 1989; 257:105–109.
31. Yasunami M, Chen C-S, Yoshida A: A human alcohol dehydrogenase gene (ADH6) encoding an additional class of isozyme. *Proc Natl Acad Sci USA* 1991; 88:7610–7614.
32. Chen C-S, Yoshida A: Enzymatic properties of the protein encoded by newly cloned human alcohol dehydrogenase ADH6 gene. *Biochem Biophys Res Comm* 1991; 181:743–747.
33. Bosron WF, Li T-K: Genetic polymorphism of human liver alcohol and aldehyde dehydrogenase, and their relationship to alcohol metabolism and alcoholism. *Hepatology* 1986; 6:502–510.
34. Hanna JM: Metabolic responses of Chinese, Japanese, and Europeans to alcohol. *Alcohol Clin Exp Res* 1978; 2:89–92.
35. Couzigou P, Fleury B, Groppi A, et al: Role of alcohol dehydrogenase polymorphism in ethanol metabolism and alcohol-related diseases. *Adv Exp Biol Med* 1990; 284:263–270.
36. Thomasson HR, Edenberg HJ, Crabb DW, et al: Alcohol and aldehyde dehydrogenase genotypes and alcoholism in Chinese Men. *Am J Hum Genet* 1991; 48:677–681.
37. Poupon RE, Nalpas B, Coutelle C, et al: Polymorphism of alcohol dehydrogenase, alcohol and aldehyde dehydrogenase activities: Implication in alcoholic cirrhosis in white patients. *Hepatology* 1992; 15:1017–1022.
38. Day CP, Bashir R, James OFW, et al: Investigation of the role of polymorphisms at the alcohol and aldehyde dehydrogenase loci in genetic predisposition to alcohol-related end-organ damage. *Hepatology* 1991; 14:798–801.

39. Yoshida A, Hsu LC, Yasunami M: Genetics of human alcohol-metabolizing enzymes. *Prog Nuc Acid Res* 1991; 40:255–287.
40. Anonymous: Nomenclature of Mammalian Aldehyde Dehydrogenases. *Prog Clin Biol Res* 1989; 290:xix–xxi.
41. Tipton KF, Henehan GTM, Harrington MC: Cellular and intracellular distribution of aldehyde dehydrogenase, in Crow KE, Batt RD (eds): *Human Metabolism of Alcohol,* vol 2. Boca Raton, Fla, CRC Press, 1989, pp 105–116.
42. *Seventh Special Report to the U.S. Congress on Alcohol and Health.* Rockville, Md, U.S. Dept. of Health and Human Services, 1990, pp 266–267.
43. Kitson TM: Reactions of aldehyde dehydrogenase with disulfiram and related compounds, in Crow KE, Batt RD (eds): *Human Metabolism of Alcohol,* vol 2. Boca Raton, Fla, CRC Press, 1989, pp 117–132.
44. Bartle WR, Fisher MM, Kerenyl N: Disulfiram-induced hepatitis. Report of two cases and review of the literature. *Dig Dis Sci* 1985; 30:834.
45. Harada S, Agarwal DP, Goedde HW: Electrophoretic and biochemical studies of human aldehyde dehydrogenase isozymes in various tissues. *Life Sci* 1980; 26:1773–1780.
46. Goedde HW, Agarwal DP, Fritze G, et al: Distribution of ADH_2 and $ALDH_2$ genotypes in different populations. *Hum Genet* 1992; 88:344–346.
47. Mizoi Y, Fukunaga T, Adachi J: The flushing syndrome in orientals, in Crow KE, Batt RD (eds): *Human Metabolism of Alcohol,* vol 2. Boca Raton, Fla, CRC Press, 1989, pp 219–230.
48. Harada S, Agarwal DP, Goedde HW, et al: Aldehyde dehydrogenase isozyme variation and alcoholism in Japan. *Pharmacol Biochem Behav* 1983; 18(suppl 1):151–153.
49. Orme-Johnson WH, Ziegler DM: Alcohol mixed function oxidase activity of mammalian liver microsomes. *Biochem Biophys Res Commun* 1965; 21:78–82.
50. Lieber CS, DeCarli LM: Ethanol oxidation by hepatic microsomes: adaptive increases after ethanol feeding. *Science* 1968; 162:917–918.
51. Koop DR: Minor pathways of ethanol metabolism, in Crow KE, Batt RD (eds): *Human Metabolism of Alcohol,* vol 2. Boca Raton, Fla, CRC Press, 1989, pp 133–146.
52. Koop DR, Nordblom GD, Coon MJ: Immunochemical evidence for a role of cytochrome P-450 in liver microsomal ethanol oxidation. *Arch Biochem Biophys* 1984; 235:228–238.
53. Morgan ET, Koop DR, Coon MJ: Catalytic activity of cytochrome P-450 isoenzyme 3a isolated from liver microsomes of ethanol-treated rabbits. *J Biol Chem* 1982; 257:13951–13957.
54. Nomura F, Pikkarainen PH, Jauhonen P, et al: Effect of ethanol administration on the metabolism of ethanol in baboons. *J Pharmacol Exp Ther* 1983; 227:78–83.
55. Holtzman JL, Gebhard RL, Eckfeldt JH, et al: The effects of several weeks of ethanol consumption on ethanol kinetic in normal men and women. *Clin Pharmacol Ther* 1985; 38:157–163.
56. Abernethy DR, Greenblatt DJ, Divoll M, et al: Differential effect of cimetidine on drug oxidation (antipyrine and diazepam) vs. conjungation (acetaminophen and lorazepam): Prevention of acetaminophen toxicity by cimeitidine. *J Pharmacol Exp Ther* 1983; 234:508–513.
57. Leist MH, Gluskin LE, Payne JA: Enhanced toxicity of acetaminophen in alcoholics: Report of three cases. *J Clin Gastroenterol* 1985; 7:55–59.
58. Seeff LB, Cuccherini BA, Zimmerman HJ, et al: Acetaminophen hepatotox-

icity in alcoholics. A therapeutic misadventure. *Ann Intern Med* 1986; 104:399–404.
59. Chance B, Sies H, Boveris A: Hydroperoxide metabolism in mammalian organs. *Physiol Rev* 1979; 59:527–605.
60. Feierman DE, Winston GW, Cederbaum AI: Ethanol oxidation by hydroxyl radicals: Role of iron chelates, superoxides, and hydrogen peroxide. *Alcohol Clin Exp Res* 1985; 9:95–102.
61. Morgelson S, Lange LG: Nonoxidative ethanol metabolism in rabbit myocardium: Purification to homogeneity of fatty acyl ethyl ester synthase. *Biochemistry* 1984; 23:4075–4081.
62. Laposata EA, Lange LG: Presence of nonoxidative ethanol metabolism in human organs commonly damaged by ethanol abuse. *Science* 1986; 231:497–499.
63. Lange LG, Sobel BE: Myocardial metabolites of ethanol. *Circ Res* 1983; 52:479–482.
64. Lieber CS: Biochemical and molecular basis of alcohol-induced injury to the liver and other tissues. *N Engl J Med* 1988; 319:1639–1650.
65. Tsukamoto H, Gaal K, French SW: Insights into the pathogenesis of alcoholic liver necrosis and fibrosis: Status report. *Hepatology* 1990; 12:599–608.
66. Rubin E, Lieber CS: Fatty liver, alcoholic hepatitis, and cirrhosis produced by alcohol in primates. *N Engl J Med* 1974; 298:128–135.
67. Lieber CS, DeCarli LM, Rubin E: Sequential production of fatty liver, hepatitis, and cirrhosis in sub-human primates fed ethanol with adequate diets. *Proc Natl Acad Sci USA* 1975; 72:437–441.
68. Porto LC, Chevallier M, Grimaud J-A: Morphometry of terminal hepatic veins. 2. Follow up in chronically alcohol-fed baboons. *Virchows Arch A Pathol Anat Histopathol* 1989; 414:299–307.
69. Ainley C, Senapati A, Brown IMH, et al: Is alcohol hepatotoxic in the baboon? *J Hepatol* 1988; 7:85–92.
70. Taraschi RF, Rubin E: Effects of ethanol on the chemical and structural properties of biologic membranes. *Lab Invest* 1985; 52:120–131.
71. Goldstein DB: Ethanol-induced adaptation in biological membranes. *Ann NY Acad Sci* 1987; 492:103–111.
72. Chin JH, Goldstein DB: Cholesterol blocks the disordering effects of ethanol in biomembranes. *Lipids* 1984; 19:929–935.
73. Taraschi RF, Ellingson JS, Wu A, et al: Phosphatidylinositol from ethanol-fed rats confers membrane tolerance to ethanol. *Proc Natl Acad Sci USA* 1986; 83:9398–9402.
74. Rottenberg H, Bittman R, Li H-L: Resistance to ethanol disordering of membranes from ethanol-fed rats is conferred by all phospholipid classes. *Biochim Biophys Acta* 1992; 1123:282–290.
75. Polokoff MA, Simon TJ, Harris RA, et al: Chronic ethanol increases liver plasma membrane fluidity. *Biochemistry* 1985; 24:3114–3120.
76. Sorrell MF, Tuma DJ: Hypothesis: alcoholic liver injury and the covalent binding of acetaldehyde. *Alcohol Clin Exp Res* 1985; 9:306–309.
77. Dianzani MU: Lipid peroxidation in ethanol poisoning: a critical reconsideration. *Alcohol* 1985; 20:161–173.
78. Barry RE, McGivan JD: Acetaldehyde alone may initiate hepatocellular damage in acute alcoholic liver disease. *Gut* 1985; 26:1065–1069.
79. Lauterberg BH, Bilzer M: Mechanisms of acetaldehyde hepatotoxicity. *J Hepatology* 1988; 7:384–390.

80. Jennett RB, Tuma DJ, Sorrell MF: Effects of acetaldehyde on hepatic proteins. *Prog Liver Dis* 1990; 9:325–333.
81. Kenney WC: Formation of Schiff base adduct between acetaldehyde and rat liver phosphatidylethanolamine. *Alcohol Clin Exp Res* 1984; 8:551–555.
82. Ristow H, Obe G: Acetaldehyde induces cross-links in DNA and causes sister-chromatid exchanges in human cells. *Mutation Res* 1978; 58:115–119.
83. Stevens VJ, Fantl WJ, Newman CB, et al: Acetaldehye adducts with hemoglobin. *J Clin Invest* 1981; 67:361–369.
84. San George RC, Hoberman HD: Reaction of acetaldehyde with hemoglobin. *J Biol Chem* 1986; 261:6811–6821.
85. Tuma DJ, Donohue TM, Medina VA, et al: Enhancement of acetaldehyde-protein adduct formation by L-ascorbate. *Arch Biochim Biophys* 1984; 234:377–381.
86. Lin RC, Lumeng L, Shahidi S, et al: Protein-acetaldehyde adducts in serum of alcoholic patients. *Alcohol Clin Exp Res* 1990; 14:438–443.
87. Nomura F, Lieber CS: Binding of acetaldehyde to rat liver microsomes: Enhancement after chronic alcohol consumption. *Biochim Biophys Res Comm* 1981; 100:131–137.
88. Barry RE, Williams AJK, McGivan JD: The detection of acetaldehyde/liver plasma membrane protein adduct formed in vivo by alcohol feeding. *Liver* 1987; 7:364–368.
89. Mauch TJ, Donohue TM, Zetterman RK, et al: Covalent binding of acetaldehyde selectively inhibits the catalytic activity of lysine-dependent enzymes. *Hepatology* 1986; 6:263–269.
90. Mauch TJ, Tuma DJ, Sorrell MF: The binding of acetaldehyde to the active site of ribonuclease: Alterations in the catalytic activity and effects of phosphate. *Alcohol Alcohol* 1987; 22:103–112.
91. Xu DS, Jennett RB, Smith SL, et al: Covalent interactions of acetaldehyde with the actin/microfilament system. *Alcohol Alcohol* 1989; 24:281–289.
92. Tuma DJ, Smith SL, Sorrell MF: Acetaldehyde and microtubules. *Ann NY Acad Sci* 1991; 625:786–792.
93. Jennett RB, Saffari-Fard A, Sorrell MF, et al: Increased covalent binding of acetaldehyde to calmodulin in the presence of calcium. *Life Sciences* 1989; 24:281–289.
94. Tuma DJ, Newman MR, Donohue TM, et al: Covalent binding of acetaldehyde to proteins: Participation of lysine residues. *Alcohol Clin Exp Res* 1987; 11:579–584.
95. Farbiszewski R, Chwiecko M, Holownia A, et al: Changes in sulfhydryl compounds in plasma, liver, and brain after acute and chronic acetaldehyde administration in rats. *Drug Alcohol Depend* 1988; 22:79–82.
96. Donohue TM, Tuma DJ, Sorrell MF: Binding of metabolically derived acetaldehyde to hepatic proteins in vitro. *Lab Invest* 1983; 49:226–229.
97. Medina VA, Donohue TM, Sorrell MF, et al: Covalent binding of acetaldehyde to hepatic proteins during ethanol oxidation. *J Lab Clin Med* 1985; 105:5–10.
98. Lumeng L, Minter RG: Formation of acetaldehyde-adducts in vivo demonstrated by high-performance liquid chromatography. *Alcohol Clin Exp Res* 1985; 9:209.
99. Behrens UJ, Hoerner M, Lasker JM, et al: Formation of acetaldehyde adducts with ethanol-inducible P450IIE1 in vivo. *Biochim Biophys Res Comm* 1988; 154:584–590.

100. Lin RC, Fillenwarth MJ, Minter R, et al: Formation of the 37-kD protein-acetaldehyde adduct in primary cultured rat hepatocytes exposed to alcohol. *Hepatology* 1990; 11:401–407.
101. Lumeng L, Lin RC: Formation of a 37 kildalton liver protein-acetaldehyde adduct in vivo and in liver cell culture during chronic alcohol exposure. *Ann NY Acad Sci* 1991; 625:793–801.
102. Israel Y, Hurwitz E, Niemela O, et al: Monoclonal and polyclonal antibodies against acetaldehyde-containing epitopes in acetaldehyde-protein adducts. *Proc Natl Acad Sci USA* 1986; 83:7923–7927.
103. Sillanaukee P, Seppa K, Koivula T, et al: Acetaldehyde-modified hemoglobin as a marker of alcohol consumption: Comparison of two new methods. *J Lab Clin Med* 1992; 120:42–47.
104. Feldmann G: The cytoskeleton of the hepatocyte. *J Hepatology* 1989; 8:380–386.
105. Phillips MJ, Satir P: The cytoskeleton of the hepatocyte: Organization, relationships, and pathology, in Arias IM, Jakoby W, Popper D et al (eds): *The Liver: Biology and Pathobiology,* ed 2. New York, Raven Press, 1988, pp 11–27.
106. Osborn M, Weber K: Intermediate filament proteins: A multigene family distinguishing major cell lineages. *Trends in Biochem Sci* 1986; 11:469–472.
107. Katsuma Y, Swierenga SH, Khettry U, et al: Changes in the cytokeratin intermediate filament cytoskeleton associated with Mallory body formation in mouse and human liver. *Hepatology* 1987; 7:1215–1223.
108. Worman HJ: Cellular intermediate filament networks and their derangement in alcoholic hepatitis. *Alcoholism Clin Exp Res* 1990; 14:789–804.
109. Szasz J, Yaffe MB, Elzinga M, et al: Microtubule assembly is dependent on a cluster of basic residues in α-tubulin. *Biochemistry* 1986; 25:4572–4582.
110. Jennett RB, Sorrell MF, Johnson EL, et al: Covalent binding of acetaldehyde to tubulin: Evidence for a preferential binding to the α-chain. *Arch Biochem Biophys* 1987; 256:10–18.
111. Smith SL, Jennett RB, Sorrell MF, et al: Acetaldehyde sub stoichiometrically inhibits bovine neurotubulin polymerization. *J Clin Invest* 1989; 84:337–341.
112. Tuma DJ, Zetterman RK, Sorrell MF: Inhibition of glycoprotein secretion by ethanol and acetaldehyde in rat liver slices. *Biochem Pharmacol* 1980; 29:35–38.
113. Volentine GD, Ogden KA, Kortje DK, et al: Role of acetaldehyde in the ethanol induced impairment of hepatic glycoprotein secretion in the rat in vivo. *Hepatology* 1987; 7:490–495.
114. Baraona E, Lieber CS: Effects of alcohol on hepatic transport of proteins. *Annu Rev Med* 1982; 33:281–292.
115. Israel Y, Orrego H, Niemela O: Immune responses to alcohol metabolites: Pathogenic and diagnostic implications. *Sem Liver Dis* 1988; 8:81–90.
116. Worrall S, DeJersey J, Shanely BC, et al: Antibodies against acetaldehyde-modified epitopes: An elevated IgA response in alcoholics. *Eur J Clin Invest* 1991; 21:90–95.
117. Niemela O, Klajner F, Orrego H, et al: Antibodies against acetaldehyde-modified protein epitopes in human alcoholics. *Hepatology* 1987; 7:1210–1214.
118. Koskinas J, Kenna JG, Bird GL, et al: Immunoglobulin A antibody to a 200-kilodalton cytosolic acetaldehyde adduct in alcoholic hepatitis. *Gastroenterology* 1992; 103:1860–1867.

119. Peterson CM, Scott BK, Jovanovic-Peterson L: Hemoglobin associated acetaldehyde correlates with the self-administered alcoholism screening test but not glycated hemoglobin in type II diabetes mellitus. *Alcohol* 1991; 8:183–185.
120. Niemela O, Israel Y: Hemoglobin-acetaldehyde adducts in human alcohol abusers. *Lab Invest* 1992; 67:246–252.
121. Niemela O, Juvonen T, Parkila S: Immunohistochemical demonstration of acetaldehyde-modified epitopes in human liver after alcohol consumption. *J Clin Invest* 1991; 87:1367–1374.
122. Sillanaukee P, Koivula T: Detection of a new acetaldehyde-induced hemoglobin fraction HbA_{1ach} by cation exchange liquid chromatography. *Alcohol Clin Exp Res* 1990; 14:842–846.
123. Deleve LD, Kaplowitz N: Importance and regulation of hepatic glutathione. *Sem Liver Dis* 1990; 10:251–266.
124. Meister A, Anderson A: Glutathione. *Annu Rev Biochem* 1983; 52:711–760.
125. Speisky H, MacDonald A, Giles G, et al: Increased loss and decreased synthesis of hepatic glutathione after acute ethanol administration. Turnover studies. *Biochem J* 1985; 225:565–572.
126. Vina J, Estela JM, Guerri C, et al: Effect of ethanol on glutathione concentration in isolated hepatocytes. *Biochem J* 1980; 188:549–552.
127. Fernandez-Checa JC, Ookhtens M, Kaplowitz N: Effects of chronic ethanol feeding on rat hepatocytic glutathione. *J Clin Invest* 1989; 83:1247–1252.
128. Fernandez-Checa JC, Garcia-Ruiz C, Ookhtens M, et al: Impaired uptake of glutathione by hepatic mitochondria from chronic ethanol-fed rats: Tracer kinetic studies in vitro and in vivo and susceptibility to oxidant stress. *J Clin Invest* 1991; 87:397–405.
129. Lelbach WK: Epidemiology of alcoholic liver disease. *Prog Liver Dis* 1976; 5:494–515.
130. Hrubec Z, Omenn G: Evidence of genetic predisposition to alcoholic cirrhosis and psychosis: Twin concordances for alcoholism and its biological endpoint by zygosity among male veterans. *Alcohol Clin Exper Res* 1981; 5:207–215.
131. Robins LN, Helzer JE, Weissman MM, et al: Lifetime prevalence of specific psychiatric disorders in three sites. *Arch Gen Psychiatry* 1984; 41:949–958.
132. Tuyns AJ, Pequignot G. Greater risk of ascitic cirrhosis in females in relation to alcohol consumption. *Int J Epidem* 1984; 13:53–57.
133. Morgan MY, Sherlock S: Sex-related differences among 100 patients with alcoholic liver disease. *Br Med J* 1977; 1(6066):939–941.
134. Fausto N, Mead JE, Guppuso PA, et al: Effects of TGF-βs in the liver: Cell proliferation and fibrogenesis. *Ciba Found Symp* 1991; 157:165–177.
135. McClain CJ, Cohen DA: Increased tumor necrosis factor production by monocytes in alcoholic hepatitis. *Hepatology* 1989; 9:349–351.
136. Bird GLA, Sheron N, Goka J, et al: Increased plasma tumor necrosis factor in severe alcoholic hepatitis. *Ann Intern Med* 1990; 112:917–920.
137. Felver ME, Mezey E, McGuire M, et al: Plasma tumor necrosis factor α predicts decreased long-term survival in severe alcoholic hepatitis. *Alcohol Clin Exp Res* 1990; 14:255–259.
138. Shedlofsky SI, McClain CJ: Hepatic dysfunction due to cytokines, in Kimball ES (ed): *Cytokines and Inflammation*. Boca Raton, Fla, CRC Press, 1991, pp. 235–273.
139. Weiner FR, Eskreis DS, Compton KV, et al: Haplotype analysis of a type I

collagen gene and its association with alcoholic cirrhosis in man. *Mol Aspects Med* 1988; 10:159–162.

140. Christa L, Zarski JP, Nalpas B, et al: Nested polymerase chain reaction on cellular DNA in plasma: A rapid method to investigate the collagen type I A2 MspI polymorphic restriction site in alcoholic patients. *Hum Genet* 1992; 88:537–540.
141. Holt K, Bennett M, Chojkier M: Acetaldehyde stimulates collagen and non-collagen protein production by human fibroblasts. *Hepatology* 1984; 4:843–848.
142. Brenner D, Chojkier M: Acetaldehyde increases collagen gene transcription in cultured human fibroblasts. *J Biol Chem* 1987; 262:17690–17695.
143. Savolainen E-R, Leo MA, Timpl R, et al: Acetaldehyde and lactate stimulate collagen synthesis of cultured baboon liver myofibroblasts. *Gastroenterology* 1984; 87:777–787.
144. Shiratori Y, Ichida T, Kawase T, et al: Effect of acetaldehyde on collagen synthesis by fat-storing cells isolated from rats treated with carbon tetrachloride. *Liver* 1986; 6:246–251.
145. Moshage H, Casini A, Lieber CS: Acetaldehyde selectively stimulates collagen production in cultured rat liver fat-storing cells but not in hepatocytes. *Hepatology* 1990; 12:511–518.
146. Casini A, Cunningham M, Rojkind M, et al: Acetaldehyde increases procollagen Type I and fibronectin gene transcription in cultured rat fat-storing cells through a protein synthesis-dependent mechanism. *Hepatology* 1991; 13:758–765.
147. Chojkier M, Houglum K, Solis-Jerruzo J, et al: Stimulation of collagen gene expression by ascorbic acid in cultured human fibroblasts. *J Biol Chem* 1989; 264:16957–16962.
148. Dicks LR, Sherry AD, Newkirk MM, et al: Reductive methylation and ^{13}C NMR studies of lysyl residues of fd gene 5 protein. *J Biol Chem* 1988; 263:18864–18872.
149. Anderson RA, Nakashima Y, Coleman JE: Chemical modifications of functional residues of fd gene 5 DNA-binding protein. *Biochemistry* 1975; 14:907–917.
150. Theodossi A, Eddleston ALWF, Williams R: Controlled trial of methylprednisolone therapy in severe acute alcoholic hepatitis. *Gut* 1982; 23:75–79.
151. Carithers RL, Jr: Alcoholic hepatitis and cirrhosis, in Kaplowitz N (ed): *Liver and Biliary Diseases,* Baltimore, Williams and Wilkins, 1992, pp 334–346.
152. Borowsky SA, Strome S, Lotte E: Continued heavy drinking and survival in alcoholic cirrhotics. *Gastroenterology* 1981; 80:1405–1409.
153. Powell WJ, Klatskin G: Duration and survival in patients with Laennec's cirrhosis. *Am J Med* 1968; 44:406–420.
154. Marsano L, McClain CJ: Nutrition and alcoholic liver disease. *JPEN* 1991; 15:337–344.
155. Tavill AS, McCullough AJ: Nutrition and the liver. *Sem Liver Dis* 1991; 11:265–348.
156. Achord JL: A prospective randomized clinical trial of peripheral amino acid-glucose supplementation in acute alcoholic hepatitis. *Am J Gastroenterol* 1987; 82:871–875.
157. Diehl AME, Mitchell MC, Herlong HF, et al: Changes in plasma amino acids during sobriety in alcoholic patients with and without liver disease. *Am J Clin Nutr* 1986; 44:453–460.

158. Porayko MK, DiCecco S, O'Keefe SJD: Impact of malnutrition and its therapy on liver transplantation. *Sem Liver Dis* 1991; 11:305–314.
159. Fischer JE, Funovics JM, Aguirre A, et al: The role of plasma amino acids in hepatic encephalopathy. *Surgery* 1975; 78:276–290.
160. Muñoz SJ: Nutritional therapies in liver disease. *Sem Liver Dis* 1991; 11:278–291.
161. Naylor DC, O'Rourke K, Detsky AS, et al: Parenteral nutrition with branched-chain amino acids in hepatic encephalopathy. A meta-analysis. *Gastroenterology* 1989; 97:1033–1042.
162. Berlin JA, Chalmers TC: Meta-analysis of branched-chain amino acids in hepatic encephalopathy. *Gastroenterology* 1989; 97:1043–1051.
163. Farivar M, Wands JR, Isselbacher KJ, et al: Effect of insulin and glucagon on fulminant murine hepatitis. *N Engl J Med* 1976; 295:1517–1519.
164. Fehér J, Cornides A, Romány A, et al: A prospective multicenter study of insulin and glucagon infusion therapy in acute alcoholic hepatitis. *J Hepatology* 1987; 5:224–231.
165. Baker AL, Jaspan JB, Haines NW, et al: A randomized clinical trial of insulin and glucagon infusion for treatment of alcoholic hepatitis: Progress report in 50 patients. *Gastroenterology* 1981; 80:1410–1414.
166. Bird G, Lau JYN, Koskinas J, et al: Insulin and glucagon infusion in acute alcoholic hepatitis: A prospective randomized controlled trial. *Hepatology* 1991; 14:1097–1101.
167. Trinchet J-C, Balkau B, Poupon RE, et al: Treatment of severe alcoholic hepatitis by infusion of insulin and glucagon: A multicenter sequential trial. *Hepatology* 1992; 15:76–81.
168. Uribe M, Schalm SW, Summerskill WHJ, et al: Oral prednisone for chronic active liver disease: Dose responses and bioavailability studies. *Gut* 1978; 19:1131–1135.
169. Helman RA, Temko MH, Nye SW, et al: Alcoholic hepatitis. Natural history and evaluation of prednisolone therapy. *Ann Intern Med* 1971; 74:311–321.
170. Porter HP, Simon FR, Pope CE, et al: Corticosteroid therapy in severe alcoholic hepatitis. *N Engl J Med* 1971; 284:1350–1355.
171. Zakim D, Boyer TD, Montgomery C: Alcoholic liver disease, in Zakim D, Boyer TD (eds): *Hepatology. A textbook of liver disease.* ed 2. Philadelphia, WB Saunders, 1990. pp 821–869.
172. Imperiale TF, McCullough AJ: Do corticosteroids reduce mortality from alcoholic hepatitis? A meta-analysis of the randomized trials. *Ann Intern Med* 1990; 113:299–307.
173. Reynolds TB, Benhamou JP, Blake J, et al: Treatment of acute alcoholic hepatitis. *Gastroenterol Int* 1989; 2:208–216.
174. Daures JP, Peray P, Bories P, et al: Corticoid therapy in the treatment of acute alcoholic hepatitis. Results of a meta-analysis. *Gastroenterol Clin Biol* 1991; 15:223–228.
175. Ramond MJ, Poynard T, Rueff B, et al: A randomized trial of prednisolone in patients with severe alcoholic hepatitis. *N Engl J Med* 1992; 326:507–512.
176. Carithers RL Jr., Herlong HF, Diehl AM, et al: Methylprednisolone therapy in patients with severe alcoholic hepatitis. A randomized multicenter trial. *Ann Intern Med* 1989; 110:685–690.
177. Kershenobich D, Alcocer J, Quiroga A, et al: Effect of colchicine on immunoregulatory T-lymphocytes and monocytes in patients with primary biliary cirrhosis (abstract). *Clin Res* 1984; 32:496.

178. Ehrlich HP, Ross R, Bornstein P: Effects of antimicrotubular agents on the secretion of collagen. A biochemical and morphological study. *J Cell Biol* 1974; 62:390–405.
179. Harris ED, Krane SM: Effects of colchicine on collagenase in cultures of rheumatoid synovium. *Arthritis Rheum* 1971; 14:669–684.
180. Mourelle M, Billalon C, Amezcua JL: Protective effect of colchicine on acute liver damage induced by carbon tetrachloride. *J Hepatol* 1988; 6:337–342.
181. Kersenobich D, Vargas F, Garcia-Tsao G, et al: Colchicine in the treatment of cirrhosis of the liver. *N Engl J Med* 1988; 318:1709–1713.
182. Pinto HC, Alexandrino P, Santos PM, et al: Colchicine in alcoholic cirrhosis: Preliminary results of a double-blind randomized trial (abstract 739). *Hepatology* 1992; 16:229A.
183. Trinchet J-C, Beaugrand M, Callard P, et al: Treatment of alcoholic hepatitis with colchicine. Results of a randomized double blind trial. *Gastroenterol Clin Biol* 1989; 13:551–555.
184. Akrividis EA, Steindel H, Pinto PC, et al: Failure of colchicine to improve short-term survival in patients with alcoholic hepatitis. *Gastroenterology* 1990; 99:811–818.
185. Kaplowitz N: Propylthiouracil treatment for alcoholic hepatitis: Should it and does it work? *Gastroenterology* 1982; 82:1468–1472.
186. Israel Y, Kalant H, Orrego H, et al: Experimental alcohol-induced hepatic necrosis: Suppression by propylthiouracil. *Proc Nat Acad Sci USA* 1975; 72:1137–1141.
187. Shanbhogue RL, Bistrian BR, Jenkins RL, et al: Resting energy expenditure in patients with end-stage liver disease and in normal population. *JPEN* 1987; 11:305–308.
188. John WJ, Phillips R, Ott L, et al: Resting energy expenditure in patients with alcoholic hepatitis. *JPEN* 1989; 13:124–127.
189. Schneeweiss B, Braninger W, Ferenci P, et al: Energy metabolism in patients with acute and chronic liver disease. *Hepatology* 1990; 11:387–393.
190. Heymsfield SB, Waki M, Reinus J: Are patients with chronic liver disease hypermetabolic? *Hepatology* 1990; 11:502–505.
191. Orrego H, Kalant H, Israel Y, et al: Effect of short-term therapy with propylthiouracil (PTU) in patients with alcoholic liver disease. *Gastroenterology* 1979; 76:105–115.
192. Hallé P, Paré P, Kaptein E, et al: Double-blind, controlled trial of propylthiouracil in patients with severe acute alcoholic hepatitis. *Gastroenterology* 1982; 82:925–931.
193. Orrego H, Blake JE, Blendis LM, et al: Long-term treatment of alcoholic liver disease with propylthiouracil. *N Engl J Med* 1988; 317:1421–1427.
194. Orrego H, Israel Y, Blake JE, et al: Assessment of prognostic factors in alcoholic liver disease: Toward a global quantitative expression of severity. *Hepatology* 1983; 3:896–905.
195. Orrego H, Blake JE, Blendis LM, et al: Prospective validation of the relationship of the combined clinical and laboratory index, the CCLI, with mortality in alcoholic liver disease (abstract). *Hepatology* 1987; 7:1083.
196. Pugh RNH, Murray-Lyon IM, Dawson JL, et al: Transection of the oesophagus for bleeding oesophageal varices. *Br J Surg* 1973; 60:646–649.
197. Howard TK, Podesta LG, Sher LS, et al: Liver Transplantation, in Kaplowitz N (ed): *Liver and Biliary Diseases.* Baltimore, Williams and Wilkins, 1992, pp 566–586.

198. Schenker S, Perkins HS, Sorrell MF: Should patients with end-stage alcoholic liver disease have a new liver? *Hepatology* 1990; 11:314–319.
199. Moss AH, Siegler M: Should alcoholics compete equally for liver transplantation? *JAMA* 1991; 265:1295–1298.
200. Cohen C, Benjamin M, The Ethics and Social Impact Committee of the Transplant and Health Policy Center, Ann Arbor, Michigan: Alcoholics and liver transplantation. *JAMA* 1991; 265:1299–1301.
201. Scharschmidt BF: Human liver transplantation: Analysis of data of 540 patients from four centers. *Hepatology* 1984; 4(Suppl 1):95S–101S.
202. Bird GLA, O'Grady JG, Harvey FAH, et al: Liver transplantation in patients with alcoholic cirrhosis: Selection criteria and rates of survival and relapse. *Br Med J* 1990; 301:15–17.
203. Kumar S, Stauber RE, Gavaler JS, et al: Orthotopic liver transplantation for alcoholic liver disease. *Hepatology* 1990; 11:159–164.
204. Lucey MR, Merion RM, Henley KS, et al: Selection for and outcome of liver transplantation in alcoholic liver disease. *Gastroenterology* 1992; 102:1736–1741.
205. Doffoël M, Fratte S, Vanlemmens C, et al: Results of liver transplantation (LT) in 75 French patients with alcoholic cirrhosis (AC). Comparison with a nonalcoholic cirrhotic group (abstract 22). *Hepatology* 1992; 16:50A.
206. Kumar S, Pound D, Van Thiel DH: Long-term survival following liver transplantation in patients with alcoholic liver disease (abstract). *Gastroenterology* 1992; 102:A837.
207. National Institutes of Health Consensus Development Conference Statement: Liver Transplantation—June 20–23, 1983. *Hepatology* 1984; 4(suppl 1):107S–110S.
208. Donovan J: Transplantation in alcoholic liver disease: Selection and post-operative management, in *Newer Aspects of Alcohol, Nutrition, and Hepatic Encephalopathy*. American Association for the Study of Liver Disease, 1992 Postgraduate Course Syllabus, pp 186–201.
209. Beresford TP, Turcotte JG, Merion R, et al: A rational approach to liver transplantation for the alcoholic patient. *Psychosomatics* 1990; 31:241–254.
210. Gish RG, Lee AH, Rome H, et al: Abstract 941. *Hepatology* 1992; 16 :280A.
211. Flavin DK, Niven RG, Kelsey JE: Alcoholism and orthotopic liver transplantation. *JAMA* 1988; 259:1546–1547.
212. Schenker S: Medical treatment vs. transplantation in liver disorders. *Hepatology* 1984; 4(suppl 1):102S–106S.
213. Baddour N, Demetris AJ, Shah G, et al: The prevalence, rate of onset and spectrum of histologic disease in alcohol abusing liver allograft recipients (abstract). *Gastroenterology* 1992; 102:A777.
214. Horn W: General pharmacology, toxicology, and future clinical development of HOE 077. *J Hepatol* 1991; 13(suppl 3):S63–S65.
215. Pihlajaniemi T, Myllylá R, Kivirikko KI: Prolyl 4-hydroxylase and its role in collagen synthesis. *J Hepatol* 1991; 13(suppl 3):S2–S7.
216. Hanauske-Abel HM: Prolyl 4-hydroxylase, a target enzyme for drug development. *J Hepatol* 1991; 13(suppl 3):S8–S16.
217. Bickel M, Baader E, Brocks DG, et al: Beneficial effects of inhibitors of prolyl 4-hydroxylase in $CC1_4$-induced fibrosis of the liver in rats. *J Hepatol* 1991; 13(suppl 13):S26–S34.
218. Ghosh MK, Cohen JS: Oligodeoxynucleotides as antisense inhibitors of gene expression. *Prog Nucleic Acid Res Mol Biol* 1992; 42:79–126.

219. Weintraub HM: Antisense RNA and DNA. *Sci Am* 1990; 262:40–46.
220. Wu CH, Walton CM, Tangco MV, et al: Targeted antisense DNA oligonucleotides specifically inhibit procollagen synthesis in cultured fibroblasts (abstract 340). *Hepatology* 1992; 16(part 2):129A.
221. Wu GY, Wu CH: Receptor-mediated in vitro gene transformation by a soluble DNA carrier. *J Biol Chem* 1987; 262:4429–4432.
222. Wu GY, Wilson JM, Shalaby F, et al: Receptor-mediated gene delivery in vivo. Partial correction of genetic analbuminemia in Nagase rats. *J Biol Chem* 1991; 266:14338–14342.
223. Makdisi WJ, Wu CH, Wu GY: Methods of gene transfer into hepatocytes: Progress toward gene therapy. *Prog Liver Dis* 1992; 10:1–37.
224. Post JJ, Benton B, Breakstone R, et al: The effects of diet and choline on fatty infiltration of the human liver. *Gastroenterology* 1952; 20:403–410.
225. Rubin E, Lieber CS: Alcohol induced hepatic injury in nonalcoholic volunteers. *N Engl J Med* 1968; 278:869–876.
226. Lieber CS, Leo MA, Mak KM, et al: Choline fails to prevent liver fibrosis in ethanol-fed baboons but causes toxicity. *Hepatology* 1985; 5:561–575.
227. Duce AM, Ortiz P, Cabrero C, et al: S-adenosyl-L-methionine synthetase and phospholipid methyltransferase are inhibited in human cirrhosis. *Hepatology* 1988; 8:65–68.
228. Lieber CS, DeCarli LM, Mak KM, et al: Attenuation of alcohol-induced hepatic fibrosis by polyunsaturated lecithin. *Hepatology* 1990; 12:1390–1398.
229. Chawla RK, Bonkovsky HL, Galambos JT: Biochemistry and pharmacology of S-adenosyl-L-methionine and rationale for its use in liver disease. *Drugs* 1990; 40(suppl 3):98–110.
230. Almasio P, Bortolini M, Pagliaro L, et al: Role of S-adenosyl-L-methionine in the treatment of intrahepatic cholestasis. *Drugs* 1990; 40(suppl 3):111–123.
231. Lieber CS, Casini A, DeCarli LM, et al: S-adenosyl-L-methionine attenuates alcohol-induced liver injury in the baboon. *Hepatology* 1990; 11:165–172.
232. Vendemiale G, Altomare E, Trizio T, et al: Effects of oral S-adenosyl-L-methionine on hepatic glutathione in patients with liver disease. *Scand J Gastroenterol* 1989; 24:407–415.

Genetic Mechanisms of Solid Tumor Oncogenesis*

Michael J. Kelley, M.D.

Medical Staff Fellow, Navy Medical Oncology Branch, National Cancer Institute, National Naval Medical Center, Bethesda, Maryland

Bruce E. Johnson, M.D.

Chief, Lung Cancer Biology Section, Navy Medical Oncology Branch, National Cancer Institute, National Naval Medical Center, Bethesda, Maryland

Cancer is the second most common cause of death in the United States with an annual incidence of more than 1,100,000 and a mortality rate of nearly 500,000 in 1993.[1] Human malignancy occurs after a multistep process disrupts the normal control of cellular growth and causes malignant transformation and unchecked proliferation.[2] In normal cells, cellular growth and division are controlled by biochemical pathways that process signals from inside and outside the cell (Fig 1). Disrupted control can be caused by genetic alterations of growth-controlling genes, viral infections, increased stimulation by growth factors, or a combination of these factors.

Genetic changes associated with malignancy were initially identified by studies of the chromosomal changes found in hematologic malignancies.[3] This led to the initial identification of chromosomal translocations involving c-*myc*, c-*abl*, and *bcl*-2 in the development of Burkitt's lymphoma, chronic myelogenous leukemia, and follicular lymphomas, respectively.[4–6]

Increased ability to perform karyotypic studies of solid tumors, the development of restriction fragment length polymorphism mapping techniques and the identification of tumor suppressor genes and additional proto-oncogenes has allowed characterization of the multiple genetic events that occur in solid tumor oncogenesis. In addition to increasing our understanding of the biology of malignancy, the discovery of these genetic changes may, in the future, lead to detection of premalignant lesions, improved oncologic diagnosis, identification of factors associated with different patient outcomes, and the development of novel strategies for treatment and prevention.

*The opinions or assertions contained herein are the private views of the authors and are not to be construed as official or as reflecting the views of the Department of the Navy or the Department of Defense. This is a U.S. government work. There are no restrictions on its use.

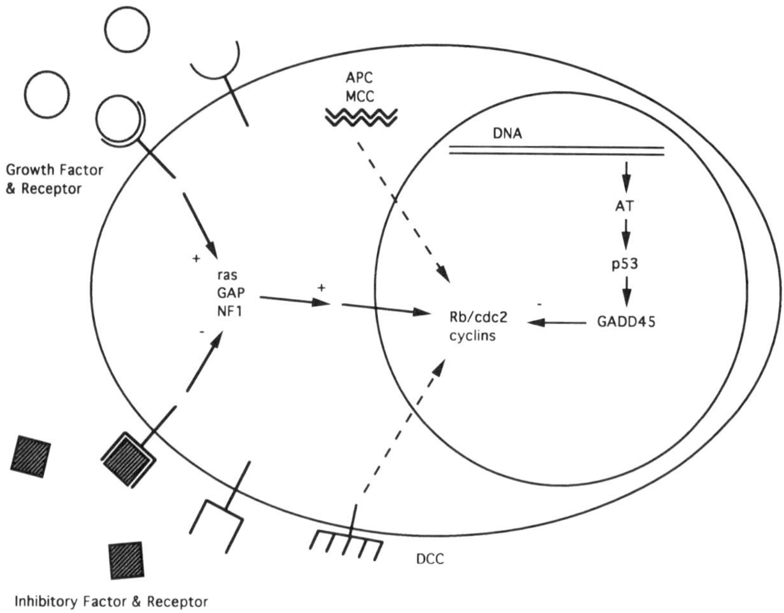

FIG 1.
Control of cellular growth and division. The biochemical pathways of cellular growth and division are shown schematically with the subcellular localization of gene products implicated in human oncogenesis. *Arrows* indicate the direction of information flow. Abbreviations are explained in the text.

Tumor Suppressor Genes and Proto-oncogenes

Genetic alterations found in human solid tumors occur in genes that can be grouped into two broad categories, tumor suppressor genes and proto-oncogenes. Tumor suppressor genes normally function to maintain the nonmalignant phenotype by limiting growth, invasiveness, and other properties found in malignant cells. Loss of this normal function, often caused by genetic alteration, leads to unregulated growth and/or tumor progression. Tumor suppressor gene mutations are usually recessive; that is, inactivation of both normal copies of the gene must occur before an alteration in the phenotype of the cell occurs (the two-hit hypothesis) (Fig 2). The existence of tumor suppressor genes was initially suspected by the loss of malignant characteristics in cellular hybrids formed between malignant and normal cells. Cytogenetic observations of consistently deleted chromosomal segments and detection of the loss of heterozygosity at specific loci detected by using restricted fragment length polymorphisms (Fig 3) led to their localization within the genome and subsequent isolation.

The second group of malignancy-associated genes, proto-oncogenes, were originally identified as the normal cellular homologues of the viral on-

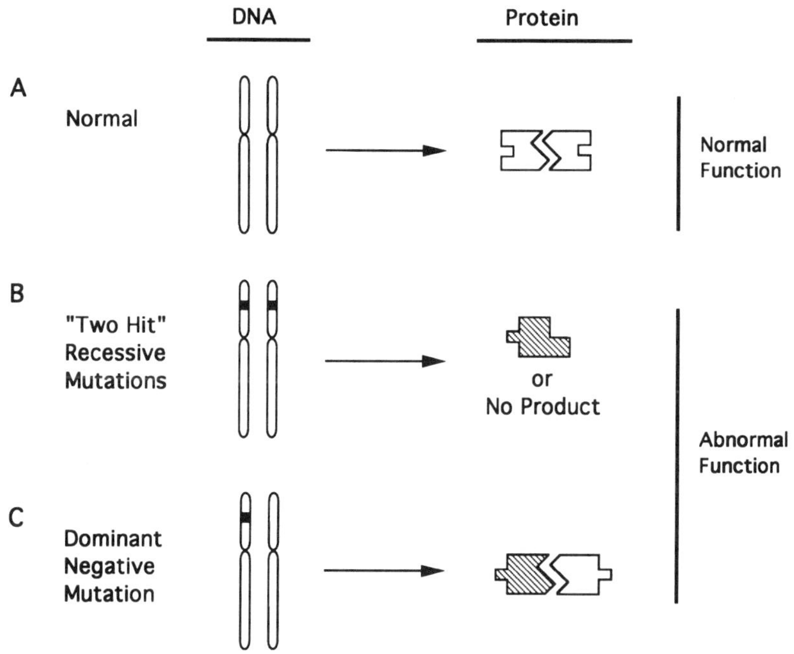

FIG 2.
Alterations of tumor suppressor genes commonly found in human malignancies. Mutated gene products are shaded. **(A)** Two normal alleles produce normally functioning protein. **(B)** The two-hit hypothesis for inactivation of tumor suppressor genes. The first mutation, leading to inactivation of one allele, does not alter the ability of the remaining normal allele to provide normal growth regulating function. After a second genetic alteration, frequently complete loss of the normal allele, normal function is lost. **(C)** Dominant negative inactivation of tumor suppressor genes. Genetic alteration of a single allele produces a mutant protein that interacts with the normal protein, altering its conformation and thereby abolishing its ability to limit cell growth.

cogenes of acutely transforming retroviruses. Proto-oncogenes have been implicated in oncogenesis because a gain or increase in their function leads to stimulation of growth or development of the malignant phenotype. Proto-oncogenes are commonly dominant, requiring only one genetic alteration to result in an increase in abnormal function.

Several mechanisms leading to the alteration of tumor suppressor gene and proto-oncogene function have been observed in human cancers (Table 1). A common genetic alteration of these genes in cancers is a point mutation. Point mutations occur by endogenous or exogenous mechanisms and result in characteristic patterns of base pair changes (Table 2). Endogenous mechanisms are those that result from alterations in normal cellular processes, while exogenous mechanisms result from the influence of agents external to the cell. One type of endogenous mechanism is

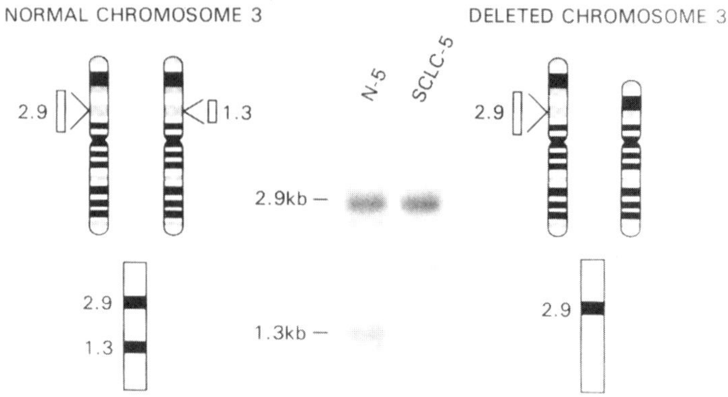

FIG 3.
Restriction fragment length polymorphism. Southern blots of normal DNA and DNA from a small cell lung cancer *(SCLC)* with an interstitial deletion of the short arm of chromosome 3 are compared after being hybridized to a DNA fragment *(D3S2)* which recognizes a restriction fragment length polymorphism on the short arm of chromosome 3. The copy of the gene on one chromosome gives rise to a band at 2.9 kb on a Southern blot hybridization of DNA digested with the restriction endonuclease Msp I. The copy of the gene on the other chromosome gives rise to a band of 1.3 kb on the same Southern blot, giving two bands. This is recognized by the two bands under N-5. An interstitial deletion of one of the two arms of chromosome 3 causes the loss of one of the two bands (1.3 kb) so the small cell lung cancer tissue from the same patient has a single band. This is referred to as *loss of heterozygosity*. In this way, the study of tumor and normal tissue can document the allelic loss of loci on specific parts of a chromosome.

deamination of 5-methylcytosine to thymidine at CG dinucleotides.[7] This C to T transition (a transition is a change from one pyrimidine [C or T] to the other pyrimidine or a change from one purine to the other, while a transversion is a change from a purine to a pyrimidine or vice versa) is accompanied by a G to A transition on the opposite strand of DNA. Methylation of cytosine residues at CG dinucleotides is thought to be a mechanism regulating the expression of nearby genes. Exogenous mechanisms result in mutagen-specific base pair changes. These latter mutations occur at DNA sequences that may also be mutagen specific.

The p53 Gene

p53 Gene Function.—The p53 gene, located on chromosome 17p13, encodes a 393–amino acid phosphoprotein capable of forming a homo-oligomer that has recently been shown to bind to specific DNA sequences,[8, 9] and act as a transcription factor.[10] In normal cells, a variety of insults to cellular DNA, such as exposure to ultraviolet (UV) light, radiomimetic drugs, or γ-irradiation, result in increased levels of the p53 protein as the result of posttranslational stabilization.[11, 12] An increased level of p53

TABLE 1.
Described Mechanisms of Alterations of Tumor Suppressor Genes and Proto-oncogenes in Human Cancers

Tumor suppressor genes
Inactivating mutation and loss of normal allele
Dominant negative mutation
Binding of gene product
Increased degradation
Proto-oncogenes
Activating mutation
Gene amplification
Chromosomal rearrangement
Insertion of viral DNA sequences

TABLE 2.
Mutations Found as the Result of Endogenous and Exogenous Mechanisms of Mutation

Mechanism of Mutation	Mutation
Endogenous	
Deamination of 5-methylcytosine	G to A at CG dinucleotides
DNA polymerase infidelity	Transitions*
Exogenous	
Tobacco smoke (benzo[a]pyrene)	G to T
Aflatoxin B_1	G to T
Ultraviolet light	C to T at dipyrimidines CC to TT

*Transitions are substitution of one purine (A or G) for the other or one pyrimidine (C or T) for the other.

leads to arrest of the cell cycle in the G1 phase (the growth phase of the cell cycle after mitosis and prior to DNA synthesis), allowing for repair of induced or spontaneously occurring DNA damage prior to replication of the DNA in the S phase of the cell cycle.[12] If DNA repair cannot be accomplished, programmed cell death (apoptosis) may occur.[13, 14] Thus, p53 is thought to ensure genomic integrity. The p53 gene does not directly establish integrity of the genome but rather acts as a transcription factor to increase expression of other genes. The growth arrest and DNA damage (GADD45) gene has recently been recognized as one of these p53-induced genes.[15] Lack of p53 function in tumor cells is thought to be responsible for the observed genomic instability of these cells as manifested by aneuploidy and the ability to undergo gene amplification.[16] The tumorigenicity in athymic nude mice of lung, breast, and colon tumor cell lines with abnormal p53 function is ablated by replacement of normal p53 function, thereby confirming its role as a tumor suppressor gene.[17–19]

p53 and Ataxia-Telangiectasia.—Induction of p53 levels following γ-irradiation requires the function of the gene(s) responsible for the autosomal-recessive disorder, ataxia-telangiectasia, located on chromosome 11q.[15] The lack of induction of p53 in response to DNA damage in patients with ataxia-telangiectasia causes genomic instability and explains two main features of the disorder: radiosensitivity and increased risk of cancer. Persons heterozygous for ataxia-telangiectasia (about 1% of the U.S. population) may be at increased risk for the development of cancer.[20] Furthermore, it has been suggested that low-dose radiation exposure such as that received from fluoroscopic diagnostic procedures (less than 2 cGy) increases the risk of breast cancer in women by about fivefold.[20] If confirmed, this finding would have important implications for cancer risk assessment and screening programs.

p53 Gene Alterations.—Mutation of the p53 gene is the most frequently identified genetic abnormality in human cancers (Table 3).[21] In addition to the mutation of the p53 gene, inactivation of p53 function can occur by other mechanisms, including inactivation of p53 by binding to another protein or increased degradation of p53. Mutation of p53 is the most common mechanism of inactivation of p53 function. The most common type of mutation in the p53 gene is a single base pair change (point mutation) resulting in an amino acid change (missense mutation) or truncation of the coding region by creation of a stop colon (nonsense mutation). Deletion and insertion mutations also occur as do mutations affecting splicing of precursor RNA to mature mRNA. The mutations in the p53 gene are concentrated in the evolutionarily conserved areas of exons 4 to 8 (Fig 4); however, mutations have been reported at sites that comprise more than one fourth of the coding sequence. Many missense mutations of p53, unlike mutations in most tumor suppressor genes, are dominant negative mutations (Fig 2,C). A dominant negative p53 gene mutation produces mutant p53 that forms a hetero-oligomeric complex with the normal p53 (i.e., a complex containing both normal and mutant forms of p53). This complex, unlike that composed solely of normal p53, is not able to function as

TABLE 3.
Characteristics of p53 Mutations in Selected Human Malignancies

Tumor Type	% With p53 Mutations	Predominant Mutation
Lung, small cell[22]	77–100	G to T
Lung, non–small cell[22]	49–75	G to T
Head and neck[23]	100*	G to T
Colon[24]	70	G to A at CG dinucleotides
Breast[25]	12–38	G to A at CG dinucleotides†
Ovarian[26]	29–71	G to A at CG dinucleotides
Gastric[27, 28]	20–38	‡
Skin, squamous[29]	58	C to T
Hepatocellular§[30–32]	50	G to T at codon 249

*Tumor cell lines.
†May vary with study population.
‡Insufficient number of mutations reported to determine predominant type.
§Associated with aflatoxin B_1 exposure.

a transcription factor and impede cell growth. These dominant mutants result in immunologically detectable cellular p53, in contrast to the normal p53 gene and p53 gene mutants of the nonsense or frameshift type. Nonsense and frameshift mutations result in truncated forms of p53 that have lost the binding domain at the C-terminus required for oligimerization and thus are necessarily recessive.

Patterns of p53 Gene Mutations.—The most frequent type of p53 point mutation found in lung cancers and squamous cell cancers of the

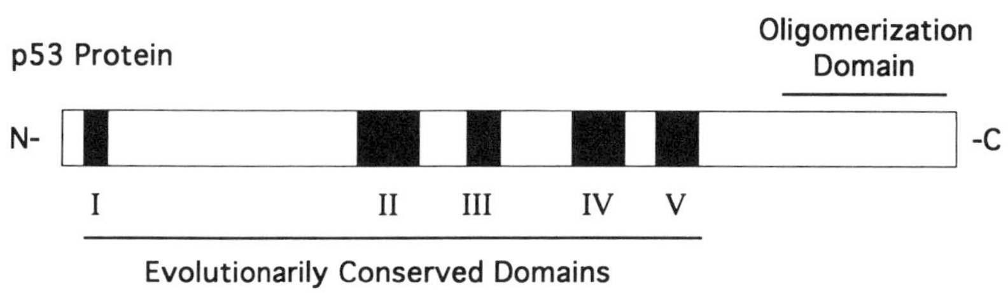

FIG 4.
The p53 protein showing areas most conserved across species *(solid boxes I to V)*. Domains II to V are most frequently found to be mutated ("hot spots"). The C-terminal domain required for oligomerization is also shown.

head and neck, both cancers strongly associated epidemiologically with tobacco smoking, are G to T transversions.[22, 23] This suggests that mutation of p53 in these tumors is occurring as the result of exposure to mutagens in tobacco smoke, such as benzo*[a]*pyrene. Benzo*[a]*pyrene has been shown to predominantly cause G to T mutations in tissue culture.[33] In contrast, among 19 lung cancers in uranium miners, none of the nine p53 mutations were of this type.[34] In these tumors the suspected carcinogen was ionizing radiation resulting from the decay of inhaled radon and its daughters. The mutations were mostly transversions other than G to T as well as two deletion mutations. This suggests an exogenous mechanism of mutation and is consistent with mutations induced by ionizing radiation.[35]

Squamous cell carcinomas of the skin, tumors associated with exposure to sunlight, have p53 mutations in about 50% of the tumors.[29] Some of these mutations result from the unusual change of a CC dinucleotide to a TT dinucleotide.[29] This mutation is only known to occur as a result of UV light exposure; furthermore, no internal malignancy has been found to have this mutation. Other mutations found in squamous cell carcinoma of the skin are C to T transitions at dipyrimidines that are also characteristic of UV light–induced mutations.[29]

Hepatocellular carcinoma (HCC) is associated with chronic viral hepatitis infections, and, in some geographic areas, aflatoxin B_1 exposure. In China and South Africa, where a high incidence of aflatoxin B_1 exposure occurs, mutations of p53 have been found in approximately 50% of HCC.[30–32] Interestingly, about 85% of these mutations were G to T transversions at codon 249. Studies from other geographic regions where aflatoxin B_1 contamination of the diet is not prevalent, including Japan, Germany, and Taiwan, p53 mutations in HCC were primarily G to T transversions but did not occur predominantly at codon 249.[36–39] In vitro experimental mutagenesis studies have shown that aflatoxin B_1 not only causes G and T transversions, but also causes mutations specifically at codon 249 of the p53 gene.[40] These observations, which support the epidemiologic relationship between HCC and aflatoxin B_1, demonstrate a precise causal mechanism for this relationship, a site-specific mutational inactivation of p53 function.

Approximately two thirds of missense mutations found in colon cancers are G to A transitions at CG dinucleotides, suggesting that the endogenous mechanism of deamination of methylated cytosine residues is involved in the pathogenesis of this common tumor. The pattern of p53 mutations in breast cancers appears to vary based on geographic location; transitions at CG dinucleotides are most common in the midwestern United States[41] and mutations consistent with exogenous mechanisms are most common in populations from North Carolina[42, 43] and Scotland.[44] While this may be artifactual because of sampling errors, it suggests that different mechanisms of mutation or differences in host susceptibility may result in pathologically similar tumors. To date, no specific mutagens have been linked by epidemiologic studies to the occurrence of breast cancer to explain the occurrence of exogenous mechanisms.

Li-Fraumeni Syndrome.—Persons with the autosomal-dominant Li-Fraumeni syndrome are at increased risk for the development of breast cancers, sarcomas, and other tumors. Clinical diagnosis of the syndrome requires (1) an individual diagnosed with sarcoma before 45 years of age; (2) a first-degree relative with cancer before 45 years of age; and (3) another first- or second-degree relative with either a sarcoma diagnosed at any age or any cancer diagnosed before 45 years of age.[45] Germline p53 mutations have been found in 17 kindreds of persons with the Li-Fraumeni syndrome.[46–48] These persons develop normally but are at increased risk for developing a malignancy associated with the Li-Fraumeni syndrome. The tumors of patients with this syndrome have lost the remaining normal p53 allele. Germline mutations of the p53 gene tend to be located in the conserved regions of the gene, similar to somatic mutations. Mutations of the germline p53 gene is rarely found in patients under 40 years of age with sporadic breast cancer (1 of 136)[25] or patients with sarcomas (3 of 181).[49] However, germline p53 mutations were found in 4 of 59 (7%) children and young adults with at least two primary cancers.[50] Less than 15% of germline p53 gene mutations arise de novo, the majority being inherited. Mutations of the p53 gene in this familial syndrome are distributed in the areas commonly affected by sporadic mutations and are also predominantly missense. The pattern of mutations is more consistent with an endogenous mechanism of mutation caused by deamination of methylcytosine at CG dinucleotides or DNA polymerase infidelity.

p53 Inactivation by Binding Oncoproteins.—p53 can also be inactivated by interaction with other proteins. In the case of the DNA tumor virus oncoproteins, this occurs with proteins that are not normally found in the cell. The E1B protein of adenovirus binds to p53 and prevents p53-activated transcription. The E6 protein of some types of human papilloma virus (HPV) binds to p53, causing p53 to be marked for degradation by covalent linkage to ubiquitin.[51] Thus, HPV infection can lead to increased p53 degradation.[51, 52] Only E6 proteins from those strains of HPV that have been strongly associated with anogenital cancers (HPV 16 and HPV 18 are most common) result in accelerated p53 degradation.

Another mechanism by which p53 is inactivated is interaction with endogenous cellular proteins. In about a third of human sarcomas, there is gene amplification of the *MDM2* gene, located at chromosome 12q13-14 (a frequently noted location of cytogenetic abnormalities in sarcomas[53]), resulting in high levels of its 90-kd nuclear protein product.[54] Binding of the *MDM2* protein to p53 is thought to inactivate its transcriptional activity.[54]

Timing of p53 Inactivation.—The temporal sequence of inactivation of p53 during oncogenesis is not the same for tumors arising in different organs. In sporadic and familial adenomatous polyposis–associated colorectal neoplasms, p53 is inactivated by mutation in malignant invasive lesions but not in benign preinvasive adenomas.[24] In contrast, there is evidence for the existence of mutant p53 in premalignant lesions of the esophagus (Barrett's esophagus, squamous dysplasia, and carcinoma in situ)[55, 56] and lung (bronchial epithelial dysplasia).[34, 57] These findings will have important implications for the development of early-detection screening strategies that are based on detection of altered p53.

p53 as a Prognostic Factor.—Altered p53 function, as determined by p53 mutation or immunohistochemical staining, has been examined as a potential prognostic factor in a variety of cancers. In early-stage, resectable, non–small cell lung cancer, two retrospective studies have found a significant association between altered p53 in tumor specimens and shortened survival. The first study, which examined lung tumors from 71 patients (48 with stage I or II) for p53 mutations, showed that this association with shortened survival was significant and independent of other known prognostic factors in a multivariate analysis.[58] The relative risk of death among patients whose tumors contained a detectable p53 mutation was 3.5.[58] The second study, utilizing the less sensitive but more clinically feasible technique of immunohistochemical staining for p53 protein accumulation in 114 stage I or II tumors, also detected this adverse association but a multivariate analysis was not reported.[59] An earlier study that examined 77 tumor cell lines from patients undergoing resection of non–small cell lung cancer and did not detect an adverse prognostic effect of p53 gene mutations[60] may not have been representative of all patients that undergo resection. Specifically, the establishment of a tumor cell line from a non–small cell lung cancer, a known adverse prognostic factor, is more likely to be successful from tumors with altered p53 function.

In breast cancer, the finding of an association between p53 immunohistochemical staining and adverse prognostic factors such as late stage, metastatic spread, and low progesterone receptor content[61] led to investigation of p53 immunohistochemical staining as a potential prognostic factor for patients with breast cancer. Of 151 patients with various stages of sporadic breast cancer, p53 immunohistochemical staining was found in 32 (21%) and was associated with a shortened survival (69% vs. 46% at 6 years) in a univariate analysis.[62] Immunohistochemical staining for p53 was also associated with shortened survival among the subset of 108 untreated individuals without tumor involvement of the axillary lymph nodes (some of whom had a family history of breast cancer), but this association did not reach statistical significance. In a multivariate analysis, p53 immunohistochemical staining was significantly associated with shortened metastasis-free survival (relative risk of death, 1.68; P = .039) but was only marginally significant for association with shorter survival (relative risk of death, 1.67; P = .052). A subgroup of 15 tumors showed 100% concordance between p53 immunohistochemical staining and p53 mutations, similar to results of earlier studies.[63]

It has been suggested that prognostic factors, other than stage, be used to guide the use of systemic adjuvant therapy for node-negative breast cancer. Therefore, a retrospective study of p53 immunohistochemical staining in 289 such patients who had received only local therapies was performed.[64] The survival of the 41 patients (14%) with p53 immunohistochemical staining was shorter than those without this staining (relative risk of death, 2.7). This finding was independent of menopausal status, tumor size, histologic grade, mitotic rate, estrogen or progesterone receptor content, c-*erb*B-2 overexpression, and DNA index. However, the S-phase fraction was more significantly associated. Further studies are needed to establish the role of p53 immunohistochemical staining in determining adjuvant systemic therapies for patients with node-negative breast cancer.

Implications of p53 Function in Cancer Therapy.—The role of p53 in carcinogenesis provides a new rationale for understanding the efficacy, however limited, of some current anticancer therapies and has suggested approaches to develop new ones. Tumor cells are sensitive to irradiation and DNA-damaging chemotherapeutic agents, at least in part because of defective p53 function that results in progression through the cell cycle despite lethal, potentially repairable genetic damage. The development of resistance to some therapies occurs by gene amplification that is possible because of the genomic instability of cells with defective p53 function. Replacement of normal p53 function results in decreased tumorigenicity of tumor cell lines derived from lung, breast and colorectal carcinomas.[17–19] This remains true, at least for colorectal cancer cell lines, even if there are multiple genetic abnormalities other than loss of p53 function.[65] These in vitro experiments utilizing gene transfer techniques are not readily amenable for use in whole organisms. Further understanding of the biochemical role in p53 may reveal clinically feasible techniques to replace p53 function.

The *ras* Gene Family

The three members of the human *ras* gene family, K-*ras*, H-*ras*, and N-*ras*, encode 21-kd proteins located on the inner surface of the plasma membrane that have been implicated in signal transduction from membrane receptors.[66] The *ras* proteins are converted from an active form to an inactive form by hydrolysis of *ras*-bound guanosine triphosphate to guanosine diphosphate by inherent guanosine triphosphatase activity. A guanosine triphosphatase–activating protein binds to *ras*, stimulates this guanosine triphosphatase activity and has also been implicated in signal transduction. The *ras* proteins containing mutations in codons 12, 13, and 61 cannot bind guanosine triphosphatase–activating protein and are constitutively activated.

***ras* Gene Mutations in Gastrointestinal Cancers.**—The *ras* genes are the most frequently mutated proto-oncogene found in human cancers.[67] In pancreatic cancer, a *ras* gene mutation has been detected in between 75% and 95% of the more than 150 tumors studied.[67] Approximately 90% of these are mutated in K-*ras* at codon 12. [67] There has been no association between the presence of *ras* mutations and either tumor characteristics (such as degree of differentiation) or clinical characteristics (stage or survival) of patients with pancreatic carcinoma. However, the number of tumors without *ras* mutations is rather limited and larger studies may yet show an association with patient characteristics and outcome.

Mutations of the *ras* gene have also been found in about 40% to 50% of colon carcinomas.[67] As with pancreatic cancer, mutations in colon cancer are most common in the K-*ras* gene (about 90%) and at codon 12 (about 90% of K-*ras* mutations). Interestingly, *ras* mutations are found in a similar proportion (approximately 50%) of adenomas larger than 1 cm, suggesting that, when *ras* mutations occur, they occur early in the sequence of events leading to colon cancer.[68]

This observation has suggested strategies to detect colonic neoplasms by detection of a mutated *ras* gene. In one such study, *ras* gene mutations were found in the stool from 8 of 9 (89%) patients with resectable colorectal neoplasms that contained a mutated *ras* gene, including both patients with adenomas.[69] Such an analysis could be used as part of a screening strategy to detect cancers at a time when they are more amenable to surgical resection. Although the incidence of K-*ras* gene mutations in colorectal carcinomas occurring in patients with ulcerative colitis is lower (24% of 33 patients in one study[70]) than in the sporadically occurring variety, it appears that preneoplastic areas of dysplasia can also contain mutated *ras* genes[71] and might be targets of early diagnosis in these patients at high risk for colorectal cancer development. No association has been found between clinical behavior of colorectal tumors and the occurrence of *ras* gene mutations.

***ras* Gene Mutations in Lung and Endometrial Cancers.**—*ras* gene mutations are found in more than 30% of adenocarcinomas of the lung.[72] The other histologic types of lung cancer, squamous cell, large cell and small cell lung cancer, have less than 10% incidence of *ras* mutations.[72] This suggests that *ras* may be involved in the type of differentiation. Experimental evidence to support this suggestion comes from the finding that expression of a mutated *ras* gene in small cell lung cancer cells results in tumor cells that develop the morphology of adenocarcinoma cells.

It should be noted, however, that *ras* gene mutations are not present in all adenocarcinomas, regardless of the body site of origin; less than 1% of breast or ovarian carcinomas have been found to have a mutated *ras* gene.[67] Furthermore, among the uncommon bronchoalveolar type of lung cancer that has glandular characteristics, *ras* gene mutation occurred in only 2 of 20 (10%) tumor specimens.[73] Adenocarcinomas of the lung among persons who smoke are about three times more likely to have a *ras* mutation than adenocarcinomas of the lung among persons who have not smoked.[72] This suggests that the *ras* mutation is caused by mutagens in tobacco smoke. In addition, *ras* gene mutations are uncommon in the lung cancers of uranium miners, most of whom also smoked cigarettes.[34] Approximately 90% of *ras* gene mutations in lung cancers are in K-*ras*, and 85% of these are in codon 12 of K-*ras*. Retrospective studies have indicated that the occurrence of a *ras* gene mutation in adenocarcinoma of the lung is associated with a shortened survival.[72, 74, 75] If these results are confirmed in prospective studies, *ras* gene mutations may identify patients that are most likely to benefit from adjuvant therapy following surgical resection.

Mutation of the K-*ras* gene is found in approximately 15% of endometrial carcinomas. In one retrospective study of 49 patients with endometrial cancer, the presence of a K-*ras* gene mutated in codon 12 was an adverse prognostic factor and, in a multivariate analysis, was associated with a ninetyfold increased risk of death.[76] This will need to be confirmed in additional studies.

Pattern of *ras* Gene Mutations.—The number of different sites at which *ras* gene mutations have been described in human cancers is significantly smaller than the number of sites found mutated in the p53 gene. Therefore, the pattern of *ras* gene mutations may be constrained by the limited number of possible activating mutations of *ras* and may less accurately reflect the mutagenic properties of associated carcinogens than the pattern of the more widespread mutations found in the p53 gene. The mutational spectrum found in the *ras* genes in pancreatic, colon, and lung cancers is shown in Table 4. The pattern of mutations in pancreatic and colon cancer is a predominance of G to A transitions, frequently at CG dimers. In contrast, the most common base pair change in the *ras* gene of adenocarcinomas of the lung is a G to T transversion. This difference strongly suggests that the mechanism of mutation in these two groups of cancers is different, the former caused by endogenous mechanisms while the latter is likely to be due to the effects of an exogenous mutagen found in tobacco smoke. For colon and lung cancer, the nucleotide changes in the *ras* gene mutations are similar to those found in the p53 gene. To date, all *ras* gene mutations found in human cancers have been somatically acquired and none have been found in the germline.

The Adenomatous Polyposis Coli Gene

The Familial Adenomatous Polyposis Syndrome.—The familial adenomatous polyposis (FAP) syndrome, an autosomal-dominant inherited condition with high penetrance, is manifested by the occurrence of a large number (hundreds to thousands) of colonic and rectal polyps. Af-

TABLE 4.
Characteristics of K-*ras* Gene Mutations Found in Selected Human Malignancies

Tumor	Approximate % Mutated	Predominant Mutation
Pancreas[67]	90	Transition at CG dinucleotides
Colon, sporadic[67]	50	Transition at CG dinucleotides
Lung, adeno[22]	30	G to T transversion
Endometrium[77]	15	*

*Insufficient number of mutations reported to determine predominant type.

flicted patients are at high risk for the development of colorectal cancer at a young age if they do not undergo prophylactic colectomy and are also at increased risk for the development of other neoplastic diseases, including osteomas; carcinoma of the stomach, gall bladder, bile ducts, and duodenum; and papillary thyroid carcinoma.

Genetic and cytogenetic studies have linked this syndrome, which occurs in about 1 of 5,000 Americans, to chromosome 5q21. This allowed the identification of a gene, adenomatous polyposis coli (APC), at this locus that is responsible for the FAP syndrome.[78, 79] This gene contains 15 coding exons that predict for a 2,843–amino acid protein. The primary sequence of the protein has heptad repeats that are predicted to form a coiled coil structure. This structure is found in structural proteins, such as myosins and keratins, and is thought to be important for formation of homo- or hetero-oligomers. It is not known if mutations of the APC gene are recessive, dominant negative, or codominant (a quantitative effect) at the cellular level. In the first instance, a second genetic event would be needed prior to loss of function, while in the latter two situations no further events would be needed. Replacement of APC function by transfer of a normal chromosome 5 into a colorectal tumor cell line markedly decreases the tumorigenicity of the cell line in athymic nude mice, further supporting the theory that APC is a tumor suppressor gene.[65]

Germline APC gene mutations have been identified in 53 of 79 (67%),[80] 5 of 40 (13%),[81] and 5 of 61 (8%)[79] individuals in FAP kindreds. More than 90% of all germline APC gene mutations identified result in truncation of the predicted protein product because of nonsense point mutations or, more commonly, frameshift mutations resulting from small insertions or deletions that cause a stop codon, resulting in premature termination. Thus it appears that the C-terminus of the APC protein is important for its function and that APC is a putative tumor suppressor gene. The location of the mutation within the APC gene appears to determine whether affected patients within a kindred will have the profuse or sparse variant of FAP.[82] The profuse variant, characterized by more than 5,000 polyps and an average age of development of colorectal cancer of 34 years, occurs if the mutation is between codons 1250 and 1464 while the sparse variant, with 1,000 to 2,000 polyps and the mean age of onset of cancer of 42 years, occurs if the mutation is outside this region. It is unknown whether all patients with FAP will ultimately be found to have abnormalities that affect the APC gene or whether defects in another gene is responsible for the development of FAP in a portion of kindreds. For those kindreds in which a mutation of APC can be identified, presymptomatic and even prenatal diagnosis is now possible with a high degree of accuracy. Genetic alterations of the APC gene have been excluded as the etiology of another hereditary syndrome predisposing to colorectal carcinoma, hereditary nonpolyposis colorectal carcinoma.[83]

The APC Gene in Sporadic Colon Cancer.—Mutations of the APC gene have also been found in sporadic colorectal carcinomas. Among 25 such cancers, 15 (60%) were found to have APC gene mutations by sequencing of the entire coding region.[84] Interestingly, mutations were also found in 10 of 16 (63%) colorectal adenomas, some as small as 0.5 cm, suggesting that mutation of the APC gene occurs early in sporadic colorectal carcinogenesis.[84] Furthermore, only 1 of 5 polyps smaller than 1 cm had a mutated *ras* gene, consistent with the fact that *ras* mutations occur later in the multistep process of colorectal oncogenesis. Similar to germline mutations found in patients with FAP, the somatically acquired mutations of sporadic colorectal neoplasms result in truncation of the predicted protein product in most cases (24 of 25). The distribution of APC gene mutations in these sporadic colorectal neoplasms was also similar to that found in FAP patients. Ninety percent of mutations were in the initial codon 1554 and 50% between codons 1281 and 1554. In addition, about 10% occurred by the deletion of the same five base pairs at codon 1309; the same mutation had also been found in 10 of 53 FAP patients. Correlation between the location of the APC mutation and clinical behavior of sporadic colorectal neoplasms (e.g., invasiveness, stage at presentation, or survival) has not been examined. The early occurrence of APC mutations in sporadic colorectal neoplasms makes this an attractive target for screening for these tumors. Among the point mutations in the APC gene identified in patients with sporadic colorectal neoplasms, most (9 of 17) occurred at CG dinucleotides, suggesting an endogenous mechanism of mutation such as deamination of 5-methylcytosine.[84]

APC Gene Mutations in Other Tumors.—Expression of the APC gene has been found in many tissues other than normal colonic mucosa. This, together with cytogenetic and linkage analyses indicating a loss of portions of the long arm of chromosome 5 in noncolonic tumors, has led to a search for mutations of the APC gene in tumors arising from sites other than the large intestine. Somatic mutations of the APC gene have been reported in 4 of 10 (40%) pancreatic carcinomas[85] and in 3 of 44 gastric carcinomas.[86] It has been suggested that the loss of the function of the APC gene product may be a common early step in oncogenesis in cancers arising in the gastrointestinal tract.[87] No APC gene mutations were detected among 55 lung cancers.

In addition to the discovery of mutations of the APC gene in colorectal, pancreatic, and gastric cancers, the APC gene or adjacent genes have been implicated in the development of other tumors by detection of allelic loss. Loss of heterozygosity at the APC/MCC (see later) loci occurs very commonly in small cell lung cancer (21 of 23 [91%] samples) and at a lesser frequency in non–small cell lung cancer (2 of 5 [40%]).[88] Loss of heterozygosity has also been described in esophageal cancers[89] and in dysplastic and malignant lesion of the colon of patients with ulcerative colitis.[90] Thus, loss of function of the APC gene product and/or another tumor suppressor gene located on chromosome 5q has been implicated in a wide variety of human neoplasms.

The Mutated in Colorectal Cancer Gene

The mutated in colorectal cancer (MCC) gene, located only 150 kilobases from the APC gene on chromosome 5q21, was identified prior to the APC gene during the search for the gene responsible for FAP. This gene, transcribed in the opposite direction as the APC gene, is predicted to encode a protein with coiled coil motifs similar to those of APC. The MCC gene was found to be mutated in 3 of 100 sporadic colorectal carcinomas,[91] implicating it in the development of this tumor. However, no germline mutation of the MCC gene has been detected in patients with FAP.[79] As noted, loss of heterozygosity has been detected at the MCC locus at 5q21 in esophageal, small cell and non–small cell lung cancers in addition to colorectal neoplasms. It is not clear if loss of heterozygosity at the MCC locus contributes to the neoplastic phenotype or occurs as a result of the proximity of MCC to APC or other tumor suppressor genes.

The Retinoblastoma Gene

The retinoblastoma gene, spread over more than 200 kilobases on chromosome 13q14, produces a ubiquitously expressed 4.7-kb mRNA that encodes a 928–amino acid nuclear phosphoprotein, rb,[92] which is thought to regulate progression through the cell cycle. The degree to which rb is phosphorylated oscillates during the cell cycle; it is hypophosphorylated during G1 and hyperphosphorylated in the S and G2 phases.[93] The $p34^{cdc2}$ serine-threonine protein kinase, which is also involved in cell cycle regulation, is thought to phosphorylate rb after stimulation of the cell with mitogens such as growth factors.[94] The underphosphorylated form of rb prevents progression of the cell cycle from G1 to S while the hyperphosphorylated form permits this transition. The phosphoprotein rb mediates its function by interaction with nuclear transcription factors, including c-*myc*, N-*myc*, and E2F.[95, 96] It has been demonstrated to be a tumor suppressor gene by its ability to suppress the tumorigenicity in athymic nude mice of tumor cell lines derived from retinoblastomas, osteosarcomas, and prostate bladder cancers.[97–99]

The ability of rb to limit cell cycle progression can be disrupted by at least three mechanisms: (1) binding of rb by viral oncoproteins; (2) decreased or absent rb protein; or (3) expression of abnormal rb protein. The E1A protein of adenovirus and the E7 protein of human papilloma virus bind to and inactivate the tumor suppressor function of rb.[100, 101] Human papillomavirus has been implicated in the development of cervical cancer. Genetic alteration of the retinoblastoma gene, including deletions and point mutations, can result in an insufficient amount or an aberrant form of the rb protein.

Retinoblastomas occurs in two clinical settings: (1) hereditary retinoblastoma, characterized by multifocal tumors with a median age of onset of 11 months and increased risk for the development of osteosarcomas and other tumors at a later age[102]; and (2) sporadic retinoblastoma, developing at the later median age of 2 years and usually unifocal. Persons with hereditary retinoblastoma have germline alterations (either deletions or mutations) of the retinoblastoma gene, while those with sporadic retinoblastoma do not. However, examination of both hereditary and sporadic tumors has shown 100% loss of function of both alleles. Thus patients with hereditary retinoblastoma need lose only the one remaining functional retinoblastoma allele while patients with sporadic retinoblastoma must lose both alleles. Osteosarcomas and other tumors developing in patients with hereditary retinoblastoma have also lost functional rb.[103]

Loss of rb function has been implicated in a number of solid tumors other than retinoblastoma (Table 5). One study of the potential predictive value of loss of rb failed to show an association between loss of rb protein and survival in 197 patients with breast cancer.[104] However, in bladder cancer, two retrospective studies have shown prognostic value for loss of rb protein detected by immunohistochemical staining. The first detected altered rb protein staining in 16 of 43 (37%) locally advanced bladder cancers.[105] Of these 16, only 3 (19%) were alive and cancer free at 3 years compared to 12 of 23 (52%) with normal rb protein staining ($P = .04$). Similar results were found in the second study of 48 patients by using a different antibody to detect rb protein.[106] There was a statistically significant trend toward shorter survival among the 14 patients (29%) whose tumors had decreased or absent rb staining compared to the 36 patients (71%) whose tumors had normal rb staining ($P < .001$). Further studies will be required to confirm these findings as well as to study the potential predictive value of rb protein loss in other tumors.

The Deleted in Colon Cancer Gene

The deleted in colon cancer (DCC) gene, located on chromosome 18q21, produces a 12-kb mRNA that encodes a candidate tumor suppressor gene and has sequence similarity to cell adhesion molecules.[107] Cell adhesion molecules, which include neural-cell adhesion molecule (N-CAM) and carcinoembryonic antigen (CEA), are transmembrane proteins whose extra-

TABLE 5.
Frequency of Retinoblastoma Gene Aberrations in Human Tumors and Cell Lines

	DNA	RNA	Protein
Retinoblastoma[92, 109]	100%		100%
Small cell lung cancer[109–113]	21%	55%	70%
Bladder cancer[109]			31%
Prostate cancer[114]			29%
Breast cancer[115–117]	17%		27%
Sarcomas[103]	21%		
Colon cancer[109]			0%
Melanoma[109]			0%

cellular domains contain regions with sequence similarity to the immunoglobulin superfamily of genes. They are thought to be involved in cell-surface interactions such as adhesions and transmission of signals regulating cellular differentiation and proliferation.[108]

The DCC Gene in Colon Cancer.—One allele of the DCC locus was found to be lost in 29 of 41 (71%) of colon cancers,[107] suggesting that it may be a tumor suppressor gene. Furthermore, the DCC mRNA, which is normally found in most human tissues, including normal colonic epithelium, was found to be present at lower levels or completely absent in 15 of 17 colon carcinoma cell lines.[107] Loss of DCC expression appears to be a late event in the multistep process of colorectal carcinogenesis, because normal levels of DCC mRNA were found in one moderate-to-severe adenoma, five carcinoma-in-adenomas, and four intramucosal carcinomas while these levels were very low or undetectable in 13 of 16 invasive carcinomas.[118] In addition, mutations have been detected within the DCC gene in 12 of 94 (13%) colorectal carcinomas.[107] Further support for the role of DCC as a tumor suppressor gene was found by the suppression of tumorigenicity of human colon carcinoma cell lines in athymic nude mice by the introduction of a normal chromosome 18.[65, 119] Thus, it has been proposed that colorectal epithelial cells lose DCC-mediated contact inhibition late in oncogenesis, allowing the malignant-appearing cells of intramucosal carcinomas to invade and metastasize.[118] Whether genetic alterations in and near the DCC gene or alterations in other genes controlling DCC gene expression is the predominant mechanism of inactivation of the DCC gene remains to be determined.

The chromosomal localization of the DCC gene to the long arm of chromosome 18 combined with its postulated role as a tumor suppressor gene in human colorectal carcinoma raised the possibility that it was a genetic locus responsible for hereditary nonpolyposis colorectal carcinoma (also known as the Lynch syndrome), which is characterized by (1) a minimum of three affected first-degree relatives in at least two generations; (2) mean age of onset of about 45 years; and (3) multifocality and multiplicity of primary cancers, particularly in the right side of the colon but also in the endometrium and other intraabdominal organs,[120] and a form of which had been genetically mapped to chromosome 18q.[121] However, further linkage analysis has excluded DCC as a candidate for the locus of hereditary nonpolyposis colorectal carcinoma.[122] Germline mutations of DCC have not been described to date, although the large area over which the gene is spread (more than 370 kb) has limited the search for such mutations.

DCC in Other Gastrointestinal Cancers.—Loss of expression of the DCC gene has also been implicated in the development of other gastrointestinal tumors. The mRNA of the DCC gene was markedly reduced or absent in 8 of 11 (73%) pancreatic tumor cell lines and in 4 of 8 (50%) pancreatic tumors.[123] Among the pancreatic tumor cell lines, loss of DCC gene expression was found only in those that were poorly differentiated or undifferentiated but was preserved in the differentiated cell lines, thus suggesting a possible role of DCC in pancreatic tumor tissue morphology. In gastric cancer, loss of one allele of DCC was found in 14 of 23 (61%) tumors.[124] This loss occurred in similar proportions of tumors invading only into the submucosa and muscularis propria and tumors invading beyond the muscularis propria. However, no preinvasive cancerous lesions were studied, preventing a comparison to the timing of loss of DCC expression found in colon cancer. Loss of heterozygosity at the DCC locus has also been reported in 8 of 30 (27%) breast[125] and in 15 of 34 (44%) ovarian carcinomas.[126]

Putative tumor suppressor gene(s) on chromosome 3p

A variety of studies have provided evidence for the existence of at least one tumor suppressor gene on the short arm of chromosome 3 (Fig 5). Evidence is strongest for small cell lung cancer and renal cell carcinoma but this chromosomal region has also been implicated in a number of other human malignancies, including non–small cell lung cancer[127] and testicular cancer.[128]

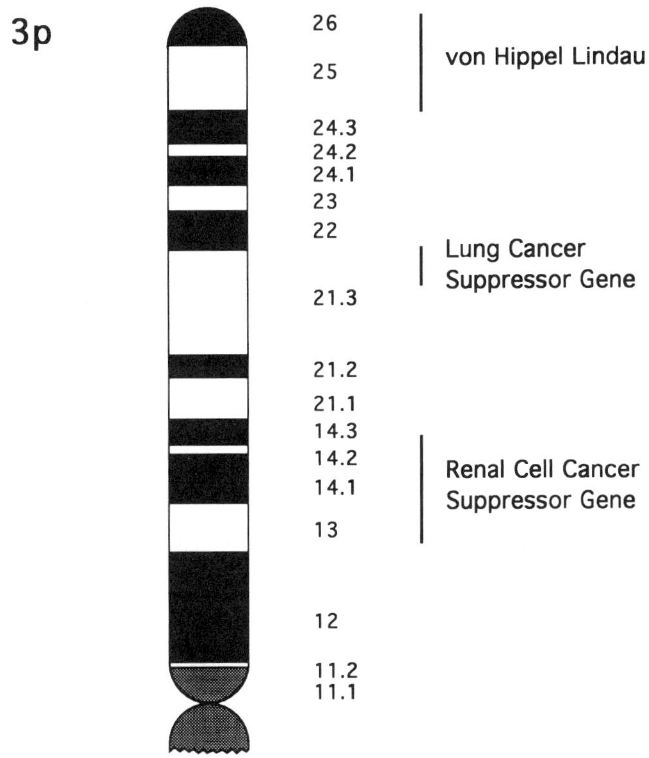

FIG 5.
Short arm of chromosome 3. The suspected locations of the putative tumor suppressor genes are shown.

Chromosome 3p and Lung Cancer.—A loss of part or all of at least one of the short arms of chromosome 3 is the most common cytogenetic abnormality in tumors and tumor cell lines from patients with small cell lung cancer. Different studies found this cytogenetic abnormality in 20% to 100% of small cell lung cancer tumors and tumor cell lines. However, more sensitive molecular biologic assays that used restriction fragment length polymorphisms mapping to loci on chromosome 3p were able to detect loss of heterozygosity in 48 of 50 (96%) of small cell lung cancer tumors or tumor cell lines.[127, 129] An intensive search for the specific tumor suppressor gene(s) is currently ongoing. More than 800 probes covering the approximately 100 megabases of the short arm of chromosome 3 have been identified,[130] which has narrowed the region containing the putative chromosome 3p tumor suppressor gene of small cell lung cancers to between bands 3p21 and 3p23, a region covering about 40 megabases. Several genes located in or near this area of chromosome 3p, including aminoacylase,[131] protein-tyrosine phosphatase γ,[132] and an unnamed gene with low mRNA expression in small cell lung cancers,[133] have been proposed as candidates for tumor suppressor genes. However, none has yet been proved to be a tumor suppressor gene. It has recently been shown that transfer of a normal chromosome 3 into the tumor cell line can reduce in vivo tumorigenicity in athymic nude mice, confirming the presence of at least one tumor suppressor gene on this chromosome.[134] Furthermore, the region responsible for this diminution of in vivo tumorigenesis was able to be narrowed to a 2-megabase area in the 3p21-22 region.[134]

Chromosome 3p and Renal Cell Cancer.—Cytogenetic analysis of renal cell carcinoma tumors and tumor cell lines has also resulted in the frequent detection of nonrandom loss of the short arm of chromosome 3.[135] Further cytogenetic support for the involvement of genes on 3p in the development of renal cell carcinoma comes from kindreds with hereditary renal cell carcinoma. Genetic and cytogenetic analysis of these kindreds reveal segregation of a balanced germline translocations at 3p13-14 with the development of renal cell carcinoma,[136–138] thus implicating a gene at this site in the development of renal cell carcinomas. Restriction fragment length polymorphism analysis in sporadic renal cell carcinomas has shown loss of heterozygosity between 3p14 and 3p21 in 65% to 75% of tumors.[139, 140] The results of some studies have suggested the presence of two tumor suppressor genes within this span, one at 3p13-14.3 (consistent with findings in hereditary renal cell carcinoma kindreds) and another at 3p21.3 (close to the 3p tumor suppressor gene of small cell lung cancers), that are involved in the development of renal cell carcinoma.[141] Interestingly, 17 of 25 renal cell cancers with retention of heterozygosity at chromosome 17p had loss of heterozygosity on chromosome 3p and 0 of 5 renal cell cancers with allelic loss at chromosome 17p had loss of heterozygosity at chromosome 3p.[142] This suggests that one of the putative tumor suppressor genes on chromosome 3 that have been implicated in renal cell carcinoma development may have tumor suppressive properties similar to those of p53. The in vivo tumorigenicity of a renal cell carcinoma cell line in athymic nude mice can be diminished by the addition of a normal chromosome 3, thus demonstrating the tumor suppression properties of the putative 3p tumor suppressor gene in renal cell carcinoma.[143]

von Hippel–Lindau Disease.—A third locus on the short arm of chromosome 3 has been implicated in human oncogenesis by association with the von Hippel–Lindau disease. This autosomal-dominant hereditary disorder is characterized by central nervous system neoplasms (hemangioblastomas in the cerebellum, retina, and spinal cord), pheochromocytomas, bilateral and multifocal renal cell carcinomas, pancreatic tumors, and cysts of the kidney, pancreas, epididymis, and other organs. Genetic studies have assigned the locus for von Hippel–Lindau disease to chromosome 3p25-26.[144] Tumors from patients with this syndrome show a high frequency of loss of chromosome 3 sequences by cytogenetics and restriction fragment length polymorphism analysis.

The NF1 Gene

The NF1 gene, located at chromosome 17q11.2, encodes a 2,819–amino acid protein called neurofibrin. Neurofibrin contains a region with homology to the guanosine triphosphatase–activating protein of *ras* and is thought to regulate *ras*,[145, 146] and may also be involved in signal transduction. Germline point mutations or deletions in this gene are responsible for neurofibromatosis (von Recklinghausen's disease) type 1,[147, 148] which is characterized by the development of numerous benign neuromas that may progress to malignancies, such as neurofibromasarcomas and optic gliomas, as well as by other nonneoplastic features. Studies of the mutations of the NF1 gene in patients with this disorder show that the gene is disrupted by a variety of genetic alterations, suggesting that it may be a tumor suppressor gene and that it is recessive at the cellular level. These genetic alterations result in a marked decrease in the ability of neurofibrin to stimulate *ras* guanosine triphosphatase activity. Initial studies of one of the 45 exons of the NF1 gene to detect somatically acquired mutations in tumors not associated with neurofibromatosis has detected mutations in one specimen each of 22 colon adenocarcinomas, 28 samples from patients with myelodysplastic syndrome, and 10 astrocytomas.[135] Interestingly, all three mutations occurred at codon 1423, an evolutionarily conserved residue within the guanosine triphosphatase–activating protein–related domain of neurofibrin, and result in a marked decreased ability of neurofibrin to activate the *ras* guanosine triphosphatase activity.[149] Further studies will be needed to determine the frequency of mutations of the NF1 gene in sporadic malignancies.

Summary

The study of the genetic alterations of tumor suppressor genes and proto-oncogenes in solid tumors has greatly increased our understanding of cancer biology. These findings have extended epidemiologic associations of carcinogens with certain tumors. Further analysis of patterns of genetic changes may implicate carcinogenic substances in cases where epidemiology has not been able to do so. Identification of germline mutations in p53, APC, and NF1 has provided improved diagnosis and presymptomatic screening in cancer kindreds. The identification of additional alterations in tumor suppressor genes may further improve the ability to predict inherent cancer risk. Screening strategies based on detection of genetic abnormalities of preinvasive cancerous lesions, such as mutant *ras* in colonic polyps, may improve early diagnosis. Finally, strategies to replace lost tumor suppressor function may provide a future therapeutic modality.

References

1. Boring CC, Squires TS, Tong T: Cancer Statistics, 1993. *CA* 1993; 43:7–26.
2. Fearon ER, Vogelstein B: A genetic model for colorectal tumorigenesis. *Cell* 1990; 61:759–767.
3. Gauwerky CE, Croce CM: Molecular biology of leukemias and lymphomas, in Broder S (ed) *Molecular Foundations of Oncology*. Baltimore, Williams & Wilkins, 1991, pp 295–310.
4. Dalla FR, Bregni M, Erikson J, et al: Human c-*myc* onc gene is located on the region of chromosome 8 that is translocated in Burkitt lymphoma cells. *Proc Natl Acad Sci USA* 1982; 79:7824–7827.
5. Collins SJ, Groudine MT: Rearrangement and amplification of c-abl sequences in the human chronic myelogenous leukemia cell line K-562. *Proc Natl Acad Sci USA* 1983; 80:4813–4817.
6. Tsujimoto Y, Cossman J, Jaffe E, et al: Involvement of the bcl-2 gene in human follicular lymphoma. *Science* 1985; 228:1440–1443.
7. Sved J, Bird A: The expected equilibrium of the CpG dinucleotide in vertebrate genomes under a mutation model. *Proc Natl Acad Sci USA* 1990; 87:4692–4696.
8. Kern SE, Kinzler KW, Bruskin A, et al: Identification of p53 as a sequence-specific DNA-binding protein. *Science* 1991; 252:1708–1711.
9. Bargonetti J, Friedman PN, Kern SE, et al: Wild-type but not mutant p53 immunopurified proteins bind to sequences adjacent to the SV40 origin of replication. *Cell* 1991; 65:1083–1091.
10. Farmer G, Bargonetti J, Zhu H, et al: Wild-type p53 activates transcription in vitro. *Nature* 1992; 358:83–86.
11. Maltzman W, Czyzyk L: UV irradiation stimulates levels of p53 cellular tumor antigen in nontransformed mouse cells. *Mol Cell Biol* 1984; 4:1689–1694.
12. Kastan MB, Onyekwere O, Sidransky D, et al: Participation of p53 protein in the cellular response to DNA damage. *Cancer Res* 1991; 51:6304–6311.
13. Yonish RE, Resnitzky D, Lotem J, et al: Wild-type p53 induces apoptosis of myeloid leukaemic cells that is inhibited by interleukin-6. *Nature* 1991; 353:345–347.
14. Shaw P, Bovey R, Tardy S, et al: Induction of apoptosis by wild-type p53 in a human colon tumor-derived cell line. *Proc Natl Acad Sci USA* 1992; 89:4495–4499.
15. Kastan MB, Zhan Q, el DW, et al: A mammalian cell cycle checkpoint path-

way utilizing p53 and GADD45 is defective in ataxia-telangiectasia. *Cell* 1992; 71:587–597.
16. Livingstone LR, White A, Sprouse J, et al: Altered cell cycle arrest and gene amplification potential accompany loss of wild-type p53. *Cell* 1992; 70:923–935.
17. Takahashi T, Carbone D, Takahashi T, et al: Wild-type but not mutant p53 suppresses the growth of human lung cancer cells bearing multiple genetic lesions. *Cancer Res* 1992; 52:2340–2343.
18. Casey G, Lo HM, Lopez ME, et al: Growth suppression of human breast cancer cells by the introduction of a wild-type p53 gene. *Oncogene* 1991; 6:1791–1797.
19. Baker SJ, Markowitz S, Fearon ER, et al: Suppression of human colorectal carcinoma cell growth by wild type p53. *Science* 1990; 249:912–915.
20. Swift M, Morrell D, Massey RB, et al: Incidence of cancer in 161 families affected by ataxia-telangiectasia. *N Engl J Med* 1991; 325:1831–1836.
21. Hollstein M, Sidransky D, Vogelstein B, et al: p53 mutations in human cancers. *Science* 1991; 253:49–53.
22. Johnson BE, Kelley MJ: Overview of genetic and molecular events in the pathogenesis of lung cancer. *Chest* 1993; 100:1S–3S.
23. Somers KD, Merrick MA, Lopez ME, et al: Frequent p53 mutations in head and neck cancer. *Cancer Res* 1992; 52:5997–6000.
24. Baker SJ, Preisinger AC, Jessup JM, et al: p53 gene mutations occur in combination with 17p allelic deletions as late events in colorectal tumorigenesis. *Cancer Res* 1990; 50:7717–7722.
25. Coles C, Condie A, Chetty U, et al: p53 mutations in breast cancer. *Cancer Res* 1992; 52:5291–5298.
26. Kihana T, Tsuda H, Teshima S, et al: High incidence of p53 gene mutation in human ovarian cancer and its association with nuclear accumulation of p53 protein and tumor DNA aneuploidy. *Jpn J Cancer Res* 1992; 83:978–984.
27. Seruca R, David L, Holm R, et al: P53 mutations in gastric carcinomas. *Br J Cancer* 1992; 65:708–710.
28. Kim JH, Takahashi T, Chiba I, et al: Occurrence of p53 gene abnormalities in gastric carcinoma tumors and cell lines. *J Natl Cancer Inst* 1991; 83:938–943.
29. Brash DE, Rudolph JA, Simon JA, et al: A role for sunlight in skin cancer: UV-induced p53 mutations in squamous cell carcinoma. *Proc Natl Acad Sci USA* 1991; 88:10124–10128.
30. Hsu IC, Metcalf RA, Sun T, et al: Mutational hotspot in the p53 gene in human hepatocellular carcinomas. *Nature* 1991; 350:427–428.
31. Bressac B, Kew M, Wands J, et al: Selective G to T mutations of p53 gene in hepatocellular carcinoma from southern Africa. *Nature* 1991; 350:429–431.
32. Scorsone KA, Zhou YZ, Butel JS, et al: p53 mutations cluster at codon 249 in hepatitis B virus-positive hepatocellular carcinomas from China. *Cancer Res* 1992; 52:1635–1638.
33. Mazur M, Glickman BW: Sequence specificity of mutations induced by benzo[a]pyrene-7,8-diol-9,10-epoxide at endogenous aprt gene in CHO cells. *Somatic Cell Mol Genetics* 1988; 14:393–400.
34. Vähäkangas KH, Samet JM, Metcalf RA, et al: Mutations of p53 and ras genes in radon-associated lung cancer from uranium miners, *Lancet* 1992; 339:576–580.
35. Grosovsky AJ, de BJ, de JP, et al: Base substitutions, frameshifts, and small

deletions constitute ionizing radiation-induced point mutations in mammalian cells. *Proc Natl Acad Sci USA* 1988; 85:185–188.
36. Oda T, Tsuda H, Scarpa A, et al: p53 gene mutation spectrum in hepatocellular carcinoma. *Cancer Res* 1992; 52:6358–6364.
37. Kress S, Jahn UR, Buchmann A, et al: p53 Mutations in human hepatocellular carcinomas from Germany. *Cancer Res* 1992; 52:3220–3223.
38. Nichida N, Fukuda Y, Kokuryu H, et al: Role and mutational heterogeneity of the p53 gene in hepatocellular carcinoma. *Cancer Res* 1993; 53:368–372.
39. Sheu J-C, Huang G-T, Lee P-H, et al: Mutation of p53 gene in hepatocellular carcinoma in Taiwan. *Cancer Res* 1992; 52:6098–6100.
40. Puisieux A, Lim S, Groopman J, et al: Selective targeting of p53 gene mutational hotspots in human cancers by etiologically defined carcinogens. *Cancer Res* 1991; 51:6185–6189.
41. Sommer SS, Cunningham J, McGovern RM, et al: Pattern of p53 gene mutations in breast cancers of women of the midwestern United States. *J Natl Cancer Inst* 1992; 84:246–252.
42. Davidoff AM, Humphrey PA, Iglehart JD, et al: Genetic basis for p53 overexpression in human breast cancer. *Proc Natl Acad Sci USA* 1991; 88:5006–5010.
43. Davidoff AM, Kerns BJ, Iglehart JD, et al: Maintenance of p53 alterations throughout breast cancer progression. *Cancer Res* 1991; 51:2605–2610.
44. Prosser J, Thompson AM, Cranston G, et al: Evidence that p53 behaves as a tumour suppressor gene in sporadic breast tumours, *Oncogene* 1990; 5:1573–1579.
45. Li FP, Fraumeni JF, Mulvihill JJ, et al: A cancer family syndrome in twenty-four kindreds. *Cancer Res* 1988; 48:5358–5362.
46. Malkin D, Li FP, Strong LC, et al: Germ line p53 mutations in a familial syndrome of breast cancer, sarcomas, and other neoplasms. *Science* 1990; 250:1233–1238.
47. Srivastava S, Zou ZQ, Pirollo K, et al: Germ-line transmission of a mutated p53 gene in a cancer-prone family with Li-Fraumeni syndrome. *Nature* 1990; 348:747–749.
48. Barnes DM, Hanby AM, Gillett CE, et al: Abnormal expression of wild type p53 protein in normal cells of a cancer family patient. *Lancet* 1992; 340:259–263.
49. Toguchida J, Yamaguchi T, Dayton SH, et al: Prevalence and spectrum of germline mutations of the p53 gene among patients with sarcoma. *N Engl J Med* 1992; 326:1301–1308.
50. Malkin D, Jolly KW, Barbier N, et al: Germline mutations of the p53 tumor-suppressor gene in children and young adults with second malignant neoplasms. *N Engl J Med* 1992; 326:1309–1315.
51. Scheffner M, Werness BA, Huibregtse JM, et al: The E6 oncoprotein encoded by human papillomavirus types 16 and 18 promotes the degradation of p53. *Cell* 1990; 63:1129–1136.
52. Crook T, Tidy JA, Vousden KH: Degradation of p53 can be targeted by HPV E6 sequences distinct from those required for p53 binding and trans-activation. *Cell* 1991; 67:547–556.
53. Smith SH, Weiss SW, Jankowski SA, et al: SAS amplification in soft tissue sarcomas. *Cancer Res* 1992; 52:3746–3749.
54. Oliner JD, Kinzler KW, Meltzer PS, et al: Amplification of a gene encoding a p53-associated protein in human sarcomas. *Nature* 1992; 358:80–83.

55. Casson AG, Mukhopadhyay T, Cleary KR, et al: p53 gene mutations in Barrett's epithelium and esophageal cancer. *Cancer Res* 1991;51: 4495–4499.
56. Bennett WP, Hollstein MC, Metcalf RA, et al: p53 mutation and protein accumulation during multistage human esophageal carcinogenesis. *Cancer Res* 1992; 52:6092–6097.
57. Sozzi G, Miozzo M, Donghi R, et al: Deletions of 17p and p53 mutations in preneoplastic lesions of the lung. *Cancer Res* 1992; 52:6079–6082.
58. Horio Y, Takahashi T, Kuroishi T, et al: Prognostic significance of p53 mutations and 3p deletions in primary resected non-small cell lung cancer. *Cancer Res* 1993; 53:1–4.
59. Quinlan DC, Davidson AG, Summers CL, et al: Accumulation of p53 protein correlates with a poor prognosis in human lung cancer. *Cancer Res* 1992; 52:4828–4831.
60. Mitsudomi T, Steinberg SM, Nau MM, et al: p53 gene mutations in non-small-cell lung cancer cell lines and their correlation with the presence of *ras* mutations and clinical features. *Oncogene* 1992; 7:171–180.
61. Davidoff AM, Herndon J2, Glover NS, et al: Relation between p53 overexpression and established prognostic factors in breast cancer. *Surgery* 1991; 110:259–264.
62. Thor Ad, Moore DI, Edgerton SM, et al: Accumulation of p53 tumor suppressor gene protein: an independent marker of prognosis in breast cancers. *J Natl Cancer Inst* 1992; 84:845–855.
63. Bartek J, Iggo R, Gannon J, et al: Genetic and immunochemical analysis of mutant p53 in human breast cancer cell lines. *Oncogene* 1990; 5:893–899.
64. Isola J, Visakorpi T, Holli K, et al: Association of overexpression of tumor suppressor protein p53 with rapid cell proliferation and poor prognosis in node-negative breast cancer patients. *J Natl Cancer Inst* 1992; 84:1109–1114.
65. Goyette MC, Cho K, Fasching CL, et al: Progression of colorectal cancer is associated with multiple tumor suppressor gene defects but inhibition of tumorigenicity is accomplished by correction of any single defect via chromosome transfer. *Mol Cell Biol* 1992; 12:1387–1395.
66. Hall A: The cellular functions of small GTP-binding proteins. *Science* 1990; 249:635–640.
67. Bos JL: *ras* oncogenes in human cancer: A review. *Cancer Res* 1989; 49:4682–4689.
68. Vogelstein B, Fearon ER, Hamilton SR, et al: Genetic alterations during colorectal-tumor development. *N Engl J Med* 1988; 319:525–532.
69. Sidransky D, Tokino T, Hamilton SR, et al: Identification of *ras* oncogene mutations in the stool of patients with curable colorectal tumors. *Science* 1992; 256:102–105.
70. Bell SM, Kelly SA, Hoyle JA, et al: c-Ki-*ras* gene mutations in dysplasia and carcinomas complicating ulcerative colitis. *Br J Cancer* 1991; 64:174–178.
71. Chen J, Compton C, Cheng E, et al: c-Ki-*ras* mutations in dysplastic fields and cancers in ulcerative colitis. *Gastroenterology* 1992; 102:1983–1987.
72. Rodenhuis S, Slebos RJ: Clinical significance of *ras* oncogene activation in human lung cancer. *Cancer Res* 1992; 52:2665S-2669S.
73. Rusch VW, Reuter VE, Kris MG, et al: Ras oncogene point mutation: an infrequent event in bronchoalveolar cancer. *J Thorac Cardiovasc Surg* 1992; 104:1465–1469.
74. Mitsudomi T, Steinberg SM, Oie HK, et al: *ras* gene mutations in non-small

cell lung cancers are associated with shortened survival irrespective of treatment intent. *Cancer Res* 1991; 51:4999–5002.
75. Sugio K, Ishida T, Yokoyama H, et al: *ras* gene mutations as a prognostic marker in adenocarcinoma of the human lung without lymph node metastasis. *Cancer Res* 1992; 52:2903–2906.
76. Mizuuchi H, Nasim S, Kudo R, et al: Clinical implications of K-*ras* mutations in malignant epithelial tumors of the endometrium. *Cancer Res* 1992; 52:2777–2781.
77. Imamura T, Arima T, Kato H, et al: Chromosomal deletions and K-*ras* gene mutations in human endometrial carcinomas. *Int J Cancer* 1992; 51:47–52.
78. Kinzler KW, Nilbert MC, Su LK, et al: Identification of FAP locus genes from chromosome 5q21. *Science* 1991; 253:661–665.
79. Groden J, Thliveris A, Samowitz W, et al: Identification and characterization of the familial adenomatous polyposis coli gene. *Cell* 1991; 66:589–600.
80. Miyoshi Y, Ando H, Nagase H, et al: Germ-line mutations of the APC gene in 53 familial adenomatous polyposis patients. *Proc Natl Acad Sci USA* 1992; 89:4452–4456.
81. Cottrell S, Bicknell D, Kaklamanis L, et al: Molecular analysis of APC mutations in familial adenomatous polyposis and sporadic colon carcinomas. *Lancet* 1992; 340:626–630.
82. Nagase H, Miyoshi Y, Horii A, et al: Correlation between the location of germ-line mutations in the APC gene and the number of colorectal polyps in familial adenomatous polyposis patients. *Cancer Res* 1992; 52:4055–4057.
83. Peltomäki P, Sistonen P, Mecklin JP, et al: Evidence that the MCC-APC gene region in 5q21 is not the site for susceptibility to hereditary nonpolyposis colorectal carcinoma. *Cancer Res* 1992; 52:4530–4533.
84. Powell SM, Zilz N, Beazer BY, et al: APC mutations occur early during colorectal tumorigenesis. *Nature* 1992; 359:235–237.
85. Horii A, Nakatsuru S, Miyoshi Y, et al: Frequent somatic mutations of the APC gene in human pancreatic cancer. *Cancer Res* 1992; 52:6696–6698.
86. Horii A, Nakatsuru S, Miyoshi Y, et al: The APC gene, responsible for familial adenomatous polyposis, is mutated in human gastric cancer. *Cancer Res* 1992; 52:3231–3233.
87. Neuman WL, Wasylyshyn ML, Jacoby R, et al: Evidence for a common molecular pathogenesis in colorectal, gastric, and pancreatic cancer. *Genes Chromosoml Cancer* 1991; 3:468–473.
88. D'Amico D, Carbone DP, Johnson BE, et al: Polymorphic sites within the MCC and APC loci reveal very frequent loss of heterozygosity in human small cell lung cancer. *Cancer Res* 1992; 52:1996–1999.
89. Miki Y, Nishisho I, Horii A, et al: Disruption of the APC gene by a retrotransposal insertion of L1 sequence in a colon cancer. *Cancer Res* 1992; 52:643–645.
90. Greenwald BD, Harpaz N, Yin J, et al: Loss of heterozygosity affecting the p53, rb, and mcc/apc tumor suppressor gene loci in dysplastic and cancerous ulcerative colitis. *Cancer Res* 1992; 52:741–745.
91. Kinzler KW, Nilbert MC, Vogelstein B, et al: Identification of a gene located at chromosome 5q21 that is mutated in colorectal cancers. *Science* 1991; 251:1366–1370.
92. Friend SH, Bernards R, Rogelj S, et al: A human DNA segment with properties of the gene that predisposes to retinoblastoma and osteosarcoma. *Nature* 1986; 323:643–646.

93. Buchkovich K, Duffy LA, Harlow E: The retinoblastoma protein is phosphorylated during specific phases of the cell cycle. *Cell* 1989; 58:1097–1105.
94. Lin BT, Gruenwald S, Morla AO, et al: Retinoblastoma cancer suppressor gene product is a substrate of the cell cycle regulator cdc2 kinase. *EMBO J* 1991; 10:857–864.
95. Rustgi AK, Dyson N Bernards R: Amino-terminal domains of c-myc and N-myc proteins mediate binding to the retinoblastoma gene product. *Nature* 1991; 352:541–544.
96. Chellappan SP, Hiebert S, Mudryj M, et al: The E2F transcription factor is a cellular target for the RB protein. *Cell* 1991; 65:1053–1061.
97. Huang HJ, Yee JK, Shew JY, et al. Suppression of the neoplastic phenotype by replacement of the RB gene in human cancer cells. *Science* 1988; 242:1563–1566.
98. Bookstein R, Shew JY, Chen PL, et al: Suppression of tumorigenicity of human prostate carcinoma cells by replacing a mutated RB gene. *Science* 1990; 247:712–715.
99. Takahashi R, Hashimoto T, Xu HJ, et al: The retinoblastoma gene functions as a growth and tumor suppressor in human bladder carcinoma cells. *Proc Natl Acad Sci USA* 1991; 88:5257–5261.
100. Whyte P, Buchkovich KJ, Horowitz JM, et al: Association between an oncogene and an anti-oncogene: The adenovirus E1A proteins bind to the retinoblastoma gene product. *Nature* 1988; 334:124–129.
101. Dyson N, Howley PM, Munger K, et al: The human papilloma virus-16 E7 oncoprotein is able to bind to the retinoblastoma gene product. *Science* 1989; 243:934–937.
102. Abramson DH, Ellsworth RM, Kitchin FD, et al: Second nonocular tumors in retinoblastoma survivors. Are they radiation-induced? *Ophthalmology* 1984; 91:1351–1355.
103. Friend SH, Horowitz JM, Gerber MR, et al: Deletions of a DNA sequence in retinoblastomas and mesenchymal tumors: Organization of the sequence and its encoded protein. *Proc Natl Acad Sci USA* 1987; 84:9059–9063.
104. Sawan A, Randall B, Angus B, et al: Retinoblastoma and p53 gene expression related to relapse and survival in human breast cancer: An immunohistochemical study. *J Pathol* 1992; 168:23–28.
105. Logothetis CJ, Xu HJ, Ro JY, et al: Altered expression of retinoblastoma protein and known prognostic variables in locally advanced bladder cancer. *J Natl Cancer Inst* 1992; 84:1256–1261.
106. Cordon-Cardo C, Wartinger D, Petrylak D, et al: Altered expression of the retinoblastoma gene product: Prognostic indicator in bladder cancer. *J Natl Cancer Inst* 1992; 84:1251–1256.
107. Fearon ER, Cho KR, Nigro JM, et al: Identification of a chromosome 18q gene that is altered in colorectal cancers. *Science* 1990; 247:49–56.
108. Johnson JP: Cell adhesion molecules of the immunoglobulin supergene family and their role in malignant transformation and progression to metastatic disease. *Cancer Metastasis Rev* 1991; 10:11–22.
109. Horowitz JM, Park SH, Bogenmann E, et al: Frequent inactivation of the retinoblastoma anti-oncogene is restricted to a subset of human tumor cells. *Proc Natl Acad Sci USA* 1990; 87:2775–2779.
110. Harbour JW, Lai SL, Whang PJ, et al: Abnormalities in structure and expression of the human retinoblastoma gene in SCLC. *Science* 1988; 241:353–357.

111. Yokota J, Akiyama T, Fung YK, et al: Altered expression of the retinoblastoma (RB) gene in small-cell carcinoma of the lung. *Oncogene* 1988; 3:471–475.
112. Rygaard K, Sorenson GD, Pettengill OS, et al: Abnormalities in structure and expression of the retinoblastoma gene in small cell lung cancer cell lines and xenografts in nude mice. *Cancer Res* 1990; 50:5312–5317.
113. Hensel CH, Hsieh CL, Gazdar AF, et al: Altered structure and expression of the human retinoblastoma susceptibility gene in small cell lung cancer. *Cancer Res* 1990; 50:3067–3072.
114. Bookstein R, Rio P, Madreperla SA, et al: Promoter deletion and loss of retinoblastoma gene expression in human prostate carcinoma. *Proc Natl Acad Sci USA* 1990; 87:7762–7766.
115. Lee EY, To H, Shew JY, et al: Inactivation of the retinoblastoma susceptibility gene in human breast cancers. *Science* 1988; 241:218–221.
116. T'Ang A, Varley JM, Chakraborty S, et al: Structural rearrangement of the retinoblastoma gene in human breast carcinoma. *Science* 1988; 242:263–266.
117. Varley JM, Armour J, Swallow JE, et al: The retinoblastoma gene is frequently altered leading to loss of expression in primary breast tumours. *Oncogene* 1989; 4:725–729.
118. Kikuchi-Yanoshita R, Konishi M, Fukunari H, et al: Loss of expression of the DCC gene during progression of colorectal carcinomas in familial adenomatous polyposis and non-familial adenomatous polyposis patients. *Cancer Res* 1992; 52:3801–3803.
119. Tanaka K, Oshimura M, Kikuchi R, et al: Suppression of tumorigenicity in human colon carcinoma cells by introduction of normal chromosome 5 or 18. *Nature* 1991; 349:340–342.
120. Lynch HT, Kimberling W, Albano WA, et al: Hereditary nonpolyposis colorectal cancer (Lynch syndromes I and II). I. Clinical description of resource. *Cancer* 1985; 56:934–938.
121. Boman BM, Lynch HT, Kimberling WJ, et al: Reassignment of a cancer family syndrome to chromosome 18. *Cancer Genet Cytogenet* 1988; 34:153–154.
122. Peltomäki P, Sistonen P, Mecklin JP, et al: Evidence supporting exclusion of the DCC gene and a portion of chromosome 18q as the locus for susceptibility to hereditary nonpolyposis colorectal carcinoma in five kindreds. *Cancer Res* 1991; 51:4135–4140.
123. Höhne MW, Halatsch ME, Kahl GF, et al: Frequent loss of expression of the potential tumor suppressor gene DCC in ductal pancreatic adenocarcinoma. *Cancer Res* 1992; 52:2616–2619.
124. Uchino S, Tsuda H, Noguchi M, et al: Frequent loss of heterozygosity at the DCC locus in gastric cancer. *Cancer Res* 1992; 52:3099–3102.
125. Devilee P, van VM, Kuipers DN, et al: Somatic genetic changes on chromosome 18 in breast carcinomas: Is the DCC gene involved? *Oncogene* 1991; 6:311–315.
126. Chenevix-Trench G, Leary J, Kerr J, et al: Frequent loss of heterozygosity on chromosome 18 in ovarian adenocarcinoma which does not always include the DCC locus. *Oncogene* 1992; 7:1059–1065.
127. Brauch H, Johnson B, Hovis J, et al: Molecular analysis of the short arm of chromosome 3 in small-cell and non-small-cell carcinoma of the lung. *N Engl J Med* 1987; 317:1109–1113.

128. Lothe RA, Fossa SD, Stenwig AE, et al: Loss of 3p or 11p alleles is associated with testicular cancer tumors. *Genomics* 1989; 5:134–138.
129. Johnson BE, Sakaguchi AY, Gazdar AF, et al: Restriction fragment length polymorphism studies show consistent loss of chromosome 3p alleles in small cell lung cancer patients' tumors. *J Clin Invest* 1988; 82:502–507.
130. Lerman MI, Latif F, Glenn GM, et al: Isolation and regional localization of a large collection (2,000) of single-copy DNA fragments on human chromosome 3 for mapping and cloning tumor suppressor genes. *Hum Genet* 1991; 86:567–577.
131. Miller YE, Minna JD, Gazdar AF: Lack of expression of aminoacylase-1 in small cell lung cancer. Evidence for inactivation of genes encoded by chromosome 3p. *J Clin Invest* 1989; 83:2120–2124.
132. LaForgia S, Morse B, Levy J, et al: Receptor protein-tyrosine phosphatase gamma is a candidate tumor suppressor gene at human chromosome region 3p21. *Proc Natl Acad Sci USA* 1991; 88:5036–5040.
133. Carritt B, Kok K, van den Berg A, et al: A gene from human chromosome region 3p21 with reduced expression in small cell lung cancer. *Cancer Res* 1992; 52:1536–1541.
134. Killary AM, Wolf ME, Giambernardi TA, et al: Definition of a tumor suppressor locus within human chromosome 3p21–p22. *Proc Natl Acad Sci USA* 1992; 89:10877–10881.
135. Kovacs G, Szucs S, De RW, et al: Specific chromosome aberration in human renal cell carcinoma. *Int J Cancer* 1987; 40:171–178.
136. Cohen AJ, Li FP, Berg S, et al: Hereditary renal-cell carcinoma associated with a chromosomal translocation. *N Engl J Med* 1979; 301:592–595.
137. Pathak S, Strong LC, Ferrell RE, et al: Familial renal cell carcinoma with a 3;11 chromosome translocation limited to tumor cells. *Science* 1982; 217:939–941.
138. Kovacs G, Frisch S: Clonal chromosome abnormalities in tumor cells from patients with sporadic renal cell carcinomas. *Cancer Res* 1989; 49:651–659.
139. Kovacs G, Erlandsson R, Boldog F, et al: Consistent chromosome 3p deletion and loss of heterozygosity in renal cell carcinoma. *Proc Natl Acad Sci USA* 1988; 85:1571–1575.
140. Bergerheim U, Nordenskjold M, Collins VP: Deletion mapping in human renal cell carcinoma. *Cancer Res* 1989; 49:1390–1396.
141. Yamakawa K, Morita R, Takahashi E, et al: A detailed deletion mapping of the short arm of chromosome 3 in sporadic renal cell carcinoma. *Cancer Res* 1991; 51:4707–4711.
142. Ogawa O, Kakehi Y, Ogawa K, et al: Allelic loss at chromosome 3p characterizes clear cell phenotype of renal cell carcinoma. *Cancer Res* 1991; 51:949–953.
143. Shimizu M, Yokota J, Mori N, et al: Introduction of normal chromosome 3p modulates the tumorigenicity of a human renal cell carcinoma cell line YCR. *Oncogene* 1990; 5:185–194.
144. Seizinger BR, Smith DI, Filling KM, et al: Genetic flanking markers refine diagnostic criteria and provide insights into the genetics of von Hippel-Lindau disease. *Proc Natl Acad Sci USA* 1991; 88:2864–2868.
145. DeClue JE, Cohen BD, Lowy DR: Identification and characterization of the neurofibromatosis type 1 protein product. *Proc Natl Acad Sci USA* 1991; 88:9914–9918.

146. Gutmann DH, Wood DL, Collins FS: Identification of the neurofibromatosis type 1 gene product. *Proc Natl Acad Sci USA* 1991; 88:9658–9662.
147. Cawthon RM, Weiss R, Xu GF, et al: A major segment of the neurofibromatosis type 1 gene: cDNA sequence, genomic structure, and point mutations. *Cell* 1990; 62:193–201.
148. Viskochil D, Buchberg AM, Xu G, et al: Deletions and a translocation interrupt a cloned gene at the neurofibromatosis type 1 locus. *Cell* 1990; 62:187–192.
149. Li Y, Bollag G, Clark R, et al: Somatic mutations in the neurofibromatosis 1 gene in human tumors. *Cell* 1992; 69:275–281.

Molecular Genetic Studies of the Adenoma-Carcinoma Sequence

Eric R. Fearon, M.D., Ph.D.

Assistant Professor of Pathology and Biology, Boyer Center for Molecular Medicine, Yale University School of Medicine, New Haven, Connecticut

The factors and mechanisms underlying the development of colon and rectal cancers are varied and complex, and include environmental and dietary factors and both inherited and somatic mutations. Although therapy for and management of patients with colorectal tumors remain difficult, these tumors have proven to be an excellent experimental system for the study of the molecular lesions that underlie their development and progression. Studies over the past decade, utilizing recombinant DNA techniques, have provided direct evidence that cancer, specifically colorectal cancer, is indeed a genetic disease.[1–5] In colon and rectal cancers, specific alterations in both oncogenes and tumor suppressor genes have been identified. Wild-type alleles of cellular oncogenes and tumor suppressor genes function in the normal regulation of development, tissue differentiation, cell cycle control, and cell proliferation. Activated alleles of cellular oncogenes can function in a dominant fashion to promote tumorigenesis; activation of an allele of a cellular oncogene can result from specific mutations in the gene or from deregulation of gene expression through chromosomal rearrangement or gene amplification.[1, 2] In contrast, tumor suppressor genes are thought to regulate cell proliferation in a negative fashion, either directly or, perhaps more likely, by transducing growth regulatory from the environment. Inactivation of tumor suppressor gene function by either inherited or somatic mutations can result in loss of normal growth control and subsequent tumor formation.[3, 6, 7]

In this chapter, the molecular alterations that have been observed in colon and rectal tumors of various stages will be reviewed. It is important to relate the alterations observed to the multistep process, or natural history, of colorectal tumorigenesis that has been documented in a large number of clinical and histopathologic studies. Therefore, the clinical and pathologic features of colorectal cancer that are relevant to the molecular genetic studies will be considered first. The molecular alterations, both inherited and somatic, that are believed to underlie the development and progres-

Advances in Internal Medicine®, vol 39

sion of colorectal adenomas and carcinomas will then be considered. Finally, the data obtained from the molecular genetic studies of colorectal tumorigenesis suggest that a number of future possibilities exist for improving the diagnosis and clinical management of patients with colorectal tumors, and some of these possibilities will be outlined.

Natural History of Colon and Rectal Cancer

Clinical and Histopathological Studies

In the United States, approximately 157,000 cases of colon and rectal cancer were diagnosed in 1991; about 70% of those were colon cancers, and about 40% to 45% of patients with colorectal cancer will die of their disease.[8] Thus, colon and rectal cancers represent a significant number of the cancer cases diagnosed annually. In addition, the adenomatous polyp or adenoma is believed to be a precursor lesion to cancer, and the number of patients with adenomatous polyps is estimated to be perhaps even tenfold greater than the number with colorectal cancers. The prevalence of adenomas in asymptomatic individuals older than 40 years of age has been estimated at 8% to 17%.[9]

At least three independent lines of evidence support the proposal that the majority of colorectal cancers arise from adenomatous polyps. First, several longitudinal studies have assessed the risk of subsequent cancer development in patients with adenomas. In a study by Murakami et al.,[10] a sizable cohort of patients with polyps either was treated with primary excision of the polyps or underwent a biopsy of the polyps and had the polyps left in situ for the duration of the study. All patients with polyps and a similar-sized cohort of patients with polyps were then followed. Those patients whose polyps were excised at the initiation of the study did not have a risk of cancer significantly different from that of the control group. Those patients whose polyps were not excised had approximately an eightfold increase in their risk of cancer. The results of a large study by Gilbertsen[11] and recent findings from the National Polyp Study[12] have also established that removal of adenomatous polyps in patients significantly reduces the incidence of subsequent cancer development. Second, the presence of foci of carcinoma arising in adenomatous polyps, as well as the presence of residual adenomatous cells in cancer specimens, suggests that carcinomas arise from preexisting adenomas.[13–15] Third, individuals with the familial adenomatous polyposis (FAP) syndrome often develop hundreds and even thousands of adenomatous polyps by 30 to 40 years of age.[16, 17] These individuals invariably develop colorectal cancers by the fourth to fifth decades of life if their colons are not removed, providing additional support for the relevance of the adenoma-carcinoma sequence in the development of colorectal cancer.

Although polyps other than adenomatous polyps, such as hyperplastic polyps, can be frequently detected in the colon, and some studies have suggested that the presence of hyperplastic polyps may be associated with increased risk of adenomatous polyp and cancer development, present data suggest that only adenomatous polyps are susceptible to progression to cancer.[13–15] The adenomatous polyp, which arises from the glandular epithelium, is characterized by the failure of the cells in the lesion to differentiate appropriately and by unrestricted cell division in the lesion. Adenomas can be distinguished on the basis of their gross and histopathologic appearances. Grossly, the lesions are described as sessile (flat), pedunculated (with a stalk), or semisessile. With regard to histopathologic classification, a number of features can be used to distinguish adenomas, and these features may predict the likelihood that the adenoma either will contain a focus of cancer or will eventually progress to cancer. In tubular adenomas the normal configuration of intestinal glands is maintained; however the crypts are elongated and the cells in the glands are incompletely differentiated columnar cells with pseudostratified nuclei. In contrast, the glands in villous adenomas consist of fingerlike processes extending outward from the surface of the adenoma. Many adenomas actually represent the continuum between tubular and villous adenomas, and regions of tubular and villous architecture often can be observed in a single adenoma (tubulovillous adenoma). In general, tubular adenomas are smaller, better differentiated, and contain less cellular atypia than do tubulovillous or villous adenomas, although exceptions to these generalizations are common.[13–15]

Although little is known about whether all colonic epithelial cells or only a subset are susceptible to neoplastic transformation, it is presumed that a small adenomatous polyp of low malignant potential can arise from normal mucosa cells or perhaps from areas of mucosa with hyperproliferative features of abnormal tissue architecture.[18, 19] Some of these polyps may then progress with increases in size and cellular atypia to a larger adenoma with increased malignant potential or to an intraepithelial neoplasia or carcinoma in situ. Finally, a subset of these lesions may progress further to invasive and metastatic cancer. This multistep process probably occurs over a period measured in years or even decades. Although clinical and histopathologic features can be used to classify tumors into relatively discrete stages, the biologic processes of clonal evolution and outgrowth that underlie adenoma formation and subsequent progression to carcinoma are likely to be continuous.

Inherited Syndromes Predisposing to Colorectal Cancer

It is estimated that 10% or more of colorectal cancer cases result, at least in part, from an inherited predisposition to the disease.[20] Several of the predisposition syndromes can readily be distinguished from one another. Familial adenomatous polyposis is an autosomal-dominant syndrome that is estimated to affect approximately 1 in 10,000 individuals in the United States.[16, 17, 20] In affected individuals, hundreds or even a thousand or more adenomas develop in the colon and rectum by the end of the third and fourth decades of life (Fig 1). A small percentage of these adenomas degenerate or progress to cancer, necessitating the prophylactic removal of the patient's colon. Several variants of FAP have been described in which

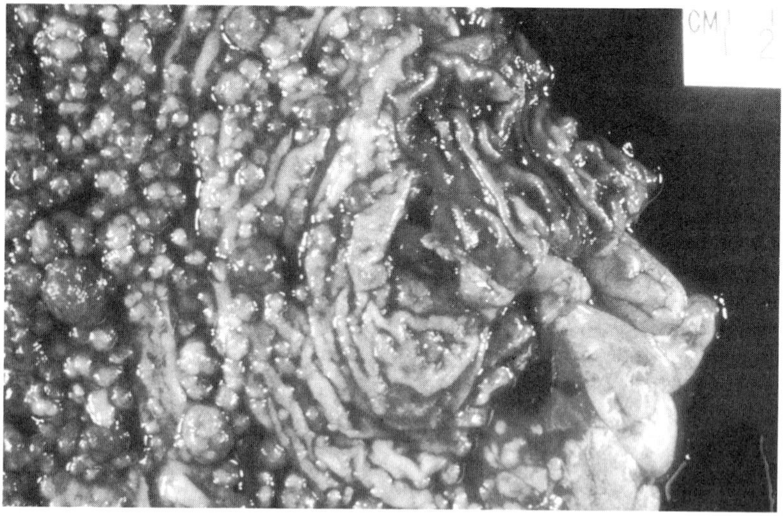

FIG 1.
Surgical resection specimen from a patient with familial adenomatous polyposis. Perhaps 100 or more adenomatous polyps are present in the specimen. Some of these polyps will inevitably progress to cancer if the patient's colon is not removed prophylactically. (Courtesy Dr. David Rimm, Yale University School of Medicine.)

tumors also develop in organs other than the colon (Table 1). These variants include Gardner's syndrome, in which affected individuals often manifest epidermoid cysts, desmoid tumors, and osteomas in addition to polyposis, and Turcot syndrome, in which brain tumors occur.[16, 17, 20] The gene responsible for FAP and Gardner's syndrome has been mapped to chromosome 5q, and recent studies have identified this predisposition gene, now termed the *adenomatous polyposis coli (APC) gene.*[21–24] The

TABLE 1.
Genetics of Inherited Colorectal Tumor Syndromes*

Syndrome	Features	Gene/Chromosome
Familial adenomatous polyposis	Multiple adenomatous polyps (>100) of the large intestine; occasionally gastric polyps	APC gene/chromosome 5q
Gardner's syndrome	Same as FAP; also, desmoid tumors, osteomas, retinal pigmentation changes	APC gene/chromosome 5q
Turcot syndrome	Same as FAP; also brain tumors	APC gene/chromosome 5q

Continued.

TABLE 1 (cont.).

Syndrome	Features	Gene/Chromosome
Attenuated adenomatous polyposis coli	Same as FAP, except marked variation in polyp number (from 10 to >100)	APC gene/chromosome 5q (at least some kindreds)
Heritable nonpolyposis colorectal cancer		
Lynch type I	Colorectal cancer without extensive polyposis	?
Lynch type II	Colorectal cancer, stomach cancer, endometrial cancer, urothelial cancer	Chromosome 18q (some kindreds)? Other kindreds?/no evidence for linkage to chromosomes 5q or 18q
Peutz-Jeghers syndrome	Hamartomatous polyps throughout the gastrointestinal tract; mucocutaneous pigmentation; estimated ninefold to thirteenfold increased risk of gastrointestinal and non–gastrointestinal cancers	?
Juvenile polyposis	Multiple hamartomatous/ juvenile polyps; increase in gastrointestinal cancer risk is poorly defined	?
Cowden's syndrome	Hamartomas of all three embryonal layers; thyroid disease—adenomas, goiter, and cancer; breast cancer; increase in gastrointestinal cancer risk is poorly defined	?

*APC = adenomatous polyposis coli; FAP = familial adenomatous polyposis.

identification of the APC gene and the role of inherited and sporadic mutations in the APC gene in colorectal cancer will be discussed in detail in the next section. It should be noted that other polyposis syndromes that manifest predominantly nonneoplastic polyps, such as Peutz-Jeghers syndrome, juvenile polyposis syndrome, and Cowden's syndrome, have not been shown to involve chromosome 5q or the APC gene and are thought to be distinct, on the basis of the clinical features, from the (neoplastic) FAP syndromes.

Utsonomiya and Lynch and their colleagues[20] have described, in addition to the FAP syndromes, several forms of inherited colorectal cancer not associated with extensive polyposis (see Table 1). Presumably, cancers in individuals with these syndromes also arise from adenomas through a multistep process, although more rapid progression from a small adenoma to carcinoma may be a feature of these syndromes. The majority of cases of colorectal cancer are termed *sporadic,* because no obvious inherited genetic component can be demonstrated. However, it has been suggested by some investigators that even these cases may not truly be sporadic. Studies by Burt, Cannon-Albright, and colleagues[25] have suggested that a large number of the colorectal cancer cases in the general population may be due, in part, to a dominantly inherited predisposition to the development of adenomas. It has been proposed that the frequency of alleles predisposing to increased rates of adenoma formation may be nearly 20% in the white population in North America. Environmental and dietary influences might contribute to variations in the number of adenomas that develop, as well as the rate at which these adenomas progress to cancer, among individuals who carry the predisposition alleles. Based on the proposed frequency of the predisposition alleles in the population and the frequency of colorectal cancer in the population, it would be predicted that, as in FAP, only a small subset of the adenomas that arise may progress to cancer.

The Genetics of Inherited Colorectal Cancer

Familial Polyposis and the APC Gene

An observation that was critical to the identification of the gene predisposing to the FAP syndrome was the demonstration in 1986 by Herrera et al.[26] of an interstitial deletion on chromosome 5q, affecting chromosomal band 5q21, in a patient with mental retardation and hundreds of adenomatous polyps in his colon. Subsequent linkage studies by other research teams confirmed that the disease phenotype segregated with DNA markers near 5q21 in multiple kindreds with either FAP or Gardner's syndrome.[27, 28] Additional molecular genetic studies over the subsequent 4 years led to the identification of the APC gene in 1991.[21–24]

The APC gene is a relatively large gene with 15 exons, and it encodes a very large protein product of 2,843 amino acids. Sequence analysis of the APC gene reveals no strong similarity to previously characterized proteins and, because well-characterized sequence features are absent, the APC protein is predicted to be localized to the cytoplasm.[21, 23] However, based on the predicted structure of the APC protein, it seems likely that the association of the APC protein with itself or with other cellular proteins may be critically important for its function. To date, germline mutations have been identified in one of the two APC alleles of affected individuals in about two thirds of the families with FAP or Gardner's syndrome who have been studied.[29, 30] All inherited mutations identified in the APC gene thus far appear to result in inactivation of the gene; they include gross deletions of the gene in a few cases and more often localized mutations that cause frameshifts or create stop codons or missense mutations in the gene product (Table 2). Thus, the presence of germline mutations that inactivate the gene in patients with FAP is consistent with the proposed function of the APC gene as a tumor suppressor gene.

The germline mutations in the APC gene in patients with Gardner's syndrome (who manifest tumors outside the colon) are identical at the DNA level, at least in some patients, to those in polyposis patients without extracolonic manifestations.[24] Thus, at the present time, detailed studies of the germline APC mutations have not revealed the basis for the variation in phenotype observed between kindreds that have only polyposis and those that have the full Gardner's syndrome phenotype. Preliminary findings from studies of a number of polyposis kindreds have suggested that the relative location of the inherited mutation in the APC gene may determine the severity of the disease phenotype, in terms of the number of polyps that are present by a given age.[30] However, further studies are necessary to substantiate these findings and to determine the molecular basis for this relationship.

TABLE 2.
Nature of Mutations in the APC Gene*

Germline Mutations (n = 63)	**Somatic Mutations (n = 78)**
Point mutations	Point mutations
Nonsense: 33%	Nonsense: 39%
Missense: 8%	Missense: 4%
	Splice site: 6%
Frameshift	Frameshift
Deletion (1–5 bp): 56%	Deletion (1–31 bp): 40%
Insertion (1–2 bp): 3%	Insertion (1–4 bp): 10%

*Data on germline mutations are from Miyoshi et al.[29] and Nagase et al.[30]; data on somatic mutations are from Miyoshi et al.[60] and Powell et al.[61]

A murine model for colorectal cancer known as the *multiple intestinal neoplasia* (Min) mouse has been described recently.[31] Perhaps somewhat remarkably, the Min mouse has been found to have a mutation in one of the two murine APC alleles.[32] The mutation is predicted to result in a prematurely truncated APC protein, and presumably this alteration is responsible for the multiple intestinal tumors that arise in these mice. However, while large benign tumors of both the small and large intestines arise in Min mice, adenomatous polyps arise frequently only in the large colon and rectum in patients with polyposis (although gastric polyps and duodenal tumors are found in some patients with FAP). In addition, many of the Min mice die as the result of blood loss from their large benign tumors, rather than from invasive or metastatic colorectal cancer, which occurs in untreated individuals with FAP. Nevertheless, the Min mouse should prove to be an extremely interesting and useful model of polyposis and colorectal tumorigenesis. Recent findings from studies in which the Min mutation has been transferred to mice with different genetic backgrounds suggest that a number of other cellular genes can exert a significant influence on the number of tumors that arise in animals carrying the Min mutation.[33] Perhaps this variation in the expression of the disease phenotype in mice carrying a germline Min mutation bears some similarity to the findings reviewed previously, wherein it was suggested that an inherited genetic component might contribute to the majority of cases of colorectal cancer in humans.[25] Specifically, it was suggested that an inherited disease allele present in high frequency in the general population predisposes to an increased rate of adenoma formation, but cancer occurs in only a subset of the individuals that inherit the disease allele.

Heritable Nonpolyposis Colorectal Cancer

Heritable nonpolyposis colorectal cancer (HNPCC) has been recognized as a distinct clinical entity for more than 25 years. Utsunomiya and Lynch and their colleagues[20] have described a large number of kindreds with apparently autosomal-dominant patterns of inherited colorectal cancer, without the features of typical polyposis. In fact, the HNPCC syndromes are thought to constitute 5% to 10% of all colorectal cancers. In some kindreds with HNPCC, colorectal cancer is the sole tumor type seen (Lynch type I syndrome; see Table 1). In others, additional tumor types can be observed in affected individuals, including endometrial, stomach, hepatobiliary, and urinary tract cancers (Lynch type II syndrome). Lynch and his colleagues[34] have reported linkage of the Lynch type II disease predisposition gene to the Kidd blood group marker in several kindreds with Lynch type II syndrome; subsequent independent studies by other investigators have assigned the Kidd blood group marker to chromosome 18q.[35] However, recent studies of five unrelated Finnish kindreds, each affected by a cancer predisposition syndrome with the features of Lynch type II syndrome, have failed to establish linkage of the predisposition gene to chromosome 18q DNA markers.[36] In addition, there is no evidence that the Lynch type II syndrome can be linked to the chromosome 5q region that contains the APC gene.[37] Thus, the molecular basis of HNPCC remains obscure at the present.

A number of features of the HNPCC syndromes have led and could continue to lead to difficulties in the identification of the disease predisposition gene(s). The syndromes are heterogeneous at the phenotypic level, and this may reflect genetic heterogeneity. Indeed, inherited mutations in several different genes could produce relatively similar or overlapping disease phenotypes. In addition, the variability in expression of the disease phenotype, such as the variation in the age of onset of colorectal or other cancer, makes difficult the precise identification of affected and unaffected individuals within a kindred. The mean age of onset of cancer was 62 years in the Finnish families that were studied for evidence of linkage of the disease phenotype to chromosome 18q and 5q DNA markers.[36, 37] Furthermore, in many kindreds, affected individuals often fail to manifest any obvious prior precursor lesions (adenomas) or have died of metastatic cancer and are not available for molecular genetic studies. Nevertheless, the rapid progress made in furthering our understanding of the genetics of the polyposis syndromes indicates that additional molecular genetic studies should shed light on the genetics and pathogenesis of HNPCC.

Somatic Genetic Alterations Underlying the Adenoma-Carcinoma Sequence

Somatic Mutations and the Clonal Origin of Human Cancer Cells

Data obtained from more than two decades of cytogenetic and molecular genetic studies of human leukemias and solid tumors have provided strong support for the proposal that somatic (arising in nongerm cells during a patient's lifetime) mutations are responsible, at least in part, for tumor initiation and progression.[1, 2] Although studies to date have not provided irrefutable evidence, it is presumed that neoplastic cells arise by somatic mutation, and progression of the initiated cells is driven by additional somatic genetic alterations, with subsequent cycles of clonal expansion and evolution.[38, 39] Thus, of greatest interest are those somatic genetic alterations that are clonal in tumors, i.e., present in all or virtually all the neoplastic cells of a primary tumor at any given stage, but not present in normal cells of the patient. The basis for inferring that such clonal genetic alterations may be causal in tumorigenesis is that somatic mutations can become clonal by only a rather limited number of mechanisms. The genetic alteration itself might be selected for by providing the cell with a growth advantage and allowing it to outgrow other progeny to become the predominant cell type in the tumor (clonal expansion). Alternatively, a specific genetic alteration detected in all neoplastic cells might have arisen coincident with another, perhaps undetected, change that was actually the one responsible for clonal outgrowth. When somatic alterations at the same chromosomal region or gene are observed in a particular tumor type from many different patients, or if the specific genetic alteration can be shown to alter the growth of cells in experimental studies, it is more likely that the genetic alteration is *causal* in clonal outgrowth than that it is merely associated with tumor development.

The specific alterations that underlie the initiation of human colorectal tumors are rather poorly understood; however, several studies suggest that colorectal adenomas and carcinomas do, in fact, arise after somatic mutational events. In particular, studies of the pattern of X-chromosome inactivation in tumors from female patients have been used to assess the clonal origin of colorectal tumors.[40] Adenomas and carcinomas from female patients with either inherited or sporadic colorectal tumors have been studied, and the results suggest that even very small adenomas (3 to 4 mm in diameter) are clonal in origin. Moreover, each adenoma from a patient appears to arise from a distinct clone of cells. Similarly, studies of early dysplastic lesions and small adenomas in mice treated with dietary carcinogens suggest that the earliest observed lesions arise in a clonal fashion in this system as well.[41] In contrast, normal colonic mucosa adjacent to the tumors from patients with or without polyposis and from the mice was found to be polyclonal. These observations are consistent with the hypothesis that a somatic mutational event causes one or a small number of somatic cells from a single intestinal crypt to initiate the neoplastic process by clonal expansion. Even in patients with polyposis who inherit a mutation in the APC gene, each adenoma represents a distinct clone, and the data suggest that somatic mutations, in addition to germline mutation in the APC gene, are necessary for adenoma formation.[4]

Alterations in Oncogenes in the Adenoma-Carcinoma Sequence

Oncogenes were first identified and molecularly cloned in the mid-1970s as genes that were incorporated in the genetic material of animal tumor viruses and were responsible for the ability of the particular RNA tumor virus to form tumors in experimental animals.[1, 42] Many different oncogenes have been identified through studies of a large number of independent RNA tumor virus isolates. In all cases, the oncogene is a copy of a cellular gene present in a wide variety of mammalian species, including humans. The oncogene carried by the RNA tumor virus is altered, often subtly, from its normal cellular counterpart. Only a relatively small subset of the cellular oncogenes identified to date have been implicated for their involvement in human cancers, not by infection of humans with RNA tumor viruses carrying the oncogene, but by somatic mutations in tumors that alter or activate the function or normal expression pattern of the cellular oncogene.[1, 2]

A large number of in vitro and animal tumor model studies, as well as the presence of frequent mutations in the genes in several types of human cancer, have implicated the *ras* gene family as critical genetic targets for somatic mutations in tumor development.[43, 44] Mutations in one of the three *ras* genes can be identified in approximately 50% of colorectal carcinomas and in about 50% of colorectal adenomas greater than 1 cm in diameter.[45] In contrast, the frequency of *ras* mutations in adenomas smaller than 1 cm in diameter is approximately 10%. Studies of adenomas with various grades of dysplasia have also found that *ras* mutations are more frequently detected in tumors with increased dysplasia.[46] Thus, because the likelihood of malignant progression is greater in adenomas that have increased size and increased dysplasia, *ras* mutations may have a direct role in increasing the likelihood of malignant progression.

Present data are not sufficient for identifying with certainty the precise role of *ras* mutations in the adenoma-carcinoma sequence. Mutations in the *ras* gene may be an early or initiating event in only a subset of adenomas, but adenomas with *ras* mutations may progress more rapidly in growth and the development of dysplasia than adenomas without *ras* mutations. Alternatively, *ras* mutations may arise in one cell of a small preexisting adenoma and contribute directly to its progression to a larger and more dysplastic adenoma. Further studies of human tumors and perhaps studies of the role of *ras* mutations in rodent models of colorectal cancer will be necessary to characterize further the role of *ras* mutations in the adenoma-carcinoma sequence. In addition, a number of interesting observations regarding the spectrum of *ras* gene mutations in colorectal tumors are not yet fully understood. Mutations that activate the K-*ras* and N-*ras* genes have been detected in colorectal tumors; the majority (88%) of these mutations were present at codons 12 and 13 of K-*ras* (70% and 18%, respectively). Mutations of the N-*ras* gene are infrequent, and no H-*ras* mutations have yet been reported, despite the facts that the H-*ras* gene is expressed in colonic epithelial cells and H-*ras* appears to have similar oncogenic potency to K-*ras* and N-*ras* in a number of experimental studies.[43, 44] Further studies will be necessary to achieve insights into the role of each of the *ras* genes in the normal growth regulatory pathways of colonic epithelial cells and how mutations in the K-*ras* and N-*ras* genes, but apparently not the H-*ras* gene, alter these pathways.

Few studies have identified specific alterations in the alleles of other cellular oncogenes, in contrast to the *ras* genes, in significant percentages of colorectal tumors of any stage. In a small percentage of cases, mostly carcinomas, cellular oncogenes have been found to be amplified and the expression of the specific oncogene has been markedly increased. Examples of oncogenes affected by gene amplification include neu (HER2 or *erb* B2), c-*myc*, and *myb*[47–57] (Table 3). Similarly, although chromosomal translocation is a well-documented mechanism of deregulating gene expression in some tumor types, and chromosome translocations can be detected in many solid tumors, including colorectal cancers, only one such rearrangement has been identified and characterized at the molecular level in colorectal tumors.[52] However, a number of studies have reported consistent differences in the expression or activity of cellular oncogenes, despite the absence of concomitant mutations in the genes encoding the oncogenes. For example, the c-*myc* gene and protein are expressed at high levels in most colorectal tumors.[51, 53] It has been suggested that deregula-

TABLE 3.
Somatic Mutations in Oncogenes and Tumor Suppressor Genes in Colorectal Cancer*

Gene	Type of Mutation	Cancers with Alteration, %†
Oncogenes		
K-*ras*	Point mutation	48
N-*ras*	Point mutation	<2
neu (HER2/*erb* B2)	Amplification	<5
c-*myc*	Amplification	<5
myc	Amplification	<5
Tumor suppressor genes		
p53	Point mutation; loss of heterozygosity	75–85
APC	Point mutation; small deletion/insertion; loss of heterozygosity	>65
DCC	Loss of heterozygosity, insertion; deletion; point mutation	70–75

*APC = Adenomatous polyposis coli; DCC = deleted in colorectal cancer.
†Literature describing the data on the frequencies of the various mutations is referenced in the text.

tion of c-*myc* gene expression might be attributable to a defect in a trans-acting factor or regulatory pathway. Preliminary studies have suggested that a locus on chromosome 5q (perhaps the APC gene) might be involved in the negative regulation of c-*myc* gene expression; it has thus been proposed that inactivation of the regulatory pathway controlled by this 5q gene would lead to increased levels of c-*myc*.[54] In addition, the tyrosine kinase activity of c-*src* is elevated in many colorectal cancers, despite the absence of detectable genetic alterations at the c-*src* locus or changes in the total amount of c-*src* protein in cells.[55] Nevertheless, although deregulation of the normal expression or activity of cellular oncogenes may be an important mechanism for promoting colorectal tumor cell growth, in the absence of specific mutations affecting an oncogene locus in tumor cells, data are insufficient at the present to determine whether these alterations in expression or activity of the c-*myc*, c-*src*, and other oncogenes are causal in tumorigenesis or merely reflect the tumor phenotype.

Tumor Suppressor Gene Alterations in the Adenoma-Carcinoma Sequence

Although, based on the frequency of FAP and the polyposis syndromes, germline mutations in the APC gene appear to be uncommon in colorectal cancer, somatic mutations in the APC gene appear to play a critical role in the development of the majority of colorectal adenomas and carcinomas.

The first studies to suggest that inactivation of the APC gene was a common event in colorectal tumor development were those that demonstrated that the chromosome 5q region containing the APC gene is frequently affected by chromosome loss events in colorectal adenomas and carcinomas from patients without polyposis.[45, 56, 57] The losses have been found to involve only one of the two parental chromosome 5q sets present in normal cells; thus they are defined as allelic losses or loss of heterozygosity (LOH) events. Similar LOH events affecting chromosome 5q and often other chromosomes have now been identified in a large number of different tumor types.[3, 6] Multiple lines of evidence support the hypothesis that the LOH in tumor cells can result in inactivation of a tumor suppressor gene.[3, 6, 58] The remaining copy of a tumor suppressor gene that maps to the chromosomal region affected by LOH is often found to be inactivated by more localized mutations, such as a point mutation or small deletion. However, present data suggest that inactivation of only one of the two copies of the FAP gene may be sufficient to alter the proper growth regulation of colonic epithelial cells.[5, 59]

Recently, detailed studies of the somatic mutations present in the APC gene in colorectal adenomas and carcinomas from patients without polyposis have been carried out. The frequency and nature of the somatic mutations in the APC gene appear to be similar in adenomas and carcinomas; mutations in the APC gene have been detected in about 60% of colorectal tumors, regardless of their histopathologic status.[60, 61] Moreover, APC mutations have been identified in several adenomas of only 0.5-cm-maximum diameter.[61] Thus, it seems likely that somatic mutations in the APC gene may arise very early in the adenoma-carcinoma sequence and perhaps could be an initiating somatic genetic event in the development of many adenomas in patients without polyposis. In some cases LOH of chromosome 5q may be an early event that occurs in cells without a prior APC mutation, and the change in dosage of the APC gene might itself be sufficient to alter cell growth. In other cases, LOH of 5q may occur in one cell of a tumor in which a localized mutation in the APC gene is already present and may inactivate the remaining normal copy of the APC gene; in some tumors from patients with or without polyposis, LOH of 5q might therefore be a progression. With regard to the timing of APC mutations in the adenoma-carcinoma sequence, in one study, of five sporadic adenomas smaller than 1 cm in diameter that were found to have an APC mutation, only one of the lesions had a *ras* mutation.[61] Thus, inactivation of the APC gene often may precede *ras* mutation in colorectal tumor development.

In addition to inactivation of the APC gene and the loss of chromosome 5q sequences in colorectal tumors, the loss of other chromosomal regions can be detected very frequently with cytogenetic techniques, or more readily, with molecular genetic techniques. As for chromosome 5q, these allelic losses or LOH events are presumed to arise and be selected during tumor development, because LOH can result in the inactivation of a tumor suppressor gene within the affected chromosomal region. Among the chromosomal regions most frequently affected by LOH in colorectal tumors are chromosomes 17p and 18q.[45, 62]

The results of studies over the past few years support the proposal that the tumor suppressor gene affected by LOH of chromosome 17p in colorectal tumors is the p53 gene.[63, 64] Present studies suggest that the p53 gene is mutated in about 75% to 85% of colorectal carcinomas, but infrequently in adenomas.[65] Some studies of tumors containing regions of both adenoma and carcinoma have suggested that mutation and loss of the p53 gene may be directly associated with the progression from adenoma to carcinoma. Thus, the data at the present suggest that inactivation of the p53 gene by mutation and/or loss is frequent only in colorectal carcinomas. The normal product of the p53 gene is a nuclear phosphoprotein that is thought to be a critical regulator of cell growth; inactivation of the p53 gene by mutation or loss may result in the loss of normal growth regulation. Recent studies have suggested that the p53 protein may regulate the expression of a number of cell genes,[66, 67] and these genes may include those that are up-regulated in response to DNA damage.[68] Moreover, some studies suggest that loss of normal p53 function may promote genetic instability in cells and may lead to an increased frequency of gene amplification and perhaps other genetic alterations in tumor cells.[69, 70] Perhaps inactivation of the p53 gene is selected for during later stages of colorectal tumor development because it can promote further genetic instability and the subsequent development of invasive and metastatic tumor cells.

Loss of heterozygosity involving chromosome 18q can be detected in approximately 70% of colorectal carcinomas, in about 50% of advanced adenomas, and infrequently in early-stage adenomas.[45] A common region of LOH on 18q involving 18q21 has been identified, for which allelic loss is seen when any allelic loss involving 18q is detected. Subsequently, a candidate tumor suppressor gene from this region, termed *deleted in colorectal cancer* (DCC), has been identified.[71] The DCC gene encodes a protein that is highly related to proteins that normally mediate cellular recognition and adhesion in the nervous system. At present, fewer data are available to establish conclusively the role of the DCC gene as a tumor suppressor gene in colorectal cancer than are available for the p53 and APC genes; however, the data are consistent with the proposal that the DCC gene may function as a tumor suppressor gene.[71, 72] In addition to the frequent LOH events of chromosome 18q that involve the DCC gene, expression of the DCC gene is greatly reduced or absent in more than 80% of the colorectal cancer cell lines studied (compared with the level of DCC expression found in normal colonic mucosa), and specific genetic alterations that would be expected to inactivate the gene can be identified in a subset of cases. Little is known about the normal function of the DCC gene. Perhaps by altering the recognition of extracellular signals from either cell-cell or cell-extracellular matrix interactions, alterations of the DCC gene may lead to the loss of normal growth control and may be, in part, responsible for some of the alterations in cell adhesion, invasion, motility, and metastasis seen in cells from later stages of colorectal tumorigenesis.

A Genetic Model for the Adenoma-Carcinoma Sequence

There is abundant clinical and histopathologic evidence that the development of colorectal cancer is a multistep process. In addition, data from epidemiologic studies suggest that multiple independent events—perhaps as few as two events or as many as six to eight—determine the rate of adenoma and carcinoma formation.[73, 74] Thus, it seems reasonable to predict that several mutations in both oncogenes and tumor suppressor genes are likely to be necessary for adenoma formation, and additional mutations may contribute to the adenoma-carcinoma progression. To date, the molecular genetic studies of adenomas and carcinomas have provided results consistent with this proposal and suggest a preliminary genetic model for colorectal tumor development and progression[4, 5] (Fig 2).

The following are the salient features of the model. First, colorectal tumors appear to arise as a combined result of the mutational activation of oncogenes, such as the *ras* gene, and the mutational inactivation of tumor suppressor genes, including the APC gene, the p53 gene, and the DCC gene. Second, in a number of cases, mutations in multiple genes (five or more different genes in some cases) can be detected in all carcinoma cells of a single tumor; thus, multiple genetic alterations may be necessary for carcinoma development, while fewer mutations may be necessary for adenoma development. The particular genetic alterations have a relative preference for their temporal occurrence with respect to different stages of the adenoma-carcinoma sequence. Mutations in the APC gene and LOH of chromosome 5q appear to occur at high frequency in the earliest stages of adenoma formation; *ras* mutations may allow progression from a small adenoma of low malignant potential to a larger and more clinically dangerous one; inactivation of the DCC and p53 genes may most often occur during the progression of a large adenoma to an in situ or invasive carcinoma. Although the various genetic alterations have a preference for their time of occurrence with respect to different stages of tumorigenesis, their relative order is not invariant, and colorectal tumor cases that represent exceptions to the preferred sequence can be identified. Thus, the accumulation and interaction of the multiple genetic alterations within a tumor cell appear most important for tumor progression and may determine the phenotype and clinical behavior of the tumor cells.

Undoubtedly, other oncogenes and tumor suppressor genes that play a critical role in colorectal tumorigenesis will be identified in the future, and their role in the adenoma-carcinoma sequence will have to be considered. In addition, the present genetic model of colorectal tumorigenesis does not consider alterations in oncogene expression or activity, growth factor responsiveness, angiogenesis, or other growth properties of tumor cells that distinguish them from normal cells. Therefore, although the model accurately reflects much of our emerging knowledge about the role of a number of oncogenes and tumor suppressor genes in the adenoma-carcinoma sequence, it is incomplete and simplistic. Nevertheless, the present model

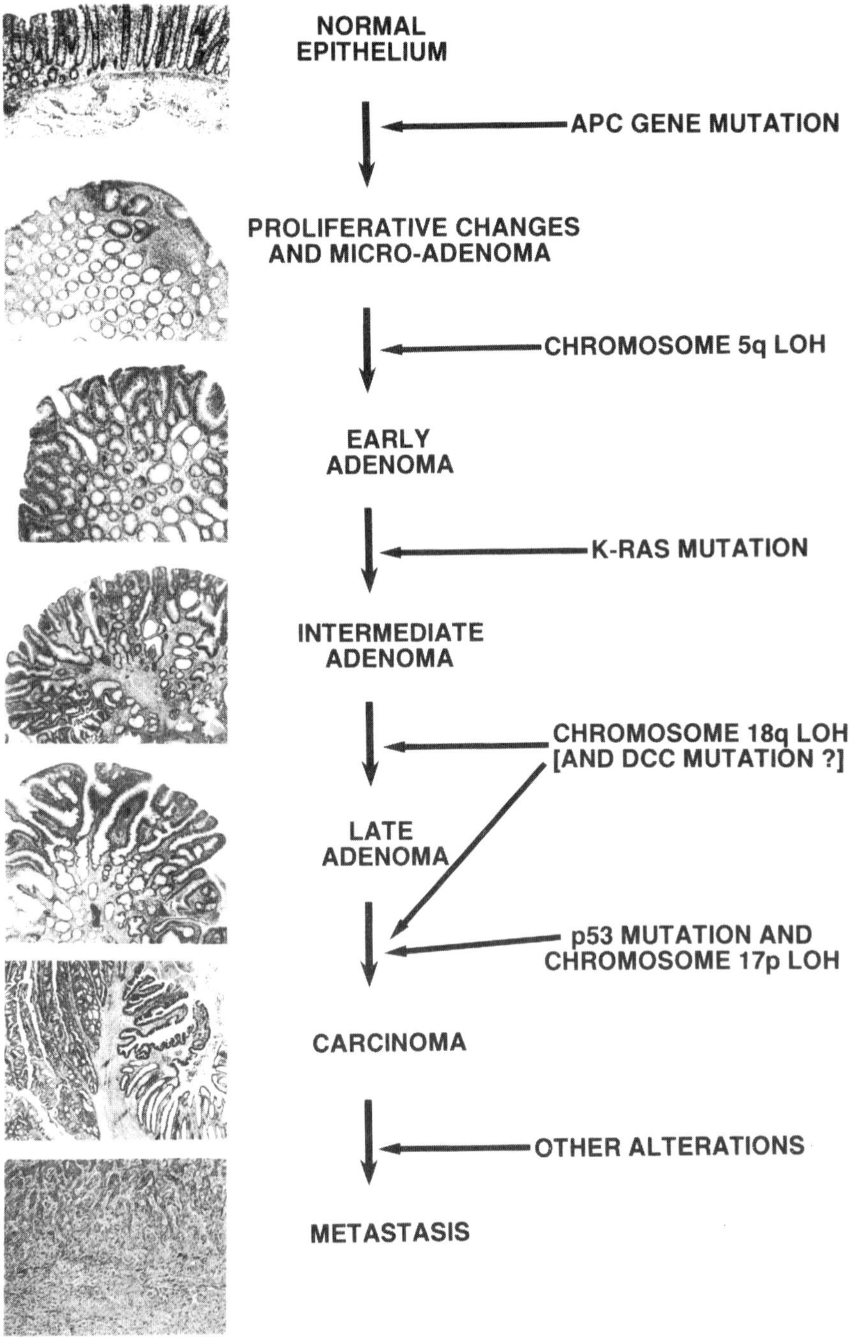

FIG 2.

A genetic model for colorectal tumorigenesis. It is believed that the majority of carcinomas arise from preexisting adenomas. In addition, several studies have suggested that proliferative changes in the mucosa and microscopic lesions may pre-

Continued.

TABLE 4.
Clinical Applications of Genetic Alterations in Colorectal Cancers*

Inherited Susceptibility/Risk Assessment	Early Detection of Tumors	Prognostic Significance
APC gene/Chromosome 5q markers	K-*ras* mutation	Chromosome 18q loss/DCC alterations
HNPCC gene(s)	N-*ras* mutation	Chromosome 17p loss/p53 mutations
Other predisposition genes	APC mutation	
	p53 mutation	Multiple chromosome losses

*APC = adenomatous polyposis coli; DCC = deleted in colorectal cancer; HNPCC = heritable nonpolyposis colorectal cancer.

does make some interesting predictions about the possible utility of using molecular techniques to detect specific genetic alterations and to improve the diagnosis and clinical care of patients and families affected by colorectal cancer (Table 4).

Clinical Applications of Molecular Genetic Studies

The identification of inherited genetic alterations that predispose an individual to the development of adenomatous polyps or carcinomas should prove useful for determining the risk of colorectal cancer development for some individuals—namely, those in kindreds affected by inherited forms of colorectal cancer. For example, the identification of the APC gene and alterations in the gene in the majority of kindreds with FAP and Gardner's syndrome provides the basis for genetic counseling of families at risk for these diseases. Individuals from polyposis kindreds who are not found to have inherited the predisposition gene will be spared anxiety and frequent colonoscopic examinations in their adolescent and early adult years. Those

FIG 2.(cont.).
cede the formation of visible adenomas, both in patients with polyposis and those without. Although multiple stages of adenoma may exist, only three are shown; in general, they represent tumors of increasing size, dysplasia, and villous content. The relative timing of the genetic events is indicated with respect to the various stages of tumor development. Although a preferred order for the genetic alterations appears to exist, the order of the changes is not invariant. (From Fearon ER, Jones PA: *FASEB J* 1992; 6:2783–2790. Used by permission.)

who have inherited the disease gene can be closely monitored and perhaps can be treated with chemopreventive regimens to delay or prevent the development of polyps. In this regard, studies by Waddell and colleagues[75] suggest that the nonsteroidal anti-inflammatory agent sulindac can cause regression of polyps in patients with FAP. Further studies will be necessary to substantiate their results, as well as to determine the basis for the effect.

At the present, it is possible to determine, with either direct or indirect detection strategies, which individuals in a polyposis kindred carry mutant APC alleles. The first step to the identification of the specific mutation in the APC gene in any kindred with polyposis requires detailed DNA sequencing studies of a copy of the gene from an affected individual from that family. Although many of the mutations in the APC gene that have been identified in polyposis patients are somewhat similar to one another, given the large size of the APC gene and the multitude of different mutations that can inactivate the function of the gene, very few unrelated kindreds have been found to have identical mutations in their APC alleles.[29, 30] However, once the specific APC mutation in a particular kindred is identified, subsequently affected family members (who must therefore carry the same mutated APC allele) can be identified presymptomatically by a direct allele-specific oligonucleotide hybridization strategy (Fig 3). Even before identification of a specific mutation in the APC gene, it is also possible to determine by more indirect linkage analysis methods whether a particular member of a kindred has inherited the disease-causing APC allele. Deoxyribonucleic acid markers from the APC gene (not the mutation in the APC gene that results in polyposis) can be used to trace the inheritance of a disease-causing APC allele in a kindred with polyposis, and individuals who have inherited the mutant APC allele can be identified presymptomatically or even prenatally. Although polyposis is a rare cause of colorectal cancer, it seems reasonable to predict that similar recombinant DNA-based strategies could be used in a more general fashion in the future to determine presymptomatically an individual's risk of colorectal cancer. In particular, such strategies would be useful for study of individuals from kindreds who have inherited genetic alterations that predispose them to heritable nonpolyposis colorectal cancer or perhaps even from kindreds with a predisposition to mildly elevated rates of adenoma formation.

FIG 3.
Determination of the inheritance of the familial adenomatous polyposis syndrome by DNA analysis. A three-generation kindred with polyposis is shown. Individuals in the kindred are denoted by generation *(I, II, III)* and number (*1, 2, 3,* etc) shown below their symbol. The age of each individual is indicated at the right above his or her symbol. Affected individuals, according to either clinical criteria or genetic diagnosis (individual III-5), are indicated by solid symbols. Dead individuals are denoted by symbols with slashes. In the upper panel, the patterns of DNA fragments detected by a region of the APC gene exhibit polymorphism or normal variation among the population. (Note: this type of variation is *not* a mutation within the

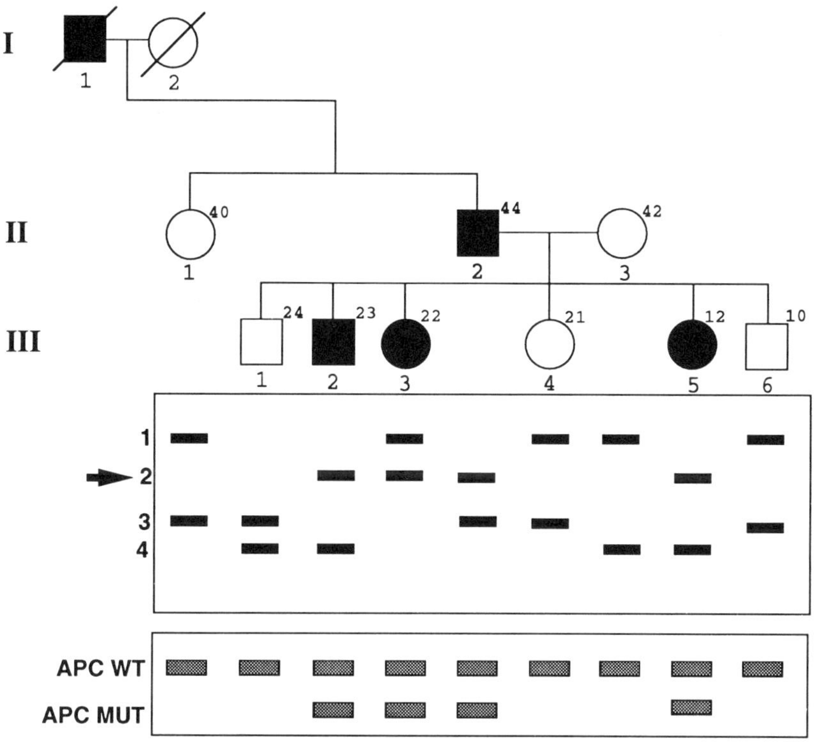

FIG. 3. (cont.).
APC gene that alters the function of the gene.) Each individual has two differently sized DNA fragments detected, corresponding to the two parental copies of chromosome 5 (and the specific APC gene) inherited—one from each parent. The father in the second generation (individual II-2) is affected by polyposis and has alleles 2 and 3. The mother (II-3), who is not affected, has alleles 1 and 4. Two children (III-2 and III-3) have polyposis, and two of the children (III-1 and III-4) have reached an age at which they would be expected to have polyps, but they have none. The affected children have inherited allele 2 from the father, and the unaffected children have inherited allele 3 from him. The other two children (III-5 and III-6) have not exhibited the polyposis phenotype, but are rather young. Thus, no firm diagnosis can be reached based on clinical criteria. Based on the observation that the affected individuals have inherited APC allele 2 from the father, the prediction would be that individual III-5 will develop polyposis because she has inherited the mutant APC allele from the father. Similarly, individual III-6 has inherited a normal APC allele from the father and is predicted to be unaffected by polyposis. Thus, the polyposis disease phenotype can be predicted presymptomatically. In the bottom panel, if the specific mutation that causes polyposis in this kindred is identified, the mutant APC allele can be detected in affected individuals by using a specific DNA oligonucleotide in an allele-specific oligonucleotide hybridization analysis (see Fig. 4). Affected individuals have both normal *(APC WT)* and mutant *(APC MUT)* APC alleles; unaffected individuals have only normal APC alleles. (Modified from Fearon ER: *Semin Colon Rectal Surg* 1991; 2:253–261. Used by permission.)

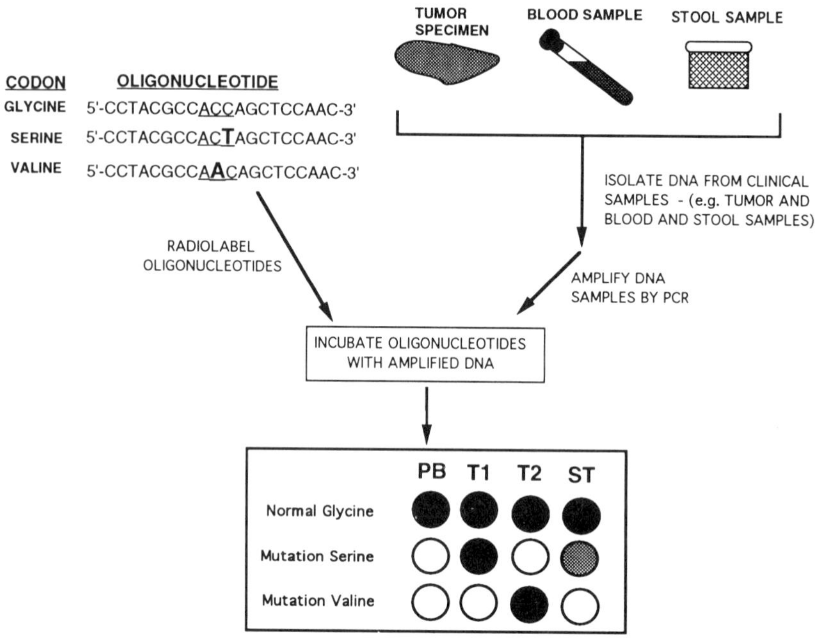

FIG 4.
Detection of mutations in the K-*ras* gene by allele-specific oligonucleotide hybridization. Deoxyribonucleic acid is isolated from a patient specimen, for example, a tumor specimen, a blood sample, or a stool sample. To greatly increase the sensitivity of the detection of *ras* mutations, the K-*ras* gene sequence of interest is amplified with respect to its copy number in total DNA using the polymerase chain reaction *(PCR)*. The amplified DNA preparations are spotted onto a nylon filter and hybridized with radiolabeled oligonucleotide that specifically recognizes either the normal glycine codon at K-*ras* codon 12 or single basepair changes that would result in a mutated serine codon or mutated valine codon. In the examples shown, the oligonucleotide detecting the normal glycine codon hybridizes to all four samples tested: peripheral blood *(PB)*, tumor specimen 1 *(T1)*, tumor specimen 2 *(T2)*, and stool specimen *(ST)*. The oligonucleotide detecting the serine mutation at codon 12 hybridizes to DNA from the tumor 1 and stool specimens, and the oligonucleotide detecting the valine mutation hybridizes to DNA from tumor 2. Although only two such examples are shown here, oligonucleotides specific for all possible amino acid substitutions at the *ras* codon under study can be prepared. Moreover, it should be noted that a strategy similar to this can be used to detect either inherited or somatic mutations in other oncogenes and tumor suppressor genes, but only when the likely position of a mutation is known. (Modified from Fearon ER: *Semin Colon Rectal Surg* 1991; 2:253–261. Used by permission.)

In addition to identifying individuals who are at elevated risk of developing colorectal tumors as a result of inherited genetic alterations, it may be possible to apply the molecular genetic studies to the early detection of colorectal tumors in the general population. It may be possible to screen for colorectal carcinomas and adenomas by identifying the mutated oncogene or tumor suppressor gene sequences in tumor cells shed into the stool or blood or perhaps by identifying antibodies made by the patient against the mutant gene products (Fig 4). Preliminary findings from studies of DNA isolated from stool samples of patients who are known to have colorectal carcinoma or advanced adenoma lesions support this proposal.[76] Indeed, if a *ras* mutation were present in the primary tumor specimen, and the tumor specimen were of sufficient size, the mutant *ras* gene sequences could readily be detected in the DNA of cells shed into the stool. The sensitivity and specificity of identifying *ras* mutations in patients with various types and sizes of colorectal tumors has not yet been determined, nor have the results obtained been confirmed in a larger study. Nevertheless, these results are encouraging given that 50% of colorectal cancers and advanced adenomas contain *ras* gene mutations. Moreover, the findings suggest that it might also be possible to design similar screening tests for the detection of mutations in other oncogenes or tumor suppressor genes.

Other possible clinical applications of the molecular genetic studies of colorectal tumorigenesis include increased and improved prognostic information about the likelihood of tumor recurrence or new tumor growth in patients. Alternatively, patients might receive varying chemotherapeutic regimens depending on the genetic alterations in their tumors. if differences are noted in response rates between patients whose tumors have different constellations of genetic alterations. Last, perhaps some of the genetic alterations may provide specific targets for new chemotherapeutic agents. Some agents might antagonize or selectively act on the products of mutated oncogenes, such as K-*ras;* other agents might suppress tumor growth by mimicking or restoring some of the normal function of tumor suppressor gene products (p53, APC, and DCC).

Summary

During the past decade, a great deal of progress has been made toward identifying some of the genetic alterations that underlie human cancer development in general, and colorectal cancer in particular. It is now clear that mutations in both oncogenes and tumor suppressor genes have an important role in the process. However, much work lies ahead before a complete understanding of the pathogenesis of colorectal tumors will be obtained. It seems reasonable to predict that additional oncogenes and tumor suppressor genes with important roles in colorectal cancer remain to be identified. Characterization of the function of these genes in normal and neoplastic cell growth will be crucial.

Unfortunately, we know little about the functions of the oncogenes and tumor suppressor genes already implicated in colorectal cancer. Undoubtedly, it will be crucial to understand the role of environmental and dietary influences on the nature and rate of mutations in colorectal tumors. Little is known about the relative significance of each of the various inherited and somatic mutations to the cancer phenotype. Moreover, although some preliminary studies have suggested possible clinical applications of the genetic studies to improved diagnosis and management of patients at risk of and harboring colorectal cancer, the scope and significance of the observations thus far are limited. Nevertheless, an optimistic view is that future molecular genetic studies not only will yield insights into the molecular basis of colorectal cancer, but also will improve the care of patients with colorectal tumors.

References

1. Bishop JM: The molecular genetics of cancer. *Science* 1987; 235:305–311.
2. Weinberg RA: Oncogenes, antioncogenes, and the molecular bases of multistep carcinogenesis. *Cancer Res* 1989; 49:3717–3721.
3. Weinberg RA: Tumor suppressor genes. *Science* 1991; 254:1138–1146.
4. Fearon ER, Vogelstein B: A genetic model for colorectal tumorigenesis. *Cell* 1990; 61:759–767.
5. Fearon ER, Jones PA: Progressing toward a molecular description of colorectal cancer development. *FASEB J* 1992; 6:2783–2790.
6. Stanbridge EJ, Cavenee WK, Heritable cancer and tumor suppressor genes: A tentative connection, in Weinberg RA (ed): *Oncogenes and the Molecular Origins of Cancer.* Cold Spring Harbor, NY, Cold Spring Harbor Laboratory Press, 1989; pp 281–306.
7. Marshall CJ: Tumor suppressor genes. *Cell* 1991; 64:313–326.
8. Boring CC, Squires TS, Ting T: Cancer statistics. *CA* 1991; 41:19, 28–29.
9. Eddy TM: Screening for colorectal cancer. *Ann Intern Med* 1990; 113:37–384.
10. Murakami R, Tsukuma H, Kanamori S, et al: Natural history of colorectal polyps and the effect of polypectomy on occurrence of subsequent cancer. *Int J Cancer* 1990; 46:159–164.
11. Gilbertsen VA: Proctosigmoidoscopy and polypectomy in reducing the incidence of rectal cancer. *Cancer* 1974; 34:936–940.
12. Winawer SJ, Zauber AG, O'Brien MJ, et al: The National Polyp Study. Design, methods and characteristics of patients with newly diagnosed polyps. The National Polyp Study Workgroup. *Cancer* 1992; 70:1236–1245.
13. Muto T, Bussey HJR, Morson BC: The evolution of cancer of the colon and rectum. *Cancer* 1975; 36:2251–2270.
14. Cohen AM, Shenk B, Friedman MA: Colorectal cancer, in DeVita VT, Hellman S, Rosenberg SA (eds): *Cancer: Principles and Practices of Oncology.* Philadelphia, Lippincott, 1989: pp 895–964.
15. Fenoglio CM, Lane N: The anatomical precursor of colorectal carcinoma. *Cancer* 1974; 34:819–823.
16. Burt RW, Samowitz WS: The adenomatous polyp and the hereditary polyposis syndromes. *Gastroenterol Clin North Am* 1988; 17:657–678.
17. Bussey HJR: *Familial Polyposis Coli: Family Studies, Histopathology, Differential Diagnosis, and Results of Treatment.* Baltimore, Johns Hopkins University Press, 1975.
18. Lipkin M: Biomarkers of increased susceptibility of gastrointestinal cancer: New application to studies of cancer prevention in human subjects. *Cancer Res* 1988; 48:235–245.
19. Tudek WR, Bird RP, Bruce WR: Foci of aberrant crypts in the colon of mice and rats exposed to carcinogens associated with foods. *Cancer Res* 1989; 49:1236–1240.

20. Utsunomiya J, Lynch HT (eds): *Hereditary Colorectal Cancer.* New York, Springer-Verlag, 1990.
21. Groden J, Thlivers A, Samowitz W, et al: Identification and characterization of the familial adenomatous polyposis coli gene. *Cell* 1991; 66:589–600.
22. Joslyn G, Carlson M, Thlivers A, et al: Identification of deletion mutations and three new genes at the familial polyposis locus. *Cell* 1991; 66:601–613.
23. Kinzler KW, Nilbert MC, Su L-K, et al: Identification of FAP locus genes from chromosome 5q21. *Science* 1991; 253:661–665.
24. Nishisho I, Nakamura Y, Miyoshi Y, et al: Mutations of chromosome 5q21 genes in FAP and colorectal cancer patients. *Science* 1991; 253:665–669.
25. Cannon-Albright LA, Skolnick MH, Bishop DT, et al: Common inheritance of susceptibility to colonic adenomatous polyps and associated colorectal cancers. *N Engl J Med* 1988; 319:533–537.
26. Herrera L, Kakati S, Gibas L, et al: Brief clinical report: Gardner syndrome in a man with an interstitial deletion of 5q. *Am J Med Genet* 1986; 25: 473–476.
27. Bodmer WF, Bailey C, Bodmer J, et al: Localization of the gene for familial polyposis on chromosome 5. *Nature* 1987; 328:614–616.
28. Leppert M, Dobbs M, Scambler P, et al: The gene for familial polyposis coli maps to the long arm of chromosome 5. *Science* 1987; 238:1411–1413.
29. Miyoshi Y, Ando H, Nagase H, et al: Germ-line mutations of the APC gene in 53 adenomatous polyposis patients. *Proc Natl Acad Sci USA* 1992; 89:4452–4456.
30. Nagase H, Miyoski, Horii A, et al: Correlation between the location of germ-line mutations in the APC gene and the number of colorectal polyps in familial adenomatous polyposis patients. *Cancer Res* 1992; 52:4055–4057.
31. Moser AR, Pitot HC, Dove WF: A dominant mutation that predisposes to multiple intestinal neoplasm in the mouse. *Science* 1990; 247:322–324.
32. Su L-K, Kinzler KW, Vogelstein B, et al: Multiple intestinal neoplasia caused by a mutation in the murine homolog of the APC gene. *Science* 1992; 256:668–670.
33. Moser A, Dove W, Drinkwater W, et al: Genetic models and multistage carcinogenesis in the gastrointestinal system of the mouse and rat, in Brugge J, Curran T, Harlow E, et al (eds): *Origins of Human Cancer: A Comprehensive Review.* Cold Spring Harbor, NY, Cold Spring Harbor Laboratory Press, 1991, pp 601–608.
34. Lynch HT, Scheulke GS, Kimberling WJ, et al: Hereditary nonpolyposis colorectal cancer (Lynch syndromes I and II): Biomarker studies. *Cancer* 1985; 56:939–951.
35. Geitvik GA, Hoyheim B, Gedde-Dahl T, et al: The Kidd (JK) blood group assigned to chromosome 18 by close linkage to a DNA-RFLP. *Hum Genet* 1987; 77:205–209.
36. Peltomaki P, Sistonen P, Mecklin J-P, et al: Evidence supporting exclusion of the DCC gene and a portion of chromosome 18q as the locus for susceptibility to hereditary non-polyposis colorectal cancer in 5 kindreds. *Cancer Res* 1991; 51:4135–4140.
37. Peltomaki P, Sistonen P, Mecklin J-P, et al: Evidence that the MCC-APC gene region in 5q21 is not the site for susceptibility to hereditary non-polyposis colorectal carcinoma. *Cancer Res* 1992; 52:4530–4533.
38. Foulds L: The natural history of cancer. *J Chronic Dis* 1958; 8:2–37.
39. Nowell P: THe clonal evolution of tumor cell populations. *Science* 1976; 194:23–28.

40. Fearon ER, Hamilton SR, Vogelstein B: Clonal analysis of human colorectal tumors. *Science* 1987; 238:193–197.
41. Ponder BAJ, Wilkinson MM: Direct examination of the clonality of carcinogen-induced colonic epithelial dysplasia in chimeric mice. *J Natl Cancer Inst* 1986; 77:967–976.
42. Bishop JM: Viral oncogenes. *Cell* 1985; 42:23–38.
43. Barbacid M: ras genes. *Ann Rev Biochem* 1987; 56:779–827.
44. Bos JL: ras oncogenes in human cancer: A review. *Cancer Res* 1989; 49:4682–4689.
45. Vogelstein B, Fearon ER, Hamilton SR, et al: Genetic alterations during colorectal tumor development. *N Engl J Med* 1988; 319:525–532.
46. Miyaki M, Seki M, Okamoto M, et al: Genetic changes and histopathological types in colorectal tumors from patients with adenomatous polyposis. *Cancer Res* 1990; 50:7166–7173.
47. Alitalo K, Schwab M, Linn CC, et al: Homogeneously staining chromosomal regions contain amplified copies of an abundantly expressed cellular oncogene (c-myc) in malignant neuroendocrine cells from a human colon carcinoma. *Proc Natl Acad Sci USA* 1983; 80:1707–1711.
48. Alitalo K, Winqvist R, Linn CC, et al: Aberrant expression of an amplified c-myb oncogene in two cell lines from a colon carcinoma. *Proc Natl Acad Sci USA* 1984; 81:4535–4538.
49. D'Emilia J, Bulovas K, D'Erole D, et al: Expression of the c-erbB-2 gene product (P-185) at different stages of neoplastic progression in the colon. *Oncogene* 1989; 4:1233–1239.
50. Ramsay RG, Thompson MA, Hayman JA, et al: Myb expression is higher in malignant human colonic carcinoma and premalignant adenomatous polyps than in normal mucosa. *Cell Growth Differ* 1992; 3:723–730.
51. Melhem MF, Meisler AI, Finley GG, et al: Distribution of cells expressing myc proteins in human colorectal epithelium, polyps, and malignant tumors. *Cancer Res* 1992; 52:5853–5864.
52. Martin-Zanca D, Hughes SH, Barbacid M: A human oncogene formed by the fusion of truncated tropomyosin and protein tyrosine kinase sequences. *Nature* 1986; 319:743–748.
53. Stewart J, Evan G, Watson J, et al: Detection of the c-myc oncogene product in colonic polyps and carcinomas. *Br J Cancer* 1986; 53:1–6.
54. Erisman MD, Scott JK, Astrin SM: Evidence that the FAP gene is involved in a subset of colon cancers with a complementable defect in c-myc regulation. *Proc Natl Acad Sci USA* 1989; 86:4264–4268.
55. Bolen JB, Veillette A, Schwartz AM, et al: Activation of pp60$^{c\text{-}src}$ protein kinase activity in human colon carcinoma. *Proc Natl Acad Sci USA* 1987; 84:2251–2255.
56. Solomon E, Voss R, Hall V, et al: Chromosome 5 allele loss in human colorectal carcinomas. *Nature* 1987; 328:616–619.
57. Ashton-Rickardt PG, Dunlop MG, et al: High frequency of APC loss in sporadic colorectal carcinoma due to breaks clustered in 5q21-22. *Oncogene* 1989; 4:1169–1174.
58. Knudson AG Jr: Hereditary cancer, oncogenes, and anti-oncogenes. *Cancer Res* 1985; 45:1437–1443.
59. Ichii S, Horii A, Nakatsuru S, et al: Inactivation of both APC alleles in an early stage of colon adenomas in a patient with familial adenomatous polyposis (FAP). *Hum Mol Genet* 1992; 6:387–390.
60. Miyoshi Y, Nagase H, Ando H, et al: Somatic mutations of the APC gene in

colorectal tumors: mutation cluster region in the APC gene. *Hum Mol Genet* 1992; 4:229–233.
61. Powell SM, Zilz N, Beazer-Barclay Y, et al: APC mutations occur early during colorectal tumorigenesis. *Nature* 1992; 359:235–237.
62. Vogelstein B, Fearon ER, Kern SE, et al: Alleotype of colorectal carcinomas. *Science* 1989; 244:207–211.
63. Baker SJ, Fearon ER, Nigro JM, et al: Chromosome 17 deletions and p53 gene mutations in colorectal carcinomas. *Science* 1989; 244:217–220.
64. Levine AJ, Momand J, Finlay CA: The p53 tumor suppressor gene. *Nature* 1991; 351:453–456.
65. Baker SJ, Preisinger AC, Jessup JM, et al: p53 gene mutations occur in combination with 17p allelic deletions as late events in colorectal tumorigenesis. *Cancer Res* 1990; 50:7717–7722.
66. Kern SE, Pietenpol JA, Thiagalingam S, et al: Oncogenic forms of p53 inhibit p53-regulated gene expression. *Science* 1992; 256:827–830.
67. Zambetti GP, Bargonetti J, Walker K, et al: Wild-type p53 mediates positive regulation of gene expression through a specific DNA sequence element. *Genes Dev* 1992; 6:1143–1152.
68. Kastan MB, Zhan Q, El-Deiry WS, et al: A mammalian cell cycle checkpoint pathway utilizing p53 and GADD45 is defective in ataxia-telangiectasia. *Cell* 1992; 71:587–597.
69. Yin Y, Tainsky MA, Bischoff FZ, et al: Wild-type p53 restores cell cycle control and inhibits gene amplification in cells with mutant p53 alleles. *Cell* 1992; 70:937–948.
70. Livingstone LR, White A, Sprouse J, et al: Altered cell cycle arrest and gene amplification potential accompany loss of wild-type p53. *Cell* 1992; 70:923–935.
71. Fearon ER, Cho KR, Nigro JM, et al: Identification of a chromosome 18q gene which is altered in colorectal cancers. *Science* 1990; 247:9–56.
72. Hedrick L, Cho K, Fearon ER, et al: The role of the DCC gene in colorectal tumorigenesis. *Cancer Res Clin* 1992; 1:90–95.
73. Armitage P, Doll R: The age distribution of cancer and a multi-stage theory of carcinogenesis. *Br J Cancer* 1954; 8:1–12.
74. Moolgavkar SH, Luebeck EG: Multistage carcinogenesis: Population-based model for colon cancer. *J Natl Cancer Inst* 1992; 84:610–618.
75. Waddell WR, Gansen GF, Cerice EJ, et al: Sulindac for polyposis of the colon. *Am J Surg* 1989; 157:175–179.
76. Sidransky D, Tokino T, Hamilton SR, et al: Identification of ras oncogene mutations in the stool of patients with curable colorectal tumors. *Science* 1992; 256:102–105.

Sexually Transmitted Diseases: Advances in Diagnosis and Treatment

Thomas C. Quinn, M.D.

Laboratory of Immunoregulation, National Institute of Allergy and Infectious Diseases, National Institutes of Health, Bethesda, Maryland; Division of Infectious Diseases, Johns Hopkins University School of Medicine, Baltimore, Maryland

Jonathan Zenilman, M.D.

Division of Infectious Diseases, Johns Hopkins University School of Medicine, Baltimore City Health Department, Sexually Transmitted Diseases Clinics, Baltimore, Maryland

Anne Rompalo, M.D.

Division of Infectious Diseases, Johns Hopkins University School of Medicine, Baltimore City Health Department, Sexually Transmitted Diseases Clinics, Baltimore, Maryland

Epidemiology

Over the past decade, sexually transmitted diseases (STDs) have continued to escalate worldwide and nationally. Currently, the World Health Organization estimates that 250 million cases of STD occur each year worldwide.[1] The annual worldwide incidence for specific diseases includes 120 million cases of trichomoniasis, 50 million cases of chlamydial infection, 30 million cases of genital warts, 25 million cases of gonorrhea, 20 million cases of genital herpes, 3.5 million cases of syphilis, 2.5 million cases of hepatitis B virus infection, two million cases of chancroid, and 11 million cases of individuals infected with the human immunodeficiency virus infection (HIV). With the escalating epidemic of HIV infection, there has been new attention focused on the public health spread of STDs in general, raising concerns about both the clinical and social consequences of these infections.[2] For example, the rate of *Chlamydia trachomatis* genital infections in the U.S. has soared (Fig 1), affecting 4 to 5 million Americans each year, thus replacing gonorrhea as the most common sexually transmitted bacterial disease.[3] In addition to causing local genital infections, chlamydia organisms have been implicated as a major cause of pelvic inflammatory disease, infertility, and ectopic pregnancy, costing an estimated

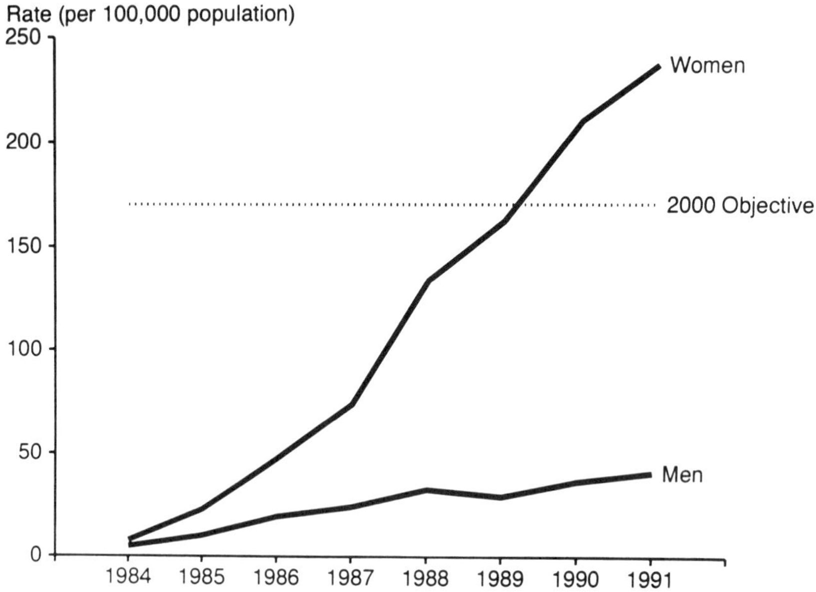

FIG 1.
Chlamydia infection rates by gender: United States, 1984–1991 and the year 2000 objective (Data from Centers for Disease Control: *Division of STD/HIV Prevention Annual Report, 1991*. Atlanta, Ga, 1992.)

5 billion in medical cost as well as significant morbidity among young, frequently adolescent women.[4, 5]

After decades of decline, the incidence of syphilis has risen sharply during the late 1980s (Fig 2).[6] In some American cities, syphilis rates have risen over 600% and now exceed post-World War II levels. Gonococcal infections, which have remained relatively stable over the past several decades, are also showing signs of increased incidence in selected populations.[5, 7] Similar to chlamydia, gonorrhea rates in teenagers actually increased between 1981 and 1989. The continuing high gonococcal rates among the teenage population may mean that gonorrhea control programs are not reaching this key high-risk group. Gonorrhea rates are now thirtyfold higher among young black Americans than among white Americans.[8] In addition, four new types of antibiotic resistance among *Neisseria gonorrhoeae* emerged during the past decade, resulting in 1.5% to 20% of reported gonococcal cases now being caused by antibiotic-resistant strains.[9] Although new and effective antibiotics have become available, antibiotic resistance continues to be a major problem in efforts to control this infection.

The cumulative burden of incurable viral STDs increased to estimates of 30 million Americans infected with herpes simplex virus type 2 (HSV-2), 40 million individuals infected with human papillomavirus (HPV), and 1.5

million infected with HIV infection.[1] The number of physician-patient consultations for genital warts and genital herpes increased more than ninefold between 1966 and 1989 (Fig 3 and 4).[5, 10] Similar to other STDs, HPV infections may be asymptomatic, or they may produce exophytic or flat condylomas, chronic persistent infections resulting in cervical intraepithelial neoplasia (CIN), and squamous carcinoma.[10, 11] Although the exact proportion of individuals with each type of clinical manifestation is not known, genital warts may represent only 10% or less of the total spectrum of genital tract HPV infections.

Fortunately, major advances have been made in the clinical recognition, microbiologic diagnosis, and treatment of many STDs. New clinical algorithms have been developed for earlier detection of pelvic inflammatory disease, urethritis, cervicitis, and vaginal infections. More sensitive and specific assays have become available for rapid diagnosis of specific etiologic agents. Rapid diagnostic tests have been developed which can determine the specific cause of an STD syndrome within 15 to 30 minutes. With the recent introduction of the polymerase chain reaction (PCR) as a diagnostic tool, it is now possible to identify early infection before clinical symptoms have developed. Molecular probes have enabled clinicians to identify asymptomatic HPV infection and to subsequently type it for strains that have been associated with cervical dysplasia. Finally, new antimicrobial agents, have markedly advanced the effective treatment of these infec-

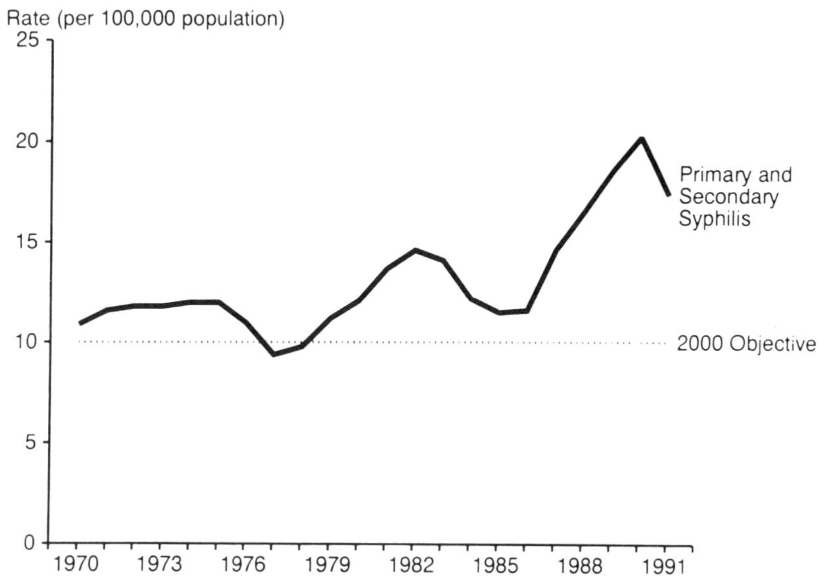

FIG 2.
Primary and secondary syphilis—Reported rates: United States, 1970–1991 and the year 2000 objective. (Data from Centers for Disease Control: *Division of STD/HIV Prevention Annual Report, 1991.* Atlanta, Ga, 1992.)

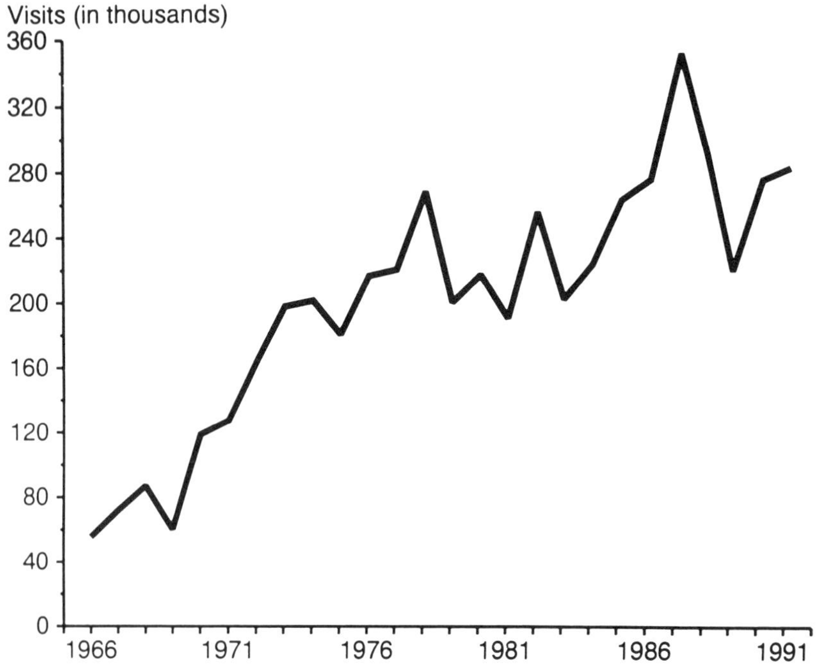

FIG 3.
Human papillomavirus (genital warts)—Initial visits to physicians' offices: United States, 1966–1991. (Data from Centers for Disease Control: *Division of STD/HIV Prevention Annual Report, 1991*. Atlanta, Ga, 1992.)

tions. New agents include acyclovir and foscarnet for the treatment and suppression of genital herpes infection,[12] azidothymidine for the early treatment of HIV infection,[13] quinolones and newer cephalosporins for the treatment of penicillin-resistant *Neisseria gonorrhoeae*,[14] and single-dose azithromycin for the treatment of chlamydia.[15] The availability of a safe and effective vaccine for hepatitis B virus has also provided another avenue for the prevention of a relatively common STD, and hope for the development of other vaccines against STDs.[16]

This chapter will review in more detail some of the major advances that have been made within the past few years for these common sexually transmitted infections, highlighting epidemiology, clinical manifestations, diagnoses, and treatment regimens for the control of these widely prevalent infections.

Chlamydia trachomatis

Genital infections caused by *C. trachomatis* are the most common bacterial sexually transmitted syndromes in the United States. Chlamydial infections are associated with a wide range of clinical disease states ranging from asymptomatic infection to urethritis, epididymitis, and proctitis in the male; cervicitis, salpingitis, and acute urethral syndrome in the female; and conjunctivitis and pneumonia in the newborn. Using gonorrhea as an index, *C. trachomatis* was estimated to cause over 2.6 million infections in women, 1.8 million in men, and 0.25 million in infants.[17] Unfortunately, these numbers do not account for the large number of people with asymptomatic infection, who sustain transmission within the community. In addition, asymptomatic infected persons are at further risk for both acute illness and serious long-term sequelae. It has been estimated that the direct and indirect costs of chlamydia exceeds $2.4 billion annually.[4]

In selected male populations, chlamydial infection occurs in 3% to 5% of asymptomatic men, 10% to 20% of men seen in STD clinics, and 13% to 15% of sexually active boys attending adolescent clinics.[18, 19] Prevalence is generally higher in the younger age group and decreases in each 5-year age period from 19 to 39 years of age. Prevalence of chlamydial infection also tends to be higher in non-whites than in whites. In one study, 19% of nonwhite males and 9% of white heterosexual males had urethral chlamydial infection.[18] Although chlamydial urethral infection is less frequent in

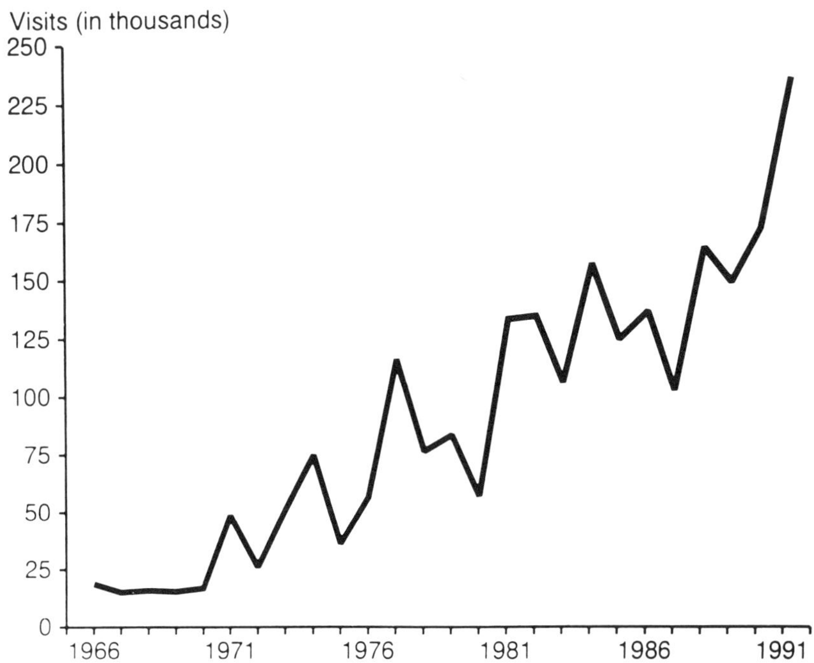

FIG 4.
Genital herpes simplex virus—Initial visits to physicians' offices: United States, 1966–1991. (Data from Centers for Disease Control: *Division of STD/HIV Prevention Annual Report, 1991*. Atlanta, Ga, 1992.)

homosexual men, it is a major cause of proctitis.[20] Pharyngeal infection with *C. trachomatis* has also been demonstrated in 3% to 6% of men and women attending STD clinics and correlates with the history of oral-genital contact.[21]

Prevalence of chlamydial infection in women has ranged from 3% to 5% in asymptomatic patients to over 20% of women seen in STD clinics.[22, 23] During pregnancy, 5% to 7% may be infected, although a 21% prevalence in inner-city black women has been reported.[24, 25] Similar to men, the proportion of sexually active women with positive cervical cultures for chlamydia has been highest for teenage women and declines thereafter.[18] The high rate of cervical infection among adolescent females is of special concern, because it is frequently asymptomatic and may persist for several months, unless routine screening tests are performed.

With repeated infections, pelvic inflammatory disease (PID) is a likely sequelae. Symptomatic PID accounts for 2.5 million outpatient visits to physicians each year.[26, 27] More than 275,000 women are hospitalized and more than 100,000 surgical procedures are performed annually because of PID.[27] Of the 1 million cases of PID diagnosed annually in the United States, approximately 50% may be caused by chlamydia.[28, 29] The proportion of women with chlamydial infection who develop infection of the upper reproductive tract such as endometritis, salpingitis, and pelvic peritonitis is poorly defined. In a recent study, an estimated 8% of women with chlamydia also had salpingitis[30]; in a second study of women with both gonococcal and chlamydial infections but treated only for gonorrhea, 40% developed salpingitis during follow-up.[31] Unfortunately, both the diagnosis and treatment of PID are unsatisfactory; approximately one in six women treated for PID will be infertile; an equal proportion will experience chronic pelvic pain as a result of their infections[31, 32]; and one in ten who conceive will have an ectopic pregnancy.[33] (See section on PID in this chapter.)

Chlamydia infection during pregnancy also poses a major health problem for the mother and infant. In 10% to 28% of pregnant women with chlamydial infection, endometritis and possibly salpingitis develop after induced abortion.[34–36] Similarly, PID may develop in the late postpartum period in 19% to 34% of infected women who deliver vaginally at term.[37, 38] Nearly two thirds of infants born vaginally to mothers with chlamydial infection become infected during delivery.[39, 40] *C. trachomatis* is the most common cause of neonatal conjunctivitis and one of the most common causes of pneumonia during the first few months of life. Even when given ophthalmia prophylaxis, including silver nitrate, tetracycline or erythromycin ointment, 15% to 25% of exposed infants still develop conjunctivitis, and 3% to 16% develop pneumonia.[41–43] Fortunately, chlamydial illness in infants generally responds to systemic treatment when the illness is recognized and treated appropriately. All postpartum and perinatal disease is readily preventable by treating the infected mother during pregnancy.

Chlamydia may also be an important cause of urinary tract symptoms in women who have experienced frequency, burning on urination, and pyuria, but have low bacterial counts on culture. This syndrome is called the acute urethral syndrome or the acute dysuria-pyuria syndrome.[44, 45] In a recent study, 65% of afebrile women presenting with dysuria or urgency who had a negative bladder urine culture for typical bacterial infection had chlamydial infection.[44] The importance of the observation is that unexplained pyuria culture-negative "cystitis" in sexually active women suggests the possibility of chlamydial infection. An important though uncommon complication of urogenital chlamydial infection is Reiter's syndrome, involving various combinations of reactive arthritis, conjunctivitis, and urethritis.[46] Chlamydial infection should be included in the differential diagnosis of arthritis in either young men or young women. This is particularly true for women because chlamydial infection is more likely to be missed in women than in men who have arthritis because of the less frequent complaint of urethritis.

Diagnosis.—Since all sexually active adolescents and young adults are at high risk for chlamydia, screening for this infection should be expanded to include all sexually active adolescents and young adults in all localities including rural, suburban and inner-city areas as well as all socioeconomic strata. Culture and nonculture methods for diagnosis of *C. trachomatis* are now widely available. Appropriate use of these diagnostic tests is strongly encouraged, especially for screening asymptomatic high-risk individuals in whom infection would otherwise be undetected. However, in clinical settings where testing for chlamydia is not routine or available, treatment is often prescribed on the basis of clinical diagnosis such as nongonococcal urethritis or mucopurulent cervicitis, or as standard cotreatment for gonorrhea.

The vast majority of female infections with chlamydia occur at the endocervix and are also frequently asymptomatic.[47] Although an early study suggested that the presence of a green or yellow mucopurulent secretion within the cervical os or ten or more polymorphonuclear leukocytes per oil immersion field of a gram-stained smear of endocervical secretions correlated with chlamydial endocervical infections,[48] subsequent investigations have found that while this might be a positive predictive indicator for chlamydia and/or gonococcal infection, the absence of such a sign does not rule out the presence of chlamydia.[49] Consequently, it has been recently recommended that all young, sexually active women be screened for chlamydia.[47] Clinicians should also consider women with endocervical mucopus or hypertrophic ectropion with inflammatory changes in their cervical cytologic specimens as being at increased risk for chlamydial infection.[50]

Currently, the laboratory standard for diagnosis of *C. trachomatis* is cell culture isolation, which has a specificity that approaches 100%. However, the sensitivity of culture has been estimated at 70% to 90% in experienced laboratories,[51] and cell culture has several other disadvantages. The method is technically difficult and requires 3 to 7 days to obtain results. Since only viable organisms are detected, special transport media must be used in transportation, and storage temperature requirements are stringent.

Finally, some specimens contain contaminating microorganisms or substances that are toxic to the cell monolayers used for isolating chlamydia.

Consequently, a wide variety of more rapid and less expensive assays has been developed for detection of chlamydia, including enzyme immunoassays (EIA) to detect chlamydial antigen in cervical secretions and urine, fluorescent monoclonal antibodies for the direct visualization of chlamydial elementary bodies on smears, rapid antigen tests designed for use in physician and STD clinics, and molecular probes including nucleic acid hybridization tests and polymerase chain reaction (PCR).[52] With the exception of PCR, most of these nonculture tests are less sensitive than culture with sensitivities ranging from 70% to 95%, and some tests may also give false-positive results (Table 1).[52, 53] Because of the possibility of false-positive results, positive test results should be interpreted cautiously as a presumptive evidence of infection. Confirmatory testing with culture or a second nonculture test is recommended in circumstances in which positive nonculture tests could lead to adverse medical, legal, social, or psychological consequences for the patient.[47]

TABLE 1.
Sensitivity of Available Diagnostic Assays for Chlamydia trachomatis

Culture	Standard*
Direct Fluorescent Antibody (DFA) Test	60%–90%
Enzyme Immunoassay (EIA) for Antigen	70%–90%
Solid Phase Rapid EIA Tests	70%–90%
Nucleic Acid Hybridization	78%-96%
Polymerase Chain Reaction	95%–100%
Ligase Chain Reaction	95%–100%
Leukocyte Esterase Test	40%–70%
Microimmunofluorescent Serology	Not recommended†

*Culture is estimated to be only 80%–90% sensitive, but it is considered to be the "gold standard" by which other tests are compared.
†Serology is not recommended for diagnosis of acute infection.

Detection of *C. trachomatis* infection in asymptomatic men had been problematic, because men were reluctant to submit to possibly painful urethral swabs in the absence of a discharge. In addition, asymptomatic men rarely attend health clinics, where they would be more likely to receive regular screening for chlamydia. New noninvasive and sensitive diagnostic tests have been able to screen male urine samples for the presence of inflammation by the leukocyte esterase tests (LET) or for chlamydia directly by EIA or PCR.[54–60] The LET is a dipstick test applied to urine specimens to screen for urinary tract infection by detecting enzymes produced by polymorphonuclear leukocytes. The LET has been demonstrated to be reasonably sensitive (46% to 100%) and specific (83% to 93%) for screening sexually active teenage males for chlamydia and gonorrhea.[54–57] Patients with positive results require specific tests for *C. trachomatis* and *N. gonorrhoeae.* Compared to urethral culture, the sensitivity of the EIA for chlamydial antigen in urines collected from asymptomatic men ranged from 75% to 90%, and for PCR, the sensitivity was 93%.[58–60] Although these results are still slightly lower than urethral culture, they provide a noninvasive technique that lends itself to the screening of large populations of men at risk for chlamydial infection.

Treatment.—The treatment for chlamydial infections consists of doxycycline, 100 mg/orally twice a day for 7 days, or tetracycline 500 mg orally 4 times a day for 7 days (Table 2).[14, 47] For pregnant women, erythromycin 500 mg orally four times a day for 7 days is substituted for tetracycline. While this treatment regimen will remain the standard because of its low cost, the development of a new drug, azithromycin (Zithromax), has made it possible to treat chlamydia with a single 1-g oral dose.[15] Azithromycin is the first azalide antibiotic which has distinctive chemical and pharmakinetic properties that differentiate it from the more common macrolide erythromycin. Recently approved by the FDA for the treatment of chlamydial genital infection, azithromycin has a serum half-life of about 68 hours and a tissue half-life of 2 to 4 days. Urinary excretion of the drug can be detected up to 7 to 10 days after a single 1-g dose.

Following in vitro susceptibility studies demonstrating the sensitivity of *C. trachomatis* to azithromycin,[61] a clinical study compared the efficacy and safety of a single 1-g dose of azithromycin with doxycycline (100 mg, twice a day in the treatment of 457 adult patients with uncomplicated genital infection with *C. trachomatis.*[15] This study was a randomized multicenter study and evaluated patients for 4 weeks following the initiation of therapy. Only 4% of those treated with azithromycin and 1% of those treated with doxycycline failed to respond clinically. None of the azithromycin-treated patients and 1% of the doxycycline-treated patients had a positive culture 21 to 35 days following treatment. Side effects were reported in 17% of patients who received azithromycin, which is comparable to the 20% side-effect rate reported for doxycycline-treated patients. The drug is classified as category B drug for use in pregnancy. This antimicrobial may prove most useful in situations in which the compliance with a 7-day regimen of

TABLE 2.
Treatment of Uncomplicated Urethral, Endocervical, or Rectal Chlamydial Infections in Adults

Recommended Treatment Regimens
- Doxycycline 100 mg, orally, 2 times a day for 7 days

  or

- Tetracycline 500 mg, orally, 4 times a day for 7 days

Alternative Treatment Regimens
- Erythromycin base 500 mg, orally, 4 times a day for 7 days*

  or

- Azithromycin 1 g, orally, once†

  or

- Ofloxacin 300 mg, orally, 2 times a day for 7 days‡
- Sulfisoxazole 500 mg, orally, 4 times a day for 10 days (or equivalent) may also be effective.

*Recommended for use in pregnancy. If not tolerated, reduce dose to 250 mg, orally, 4 times a day for 14 days.

†Azithromycin has not yet been shown to be effective in treating nongonococcal urethritis not caused by chlamydia. Therefore, in men, a specific chlamydial diagnosis is needed prior to instituting azithromycin therapy for nongonococcal urethritis. Azithromycin is not recommended for use during pregnancy.

‡Ofloxacin is effective in treating nongonococcal urethritis not caused by chlamydia. Ofloxacin is not recommended for use in adolescents aged 17 years or under, nor during pregnancy.

another antimicrobial cannot be insured. In view of the high efficacy of tetracycline, costs should also be considered when choosing among these alternatives. Azithromycin has not been shown to be effective in treating nongonococcal urethritis (NGU) not caused by chlamydia. Therefore, in men, a specific chlamydia diagnosis is recommended prior to instituting azithromycin therapy for NGU.

Another drug which has also been approved for the treatment of chlamydia infections including nonchlamydia NGU is ofloxacin (300 mg, orally, two times per day for 7 days), a quinolone which was demonstrated to have similar efficacy compared to a 7-day course of doxycycline.[62] However, because of its higher cost compared to doxycycline, its contra-indication in pregnant women, and its requirement for several-day dosing, it remains a less optimal alternative than doxycycline, azithromycin or erythromycin.

Neisseria gonorrhoeae

The epidemiology of gonococcal infections in the U.S. contrasts to that seen in other developed countries. In Sweden, infections caused by *Neisseria gonorrhoeae* have declined to a population-based rate of 14/100,000 per year,[63] whereas in the U.S., the incidence rate even after 15 years' decline, is approximately 240/100,000 cases per year[5] or 620,000 infections reported annually. An additional 2 to 3 unreported infections are estimated for every case that is reported. More importantly, gonococcal infections have increasingly become a disease of the inner city, with a very high prevalence of disease in lower-economic, inner-city populations, contrasted with lower prevalences of disease in middle-class populations. This is interesting because condom use and the number of sexual partners, both behavioral risk measures for STD, appears to be similar among both middle-class and inner-city clinic patients.[64, 65]

Studies which have confirmed the increasing localization of gonococcal disease within the inner city were recently conducted in Seattle,[66] where Rice and co-workers examined the sociodemographic distribution of gonococcal disease, demonstrating that incident gonorrhea occurred preferentially within census tracts located within the inner city. Handsfield[67] further refined and extended the concept to antibiotic-resistant infection, indicating that penicillinase-producing *N. gonorrhoeae* (PPNG) outbreak strains are located within inner-city census tracts. Zimmerman[68] in Colorado Springs demonstrated that whereas gonococcal disease clustered in the urban census tract areas, chlamydia in contrast did not cluster at all, and assumed a more diffuse distribution of disease. Upchurch and co-workers in the Baltimore City STD clinics found that men with new or casual partners were much more likely to have gonococcal disease than were men who had sex with a regular partner (odds ratio = 2.7). They further reported that 33% of patients who noted STD symptoms (i.e,. urethral discharge) continued to engage in sexual activity after the onset of symptoms.[65] Other factors highly associated with gonococcal acquisition included intravenous drug use, prostitute exposure, casual partners, and those with previous history of repeated gonorrhea. In similar studies, patients who later were diagnosed with a gonococcal infection which was resistant to antimicrobial agents (such as penicillin and tetracycline) were also classified into behavioral subgroups.[69] These individuals tended to be older, IV drug users, and had an increased number of sexual partners. In this context, patients with gonorrhea tend to be individuals who are high-risk takers compared to the rest of the general STD clinic population.

Over the past decade there have been no further developments in the understanding of the sequelae or clinical course of gonococcal infection. Asymptomatic men are increasingly understood to be major facilitators of gonococcal transmission. For example, in a large study conducted at the Grady Memorial Hospital Emergency Room in Atlanta, 3.3% of men between the ages of 18 and 25 were culture positive for *N. gonorrhoeae* despite being asymptomatic.[57] Recognition of a male reservoir for transmission, in addition to the substantial burden of asymptomatic disease in women, is necessary in order for adequate control measures to be taken.[70]

In most settings, diagnosis of gonorrhea is made most cheaply and reliably by culture. A number of selective (i.e., antibiotic-containing) culture media are available. In addition, Gram's stain diagnosis as presumptive evidence for gonococcal disease has a sensitivity greater than 95% in men and approximately 60% in women.[71, 72] Specificity in both tests is high, generally above 95%. However, the applicability of Gram's stain diagnosis in the office setting has been recently compromised by the Comprehensive Laboratory Improvement Act (CLIA). The new CLIA regulations have designated Gram's stains as "moderate complexity" procedures, which affect the ability of many practices to perform the procedure "in-office." New nonculture methods such as genetic probe techniques have become available.[73, 74] These tests offer sensitivity and specificity close to that of culture, albeit at somewhat increased cost. These techniques are especially useful in areas where specimen transport is an issue.

Treatment.—Antimicrobial resistance continues to be the major epidemiologic area of interest. Antimicrobial resistance in *N. gonorrhoeae* is due to both plasmid-mediated resistance and chromosomally mediated resistance to penicillin, tetracycline, cephalosporins, and aminocyclitols. Systematic surveillance of gonococcal resistance was reported initially by Schwarcz,[75] who described the results from the Centers for Disease Control Gonococcal Isolates Surveillance Project (GISP), which is a sentinel-site surveillance system that monitors antimicrobial resistance at 21 public health clinics in the United States. In 1990,[76] data from the GISP system demonstrated that 10.1% of isolates were PPNG (plasmid-mediated penicillinase producing *N. gonorrhoeae*), 5.8% were TRNG (plasmid-mediated tetracycline-resistant *N. gonorrhoeae*), and 1.7% were high-level PPNG and TRNG organisms (Fig 5). In addition, 3.1% had chromosomally mediated resistance to at least two antibiotics in the panel. Although quinolones are being increasingly used for antigonococcal therapy, no high-scale resistance to either quinolones or third-generation cephalosporin agents has been identified in the United States to date. However, isolates which appear to be significantly less susceptible to both quinolones and to the third-generation cephalosporins have been isolated from both Southeast Asia and from Europe.[77–80]

Current therapy recommendations for gonorrhea presume that all gonococcal isolates are resistant to former first-line drugs such as penicillin and tetracyclines. The primary treatment regimen recommended in 1993 is ceftriaxone, 125 mg, intramuscularly.[14] These regimens also include a

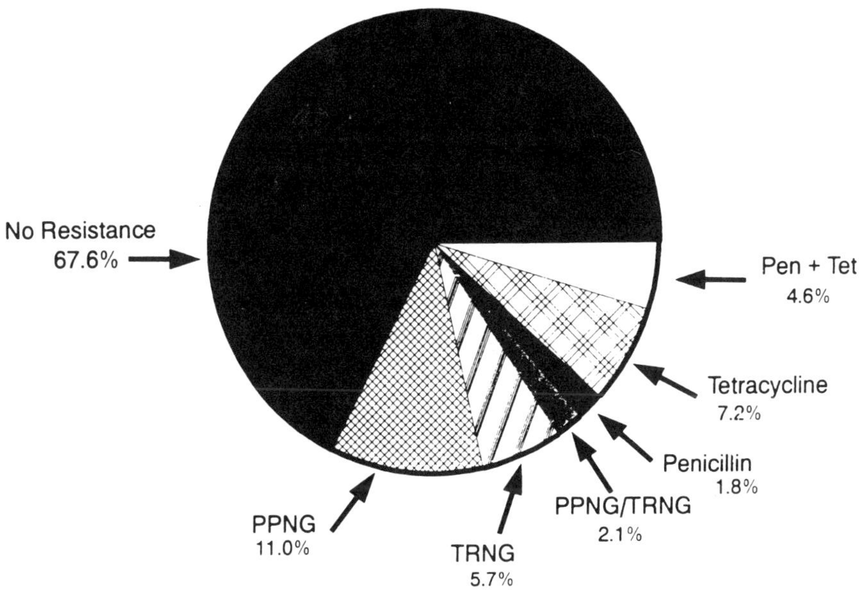

FIG 5.
Gonococcal Isolate Surveillance Project (GISP)—Percentage distribution of antimicrobial resistance in gonorrhea isolates, 1991. *Pen* and *Tet* refer to chromosomally mediated resistance to penicillin (corresponding to a minimum inhibitory concentration [MIC] of greater than or equal to 2 μ/g/mL) and tetracycline (corresponding to an MIC of greater than or equal to 2 μg/mL); *PPNG (penicillinase-producing Neisseria gonorrhoeae)* and *TRNG* (tetracycline-resistance *Neisseria gonorrhoeae*) refer to plasmid-mediated resistance to these antibiotics.

number of different oral regimens which have become available. Cefixime at both the 400-mg and 800-mg. doses has been shown to be effective in treating *N. gonorrhoeae* infection.[81] The quinolones (ciprofloxacin, norfloxacin, ofloxacin, enoxacin, and lomefloxacin) have all been shown to be effective against gonococci in U.S. patient populations (Table 3).[82–84] No significant antibiotic resistance to the quinolones has been identified in the United States, although as stated earlier, some has been seen in Europe. In our experience, quinolones have been extraordinarily safe and effective.[85] Ciprofloxacin has been the first-line therapy for gonorrhea in Baltimore since 1989. We have observed non-life-threatening anaphylactoid reactions at a rate of 1/5,000 doses, which is consistent with the reported literature.[86] Quinolones have the disadvantage of being contraindicated in pregnant women and in children. All outpatient treatment regimens for *N. gonorrhoeae* infections (urethritis, cervicitis) are single-dose regimens. In addition, they should be accompanied by cotreatment for chlamydial infection, which is present in an estimated 10% to 50% of individuals with gonorrhea. Cotreatment is cost-effective despite the overtreatment which occurs.[47, 87] The estimate of overtreatment for *C. trachomatis* infections in

TABLE 3.
Treatment Regimens for Gonorrhea*

Cephalosporin
Cefixime 400 mg, orally
Ceftriaxone 125 mg, IM
Cefotaxime 1 g, IM
Cefotetan 500 mg, IM
Ceftizioxime 500 mg, IM
Cefuroxime axetil 1 g, orally
Cefpodoxime proxetil 200 mg, orally
Quinolones
Ciprofloxacin 500 mg, orally
Norfloxacin 800 mg, orally
Ofloxacin 400 mg, orally
Enoxacin 400 mg, orally
Lomefloxacin 400 mg, orally

*All regimens are single dose. All patients treated for gonorrhea should also be treated for chlamydia.

patients treated for gonococcal disease is between 200% and 400%. However, no prospective controlled studies, using real (as opposed to estimated) data to evaluate the cost-effectiveness of these therapies have ever been performed.

Disseminated gonococcal infection (DGI) is characterized by systemic signs of disease, including fever, chills, tenosynovitis, and arthritis. Bacteremia is present in approximately half of cases of DGI. The pathophysiology of DGI is complex and beyond the scope of this review article. Furthermore, most authorities believe that the incidence of DGI has decreased over the past 10 to 15 years for reasons that are not completely clear. Despite commonly held beliefs to the contrary, antimicrobial resistance is a substantial problem in patients with disseminated gonococcal infection (DGI). We therefore recommend that all patients who are diagnosed with disseminated gonococcal infection be treated as if they have an organism which is resistant to multiple antibiotics.[88]

Pelvic Inflammatory Disease

Pelvic inflammatory disease (PID) is frequently a consequence of several bacterial STDs, which include gonorrhea, chlamydia, and mycoplasma.

Approximately 1 million women are treated for PID in the United States annually. One quarter of these women develop serious sequelae, including ectopic pregnancy, tubal infertility, and chronic pelvic pain.[27] Since the epidemiology and clinical presentation of PID are diverse, and the understanding of the pathogenesis of PID is limited, many questions concerning the diagnosis, treatment, and prevention of PID and its complications remain unanswered.

Traditionally, the clinical diagnosis of PID was based on the presence of lower abdominal pain, tenderness on bimanual examination with or without endocervical discharge, and an elevation of temperature, white blood cell count, sedimentation rate, or C-reactive protein.[89] However, recent studies indicate that approximately two thirds of women undergoing laparoscopy on the basis of these traditional criteria actually have salpingitis.[28] Furthermore, over one half of infertile women with tubal dysfunction, occlusion, or both do not report any history of PID. Many of these women may have had "silent PID," or pelvic inflammation with no notable symptoms that would trigger medical evaluation. Therefore, in an attempt to develop improved clinical algorithms to diagnose PID, several investigators have combined selective and sequential use of procedures such as pelvic- or vaginal-probe ultrasound, endometrial biopsy, and laparoscopy with routine examination and laboratory findings.

Unfortunately, syndromic approaches based on signs, symptoms, and low-cost tests often do not correlate with laparoscopic findings.[90, 91] Etiologic diagnosis, although important in partner notification, may not truly reflect the cause of PID because of the site sampled (cervix, endometrium, or fallopian tubes) or the sampling method.[91] Variable correlations are reported between cervical and intraabdominal cultures, and between culdocentesis and fallopian tube isolates.[92, 93] Laparoscopic diagnosis, the "gold standard," relies on subjective interpretation of the gross appearance of the tubes. Subtle changes of early disease may be missed, and the cost of the procedure is often prohibitive. Endometrial biopsy may provide objective histopathologic evidence of endometritis, which has been highly correlated with *C. trachomatis* infection and to a lesser degree with *N. gonorrhoeae*.[95, 95] The patchy nature of endometritis, however, limits the usefulness of this diagnostic technique. Intravaginal ultrasound has recently been used to explore a noninvasive alternative to both laparoscopy and endometrial biopsy.[95, 96] Although the ultrasound readily visualizes advanced changes in ovarian and tubal morphology, its sensitivity in diagnosing early disease is still questionable.

The most salient concern in both the diagnosis and prevention of PID is silent or subclinical PID. This entity probably accounts for the majority of tubal infertility and a significant proportion of ectopic pregnancies. This term was invoked when researchers found that more than half of women with documented tubal occlusion report no history of previous PID, despite serologic evidence of past chlamydial or gonococcal infection.[96–99] On histologic examination, women with silent salpingitis had similar degrees of distal tubal ultrastructural damage as did those women with overt salpingitis. Unfortunately, no demographic or clinical risk factors differentiate those women with silent salpingitis from those with clinical PID, making attempts at prevention of tubal dysfunction or obstruction very difficult.

In recent attempts to identify the subset of women with PID who are at particularly high risk for sequelae, host factors as well as bacterial factors are being considered. Anatomically, the cervix is the major barrier to the ascent of lower genital tract infection to the upper tract. Changes in the zone of ectopy, cervical mucus, or local immune response may determine whether infecting organisms ascend or are cleared. Hormonal factors appear to affect the cervical environment and are associated with the pathogenesis of PID.[100–105] Data, however, are conflicting. Both estrogen and progesterone may facilitate the growth and survival of chlamydial infection.[101, 104, 105] Progesterone oral contraceptives, however, reportedly thicken cervical mucus making it less penetrable to ascending infection.[100]

Specific and nonspecific host responses to bacterial infection may predispose certain women to develop PID or its sequelae. Chlamydial infection, for example, may induce a cell-mediated response to tubal epithelial antigens and may be a major contributor to tubal damage.[106, 107] Delayed hypersensitivity reaction to *C. trachomatis* 57 kd heat-shock protein may be the mechanism of chronic tubal damage.[106, 108–110] High serum titers to this antigen may be prognostic of long-term fertility problems. Tumor-associated trypsin inhibitor and a tumor-associated protein, CA-125, are being explored as markers for subclinical tubal inflammation, although these markers do not appear to be sensitive or specific to diagnose acute infection.[111] Further studies may reveal their importance as predictors for permanent tubal damage.

Treatment.—Since questions persist regarding the etiology and diagnosis of PID, the appropriate antimicrobial treatment regimen and definition of "cure" also remain controversial (Table 4). Because of the polymicrobial etiology of PID, broad spectrum empiric treatment aimed against gonorrhea, chlamydia, and the possibility of mixed aerobic and anaerobic lower genital tract organisms is usual.[14] For the selected regimen to be effective, however, it must eliminate the infecting organisms as well as the signs and symptoms of infection and interrupt the development of serious sequelae. Although many current studies address immediate treatment related issues, such as the resolution of initial signs and symptoms, no randomized studies have compared different treatment regimens with fertility as an outcome.

New compounds entering the antimicrobial market may alter the duration of therapy.[112–115] New second- and third-generation cephalosporins, quinolones, monobactams, and carbapenems are available and need to be evaluated as alternative regimens for PID. Single-dose agents, such as azithromycin, which are effective against lower tract chlamydial infection may be effective for shorter course PID therapy. The role of antiinflammatory agents or hormonal intervention to prevent or ameliorate sequelae is unknown.

TABLE 4.
Treatment of Pelvic Inflammatory Disease

Inpatient Treatment	Outpatient Treatment
Regimen A Cefoxitin 2 g (IV) every 6 hr or Cefotetan IV 2 g every 12 hr Regimen B Clindamycin IV 900 mg every 8 hr plus Gentamicin loading dose IV or IM (2 mg/kg) of body weight followed by a maintenance dose (1.5 mg/kg) every 8 hrs. Alternative Regimens Sulbactam/ampiccillin 2 g IV every 6 hr plus doxycycline 100 mg orally every 12 hr	Cefoxitin 2 g IM plus probenecid, 1 g orally, concurrently or ceftriaxone 250 mg IM or other third-generation cephalosporin (e.g., ceftizoxime or cefotaxime) plus Doxycycline 100 mg orally twice a day for 10–14 days Alternative Regimens Ofloxacin 400 mg orally twice per day plus either metronidazole 500 mg orally twice a day or clidamycin 450 mg 4 times a day for 10–14 days Amoxicillin/clavulanic acid 1.5 g 4 times a day plus doxycycline 100 mg twice a day for 10–14 days Azithromycin 2 g orally as a single dose plus metronidazole 500 mg twice a day or clindamycin 450 mg 4 times a day

Syphilis

Although it has been recognized for centuries, syphilis still remains an enigma. It continues to plague both the patient and the physician with its varied clinical manifestations, serious late complications, and diagnostic difficulties. In combination with HIV infection, the task of diagnosing and treating syphilis becomes even more complex.

Diagnosis.—Since *Treponema pallidum* cannot be cultured continuously in vitro, the diagnosis of syphilis relies on identification of clinical signs and/or detection of treponemal antibodies in sera. Syphilis, however, is characterized by episodes of active clinical disease punctuated by periods of asymptomatic, latent infection. The duration of each clinical episode may vary, stages may overlap, and not all patients progress through each stage. Nevertheless, the first clinical manifestation, or primary stage, is a painless indurated ulcer, or chancre, at the inoculation site. Approximately one half of patients with untreated syphilis will progress to the secondary, or hematogenous stage, and the rest will go directly into a latent phase of the disease.[116] With secondary syphilis, the hematogenous dissemination of the spirochetes produces widespread physical findings such as generalized rash which characteristically involves the palmar and plantar surfaces, mucous patches, or condylomata lata which are moist, wart-like lesions teeming with spirochetes. If darkfield microscopy is available, spirochetes may be visualized in the serous exudate taken from the base of the chancre or condylomata lata. Identification of these flexing, thin corkscrew-like bacterium confirms the diagnosis of early syphilis. If darkfield microscopy is not available, fluorescent microscopy of lesion exudates with monoclonal or polyclonal anti-*T. pallidum* antibody reagents is available, but also more expensive and labor intensive.[117] New tests using PCR technology to detect *T. pallidum* DNA in clinical specimens are currently being developed and tested and may provide better insight and ease in diagnosing syphilis.[118]

Without therapy, patients with primary or secondary syphilis will resolve their symptoms and signs of infection and progress into a latent phase of disease. They may remain in latency and the disease will be detected only if screening serology is done. One third of these patients, however, may progress to a tertiary phase of disease which is manifested by end-organ damage such as gummas, neurosyphilis, or cardiovascular syphilis. Diagnosis of tertiary syphilis relies on a high index of suspicion, serologic and cerebrospinal fluid findings, and pathology reports.[119]

The most widely used technique for diagnosing syphilis is serologic testing. Two tests are used in tandem: a quantitative nontreponemal or reaginic screening test, which if positive is followed by a specific treponemal test. The sensitivity and specificity of these tests vary according to the stage of syphilis.[116, 120, 121] The nontreponemal tests which are used for screening as well as for monitoring therapeutic response include the Venereal Disease Research Laboratory (VDRL) test or the Rapid Plasma Reagin (RPR) card test. Specimens reactive in either of these tests are titered using serial two-fold dilutions and then confirmed using a specific-antibody-directed test such as the fluorescent treponemal antibody-absorption test (FTA-ABS). These tests are usually done sequentially, except in some cases of early primary syphilis, in which the treponemal test may become reactive before the reaginic tests.

Results of RPR or VDRL tests are thus reported as reactive at a quantitative ratio (for example, 1:4, 1:8, or 1:16). Traditionally, the magnitude of these nontreponemal serum titers are believed to correspond with active disease. Titer decline is, therefore, used as a guide during treatment. After appropriate therapy a fourfold titer decline within a 6 month to 1-year period is indicative of cure. Titers decline more rapidly in patients with earlier stages of infection, lower titers, and without prior syphilis.[121, 122] Romanowski and coworkers recently reviewed the post-therapy decline in RPR titers and found that the rate of decline was slower with later stages of disease.[123] FTA-ABS tests, that were thought to have lifelong reactivity, became negative in 13% of early syphilis cases. Tests for detection of antitreponemal IgM antibodies have been developed.[124] These tests have potential in detecting active infection and congenital disease. Although successful in research laboratories, they have not had similar consistent results when used in diagnostic laboratories.

Treatment.—Parenteral penicillin G remains the drug of choice for all stages of syphilis in the nonallergic patient. The preparation (benzathine, aqueous procaine, or aqueous crystalline), dose, and duration of therapy depends on the stage and clinical manifestation of the disease (Table 5). The most important new challenge regarding syphilis is its diagnosis and treatment in an HIV-infected individual. Numerous reports suggest that the clinical manifestations of syphilis may be more florid and follow a more accelerated course among HIV-infected patients than among HIV-uninfected patients.[120, 125–129] Serologic manifestations of syphilis may be modified, and HIV-infected patients may present with slightly higher titers or with false-negative serologic tests.[130–132] When clinical manifestations suggest syphilis, but serologic tests are negative, alternative diagnostic techniques such as biopsy of lesions, darkfield examination, and direct fluorescent antibody staining of biopsies or lesion material should be used.[132] In general, however, serologic tests appear to be accurate and reliable for diagnosis and evaluation of treatment response in the majority of HIV-infected patients. Treatment response, nonetheless, should be monitored carefully when using currently recommended, single-dose, benzathine penicillin therapy. Treponemicidal levels are rarely attained in the cerebral spinal fluid (CSF) after single-dose benzathine penicillin therapy, thus the central nervous system may provide a shelter site for potential systemic relapse in immunologically impaired hosts. It is, therefore, not surprising that failure of early syphilis therapy in the form of early neurosyphilis and ocular disease has been reported in HIV-infected patients. Examination of CSF for evidence of neurosyphilis, therefore, should be considered in all HIV-infected individuals and should be done if any HIV-infected patient fails therapy or has neurologic signs or symptoms of central nervous system (CNS) invasion. The optimum therapy for any HIV-infected patient is a penicillin regimen, and the penicillin-allergic patient should, when possible, be desensitized and treated. Limited experience suggests that ceftriaxone 1-g intramuscularly or intravenously, daily, for 14 days may be effective for treatment of neurosyphilis. If this regimen is used, close follow-up is essential.[118]

Genital Human Papillomavirus Infections

Genital warts are caused by sexually transmitted HPVs. More than 60 HPV types have been characterized, 12 of which have been identified in the genital tract.[10, 11] The cauliflower-shaped warts often appear on the penis, vulva, cervix, vagina, or anus. Genital warts usually develop 1 to 3 months after exposure. Acute infections may be asymptomatic or may produce exophytic or flat condylomas, chronic persistent infections resulting in cer-

TABLE 5.
Treatment of Syphilis

	Early Syphilis*	**Late Syphilis†**
Regimen	Nonallergic patients Benzathine penicillin G, 2.4 million units IM, in one dose	Nonallergic patients Benzathine penicillin G, 7.2 million units total, administered as doses of 2.4 million units IM, given 1 week apart
Follow-Up	Patients should be reexamined clinically and serologically at 3 mos and 6 mos	3. Quantitative nontreponemal serologic tests repeated at 6 mos and 12 mos 4. If titers increased fourfold, or if an initially high titer $\geq$ 1:64) failed to decrease, or if the patient develops signs or symptoms attributable to syphilis, the patient should be evaluated for neurosyphilis and treated appropriately
Special Considerations	Penicillin allergy Nonpregnant patients: Doxycycline, 100 mg, orally twice a day for 2 weeks Pregnant patients: Tetracycline, 500 mg, orally 4 times a day for 2 weeks	Penicillin allergy Non-pregnant patients: Doxycycline, 100 mg. orally twice a day for 4 weeks or tetracycline, 500 mg orally 4 times a day for 4 weeks
Regimen (Pregnancy)	Penicillin regimen which is appropriate for the woman's stage of syphilis	Pencillin regimen which is appropriate for the womans stage of syphilis

*Primary and secondary and early latent (less than 1 year in duration)
†Late latent syphilis (greater than 1 year or of unknown duration), gummas, and cardiovascular syphilis, not neurosyphilis.

vical intraepithelial neoplasia, and squamous carcinoma. Although the exact proportion of individuals with each type of clinical manifestation is not known, genital warts may represent only 10% or less of the total spectrum of genital tract HPV infections.[10] Though often asymptomatic, the frequency of consultations for symptomatic genital warts is nearly threefold that for genital herpes and continues to increase.[10] In the United States, the number of physician-patient consultations for genital warts increased from 179,000 to 1.7 million between 1966 and 1989.[5] First visits also increased from 54,000 in 1966 to 480,000 in 1989 (Fig 3). Patients from 20 to 24 years of age had more frequent consultations for genital warts than did patients in other age groups; visits for women outnumbered those for men.

The role of HPV in cervical cancer has been the focus of multiple studies. The premalignant lesion, termed cervical intraepithelial neoplasia (CIN), is characterized by a lack of differentiation of stratified squamous epithelial cells and is graded from I to II in increasing severity, with CIN III exhibiting little or no differentiation. Although genital HPV types 6 and 11 are associated with benign genital warts and low-grade CIN, the HPV types 16 and 18 are associated with most CIN lesions of all grades and invasive cancer.[133–136] The viral DNA detected in premalignant CIN is episomal, freely replicating, and produces infectious virus, whereas in malignant cells, the DNA is randomly integrated into various chromosomes. It appears, therefore, that there are two groups of HPV—one group with low and one group with high oncogenic potential.

In a multicenter, case-controlled study by Reeves et al.[137] in Latin America, 759 cases of invasive cervical cancer and 1,467 randomly selected age-matched controls were studied to evaluate the possible association between infection with HPV and cervical cancer. Cervical infection with HPV 16 or 18 or both was strongly associated with cervical cancer. HPV-DNA was detected in 62% of the cases, and in 32% of the controls, and the relative risk of cancer increased from 2.1 to 9.1 with hybridization reactions of increasing strength. Although the number of sex partners, age at first intercourse, number of live births, and Pap smear history were also significant risk factors, a strong association between infection with HPV 16 or 18 or both and cervical cancer persisted after adjusting for these variables.

In another study in which 846 women with cytologic evidence of HPV infection on their Pap smear were followed over a 6-year period, carcinoma in situ developed in 30 women, compared with an expected number of 1.9 by general population incidence figures (relative risk, 15.6).[138] The risk was greatly increased in women younger than 25 years, when the cytologic diagnosis of HPV infection was made. In another study of cytologic examinations and HPV-DNA detection in 9,000 women in Germany, cervical cytology was normal in 94.2%, an additional 2.1% had cytologic changes suggestive of HPV infection (koilocytosis), and 3.7% had dysplasia or invasive carcinoma.[139] Of the patients with normal cytology, 9% were positive for HPV, whereas 35% of those with dysplasia or cancer were positive for HPV. CIN was associated with condyloma acuminata of the cervix in approximately 50% of women.

Although it is becoming increasingly accepted that some HPV types are involved in the development of premalignant disease, other factors may be necessary for progression to malignancy. One independent risk factor is smoking and another is the oral contraceptive pill, although the epidemiologic evidence for the latter is still debatable. Other infections such as HIV may also increase the oncogenic potential of HPV infection. In a recent study, the prevalence of cervical dysplasia in HIV-positive women was 8 and 11 times greater than the presence of dysplasia for women residing in two respective communities.[140] The association of HIV infection with CIN and HPV of the cervix was also prospectively investigated in 132 women attending a methadone maintenance clinic.[141] HPV infection was present in 67% of symptomatic HIV-positive women, 31% of asymptomatic HIV-positive women, and 27% of HIV-negative women. HPV was more strongly associated with CIN in symptomatic (odds ratio = 29.3) and asymptomatic (odds ratio = 8.8) HIV-seropositive women than it was in HIV-seronegative women (odds ratio = 2.3). In women who were not infected with HPV, no association was found between HIV and CIN. The findings of this investigation suggest that HIV-induced immunosuppression may predispose to HPV-mediated cervical cytologic abnormalities. Intraepithelial carcinoma has also been described in homosexual men with anal warts who have also had HIV infection.[142] Consequently, persons with anal warts should be offered screening for HIV and should receive a careful follow-up to detect any pre-neoplastic transformation.

Diagnosis.—Diagnosis of genital HPV infection is limited and in some cases requires sophisticated molecular techniques. As noted, visible genital warts constitute only a minority of genital tract HPV infections, and some clinical infections may require more specialized testing. HPV cannot be propagated or enriched from tissue specimens by cell culture, but there are now several different methods by which HPV can either be inferred or directly demonstrated.[143] In addition to gross observation, examination under magnification after the application of acetic acid may identify areas of subclinical HPV infection. Following clinical observations, a laboratory test available to all clinicians for detection of subclinical cervical HPV infection is the Pap smear. Koilocytes, large cells with a hyperchromatic nucleus and perinuclear clear ring in the cytoplasm, are highly characteristic of an HPV-induced lesion and are virtually diagnostic. However, there are many HPV-infected tissues that do not exhibit koilocytosis, therefore, a cytologic specimen that does not exhibit this change cannot be assumed to be free of HPV.

Immunologic methods can detect either specific HPV antigens or antigens common to many HPVs, but these tests are currently too insensitive to be clinically useful. Molecular detection of HPV infection is becoming increasingly available in some centers and is capable of differentiating HPV types.[144] Two methods that have been widely used for the detection of HPV in cells collected by cervical scraping or lavage are the dot-blot and the filter in situ hybridization assay.[145, 146] In these assays, cells are filtered directly onto a hybridization membrane and disrupted in situ to release the cellular DNA. The membrane is then reacted with a labeled, cloned HPV DNA, and the binding of the label is taken as evidence of HPV in the specimen. Because of its simplicity, this method can be easily used to test large numbers of specimens. However, the sensitivity and specificity of the filter in situ hybridization assay are not as good as those of the southern blot, which remains "the gold standard" for detecting and typing HPV. Unfortunately, this latter assay is slow, labor intensive, and expensive. More recently, the PCR method has been used in research studies, and it is hoped that it will be more widely available in the future for routine diagnosis.[147] This technique amplifies a small segment of HPV DNA to sufficient levels to be easily detected on a gel or by a hybridization technique, a method which is exquisitely sensitive and specific. PCR has been reported to detect as little as one viral genome in 10^5 cells.

Treatment.—No therapy has been shown to eradicate HPV infection, HPV has been demonstrated in adjacent tissue after laser treatment of HPV-associated CIN and after attempts to eliminate subclinical HPV by extensive laser vaporization of the anogenital area. The benefit of treating patients with subclinical HPV infection has not been demonstrated and recurrence is common. The goal of treatment is removal of exophytic warts and the amelioration of signs and symptoms, not the eradication of HPV.[14] Extensive, toxic therapies and procedures that result in scarring should be avoided. Sex partners should be examined for evidence of warts. Patients with anogenital warts should be made aware that they are contagious to uninfected sex partners and the use of condoms is recommended to help reduce transmission. For women with cervical warts, dysplasia must be excluded before treatment is begun. Management should be carried out in consultation with an expert in this area.

In most clinical situations, cryotherapy with liquid nitrogen or cryoprobe is the treatment of choice for external genital and perianal warts.[14] Cryotherapy is nontoxic, does not require anesthesia, and if used properly, does not result in scarring. The use of a cryoprobe in the vagina is not recommended, because of the risk of vaginal perforation and fistula formation.

For the treatment of condyloma acuminata in 572 men and women, cryotherapy eliminated visible warts in 79% of patients compared with 51% of podophyllin-treated patients.[148] Fewer treatments were required to eradicate warts in the cryotherapy group. No patient in either treatment group suffered from serious adverse effects. Patients with CIN have been treated with cryotherapy. In a study of 1,675 patients treated over an 11-year period, 94% had normal cytologic and colposcopic findings one year after completion of therapy.[149] In the patients who were available for reassessment, 89% and 85% did not have a recurrence of dysplasia at 5 and 10 years, respectively.

Podophyllin, podophyllotoxin, trichloroacetic acid (TCA), and electrodesiccation/electrocautery are alternative therapies. Treatment with interferon is not recommended because of its relatively low efficacy, high incidence of toxicity, and high cost. The carbon dioxide laser and conventional surgery are useful in the management of extensive warts, particularly for patients who have not responded to cryotherapy; these alternatives are not appropriate for limited lesions.

Podophyllin (10%–25% in a compound tincture of benzoin) is applied directly to the involved area and thoroughly washed off in 1 to 4 hours.[14] Repeat applications may be performed at weekly intervals. Mucosal warts are more likely to respond than highly keratinized warts. When possible, podophyllin should not be used on the cervix, vagina, urethral meatus, anal mucosa, or buccal mucosal.

Podophyllotoxin, a therapeutically active drug found in podophyllin resin, may be more effective than podophyllin alone. In one study comparing physician-applied podophyllin with patient-applied podophyllotoxins (0.5%), there was quicker resolution of genital warts in the podophyllin group.[150] No significant difference in the rate of local complications occurred and no patient in either group experienced a serious systemic effect.

For pregnant women, podophyllin is contraindicated and should not be used. When possible, cryotherapy with liquid nitrogen may be used. Neither routine HPV screening tests or cesarean delivery are indicated to prevent transmission of HPV infections to the newborn. In rare instances, however, cesarean delivery may be indicated for women with genital warts if the pelvic outlet is obstructed or vaginal delivery would result in excessive bleeding. Genital papillary lesions do have a tendency to proliferate and to become friable during pregnancy. Many experts advocate removal of visible warts during pregnancy, although data on this subject are limited. While HPV can cause laryngeal papillomatosis in infants, the routes of transmission are unknown, and the preventive value of cesarean delivery is unknown. The perinatal transmission rate is also unknown, although it must be relatively low given the relatively high prevalence of genital warts and the rarity of pharyngeal papillomas.

Genital Herpes

Recent studies of the epidemiology of genital herpes have focused on risk-factor assessment as well as increasing appreciation of the high prevalence of asymptomatically infected individuals. Because genital herpes simplex is a lifelong infection, individuals infected are potentially infectious to their sexual partners afterwards, because of intermittent asymptomatic shedding. The major difficulty in ascertainment of persons at risk for asymptomatic shedding from a clinical and epidemiologic standpoint is the lack of specificity of currently available commercial tests for herpes simplex immunoassay. Using the reference Western blot techniques, investigators have delineated the problem. In a study of 4,527 patients attending family planning clinics in western Pennsylvania,[151] seroprevalence of HSV-2 documented by immunoblot was 22%. HSV seropositivity was associated with patients who had more than 5 years of sexual activity, were black, had a previous history of genital infection, and had higher numbers of sexual partners. Studies in Seattle compared HSV-2 seroprevalence and shedding rates at an STD clinic and university student clinic.[152] Of 776 women evaluated in the STD clinic, 41% were seropositive for HSV-2, compared with 9% of patients evaluated at the university clinic. Furthermore, in the STD clinic setting, 8% of all women presenting to the clinic had positive HSV cultures at the time of examination; the majority were asymptomatic.

Patient history of genital herpes has also been shown to have poor sensitivity and, interestingly, specificity. In a large community-based cross-sectional study recently conducted in San Francisco,[153] seroprevalence of HSV-2 in men with self-reported genital herpes was 62%; however, only 15% of persons who are HSV-2 seropositive reported histories of genital herpes. In this study, which targeted populations at high-risk for STDs, herpes simplex virus seropositivity was associated with intravenous drug use and crack cocaine, especially in women. Underdiagnosis was confirmed in a number of different cities, including Seattle, where 22% of patients who had antibody to HSV, were asymptomatic or had histories of ulceration. Again, these studies underscore the difficulty in using patient historical data in order to evaluate risk for HSV.[154]

Sexual transmission of herpes has been studied in a number of different settings. Brock[155] studied asymptomatic shedding in recurrent HSV disease in women and found that 45% of women had asymptomatic shedding based only on viral culture results. Shedding was not related to symptoms or to their menstrual cycle.[155, 156] These data confirm previous studies, which indicate that approximately 1% of women who have been infected with HSV-2 within the past 5 years are asymptomatically shedding virus at any specific time. Another study found that 50% of women who are counseled after being diagnosed with asymptomatic HSV will identify HSV-2 lesions in the genital tract within 5 months of diagnosis.[157] These studies confirm previous studies of asymptomatic transmission in which a large proportion of patients who are source contacts, and who are herpes positive, indicated that they had had symptoms of HSV-2 disease, but were not aware that those symptoms actually represented a herpes infection. In summary, asymptomatic transmission appears to be the most common cause of transmission of HSV-2 disease at the present time.[158]

Although this review is targeted toward the practicing internist, the issues of pregnancy in individuals who have herpes does occur in internal medicine practice. When treating herpes-infected women during pregnancy, it is important to differentiate between the presence of recurrent or primary herpes infection. There are good data to suggest that the attack rate for neonatal herpes among infants who have been exposed to mothers with recurrent herpes simplex is low,[160] which is validated by the relatively low incidence rates of neonatal herpes, contrasted with the high prevalence rates of individuals who are HSV-2 positive. Women who have primary herpes (the first episode documented by both clinical and serological means) are 10 times more likely to transmit the disease to the infant than are women with recurrent disease.[161] This presents a counseling dilemma for the practitioner faced with a couple who are pregnant in which one partner has a history of herpes and the other does not. For example, Kulhanjian estimated that 10% of couples were discordant for herpes simplex by both serological and diagnostic methods, and the wife was susceptible.[162] In this situation, knowing that primary herpes simplex poses the greatest risk to the fetus, the practitioner may suggest abstinence for the remainder of pregnancy, condom use, or serologic testing in order to evaluate the couple further.

In terms of pregnancy management, it is currently recommended that women who have recurrent herpes disease (which is the most common problem) undergo clinical evaluation at delivery. If lesions are present in the birth canal, then a cesarean section is suggested; if lesions are not present, then cultures are taken at delivery. If the cultures are positive (usually within 2 to 3 days), then the infant is given a short course of acyclovir prophylaxis.[163, 164]

Diagnosis.—Diagnosis of HSV is still most commonly made by culture. Culture offers the advantages of high sensitivity and 100% specificity. Sensitivity of culture is estimated to be on the order of 80% to 90%. False-negative cultures are usually caused by inadequate samples, or by sampling late in the course of the disease after lesions are crusted. The recommended sampling technique is to sample vesicular fluid or basal or parabasal layers of the skin from the genital ulcer instead of the overlying exudate.

Direct fluorescent antibody and ELISA techniques are available for diagnosis of herpetic lesions. These techniques are highly specific; however, sensitivity is a major problem, especially late in the course of the disease. Assessment of the later outbreaks is made clinically, and there is usually no need to culture patients after a diagnosis has been made. Newer sensitive techniques for HSV diagnosis, such as PCR have been extensively used in evaluating CNS herpes (herpes encephalitis).[165] However, evaluation of the genital lesions with PCR techniques presents problems in that the asymptomatic shedding rate is very high, and therefore, it is difficult to interpret a positive genetic-probe technique or PCR result in the absence of viable virus.

Commercially available serologic techniques for diagnosis of herpes present substantial problems. Commercial serologic techniques are based on immunofluorescence of pooled antigens. Ashley has conclusively shown that commercially available serologic diagnosis presents both sensitivity and specificity problems when compared to reference Western Blot methods.[166] Outside of epidemiologic research, we recommend use of serologic techniques for clinical evaluation only in limited circumstances. Serologic techniques are only useful in differentiating primary vs. recurrent herpes. In the case of recurrent herpes, a positive result indicates only that the patient has been infected with herpes at some time in the past. These techniques are especially useful during pregnancy in differentiating recurrent vs. primary disease; however, the only techniques which we would recommend would be Western blot or the immunodot, which are based on purified herpes simplex glycoproteins. These techniques are currently available only in research laboratories.

Treatment.—Acyclovir is still the mainstay of treatment.[163] This nucleoside analog has been utilized for the past 10 years, and it has been found to be highly safe and effective. Acyclovir inhibits early DNA replication by substituting a false nucleoside for guanosine. Acyclovir has been found to shorten the course of genital herpes, shorten viral shedding time, and shorten the healing time. In addition, patients subjectively report that genital herpes when treated with acyclovir is less severe. The specific dosage schedules for acyclovir are indicated in Table 6, In our experience, systemic acyclovir (i.e., oral medication as opposed to the earlier approved topical preparations) is much more effective. Furthermore, in practice, acyclovir is much more effective when treatment is initiated early in the course of disease. Intravenous acyclovir is reserved for cases of severe mucocutaneous herpes in immunocompromised hosts, generalized herpes infections such as herpes encephalitis, herpes hepatitis, or herpes simplex meningitis, which can be part of the primary herpes syndrome.

Acyclovir has also been widely used for herpes prophylaxis. Individuals who are candidates for prophylaxis are those with more than six recurrent episodes annually. In these individuals prophylaxis with acyclovir has been found to reduce recurrences by over 90% in well-controlled studies.[167–169] Our approach is to initiate prophylactic therapy with 400 mg, twice daily, and titrate the dosage either up or down to the patient's individual requirement in order to prevent recurrent disease.

Resistance to acyclovir is rare, and has been reported mostly in immunocompromised hosts.[170–172] Acyclovir-resistant mutants have been

TABLE 6.
Treatment of Genital Herpes

First Clinical Episode
- Genital HSV:
- Acyclovir 400 mg 3 times/day
- or 800 mg 2 times/day
- HSV Proctitis:
- Acyclovir 400 mg 5 times/day
- Treatment recommended for 7–10 days, or until clinical resolution occurs (either sooner or later).
- Recurrent disease is treated at same dose, but for half the time course.

Suppressive Therapy
- Acyclovir 400 mg twice/day
- Suppression recommended for those patients with ≥ 6 recurrences/year.

found predominantly in patients co-infected with HIV and chronic mucocutaneous herpes. The most common type of viral resistance has been thymidine kinase mutants, because acyclovir needs to be phosphorylated in order to become effective. Herpes isolates which are deficient in thymidine kinase are therefore resistant to herpes. Acyclovir-resistant herpes should be suspected in patients with AIDS or other severe immunocompromised conditions and chronic herpes, which does not respond to therapy. In patients with acyclovir-resistant herpes, foscarnet is the most commonly used alternative, although vidarabine is also probably effective.

Hepatitis B Virus

In the United States, an estimated 200,000 to 300,000 new hepatitis B virus (HBV) infections occur annually,[173] and approximately 1 to 1.25 million individuals have chronic HBV infection, that is, are carriers of hepatitis B surface antigen and are potentially infectious to others. The mortality potential of HBV is reflected in the fact that 4 to 5 thousand individuals die annually from chronic liver disease and primary hepatocellular carcinoma.

In contrast to other parts of the world, such as Asia, most persons in the United States acquire the infection as adolescents or young adults. Sexual transmission of hepatitis B infection has been recognized since 1975[174] and more recently, studies conducted in the late 1970s and early 1980s have reported the risk of hepatitis B in homosexual men.[175, 176] For example, multicenter studies conducted in the early 1980s revealed that 62% of homosexual men had serologic evidence of either active hepatitis B infection (HBsAg) or prior exposure and immunity to hepatitis B infection (HB antibody).[176] With the development of hepatitis B vaccine and its approval in 1981, targeted populations for vaccination included homosexual men and health care workers, both of which groups were identified as having inordinate exposure potential to hepatitis B infection. However, during the 1980s the heterosexual transmission of HBV both increased and became increasingly apparent.[16, 176] The CDC estimated that between 1981 and 1988, hepatitis B transmission increased 38% in heterosexual men. CDC surveillance, coupled with other studies in areas of high hepatitis B prevalence, such as sexually transmitted disease clinics[180, 181] and communities with high incidence of hepatitis B, concluded that the vast majority of new hepatitis B cases were transmitted heterosexually. The risk factors for heterosexual transmission included presence of other STDs and increased number of sexual partners. In some STD clinic populations, the prevalence of HBV markers is over 50% in men and women over the age of 30 (Baltimore, 1993, unpublished data).

Although hepatitis B vaccine efficacy is over 95%, targeted vaccination of high-risk groups during the 1980s was limited as an overall public health strategy because of the following reasons[173]:

1. Hepatitis B vaccine is relatively expensive (approximately $100 per vaccination series), and patients typically in underserved groups, such as

TABLE 7.
Recommended Doses of Currently Licensed Hepatitis B Vaccines

Group	Recombivax HB		Engerix-B	
	Dose, μg	**mL**	**Dose, μg**	**mL**
Children and adolescents 11–19 years	5	0.5	20	1.0
Adults ≥ 20 years	10	1.0	20	1.0
Dialysis patients and other immunocompromised persons	40	1.0	40	2.0

heterosexual individuals in STD clinics, did not have the financial resources. Furthermore, with cutbacks in preventive medicine programs which occurred during the late 1980s, public health authorities were unable to afford HBV vaccination.

2. In some instances, even when offered vaccine, individuals who were members of high-risk groups such as IV drug users refused vaccination (Worcester Hepatitis data).

3. Logistical difficulties in arranging for follow-up of patients to complete their HBV series has often resulted in undervaccination of many individuals.

4. CDC criteria to identify pregnant women with respect to HBV failed to identify the majority of hepatitis B surface-antigen-positive mothers.[182]

Under these circumstances, the recommendations were made in early 1991 to universally vaccinate all individuals for hepatitis B as part of the routine vaccination series during early childhood. The tables for vaccination, as well as postexposure vaccination for individuals who may have been recently exposed to hepatitis B are demonstrated in Table 7.[173]

Hepatitis C Virus

Hepatitis C virus (HCV) represents one of the components of non-A, non-B hepatitis. Non-A, non-B hepatitis has been subdivided into hepatitis C, which is parenterally transmitted, and hepatitis E, which is transmitted via the orofecal route and is commonly found in developing countries. Since the development of the HCV assays, HCV transmission has been verified by blood transfusion and by organ transplantation. Blood transfusion is highly efficient in transmitting hepatitis C (greater than 90%),[183] and organ transplantation has been found to have a transmission rate of approximately 50%.[184, 185] Needlestick transmission has been well documented.[186] HCV has also been found to be the cause of the vast majority of cases of chronic hepatitis following transfusion and has also been putatively identified as a co-factor in hepatocellular carcinoma independent of HBV.[187]

Studies of the sexual transmission of HCV have indicated that sexual transmission is probably rare. A large study conducted in postsurgical National Institutes of Health (NIH) patients found that sexual transmission to partners of patients infected via blood transfusion was rare. However, that study has been criticized in that the median age of patients was 55, and sexual activity may be a variable which had not been taken into account.[188] However, studies in younger populations in STD clinics are inconclusive for sexual transmission of HCV. In populations of IV drug users, IV drug use is strongly related to HCV acquisition when controlled for in multivariate analysis; sexual transmission is not a major variable. In conclusion, HCV appears to be parenterally transmitted; if sexual transmission does occur, it probably plays a very minor role. There have been no prevention strategies which have been developed for HCV exclusive of testing of the blood supply and avoiding IV drugs.

Bacterial Vaginosis

Bacterial vaginosis (BV), formerly known as non-specific vaginitis, *Haemophilus vaginitis, Gardnerella vaginalis,* and anaerobic vaginosis is the most prevalent form of vaginal infection among reproductive-age women in the United States (Fig 6).[189] The prevalence of BV ranges from high among STD clients (32% to 64%) to relatively low among obstetric patients (10% to 26%). Women may present to their clinicians complaining of a vaginal discharge which may have a foul or "fishy" odor, but asymptomatic infections are thought to be common. This discharge is not caused by inflammation of the vaginal epithelium, but is the result of an alteration in the normal vaginal ecosystem, so that the concentrations of anaerobic and aerobic bacteria increases 100- to 1000-fold and anaerobes predominate.[190–193] Predisposing factors for BV include a lengthy history of sexual activity, a large number of sexual partners, the presence of other sexually transmitted infections and the use of an intrauterine device for contraception.[194, 195] The risk for BV has not been firmly associated with recent use of antibiotics, the diaphragm, spermicidal cream, age, and smoking. Furthermore, evidence for sexual transmission, although intuitive, is not confirmed.

Diagnosis.—Since our understanding of BV has evolved over the past 100 years and its exact cause is still unknown, the standard method for diagnosing BV is based on clinical criteria[189, 192] (Table 8). During the female reproductive period, one result of estrogen production is an increase in glycogen content of the vaginal epithelium.[196] Normal vaginal flora consists of both aerobic and anaerobic organisms, with a predominance of hydrogen peroxide-producing lactobacilli.[190, 192, 197] These lactobacilli help

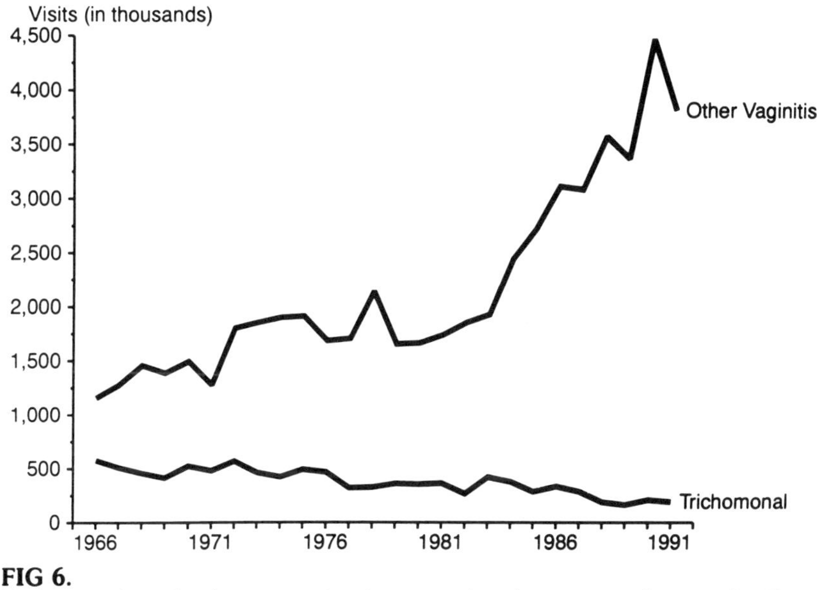

FIG 6.
Trichomonal and other vaginal infections—Initial visits to physicians' offices: United States, 1966–1991. (Data from Centers for Disease Control: *Division of STD/HIV Prevention Annual Report, 1991.* Atlanta, Ga, 1992.)

to degrade the glycogen to an end product of lactic acid, which is responsible for the normally low vaginal pH of 3.8 to 4.2. This acidic environment along with various antibacterial compounds produced by lactobacilli including H_2O_2 inhibits the growth of *G. vaginalis* and anaerobes. When the normal lactobacilli-dominated flora is replaced with a mixed flora, consisting of increased concentrations of *G. vaginalis, Mycoplasma hominis,* and a variety of anaerobes such as *Bacteroides* species, *Peptostreptococcus,* and *Mobiluncus,* then BV may result.[198–201] The resulting patient complaint is a malodorous vaginal discharge. The odor is caused by the production of amines by anaerobic bacteria. On gynecologic examination, instead of the normal viscous and floccular vaginal secretion, a thin grey or white homogeneous discharge that adheres to the vaginal walls may be seen. Examination of the vaginal discharge by light microscopy under high power (×40) should reveal "clue cells," or epithelial cells coated with large numbers of bacteria which obscure the cell border. The clinical criteria for diagnosis of BV include the detection of three of the four following signs: (1) thin, homogenous discharge that adheres to the vaginal walls; (2) an elevated vaginal pH > 4.5; (3) presence of amine odor after adding a few drops of 10% potassium hydroxide (KOH) to the vaginal secretions (positive "whiff" test); or (4) presence of $\geq 20\%$ clue cells on microscopic examination of vaginal secretion saline wet mount preparation.

In diagnosing BV by these criteria, care should be taken to sample vagina, not cervical, secretions when measuring pH. Other methods for diagnosis of BV are either unreliable or too technical for clinical application.

TABLE 8.
Differential Diagnosis of Vaginal Infections*

	Syndrome			
Diagnostic Criteria	**Normal**	**Bacterial Vaginosis**	**Candida Vulvovaginitis**	**Trichomonas Vaginitis**
Vaginal pH	3.8–4.2	≥4.5	≥4.5	≥4.5
Discharge	Clear, flocculent	Thin, homogeneous, white, yellowish, gray, adherent, often increased	White, curdy, "cottage cheese"–like, sometimes increased	Yellow, green, frothy adherent
Amine odor (KOH "whiff' test)	Absent	Present (fishy)	Absent	Present (fishy)
Microsopic	Lactobacilli	Clue cells, coccoid bacteria, no WBCs	Mycelia, budding yeast, pseudohyphae with KOH prep	Trichomonads WBCs >10/hpf
Main patient complaints	None	Discharge, bad odor—possibly worse after intercourse	Itching/burning, discharge	Frothy discharge, bad odor, vulvar pruritus, dysuria

*KOH = potassium hydroxide; WBC = white blood cell.

Cultures of vaginal secretions, for example, are laborious and unreliable. Papanicolaou smears which can detect the presence of clue cells remain controversial in the diagnosis of BV. Data are conflicting reporting diagnostic sensitivities of 25% to 90% and specificities of 58% to 97%. Gram's stain of vaginal secretions is useful to the diagnosis of BV, if it is interpreted using a scoring system developed by Nugent and co-workers which incorporates the identification and quantification of bacterial morphotypes associated with BV.[202]

Treatment.—Treatment of BV, formerly considered a minor and harmless syndrome in the context of all STDs, has become an issue because of several studies that pinpoint it as a risk factor in the development of PID, posthysterectomy infections, postabortal PID, preterm delivery, premature rupture of membranes, amniotic fluid infections, and postpartum endometritis. Currently recommended therapy consists of 500 mg of metronidazole taken orally twice a day for 1 week, or 500 mg of ampicillin given according to the same schedule as an alternative. New therapies also include metronidazole vaginal gel intravaginally twice daily for 5 days. Since a variety of serious postpartum sequelae have been associated with prevalent BV, identification of a safe therapeutic regimen during pregnancy is needed.

The issue of the sexual transmission of BV is unresolved. Since the organisms commonly associated with BV are endogenous, sexual acquisition of BV may not be necessary. However, inoculation of BV-associated organisms from the male urethra to the female vagina may precipitate the syndrome. Studies comparing cotreatment regimens of female patients and their male partners to treatment of female patients alone showed no differences in cure or relapse rates.[203, 204] Unfortunately, relapse rates range from between 10% and 30% even with the best treatment regimens.[189, 205, 206]

Trichomonas vaginalis

Diagnosis.—The mainstay of diagnosing trichomoniasis has been the saline vaginal wet preparation. Although this method is cheap, easy, and 100% specific if motile trichomonads are seen, it has a low sensitivity ranging from 45% to 60%.[207] The Pap smear may detect trichomonads, but it does not significantly improve on the sensitivity of the wet prep, and the results are not immediately available. Culture, which is the current "gold standard," has a sensitivity of 92% to 95%.[208] Unfortunately, in addition to the added cost of culture media and technician time, 3 to 7 days are required for organism growth before the diagnosis can be confirmed. New diagnostic techniques are available such as direct immunofluoresence assays (DFA), direct enzyme immunoassays (EIA), and latex agglutination tests.[209] All have sensitivities in the 90% range with excellent specificity, but all are limited in clinical use by complexity and cost.

Standard therapy is metronidazole in a 2-g oral dose.[14, 213] Metronidazole suppositories have been tried with cure rates of 30% to 60%, which may be due to the multifocal nature of the infection involving Skene's glands, the vaginal epithelium, Bartholin's glands, and the urethra. Metronidazole resistance has been reported since 1963, but has not become a major problem.[214] Since resistance to metronidazole is not an all-or-none phenomenon, longer courses of therapy have generally worked.[215, 216] Although not available in the United States to date, tinidazole may provide an alternative treatment for highly metronidazole-resistant strains. As with other STDs, treatment during pregnancy is an issue, and recent data link trichomonas to premature rupture of membranes and low birth weight. Symptomatic pregnant women can be treated with 100-mg clotrimazole suppositories daily at bedtime for 2 weeks. If prenatal intervention is necessary, the single 2-g dose of metronidazole can be given in the second or third trimester.[14]

Human Immunodeficiency Virus and Sexually Transmitted Diseases

Because many of these diseases are biologically and behaviorally linked to the spread of HIV infection, we are currently witnessing an "epidemiologic synergy" among these infections that threatens to propel further dissemination of all STDs, including HIV.[217] Several studies in the United States and in Africa have clearly demonstrated strong associations between increased seroconversion rates to HIV among high-risk individuals with genital ulcers due to chancroid, syphilis, and herpes.[217, 218] Furthermore, several studies have also suggested an increased risk of HIV acquisition among patients with nonulcerative STDs such as chlamydia, gonorrhea, and trichomoniasis.[219, 220] While behavioral activities such as unsafe sex practices, multiple sexual partners, and other factors may be responsible for these associations, the presence of inflammatory changes and/or ulcerations may influence HIV transmission by providing a portal of entry for the virus in the recipient, or by increasing the infectivity of the index case by enhanced viral shedding. Lymphocytes are the primary target cells for HIV, and lymphocytic infiltration is prominent in biopsies from genital ulcers, chancroid, syphilis and herpes. Furthermore, HIV has been isolated from the base of genital ulcers in HIV-infected prostitutes.[221] Changes of the cervix due to chlamydia, gonorrhea, or trichomoniasis may result in microulcerations, ectopy, or cervical friability, thereby increasing susceptibility to HIV transmission or infectiousness.

HIV infection itself may alter the natural history and response to therapy of many STDs, including chancroid, syphilis, genital HSV, and human papillomavirus. For example, individuals who are co-infected with *Haemophilis ducreyi* and HIV are less responsive to standard antibiotic treatment for chancroid than HIV-seronegative controls.[222] Rapid progression from early syphilis to central nervous system involvement has also been documented after an interval of months as opposed to years for HIV-infected individuals.[118] The severity and frequency of reactivation of HSV infection increases dramatically as HIV-induced immunosuppression progresses. Acyclovir-resistant mutants of HSV-2 have been most commonly reported among AIDS patients, and alternative therapy with foscarnet is often required.[170, 223] Among HIV-infected women, intraepithelial neoplasia involving the cervix in association with HPV infection appears to be increased compared to HIV-uninfected women.[140, 141] HIV control programs recognizing the strong association between STDs and HIV transmission have advocated more effective treatment regimens for traditional STDs coupled with other STD control measures such as condom use and safe sex counseling, which, it is hoped, will have a direct impact on HIV control as well as STD prevention. For these reasons, the control of STDs, particularly in those populations at high risk for HIV infection, is currently of highest priority and an integral component of AIDS control programs worldwide.

Epidemiology and Control Issues in Sexually Transmitted Diseases

Drug use, especially that of "crack" cocaine, has had a major impact on the epidemiology of STDs and the ability of public health authorities to institute adequate control measures. Crack cocaine use has been empirically associated with epidemic syphilis, especially in those cases which involve "sex for drugs" prostitution.[225] Other diseases in which crack has been implicated, but not as extensively studied, include HIV infection, chancroid, and PID. Crack cocaine has been conclusively linked to congenital syphilis, and it appears to be part of an overall behavioral phenomenon which includes sex for drugs, prostitution, no prenatal care, and large numbers of anonymous sex partners. One of the problems in the above studies is that they evaluated STD clinic patients, or others who are at inordinately high risk for STDs. One population-based, cross-sectional study which evaluated crack cocaine use among black adolescents in San Francisco found that individuals with gonorrhea were significantly more likely to have used crack cocaine, compared to those who did not have gonorrhea.[226]

Although large-scale, cross-sectional data are not available on sexual behavior, population subgroups at high risk for STDs have been particularly well studied. Kotloff in 1988 studied college students at a major mid-Atlantic university and found that 19% of men and 13% of women had had over four sexual partners in the past month.[64] Although these college students had low rates of IV drug use, they also had low rates (below 20%) of consistent condom use.

In a national, cross-sectional study conducted during 1989-1991, high school students who discussed sexual issues with their parents tended to have less sexual activity and fewer sexual partners.[227] Condom use was relatively stable across all groups studied, but fewer than half of the individuals reported consistent condom use. In comparison, 58% of intravenous drug users studied in 1991 never used condoms during vaginal intercourse,[228] which presents a substantial risk to the partners of these high-risk individuals. In an STD clinic setting in Baltimore,[65] 17% of patients reported condom use at last sexual intercourse. Only 5% of men and 6% of women in this population always used condoms, which by definition is self-selected for disease presentation. Individuals with more sexual partners and younger patients were also more likely to use condoms. What appears to be relatively consistent behavior across all groups is that individuals tend to use condoms or disease control measures with partners outside their regular partners, when they do use those measures. Individuals involved in stable relationships tend not to use disease protection measures under the assumption that their partners are "safe." Finally, there is increasing realization among the STD and behavioral research community that AIDS education and risk-reduction programs, as they have been presented during the past 5 years, have emphasized education as opposed to individual counseling. Most patients presenting in STD clinics and schools have substantial knowledge regarding STD and HIV transmission. The challenge is to translate this knowledge into action evidenced by increased condom use and lower numbers of high-risk sexual encounters.[229] Counseling models which stress interactive counseling, as opposed to educational/informational sessions, are currently being studied to determine whether they result in more, longer-term behavioral changes.[230]

References

1. Quinn TC, Cates W: Epidemiology of sexually transmitted diseases in the 1990's, in Quinn TC (ed): *Advances in Host Defense Mechanisms vol 8.* New York, Raven Press, 1992, pp 1–37.
2. Cates W, Jr: AIDS, STD and epidemiology: past lessons, present knowledge, and future opportunities. *Am J Epidemiol* 1990; 131:749–758.
3. Stamm WE, Holmes KK: *Chlamydia trachomatis* infections of the adult, to Holmes KK, Mardh PA, Sparling PF, et al (eds): *Sexually Transmitted Diseases.* New York, McGraw-Hill Co, 1990, pp 181–193.
4. Washington A, Johnson R, Sanders L: *Chlamydia trachomatis* infections in the United States. What are they costing us? *JAMA* 1978; 257:2070–2072.
5. Centers for Disease Control: *Divison of STD/HIV Prevention Annual Report, 1991.* Atlanta, Ga, 1992.
6. Rolfs RT, Nakashima AK: Epidemiology of primary and secondary syphilis in the United States, 1981 through 1989. *JAMA* 1990; 264:1432–1437.
7. Cates W, Jr: Teenagers and sexual risk taking: The best of times and the worst of times. *J Adolesc Health Care,* 1991;12:84–94.
8. Fullilove RE, Fullilove MT, Bowser BP, et al: Risk of sex ually transmitted disease among black adolescent crack users in Oakland and San Francisco, California. *JAMA* 1990; 263:851–855.
9. Whittington WL, Knapp JS: Trends in resistance of *Neisseria gonorrhoeae* to antimicrobial agents in the United States. *Sex Trans Dis* 1988; 15:202–210.
10. Koutsky LA, Galloway DA, Holmes KK: Epidemiology of genital human papillomavirus infection. *Epidemiol Rev* 1988; 10:122–163.
11. Stone KM: Epidemiologic aspects of genital HPV infection. *Clin Obstet Gynecol* 1989; 32:112–116.

12. Corey L: Genital herpes, in Holmes KK, Mardh PA, Sparling PF, et al (eds): *Sexually Transmitted Diseases.* New York, McGraw-Hill Co, 1990, pp 391–413.
13. Volberding PA, Lagakos SW, Koch MA, et al: Zidovudine in asymptomatic human immunodeficiency virus infection. *N Engl J Med* 1990; 322:941–949.
14. Centers for Disease Control: 1989 Sexually Transmitted Disease Treatment Guidelines. *MMWR* 1989; 38(No. S-5):1–43.
15. Martin DH, Mroczkowski TF, Dalu ZA, et al: A controlled trial of a single dose of azithromycin for the treatment of chlamydial urethritis and cervicitis. *N Engl J Med* 1992; 327:921–925.
16. Alter MJ, Margolis HS: The emergenc of hepatitis B as a sexually transmitted disease. *Med Clin N Amer* 1990; 74:1529–1541.
17. Washington AE, Johnson RE, Sanders LL, et al: Incidence of *Chlamydia trachomatis* infections in the United States: using reported *Neisseria gonorrhoeae* as surrogate, in Oriel D, Ridgway G, Schachter J, et al (eds): *Chlamydia Infections.* Cambridge, England, Cambridge University Press, 1986, pp 487–490.
18. Stamm WE, Koutsky LA, Benedetti JK, et al: *Chlamydia trachomatis* urethral infections in men. prevalence, risk factors, and clinical manifestations. *Ann Intern Med* 1984; 100:47–52.
19. Shafer M, Prager V, Shalwitz J, et al: Prevalence of urethral *Chlamydia trachomatis* and *Neisseria gonorrhoeae* among asymptomatic sexually active adolescent males. *J Infect Dis* 1987; 156:223–224.
20. Quinn TC, Goodell SE, Mkritchian E: *Chlamydia trachomatis* proctitis. *N Engl J Med* 1981; 305:195–200.
21. Jones RB, Rabinovitch RA, Katz BP, et al: *Chlamydia trachomatis* in the pharynx and rectum of homosexual patients at risk for genital infection. *Ann Intern Med* 1985; 102:757–762.
22. Chacko M, Lovchik J: *Chlamydia trachomatis* infection in sexually active adolescents: prevalence and risk factors. *Pediatrics* 1984; 73:836–840.
23. McCormack W, Rosner B, McComb D, et al: Infection with *Chlamydia trachomatis* in female college students. *Am J Epidemiol* 1985; 121:115–120.
24. Martin DH, Pastorek JG, Faro S: Risk factors for *Chlamydia trachomatis* in a high-risk population of pregnant women, in Oriel D, Ridgeway G, Schachter J, et al (eds): *Chlamydial Infections.* Cambridge, England, Cambridge University Press; 1986, pp 189–193.
25. Harrison HR, Alexander ER, Weinstein L, et al: Cervical *Chlamydia trachomatis* infection in university women: relationship to history, contraception, ectopy, and cervicitis. *Am J Obstet Gynecol* 1985; 153:244–251.
26. Rolfs RT, Galaid EI, Zaidi AA: Pelvic inflammatory disease: trends in hospitalization and office visits, 1979 through 1988. *Am J Obstet Gynecol* 1992; 166:983–990.
27. Centers for Disease Control: Policy guidelines for the prevention and management of pelvic inflammatory disease (PID). *MMWR* 1991; 40(RR-5):1–25.
28. Cates W, Jr, Rolfs RT, Aral SO: Sexually transmitted diseases, pelvic inflammatory disease, and infertility: an epidemiologic update. *Epidemiol Rev* 1990; 12:199–220.
29. Kiviat NB, Koutsky LA, Paavonen JA, et al: Prevalence of genital papillomavirus infection among women attending a college student health clinic or a sexually transmitted disease clinic. *J Infect Dis* 1989; 159:293–302.
30. Westrom L, Svensson L, Wolner-Hanssen P, et al: Chlamydial and gonococcal infections in a defined population of women. *Scand J Infect Dis Suppl* 1982; 32:157–162.

31. Westrom L: Effect of acute pelvic inflammatory disease on fertility. *Am J Obstet Gynecol* 1975; 121:707–713.
32. Westrom L, Mardh PA: Acute pelvic inflammatory disease (PID), in Holmes KK, Mardh P-A, Sparling PF, et al (eds): *Sexually Transmitted Diseases.* New York, McGraw-Hill Information Services Co, 1990, pp 593–613.
33. Westrom L, Joesoef R, Reynolds G, et al: Pelvic inflammatory disease and fertility: a cohort study of 1,844 women with laparoscopically verified disease and 657 women with normal laparoscopy. *Sex Trans Dis* 1993, in press.
34. Westergaard L, Philipsen T, Schiebel J: Significance of cervical *Chlamydia trachomatis* infection in postabortal pelvic inflammatory disease. *Obstet Gynecol* 1982; 60:322–325.
35. Moller BR, Ahrons S, Laurin J, et al: Pelvic infection after elective abortion associated with *Chlamydia trachomatis. Obstet Gynecol* 1982; 59:210–213.
36. Barbacci M: Post abortal endometritis and the isolation of *Chlamydia trachomatis. Obstet Gynecol* 1986; 68:686–688.
37. Plummer FA, Laga M, Brunham RC, et al: Postpartum upper genital tract infections in Nairobi, Kenya: epidemiology, etiology, and risk factors. *J Infect Dis* 1987; 156:92–98.
38. Wager GP, Martin DH, Koutsky L: Puerpal infectious morbidity: Relationship to route of delivery and to antepartum *Chlamydia trachomatis* infection. *Am J Obstet Gynecol* 1980; 138:1028–1033.
39. Bell TA, Stamm WE, Kuo CC, et al: Delayed appearance of *Chlamydia trachomatis* infections acquired at birth. *Pediatr Infect Dis J* 1987; 6:928–931.
40. Schachter J, Grossman M, Sweet RL, et al: Prospective study of perinatal transmission of *Chlamydia trachomatis* in Nairobi. *J Infect Dis* 1988; 158:524–528.
41. Bell TA, Sandstrom KI, Gravett MG, et al: Comparison of ophthalmic silver nitrate solution and erythromycin ointment for prevention of natally acquired *Chlamydia trachomatis. Sex Transm Dis* 1987; 14:195–200.
42. Hammerschlag MR, Cummings C, Roblin PM, et al: Efficacy of neonatal ocular prophylaxis for the prevention of chlamydial and gonococcal conjunctivitis. *N Engl J Med* 1989; 320:769–772.
43. Preece PM, Anderson JM, Thompson RG: *Chlamydia trachomatis* infection in infants: a prospective study. *Arch Dis Child* 1989; 64:525–529.
44. Bowie WR: Urethritis in males, in Holmes KK, Mardh P-A, Sparling PF, et al (eds): *Sexually Transmitted Diseases.* New York, McGraw-Hill Information Services Co, 1990, pp 627–639.
45. Stamm WE, Wagner KF, Amsel R, et al: Causes of the acute urethral syndrome in women. *N Engl J Med* 1980; 303:409–413.
46. Martin DH, Pollock S, Kuo C-C, et al: *Chlamydia trachomatis* infections in men with Reiter's syndrome. *Ann Intern Med* 1984; 100:203–207.
47. Centers for Disease Control: *Chlamydia trachomatis* infections: policy guidelines for prevention and control. *MMWR: Recommendations and Reports* 1985; 34:53S–74S.
48. Brunham RC, Paavonen J, Stevens CE, et al: Mucopurulent cervicitis—the ignored counterpart in women of urethritis in men. *N Engl J Med* 1984; 311:1–6.
49. Nugent RP, Berlin L, Rhoads GG, et al: Risk factors for cervicitis and *Chlamydia trachomatis* in an inner city pregnant population, in Oriel D, Ridgway G, Schachter J, et al (eds): *Chlamydia Infections.* Cambridge, England, Cambridge University Press, 1986, pp 487–490.

50. Kiviat NB, Paavonen JA, Brockway J, et al: Cytologic manifestations of cervical and vaginal infections. I. Epithelial and inflammatory cellular changes. *JAMA* 1985; 253:989–992.
51. Schachter J: Biology of *Chlamydia trachomatis,* in Holmes KK, Mardh P-A, Sparling PF (eds): *Sexually Transmitted Diseases.* New York, McGraw-Hill, 1984, pp 243–257.
52. Barnes RC: Laboratory diagnosis of human chlamydial infections. *Clin Microbiol Rev* 1989; 2:119.
53. Magder LS, Klontz KC, Bush LH, et al: Effect of patient characteristics on performance of an enzyme immunoassay for detecting cervical *Chlamydia trachomatis* infection. *J Clin Microbiol* 1990; 28:781–784.
54. O'Brien SF, Bell TA, Farrow JA: Use of a leukocyte esterase dipstick to detect *Chlamydia trachomatis* and *Neisseria gonorrhoeae* urethritis in asymptomatic adolescent male detainees. *Am J Public Health* 1988; 78:1583–1584.
55. Shafer MA, Prager V, Shalwitz J, et al: Prevalence of urethral *Chlamydia trachomatis* and *Neisseria gonorrhoeae* among asymptomatic, sexually active adolescent boys. *J Infect Dis* 1987; 156:223–224.
56. Werner MJ, Biro FM: Urinary leukocyte esterase screening method for asymptomatic sexually transmitted disease in adolescent males. *J Adolesc Health* 1991; 12:326–328.
57. McNagny SE, Parker RM, Zenilman JM, et al: Urinary leukocyte esterase test: a screening method for the detection of asymptomatic chlamydial and gonococcal infections in men. *J Infect Dis* 1992; 165:573–576.
58. Chernesky M, Castriciano S, Sellors J, et al: Detection of *Chalmydia trachomatis* antigens in urein as an alternative to swabs and cultures. *J Infect Dis* 1990; 161:124–126.
59. Schwebke JR, Clark AM, Pettinger MB, et al: Use of a urine enzyme immunoassay as a diagnostic tool for *Chlamydia trachomatis* urethritis in men. *J Clin Microbiol* 1991; 29:2446–2449.
60. Palmer HM, Gilroy CB, Thomas BJ, et al: Detection of *Chlamydia trachomatis* by the polymerase chain reaction in swabs and urine from men with nongonococcal urethritis. *J Clin Pathol* 1992; 44:321–325.
61. Slaney L, Chubb H, Ronald AR, et al: In-vitro activity of azithromycin, erythromycin, ciprofloxacin adn norfloxacin against *Neisseria gonorrhoeae, Haemophilus ducreyi,* and *Chlamydia trachomatis. J Antimicrob Chemother* 1990; 25(suppl A):1–5.
62. Toomey K, Barnes R: Treatment of *Chlamydia trachomatis* genital infection. *Rev Infect Dis* 1990; 12(Suppl 6):S645–S655.
63. Danielsson D: Gonorrhoea and syphils in Sweden—past and present. *Scand J Infect Dis* 1990; 69:69–76.
64. Kotloff KL, Tacket CO, Wasserman SS, et al: A voluntary serosurvey and behavioral risk assessment for human immunodeficiency virus infection among college students. *Sex Trans Dis* 1991; 18:223–227.
65. Upchurch DM, Ray P, Reichart C, Celentano DD, et al: Prevalence and patterns of condom use among patients attending a sexually transmitted disease clinic. *Sex Trans Dis* 1992; 19:175–180.
66. Rice RJ, Roberts PL, Handsfield HH, et al: Sociodemographic distribution of gonorrhea incidence: implications for prevention and behavioral research. *Amer J Public Health* 1991; 81:1252–1257.
67. Handsfield HH, Rich RJ, Roberts MC, et al: Localized outbreak of penicillinase-producing *Neisseria gonorrhoeae. JAMA* 1989; 261:2357–2361.

68. Zimmerman HL, Potterat JJ, Dukes RL, et al: Epidemiologic differences between chlamydia and gonorrhea. *Amer J Public Health* 1990; 80:1338–1342.
69. Hook EW, III, Brady WE, Reichart CA, et al: Determinants of emergency of antibiotic-resistant *Neisseria gonorrhoeae. J Infect Dis* 1989; 159:900–907.
70. Potterat JJ, Dukes RL, Rothenburg RB: Disease transmission by heterosexual men with gonorrhea: an empiric estimate. *Sex Transm Dis* 1987;14: 107–110.
71. Goodhart ME, Ogden J, Zaidi AA, et al: Factors affecting the performance of smear and culture tests for the detection of *Neisseria gonorrhoeae. Sex Trans Dis* 1982; 9:63–69.
72. Goh BT, Varia KB, Ayliffe PF, et al: Diagnosis of gonorrhea by gram-stained smears and cultures in men and women: role of the urethral smear. *Sex Transm Dis* 1985; 135–138.
73. Limberger RJ, Biega R, Evancoe A, et al: Evaluation of culture and the gen-probe PACE2 assay for detection of *Neisseria gonorrhoeae* and *Chlamydia trachomatis* in endocervical specimens transported to a state health laboratory. *J Clin Micro* 1992; 30:1162–1166.
74. Panke ES, Yang LI, Leist PA, et al: Comparison of Gen-Probe DNA probe test and culture for the detection of *Neisseria gonorrhoeae* in endocervical specimens. *J Clin Micro* 1991; 29:883–888.
75. Schwarcz SK, Zenilman JM, Schnell D, et al: National surveillance of antimicrobial resistance in *Neisseria gonorrhoeae. JAMA* 1990; 264:1413–1417.
76. Centers for Disease Control: Plasmid-mediated antimicrobial resistance in *Neisseria gonorrhoeae*—United States, 1988 and 1989. *MMWR* 1990; 39:284–287.
77. Wagenvoort JHT, van der Willigen AH, van Vliet HJA, et al: Resistance of *Neisseria gonorrhoeae* to enoxcin. *J Antimicro Agents Chemother* 1986; 18:429.
78. Turner A, Jephcott AE, Gough KR: Laboratory detection of ciprofloxacin resistant *Neisseria gonorrhoeae. J Clin Pathol* 1991; 44:169–170.
79. Young H, Moyes A, Tait IB, et al: Non-typable quinolone-resistant gonococci. *Lancet* 1990; 10:604.
80. Yeung KH, Dillon JR: Norfloxacin resistant *Neisseria gonorrhoeae* in North America. *Lancet* 1991; 336:759.
81. Handsfield HH, McCormack WM, Hook EW, III, et al: A comparison of single-dose cefixime with ceftriaxone as treatment for uncomplicated gonorrhea. *N Engl J Med* 1991; 325:1337–1341.
82. Bryan JP, Hira SK, Brady W, et al: Oral ciprofloxacin vs. ceftriaxone for the treatment of urethritis from resistant N. gonorrhoeae in Zambia. *Antimicro Agents Chemother* 1990; 34:819–822.
83. Smith BL, Cummings MC, Covino JM, et al: Evaluation of ofloxacin in the treatment of uncomplicated gonorrhea. *Sex Transm Dis* 1991; 18:18–20.
84. Loo PS, Ridgway GL, Oriel JD: Single dose ciprofloxacin for treating gonococcal infections in men. *Genitourin Med* 1985; 61:302–305.
85. Hooper DC, Wolfson JS: Fluoroquinolone antimicrobial agents. *N Engl J Med* 1991; 324:384–394.
86. Davis H, McGoodwin E, Reed TG: Anaphylactoid reactions reported after treatment with ciprofloxacin. *Ann Intern Med* 1989; 111:1041–1044.
87. Washington AE, Browner Ws, Korenbrot CC: Cost-effectiveness of combined treatment for endocervical gonorrhea: considering co-infection with *Chlamydia trachomatis. JAMA* 1987; 257:2056–2060.

88. Zenilman JM: Therapy of disseminated gonococcal infection, in Kass EH, Platt R (eds): *Current Therapy of Infectious Diseases*. Toronto, BC Decker, 1990.
89. Eschenback D, Harnisch JP, Holmes KK: Pathogenesis of acute pelvic inflammatory diseases: role of contraception and other risk factors. *Am J Obstet Gynecol* 1977; 128:838–850.
90. Sellors JW, Mahoney JB, Goldsmith C, et al: The diagnosis of pelvic inflammatory disease (PID): The accuracy of clinical and laparoscopic findings (abstract). *Inter Society STD Research* Sept, 1989.
91. Svennsson L, Westrom L, Ripa KT, et al: Differences in some clinical and laboratory parameters in acute salpingitis related to culture and serological findings. *Am J Obstet Gyn* 1980; 138:1017–1021.
92. Sweet RL, Mills J, Hadley KW, et al: Use of laparoscopy to determine the microbiologic etiology of acute salpingitis. *Am J Obstet Gynecol* 1979; 134:68–74.
93. Soper DE, Brockwell NJ, Dalton HP: False-positive cultures of the cul-de-sac associated with culdocentesis in patients undergoing elective laparoscopy. *Obstet Gynecol* 1991; 77:134–138.
94. Kiviat NB, Wolner-Hassen P, Eschenbach DA, et al: Endometrial histopathology in patients with culture-proven upper genital tract infection and laparoscopically diagnosed acute salpingitis. *Am J Surg Pathol* 1990; 14:167–175.
95. Paavonnen J, Aine R, Teisala K, et al: Comparison of endometrial biopsy and peritoneal fluid cytologic testing with laparoscopy in the diagnosis of acute pelvic inflammatory disease. *Am J Obstet Gynecol* 1985; 151:645–650.
96. Rosenfeld DL, Seidman SM, Bronsen RA, et al: Unsuspected chronic pelvic inflammatory disease in the infertile female. *Fertil Steril* 1983; 39:44–48.
97. Jones RB, Ardery BP, Hui SL, et al: Correlation between serum antichlamydial antibodies and tubal factor as a cause of infertility. *Fertil Steril* 1982; 38:553–557.
98. Gump DW, Gibson M, Ashikaga T: Evidence of prior pelvic inflammatory disease and its relationship to *Chlamydia trachomatis* antibody and intrauterine contraceptive device use in infertile women. *Am J Obstet Gynecol* 1983; 146:153–159.
99. Henry-Suchet J, Utzmann C, DeBrux J, et al: Microbiologic study of chronic inflammation associated with tubal factor infertility: role of *Chlamydia trachomatis*. *Fertil Steril* 1987; 47:274–277.
100. Senanayake P, Kramer DG: Contraception and the etiology of PID: New perspectives. *Am J Obstet Gynecol* 1980; 138:852.
101. Tuffrey M, Taylor-Robinson D: Progesterone as a key factor in the development of a mouse model for genital infection with *Chlamydia trachomatis*. *FEBS Lett* 1981; 12:111–115.
102. Ryden G, Fahraeus L, Molin L, et al: Do contraceptives influence the incidence of acute pelvic inflammatory disease in women with gonorrhea? *Contraception* 1979; 20:149–157.
103. Salit IE: The differential susceptibility of gonococcal opacity variants to sex hormones. *Can J Microbiol* 1982; 28:301–306.
104. Shafer M-A, Beck A, Blain B, et al: *Chlamydia trachomatis:* Important relationships to race, contraception, lower genital tract infection, and Papanicolaou smear. *J Pediatr* 1984; 104:141–146.
105. Rank RG, Barron AL: Prolonged genital infection by GPIC agent associated with immunosuppression following treatment with estradiol, in Mardh PA,

Holmes KK, Oreil JD, et al (eds): *Chlamydia Infections*. Amsterdam, Elsevier Biomedical Press, 1982, pp 391–394.

106. Morrison RP, Lyng K, Caldwell HD: Chlamydial disease pathogenesis: Ocular hypersensitivity elicited by a genus-specific 57 kD protein. *J Exp Med* 1989; 169:663–675.
107. Patton DL, Halbert SA, Kuo CC, et al: Host response to primary *Chlamydia trachomatis* infection of the fallopian tube in pig-tailed monkeys. *Fertil Steril* 1983; 40:829–840.
108. Patton DL, Kuo CC: Histopathology of *Chlamydia trachomatis* salpingitis after primary and repeated reinfections in the monkey subcutaneous pocket model. *J Reprod Fert* 1989; 85:647–656.
109. Patton DL, Kuo CC, Wang SP, et al: Distal obstruction induced by repeated *Chlamydia trachomatis* salpingeal infections in pig-tailed macaques. *J Infect Dis* 1987; 155:1292–1299.
110. Patton DL, Landers DV, Schachter J: Experimental *Chlamydia trachomatis* salpingitis in mice: Initial studies on the characterization of the leukocyte response to chlamydial infection. *J Infect Dis* 1989; 159:1105–1110.
111. Aaran RK, Lehtinen M, Kallionoemi OP, et al: Serum Ca 125 and TAT1 levels in inpatients and outpatients with pelvic inflammatory disease (abstract). *Inter Society for STD Res* Sept, 1989.
112. Crombleholme WR, Schachter J, Ohm-Smith M, et al: Efficacy of single-agent therapy for the treatment of acute pelvic inflammatory disease with ciprofloxacin. *Am J Med* 1989; 87 (suppl 5):142s–147s.
113. Crombleholme W, Landers D, Ohm-Smith M, et al: Sulbactam/ampicillin versus metronidazole/gentamicin in the treatment of severe pelvic infections. *Drugs* 1986; 3(suppl 2):11–13.
114. Dodson M, Faro S, Gentry LO: Treatment of acute pelvic inflammatory disease with aztreonam, a new monocyclic beta-lactam antibiotic, and clindamycin. *Obstet Gynecol* 1986; 67:657–662.
115. Faro S, Martens MG, Philips LE, et al: Ceftizoxime versus cefotaxime in the treatment of hospitalized patients with pelvic inflammatory disease. *Curr Ther Res* 1988; 43:349–354.
116. Hook EW, III, Marra CM: Acquired syphilis in adults. *N Engl J Med* 1991; 326:1060–1069.
117. Hook EW, III, Roddy RE, Lukehart SA, et al: Detection of *Treponema pallidum* in lesion exudate with a pathogen-specific monoclonal antibody. *J Clin Micro* 1985; 22:241–244.
118. Grimprel E, Sanchez PJ, Wendel GD, et al: Use of polymerase chain reaction and rabbit infectivity testing to detect *Treponema pallidum* in amniotic fluid, fetal and neonatal sera, and cerebrospinal fluid. *J Clin Micro* 1991; 29:1711–1718.
119. Lukehart SA, Hook EW, Baker-Zander SA, et al: Invasion of the central nervous system by *Treponema pallidum:* implications for diagnosis and treatment. *Ann Intern Med* 1988; 109:855–862.
120. Hook EW: Syphilis and HIV infection. *J Infect Dis* 1989; 160:530–534.
121. Haas JS, Bolan G, Larsen SA, et al: Sensitivity of treponemal tests for detecting prior treated syphilis during human immunodeficiency virus infection. *J Infect Dis* 1990; 162:862–866.
122. Hicks CB, Benson PM, Lupton GP, et al: Seronegative secondary syphilis in a patient infected with the human immunodeficiency virus (HIV) with Kaposi sarcoma. *Ann Intern Med* 1987; 107:492–495.

123. Romanowski B, Sutherland R, Fick GH, et al: Serologic response to treatment of infectious syphilis. *Ann Intern Med* 1991; 114:1005–1009.
124. Lefevre JC, Bertrand MA, Bauriard R: Evaluation of the captia enzyme immunassays for detection of immunoglobulins G and M to *Treponema pallidum* in syphilis. *J Clin Micro* 1990; 28:1704–1707.
125. Musher D, Hainill RJ, Baughn RE: Effect of human immunodeficiency virus infection on the course of syphilis and on the response to treatment. *Ann Intern Med* 1990; 113:872–881.
126. Radolf JD, Kaplan R: Unusual manifestations of secondary syphilis and abnormal humoral immune response to *Treponema pallidum* antigens in a homosexual man with asymptomatic human immunodeficiency virus infection. *J Am Acad Dermatol* 1988; 18:423–428.
127. Katz DA, Berger JR: Neurosyphilis in acquired immunodeficiency syndrome. *Arch Neurol* 1989; 46:895–898.
128. McLeish WM, Pulido JS, Holland S, et al: The ocular manifestations of syphilis in the human immunodeficiency virus type 1-infected host. *Ophthalmology* 1990; 97:196–203.
129. Johns DR, Tierney M, Felsenstein D: Alteration in the natural history of neurosyphilis by concurrent infection with the human immunodeficiency virus. *N Engl J Med* 1987; 316:1569–1572.
130. Hutchinson CM, Rompalo AM, Reichart CA, et al: Characteristics of patients with syphilis attending Baltimore STD clinics. *Arch Intern Med* 1991; 151:511–516.
131. Johnson PDR, Graves SR, Stewart L, et al: Specific syphilis serological tests may become negative in HIV infection. *AIDS* 1991; 5:419–423.
132. Berry CD, Hooton TM, Collier AC, et al: Neurologic relapse after benzathine penicillin therapy for secondary syphilis in a patient with HIV infection. *N Engl J Med* 1987; 316:1587–1590.
133. Campion MJ: Increased risk of cervical neoplasia in the consorts of men with penile condylomata. *Lancet* 1985; i:943–946.
134. Durst M, Kleinheinz A, Hotz M, et al: The physical state of human papillomavirus type 16 DNA in benign and malignant genital tumors. *J Gen Virol* 1985; 66:1515–1522.
135. McCance DJ, Kalache A, Ashdown K, et al: Human papillomavirus types 16 and 18 in carcinomas of the penis from Brazil. *Int J Cancer* 1986; 37:55–59.
136. Gupta J, Pilotti S, Rilke F, et al: Association of human papillomavirus type 16 with neoplastic lesions of the vulva and other genital sites by in situ hybridization. *Am J Pathol* 1987; 127:206–215.
137. Reeves WC, Brinton LA, Garcia M, et al: Human papillomavirus infection and cervical cancer in Latin America. *N Engl J Med* 1989; 320:1437–1441.
138. Mitchell H, Drake M, Medley G: Prospective evaluation of risk of cervical cancer after cytological evidence of human papillomavirus infection. *Lancet* 1986; 1:573–577.
139. de Villiers E-M, Wagner D, Schneider A, et al: Human papillomavirus infections in women with and without abnormal cervical cytology. *Lancet* 1987; ii:703–706.
140. Centers for Disease Control: Risk for cervical disease in HIV-infected women—New York City. *MMWR* 1990; 39:846–849.
141. Feingold AR, Vermund SH, Burk RD, et al: Cervical cytologic abnormalities and papillomavirus in women infected with human immunodeficiency virus. *J Acquir Immun Defic Syndr* 1990; 3:896–903.

142. Daling JR, Weiss NS, Hislop TG, et al: Sexual practices, sexually transmitted diseases, and the incidence of anal cancer. *N Engl J Med* 1987; 317:973–977.
143. Shah KV, Howley PM: Papillomaviruses, in Fields B, et al (eds): *Virology*. New York, Raven Press, 1990; pp 1625–1650.
144. de Villiers E-M: Heterogeneity of the human papillomavirus group. *J Virol* 1989; 63:4898–4903.
145. Beckmann AM, Myerson D, Daling JR, et al: Detection and localization of human papillomavirus DNA in human genital condylomas by in situ hybridization with biotinylated probes. *J Med Virol* 1985; 16:265–273.
146. Wagner D, Ikenberg H, Boehm N, et al: Identification of human papillomavirus in cervical swabs by deoxyribonucleic acid in situ hybridization. *Obstet Gynecol* 1984; 64:767–772.
147. Human papillomaviruses and the polymerase chain reaction (editorial). *Lancet* 1989; 1051.
148. Bashi SA: Cryotherapy versus podophyllin in the treatment of genital warts. *Int J Dermatol* 1985; 24:535–536.
149. Benedet JL, Miller DM, Nickerson KG, et al: The results of cryosurgical treatment of cervical intraepithelial neoplasia at one, five and ten yeras. *Am J Obstet Gynecol* 1987; 157:268–273.
150. Beutner KR, Conant MA, Friedman-Kien AE, et al: Patient-applied podofilox for treatment of genital warts. *Lancet* 1989; 831–833.
151. Breinig MK, Kingsley LA, Armstrong JA, et al: Epidemiology of genital herpes in Pittsburgh: serologic, sexual, and racial correlates of apparent and inapparent herpes simplex infections. *J Infect Dis* 1990; 162:299–305.
152. Koutsky LA, Ashley RL, Holmes KK, et al: The frequency of unrecognized type 2 herpes simplex virus infection among women. *Sex Trans Dis* 1990; 17:90–94.
153. Siegel D, Golden E, Washington E, et al: Prevalence and correlates of herpes simplex infections: the population-based AIDS in multiethnic neighborhoods study. *JAMA* 1992; 268:1702–1708.
154. Koutsky LA, Stevens CE, Holmes KK, et al: Underdiagnosis of genital herpes by current clinical and viral-isolation procedures. *N Engl J Med* 1992; 326:1533–1599.
155. Brock BV, Selke S, Benedetti J, et al: Frequency of asymptomatic shedding of herpes simplex virus in women with genital herpes. *JAMA* 1990; 263:418–420.
156. Koelle DM, Benedetti J, Langenberg A, et al: Asymptomatic reactivation of herpes simplex virus in women after the first episode of genital herpes. *Ann Intern Med* 1992; 116:433–437.
157. Langenberg A, Benedetti J, Jenkins J, et al: Development of clinically recognizable genital lesions among women previously identified as having "asymptomatic" herpes simplex virus type 2 infection. *Ann Intern Med* 1989; 110:882–887.
158. Mertz GJ, Benedetti J, Ashley R, et al: Risk factors for the sexual transmission of genital herpes. *Ann Intern Med* 1991; 116:197–202.
159. Johnson RE, Nahmias AJ, Magder LS, et al: A seroepidemiologic survey of the prevalence of herpes simplex virus type 2 infection in the United States. *N Engl J Med* 1989; 321:7–12.
160. Prober CG, Sullender WM, Yasukawa LL, et al: Low risk of herpes simplex virus infections in neonates exposed to the virus at the time of vaginal deliv-

ery to mothers with recurrent genital herpes simplex virus infections. *N Engl J Med* 1987; 316:240–244.
161. Brown ZA, Vontver LA, Benedetti J, et al: Effects on infants of a first episode of genital herpes during pregnancy. *N Engl J Med* 1987; 317:1246–1251.
162. Kulhanjian JA, Sourish V, Au DS, et al: Identification of women at unsuspected risk of primary infection with herpes simplex virus type 2 during pregnancy. *N Engl J Med* 1992; 326:916–920.
163. Whitley RJ, Gnann JW: Acyclovir: a decade later. *N Engl J Med* 1992; 327:782–789.
164. Brown ZA, Baker DA: Acyclovir therapy during pregnancy. *Obstet Gynecol* 1989; 73:526–531.
165. Yamamoto LJ, Tedder DG, Ashley R, et al: Herpes simplex virus type 1 DNA in cerebrospinal fluid of a patient with Mollaret's meningitis. *N Engl J Med* 1991; 325:1082–1085.
166. Ashley R, Cent A, Maggs V, et al: Inability of enzyme immunoassays to discriminate between infections with herpes simplex virus types 1 and 2. *Ann Interm Med* 1991; 115:520–526.
167. Kaplowitz L, Baker D, Gelb L, et al: Prolonged continuous acyclovir treatment of normal adults with frequently recurring genital herpes simplex virus infection. *JAMA* 1991; 275:747–751.
168. Lehrman SN, Douglas JM, Corey L, et al: Recurrent genital herpes and suppressive oral acyclovir therapy. *Ann Intern Med* 1986; 104:786–790.
169. Mertz GJ, Jones CC, Mills J, et al: Long-term acyclovir suppression of frequently recurring genital herpes simplex virus infection. *JAMA* 1988; 260:201–206.
170. Erlich KS, Mills J, Chatis P, et al: Acyclovir-resistant herpes simplex virus infections in patients with the acquired immunodeficiency syndrome. *N Engl J Med* 1989; 320:293–296.
171. Chatis PA, Crumpacker CS: Resistance of herpes viruses to antiviral drugs. *Antimicrob Agents Chemother* 1992; 36:1589–1595.
172. Bevilacqua F, Marcello A, Toni M, et al: Acyclovir resistance/susceptibility in herpes simplex virus type 2 sequential isolates from an AIDS patient. *J Acquir Immun Defic Syndr* 1991; 4:967–969.
173. Centers for Disease Control: Hepatitis B virus: a comprehensive strategy for eliminating transmission in the United States through universal childhood vaccination. *MMWR* 1991; 40 (No. RR-13):1–25.
174. Szmuness W, Much I, Prince AM, et al: On the role of sexual behavior in the spread of hepatitis B infection. *Ann Intern Med* 1975; 83:489–495.
175. Kryger P, Pedersen NS, Mathiesen LR, et al: Increased risk of infection with hepatitis A and B viruses in men with a history of syphilis: relation to sexual contacts. *J Infect Dis* 1982; 145:23–26.
176. Schreeder MT, Thompson SE, Hadler SC, et al: Hepatitis B in homosexual men: Prevalence of infection and factors related to transmission. *J Infect Dis* 1992; 146:7–15.
177. Rosenblum LS, Hadler SC, Castro KG, et al: Heterosexual transmission of hepatitis B virus in Belle Glade, Florida. *J Infect Dis* 1990; 161:407–411.
178. Centers for Disease Control: Changing patterns of groups at high risk for hepatitis B in the United States. *MMWR* 1988; 37 (28):429–438.
179. Shapiro CN, Margolis HS: Hepatitis B epidemiology and prevention. *Epidemiologic Reviews* 1990; 12:221.
180. Osmond DH, Padian NS, Sheppard HW, et al: Risk factors for hepatitis C virus seropositivity in heterosexual couples. *JAMA* 1993; 269:361–365.

181. Weinstock HS, Bolan G, Reingold AL, et al: Hepatitis C virus infection among patients attending a clinic for sexually transmitted diseases. *JAMA* 1993; 269:392–394.
182. Jonas MM, Schiff ER, O'Sullivan MJ, et al: Failure of Centers for Disease Control criteria to identify hepatitis B infection in a large municipal obstetrical population. *Ann Intern Med* 1987; 107:335–337.
183. Aach RD, Stevens CE, Hollinger FB, et al: Hepatitis C virus infection in post-transfusion hepatitis. *N Engl J Med* 1991; 325:1325–1329.
184. Pereira BJG, Milford EL, Kirkman RL, et al: Transmission of hepatitis C virus by organ transplantation. *N Engl J Med* 1991; 325:454–460.
185. Pereira BJG, Milford EL, Kirkman RL, et al: Prevalence of hepatitis C virus RNA in organ donors positive for hepatitis C antibody and in the recipients of their organs. *N Engl J Med* 1992; 327:910–915.
186. Kiyosawa K, Sodeyama T, Tanaka E, et al: Hepatitis C in hospital employees with needlestick injuries. *Ann Intern Med* 1991; 115:367–369.
187. Kaklamani E, Trichopoulos D, Tzonou A, et al: Hepatitis B and C viruses and their interaction in the origin of hepatocellular carcinoma. *JAMA* 1991; 265:1974–1976.
188. Everhart JE, Di Bisceglie AM, Murray LM, et al: Risk for non-A, non-B (type C) hepatitis through sexual or household contact with chronic carriers. *Ann Intern Med* 1990; 112:544–545.
189. Easmon CS, Hay PE, Ison CA: Bacterial vaginosis: a diagnostic approach. *Genitourin Med* 1992; 68:154–158.
190. Eschenback DA, Davick PR, William BL, et al: Prevalence of hydrogen peroxide-producing Lactobacillus species in normal women and women with bacterial vaginosis. *J Clin Microbiol* 1989; 27:251–256.
191. Spiegel CA: Vaginitis/Vaginosis. *Clin Lab Med* 1989; 9:525–533.
192. Amsel R, Toten PA, Spiegel CA, et al: Nonspecific vaginitis: Diagnostic criteria and microbial and epidemiological associations. *Am J Med* 1983; 74:14–22.
193. Taylor E, Blackwell AL, Barlow D, et al: *G. vaginalis,* anaerobes and vaginal discharge. *Lancet* 1982; 1:1376–1379.
194. Barbone FJ, Austin H, Lowe WC, et al: A follow-up study of methods of contraception, sexual activity, and rates of trichomoniasis, candidiasis, and bacterial vaginosis. *Am J Obstet Gynecol* 1990; 153:510–514.
195. Bhalla P, Rewald N, Chadha P: *Gardinella vaginalis* in CuT20 users. *Indian J Med Res* 1989; 89:80–86.
196. Wylie JG, Henderson A: Identity and glycogen-fermenting ability of lactobacilli isolated from the vagina of pregnant women. *J Med Microbiol* 1969; 2:363–366.
197. Larsen B, Galask RP: Vaginal microbial flora: composition and influence of host physiology. *Ann Intern Med* 1982; 96:926–930.
198. Skarin A, Sylwan F: Vaginal lactobacilli inhibition growth of *G. vaginalis, Mobiluncus* and other bacterial species cultured from vaginal content of women with bacterial vaginosis. *Acta Pathol Microbiol Immun Scand* 1987; 94:399–403.
199. Sobel JD, Cook RL: , in Horowitz, Mardh (eds): *Vaginitis and Vaginosis.* New York, Wiley-Liss, 1991, pp 46–53.
200. Hillier SI, Krohn MA, Klebanoff SJ, et al: The relationship of hydrogen peroxide-producing lactobacilli to bacterial vaginosis and genital microflora in pregnant women. *Obstet Gynecol* 1992; 79:369–373.

201. Thomason JL, Gelbart SM, Scaglione NJ: Bacterial vaginosis: current review with indications for asymptomatic therapy. *Am J Obstet Gyneco* 1991; 165:1210–1215.
202. Nugent RP, Krohn MA, Hillier SL: Reliability of diagnosing bacterial vaginosis is improved by a standardized method of gram stain interpretation. *J Clin Microbiol* 1991; 29:297–301.
203. Vejtorp M, Bollerup AC, Vejtorp L, et al: Bacterial vaginosis: a double-blind randomized trial of the effect of treatment of the sexual partner. *Br J Obstet Gynecol* 1988; 95:920–925.
204. Moi H, Erkkola R, Herve F, et al: Should male consorts of women with bacterial vaginosis be treated? *Genitourin Med* 1989; 65:253–258.
205. Jones B, Geary I, Alawattegama A, et al: In-vitro and in-vivo activity of metronidazole against *Gardinella vaginalis, Bacterioles spp.* and *Mobiluncus spp,* in bacterial vaginosis. *J Antimicrob Chemother* 1985; 16:189–197.
206. Swedberg J, Steiner JF, Deiss F, et al: Comparison of single-dose vs. one week course of metronidazole for symptomatic BV. *JAMA* 1985; 254:1046–1049.
207. Rein MF: *Trichomonas vaginalis,* in Mandel GL, Douglas RG, Jr., Bennett JE (eds): *Principles and Practice of Infectious Diseases.* New York, Churchill-Livingstone, 1990, pp 2115–2118.
208. Honigsberg BM: *Trichomonads parasitic in humans,* New York, Springer-Verlag, 1990, p 1.
209. Krieger JM, Tam MR, Stevens CE, et al: Diagnosis of trichomoniasis: comparison of conventional wet mount examination with cytolytic studies, cultures and monoclonal antibody staining of direct specimens. *JAMA* 1988; 259:1223–1227.
210. Yule A, Gellan MA, Driel JD, et al: Detection of *Trichomonas vaginalis* antigen in women by enzyme immunoassay. *J Clin Pathol* 1987; 40:566–568.
211. Watt RM, Philip A, Wos SM, et al: Rapid assay for immunological detection of *Trichomonas vaginalis. J Clin Microbiol* 1986; 24:551–555.
212. Carney JA, Unadkat P, Yule A, et al: A new rapid agglutination test for the diagnosis of *Trichomonas vaginalis* infection. *J Clin Pathol* 1988; 41:806–808.
213. Rein MF: Current therapy vulvovaginitis. *Sex Transm Dis* 1981; 8:316–320.
214. Lossick JG: Single dose metronidazole treatment for vaginal trichomoniasis. *Obstet Gynecol* 1980; 56:508–510.
215. Muller M, Lossick JG, Gorrell TE: In vitro susceptibility of *Trichomonas vaginalis* to metronidazole: treatment outcome in vaginal trichomoniasis. *Sex Transm Dis* 1988; 15:17–24.
216. Lossick JG, Muller M, Gorrell TE: In vitro drug susceptibility and doses of metronidazole required for cure in case of refractory vaginal trichomoniasis. *J Infect Dis* 1986; 153:948–955.
217. Wasserheit JN: Epidemiological synergy: interrelationships between human immunodeficiency virus infection and other sexually transmitted diseases. *Sex Trans Dis* 1992; 19:61–77.
218. Pepin J, Plummer FA, Brunham RC: The interaction of HIV infection and other sexually transmitted diseases: an opportunity for intervention. *AIDS* 1989; 3:3–9.
219. Plummer F, Cameron W, Simonsen N, et al: Cofactors in male-female transmission of HIV. *J Infect Dis* 1993, in press.
220. Laga M, Nzila N, Manoka AT, et al: High prevalence and incidence of HIV and other sexually transmitted diseases (STD) among 801 Kinshasa prosti-

tutes (abstract). *Fifth International Conference on AIDS, Montreal, Canada,* June 1989:ThAO 21.

221. Kreiss JK, Coombs R, Plummer F, et al: Isolation of human immunodeficiency virus from genital ulcers in Nairobi prostitutes. *J Infect Dis* 1989; 160:380–384.
222. Cameron DW, Plummer FA, D'Costa L, et al: Female to male transmission of human immunodeficiency virus type 1: Risk factors for seroconversion in men. *Lancet* 1989; ii:403–407.
223. Erlich KS, Jacobson MA, Koehler JE, et al: Foscarnet therapy for severe acyclovir-resistant herpes simplex virus type-2 infections in patients with the acquired immunodeficiency syndrome. *Ann Intern Med* 1989; 110:710–713.
224. Maiman M, Fruchter RG, Serur E, et al: Human immunodeficiency virus infection and cervical neoplasia. *Gynecol Oncol* 1990; 38:377–382.
225. Rolfs RT, Goldberg M, Sharrar RG: Risk factors for syphilis: cocaine use and prostitution. *Amer J Public Health* 1990; 80:853–857.
226. Schwarcz SK, Bolan GA, Fullilove M, et al: Crack cocaine and the exchange of sex for money or drugs. *Sex Trans Dis* 1992; 19:7–13.
227. Centers for Disease Control: HIV instruction and selected HIV-risk behaviors among high school students—U.S., 1989–91. *MMWR* 1992; 41:866–868.
228. Centers for Disease Control: Drug use and sexual behaviors among sex partners of injecting drug users—United States, 1988–90. *MMWR* 1991; 40:855–860.
229. Zenilman JM, Erickson B, Fox R, et al: Effect of HIV posttest counseling on STD incidence. *JAMA* 1992; 267:843–845.
230. Calsyn DA, Saxon AJ, Freeman G, Jr, et al: Ineffectiveness of AIDS education and HIV antibody testing in reducing high-risk behaviors among injection drug users. *Am J Public Health* 1992; 82:573–575.

Approach to the Patient With Rheumatoid Arthritis

Andrea T. Slotkoff, M.D.

Post Doctoral Fellow, Division of Rheumatology, Immunology and Allergy, Department of Medicine, Georgetown University Medical Center, Washington, D.C.

Paul Katz, M.D.

Professor and Vice Chairman, Department of Medicine, Chief, Division of Rheumatology, Immunology and Allergy, Georgetown University Medical Center, Washington, D.C.

Rheumatoid arthritis (RA), the prototype chronic inflammatory polyarthropathy in man, is worldwide in distribution. Women are disproportionately affected, with a threefold increase in prevalence. Although RA is most common in young to middle-aged adults, the development of disease after the age of 60 is not infrequently seen. This disease in individuals less than 16 years of age has been referred to as juvenile RA, although the similarities to the adult form are considerable.

Most problematic in the approach to this disease is therapy. As will be described, the diagnosis is generally not elusive; once the diagnosis of RA is established, this arthropathy must be treated.

Complicating the therapeutic approach to RA is the heterogeneity of this disease and the variability in disease course. Nonetheless, most patients do develop some degree of joint destruction and dysfunction. Further confounding treatment is the uncertainty about the efficacy of drug treatment. As we will outline in this chapter, considerable controversy exists about which medications should be used, when these agents should be employed, and what regimens should be utilized. Thus, there is considerable overlap between the art and science of the treatment of this disease.

We intend to present a broad-based approach to the patient with RA, initially concentrating on pathogenesis and diagnosis, but with particular emphasis on our existing knowledge regarding drug therapy. The readers should understand, however, that the treatment of RA is in evolution; as new drugs are developed and as new protocols using existing agents are employed, it is likely that therapy will change. At the present time, there is no "correct" way to treat RA. What follows is what we believe to be a rational therapeutic assessment.

Pathogenesis

The characteristic feature of RA is chronic polyarticular inflammation. Intensive research has been conducted in recent years to identify the factors that initiate and perpetuate this inflammatory response. Further clarification of the etiology, immunogenetics, and immunopathology of RA will be critical for the development of newer, more effective therapies. Although important pieces of the puzzle are still missing, the combined data provide a framework for our current understanding of the pathogenesis of RA. As in-depth analysis of the pathogenesis of RA is beyond the scope of this work, the reader is referred to excellent reviews.[1–6]

The primary cause of RA is unknown. It is thought to be triggered by the presence of an as yet unidentified antigen(s) in an immunogenetically susceptible host; the nature of the antigen responsible for the arthritic reaction in RA has yet to be clearly established. Both endogenous and exogenous agents have been proposed as potential antigenic stimuli.

Etiology

Infectious agents as possible exogenous causes of RA have been studied extensively. Although a variety of organisms, including human T-cell leukemia virus-1, rubella virus, cytomegalovirus, herpesvirus, and parvovirus have been implicated as possible pathogenic antigens, the evidence to support their role in the pathogenesis of RA is indirect and inconclusive.

Attention has been focused on Epstein-Barr virus (EBV) since the late 1970s, when EBV-associated cellular and humoral abnormalities were described in RA patients. The number of circulating B cells infected with EBV was increased, and the cytotoxic T-cell response to EBV was reduced in RA patients. EBV is known to induce a polyclonal B-cell response, often including the production of rheumatoid factor. Up to 80% of patients have antibodies to an EBV-associated antigen. However, further studies revealed that these immunologic changes were neither disease nor virus specific. In addition, circulating EBV antigens were not elevated early in the disease process, suggesting that EBV infection is not a primary cause of RA. Rather, RA may occur as the result of disordered immune regulation from another cause, leading to poor handling of the virus.

Renewed enthusiasm emerged for associating EBV and RA with the discovery that sequences of amino acids from the viral capsid of EBV (glycoprotein 110) were essentially identical to the region of HLA-DR Class II molecules responsible for genetic susceptibility to RA.[7] This molecular mimicry raises the possibility that T-cell recognition of EBV gp110 in patients with HLA susceptibility may induce or amplify the inflammatory response in RA.[8, 9] Similarities found between Epstein-Barr nuclear antigen (EBNA) protein sequences and type II collagen sequences may also play a theoretical pathogenic role by provoking anticollagen autoimmunity. Yet another intriguing mechanism of disease may be that molecular mimicry between EBV and host Class II molecules leads to immune tolerance of the virus that has been perceived as a self-antigen. This in turn allows the infection to persist and chronic inflammation to develop.

Mycobacteria have long been suspected to be pathogenic agents in RA. Since the early 1980s, observations that link these organisms with RA have been recognized. Patients with RA have a defect in IgG glycosylation that renders the immunoglobulin more adherent, possibly contributing to immune complex formation. However, this agalactosyl IgG is present in patients with tuberculosis, and the phenomenon is nonspecific, having been described in other inflammatory diseases, such as Crohn's disease and systemic lupus erythematosus (SLE).

Heat-shock proteins, located on the cell surface of mycobacteria, can induce adjuvant arthritis in Lewis rats, the animal model often used to study RA. These arthritogenic proteins are homologous to heat-shock proteins found in humans. Elevated levels of antibodies directed against, and T-cell receptors specific for, mycobacteria heat-shock proteins have been described in RA patients. The concept of molecular mimicry has been applied to hypothesize that cross-reactivity between mycobacterial heat-shock proteins and synovial heat-shock proteins may result in the development of RA. Once again, the evidence to support mycobacteria as etiologic agents is weak, since heat-shock proteins from many animals and bacteria are homologous.

Investigations of possible endogenous antigens have most frequently included type II collagen and rheumatoid factors. Type II collagen administration produces a RA model in rats. Although arthritis in mice has been produced by injection of anticollagen antibodies, and although elevated levels of antibodies to both native and denatured collagen are present in RA patients, the data have yet to support an etiologic role in humans. Current opinion is that anticollagen antibodies are a secondary immune response to degraded collagen; and since these antibodies form immune complexes within the synovium, they augment the invasive inflammatory process.

Rheumatoid factors (RF) are antibodies, usually IgM, directed against the Fc portion of IgG. These form the basis of the humoral autoimmune response in RA by creating immune complexes that activate the complement system, enhance cytokine release, and lead to inflammation. However, the stimulus for RF production is still unclear, and further study of potential viral stimuli, as well as immunogenetic causes, needs to be conducted before the role of RF in the pathogenesis of RA is fully understood.

Immunogenetics

The possible influence of genetics on RA has been underscored with the discovery of an increased incidence of HLA-DR4 expression in RA patients compared to normal populations. The HLA subregion D of chromosome 6, which includes DR, DQ, and DP alleles, is the gene locus for Class II molecules. These molecules, located on antigen-presenting cells (mainly macrophages, but also fibroblasts, B-lymphocytes, and endothelial cells), present processed antigen to T-lymphocytes. Antigen is engulfed by the cell and digested into smaller peptides; the peptides are then bound within a groove in the Class II molecule on the antigen-presenting cell surface for T-cell receptor recognition. The binding of antigen peptide to Class II molecules is allele-specific; that is, not all Class II molecules will bind all antigens. The specificity of peptide binding is determined by the Class II α and β chains that possess allelic hypervariability. The third hypervariable region of the β-1 chain contains a sequence of amino acids at positions 70-74 that is found in three subgroups of HLA-DR4 (DRw4, DRw14, and DRw15) known to confer genetic susceptibility. Two other subgroups—DRw10 and DRw13—do not have this amino acid sequence, and have not been associated with RA. All of the HLA Class II molecules associated with RA, including others such as DR1 and Dw6Dw16, share the same amino acid sequence in the third hypervariable region. The "shared epitopes" hypothesis combines these observations to state that equivalent structural features found in a variety of HLA-DR alleles are responsible for immunogenetic susceptibility in RA.[10, 11] Thus, RA may occur when a patient with the requisite Class II molecules is exposed to one or more antigens capable of being processed by these molecules and subsequently recognized by T-cell receptors.

Immunopathology

Once antigen is processed and bound to the proper Class II molecules on the antigen-presenting cell, the resulting complex interacts with specific receptors located primarily on CD4+ helper T cells. T-cell receptor analysis has attempted to further characterize the T-cell response as oligoclonal, in the hope of demonstrating a selective activation by particular antigen/antigen-presenting cell complexes, but controversy over oligoclonality still remains. Following activation, the T-cell manufactures a number of cytokines, small hormone-like proteins that allow intercellular communication and modulation. These are produced by macrophage and fibroblasts as well. Interestingly, cytokines of T-cell origin (interleukin-2, interleukin-3, interleukin-4, and interferon-γ) are found in lower concentrations in the synovial membrane than those from macrophages and fibroblasts (interleukin-1, interleukin-6, colony-stimulating factor-1, and tumor necrosis factor-α) despite the prominent role T cells are thought to play in synovial inflammation.[12] Hypotheses to explain this incongruity conjecture that macrophage cytokines suppress the expression of T-cell cytokines, and that only a limited number of antigen-specific T-cell products are required for initiating and perpetuating synovitis.[13] Regardless of which cell(s) figures more prominently in the process, the net effect of cytokine production in the synovium is inflammation. Further discussion of specific cytokines and their relation to newer therapies will follow.

T-cell and macrophage activation and subsequent cytokine production lead to endothelial cell proliferation within the synovium. Endothelial cell metalloproteinases assist in this invasion. Adhesion of lymphocytes and neutrophils to the newly formed capillaries is mediated by a number of factors including macrophage cytokines, homing receptors on T-cells, addressins on endothelial cells, and CD18 on the cell surface of neutrophils. B-cells proliferate in response to T-cell activation, and differentiate to produce RF. In addition to its other properties described above, RF complexes may precipitate on the synovial membrane promoting local destruction.

The events leading to the clinical manifestations of RA are complex, and many aspects of the process remain a mystery. The underlying cause is likely to be attributed to a variety of pathogens capable of stimulating an immune response in a genetically susceptible host through the mechanisms described above. The importance of each cytokine involved in driving the chronic inflammation of RA continues to be an area of great interest for the development of new therapies targeted at selected aspects of the inflammatory response.

Basic Approach

Diagnosis

The diagnosis of RA is primarily based on clinical grounds, although laboratory, radiologic, and pathologic findings aid in the diagnosis. Typically, the early manifestations consist of the insidious onset of fatigue, malaise, and morning stiffness. Joint pain and swelling are usually polyarticular, occurring most commonly in the metacarpophalangeal (MCP) joints, proximal interphalangeal (PIP) joints, and wrists in a symmetric distribution. The initial presentation may be asymmetric or monoarticular. Distal interphalangeal (DIP) joints are rarely involved. Laboratory studies may reveal a mild anemia, leukocytosis, and thrombocytosis, as well as an elevated erythrocyte sedimentation rate (ESR) and C-reactive protein (CRP); these parameters are not diagnostic and reflect the ongoing inflammatory process. Radiographic changes range from juxtaarticular osteoporosis early in the disease to bony erosions, deformities, and ankylosis later in the process. The synovial histopathology in RA shows marked villous hypertrophy, synovial cell proliferation, lymphocyte infiltration, and fibrin deposition.

In the early stages, RA may resemble a variety of other diseases which should be considered in the differential diagnosis, since these may have very specific therapies (Table 1). The first criteria to confirm the diagnosis of RA were established in 1958 by the American Rheumatism Association (ARA) and were subsequently revised in 1987. These criteria have been utilized mainly for epidemiologic studies and not primarily for the diagnosis of individual cases. However, they do provide a useful guideline for the practitioner to categorize an inflammatory arthropathy as RA.

The 1987 revised ARA criteria were simplified to be less costly and easier to apply than the more rigorous 1958 ARA criteria, and they have main-

TABLE 1.
Differential Diagnosis of Rheumatoid Arthritis*

Seronegative spondyloarthropathy (ankylosing spondylitis, Reiters syndrome, psoriatic arthritis, enteropathic arthritis)
Crystal-induced arthropathy (gout, pseudogout)
Diffuse connective tissue disease (systemic lupus erythematosus, polymyositis, fibromyalgia)
Infectious arthritis
Osteoarthritis
Polymyalgia rheumatica
Reactive arthritis
Hemoglobinopathies
Hemachromatosis
Lyme disease
Malignancy
Thyroid disease
Hemophilic arthropathy
Hypertrophic osteoarthritis

*Adapted from Harris ED, Jr: Clinical Features of Rheumatoid Arthritis, in Kelly WN (ed): *Textbook of Rheumatology*. Philadelphia, W.B. Saunders Co; 1989; pp 943–981.

tained a relatively high degree of sensitivity and specificity (91%–94% and 89%, respectively).[14] The 1987 revised criteria no longer classify patients as classic, definite, or probable RA based on the number of criteria satisfied, and they no longer include criteria based on synovial fluid findings or synovial histopathology. The new criteria are reproduced in Table 2. At least four of the seven criteria, plus the presence of the first four symptoms for at least six weeks, are required for the diagnosis of RA.

General Management

RA is a heterogeneous disease affecting not only joints, but the well-being and general health of the patient. The clinical course of rheumatoid disease will differ; therefore, each treatment program should be individualized. No single therapeutic regimen is applicable to all patients. Although specific therapeutic interventions may vary, the overall goals of management should be to: (1) decrease pain and inflammation; (2) preserve function;

(3) minimize drug toxicities; (4) prevent disease progression; and (5) avoid unnecessary costs. RA impacts on every aspect of life and the approach to therapy should involve the collaboration of the patient with a team of health professionals working to address the physical, emotional, and financial needs of the patient.

It is now well recognized that RA has a significant effect on mortality as well as morbidity.[15] However, lack of consensus still exists on the ideal markers for predicting outcome or monitoring disease activity. A number of clinical and laboratory features have been associated with increased severity of disease. The presence of nodules and extraarticular manifestations predict a more aggressive clinical course. Seropositive patients with high titer RF also experience more disabling disease compared to their seronegative counterparts. In particular, elevated levels of IgA RF correlate with the occurrence of subsequent bony erosions.[16]

Measurement of disease activity is typically used to indicate response to therapy. The logic for using parameters of disease activity to guide therapy is based not only on the short term goal of of relieving pain, but on the assumption that disease activity correlates with future functional loss.[17] The traditional measures of disease activity—joint tenderness, grip strength, and acute phase reactants such as ESR and CRP—continue to be the most relevant markers.[18–20] Assessment of functional ability and psychosocial status using recently developed questionnaires—the Stanford Health Assessment Questionnaire (HAQ) and the Arthritis Impact Measurement Scales (AIMS)—have shown a correlation with disease activity as evaluated by other traditional methods.[21, 22] Additional laboratory measures have been associated with increased disease activity and a less favorable progression: elevated serum levels of the complement component

TABLE 2.
The 1987 Revised American Rheumatism Association Criteria for Rheumatoid Arthritis*

1. Morning stiffness lasting at least 1 hour.
2. Swelling of 3 or more joints.
3. Arthritis of hand joints.
4. Symmetric joint swelling.
5. Rheumatoid nodules.
6. Serum rheumatoid factor.
7. Radiographic changes.

*Adapted from Arnett FC, Edworthy S, Block DA, et al: The 1987 revised ARA criteria for rheumatoid arthritis. *Arthritis Rheum* 1988; 30:S17.

C1q,[23] elevated serum levels of soluble interleukin-2 receptor,[24] and HLA-DR4 positivity.[25] Experience with these newer laboratory markers of disease activity is limited, and their clinical utility has yet to be established.

Joint imaging is another standard method of evaluating disease activity and response to therapy. Although imperfect due to reader variability, laborious scoring methods, and potential lag time between active inflammation and radiologic deterioration, radiographs have shown correlation with other traditional measures of disease progression in many studies.[26] In the future, magnetic resonance imaging (MRI) and radionuclide studies may become effective tools for documenting early articular inflammation and destruction, but their use is not currently routine.

Predictors of mortality in RA have been reviewed extensively in the literature.[27, 28] Studies have described increased mortality in RA patients who are less than 50 years old, male, and have involvement of more than 30 joints. Patients with a lower level of education and socioeconomic class have an increased risk of early death.[27, 29, 30] Studies using questionnaires that reflect disability and general health (HAQ and AIMS) have confirmed the value of functional assessments in predicting outcome.[21, 31, 32]

Early in the disease, patient education can favorably influence outcome. The patient should be presented with realistic expectations about the process. Both the possibility of complete remission and the probability of repeated flares of disease over time should be reviewed. Patient compliance with treatment can be enhanced by discussion of and agreement on management goals.

Dietary adjustments have been popular for attempting to control disease. Only recently have efforts been made to determine the benefits of dietary elimination and supplementation therapy through controlled trials. Numerous foods have been implicated in the exacerbation of arthritic symptoms; refined cereals and grains, acidic foods, dairy products, red meats, coffee and sugar have been listed most often. Theories to explain the apparent association of these foods with worsening symptoms postulate that an underlying immune mechanism of food intolerance, an increased gastrointestinal permeability to offending antigens, and/or an alteration in gut flora may be involved.[33] Dietary supplementations with ω-3 fatty acids from fish oils and γ-linolenic acid from evening primrose oil have been proposed as a means to reduce inflammation.[34] These oils potentially divert the production of prostaglandins and leukotrienes to less inflammatory forms, and improvement in symptom have been demonstrated with their use.[35] Although consistent results from scientific studies are lacking, some evidence suggests a role for dietary manipulation in a subgroup of RA patients.[33]

Both rest and exercise requirements change with the onset of RA. Complete bedrest is usually unnecessary for the local management of joint inflammation, but daily naps and a restful sleep at night are recommended to offset fatigue. An exercise plan is important for maintaining muscle strength and mobility without damaging joints. Actively inflamed joints should be rested. Splinting of the knee or wrist for a short interval can reduce inflammation and increase function.[36] When disease activity subsides, exercise should progress from passive range of motion to active assisted range of motion and subsequently to more strenuous activities such as brisk walking or swimming as the patient improves.

Physical and occupational therapy provide important adjuncts to management. The physical therapist educates the patient on methods of minimizing strain on joints, assesses ability of the patient to do daily activities of living, and provides additional therapeutic modalities such as thermal treatment and hydrotherapy. The occupational therapist instructs on the use of assisted devices to compensate for loss of function; these can tremendously enhance a patient's independence. The social worker and counselor help meet psychosocial needs by furnishing information on community resources such as support groups, educational classes, and financial assistance.

First-Line Drug Therapy

Nonsteroidal Anti-inflammatory Drugs

Nonsteroidal anti-inflammatory drugs (NSAIDS) are the pharmacologic agents selected most often for the initial drug therapy of RA. Although salicylates have been used extensively with success over the years, NSAIDS have been shown to be as effective with fewer side effects. Their convenient dosing may enhance patient compliance, and the variety of preparations allows for more flexibility of choice when a particular NSAID is unsuccessful. Since the biochemistry, pharmacology, and dosages of individual preparations have been adequately reviewed elsewhere,[37] only those characteristics common to most NSAIDS will be discussed as they relate to the treatment of RA. Classification and dosing of the frequently used NSAIDS are provided in Table 3.

NSAIDS reduce the signs and symptoms of RA, but there is no evidence to show these agents alter the course of the disease.[38] A number of hypotheses have been proposed to explain their anti-inflammatory effects. NSAIDS decrease proinflammatory prostaglandin production by inhibiting cyclo-oxygenase (prostaglandin H synthase) in the arachidonic acid cascade. In the neutrophil, NSAIDS increase cyclic adenosine monophosphate (cAMP), limiting cellular functions such as migration, aggregation, and phagocytosis. NSAIDS have also been shown to alter lymphocyte and monocyte function.[39] In addition, platelet cyclo-oxygenase inhibition leads to diminished platelet aggregation, which can interfere with hemostasis.

As NSAIDS have become more widely utilized for a variety of rheumatic diseases including RA, their side effects have been increasingly well recognized. The inhibition of prostaglandins along with the acidic nature of most NSAIDS account for the majority of adverse reactions associated with these drugs. Chronic use of NSAIDS can cause considerable mortality and morbidity from gastrointestinal (GI) mucosal damage and bleeding.[40] This

TABLE 3.
Commonly Prescribed NSAIDs

Classification	Half Life, hr	Dosage Range, mg/day
Proprionic Acid		
Ibuprofen	2	1200–3200
Naproxen	13	250–1500
Fenoprofen	2	1200–3200
Ketoprofen	1.5	100–300
Oxaprozin	40	600–1800
Phenylacetic Acid		
Diclofenac	1.5	100–150
Indoleacetic Acid		
Indomethacin	3–11	50–200
Sulindac	16	300–400
Tolmetin	1–2	600–2000
Fenamate		
Meclofenamate	2–3	200–400
Oxicam		
Piroxicam	30–86	20

effect appears to be dose related. Ulcerations can appear de novo or as an exacerbation of previous peptic ulcer disease. Significant ulcers often remain asymptomatic until bleeding develops. The population of patients at particularly high risk of serious complications from ulcerations include older patients with a previous history of upper abdominal pain, peptic ulcer disease, NSAID GI-side effects, antacid or H_2 antagonist use, and possibly concomitant use of corticosteroids.[41] Currently, misoprostol is the only proved effective prophylaxis against GI mucosal damage. NSAIDS can decrease creatinine clearance by suppressing the vasodilatory function of renal prostaglandins, particularly in patients who are elderly or have impaired renal function. Occasionally, acute interstitial nephritis, the nephrotic syndrome, and renal papillary necrosis may develop, although it is unclear if these reactions are directly related to prostaglandin inhibition. Hepatocellular toxicity with mild transaminase elevations has been related to NSAIDS. Liver function tests usually return to normal with discontinuation of the drug; only rarely is hepatic dysfunction severe.

NSAIDS have the ability to interact with a number of other drugs causing significant toxicity.[42] Most NSAIDS are highly protein-bound and may displace other protein-bound drugs from their binding sites, increasing their plasma concentration and their pharmacologic effect. Warfarin, phenytoin, sulfonamides, methotrexate, and oral hypoglycemics are among the drugs potentially affected in this manner. NSAIDS may also decrease the renal clearance of methotrexate by competition for renal tubular excretion.

Individual responses to NSAID therapy vary greatly. Neither the effectiveness nor the toxicities can be predicted for every patient taking a specific NSAID. The choice of NSAID is empiric. The highest tolerated dose should be given for a minimum of 2 weeks before substituting another preparation. Combination therapy with multiple NSAIDS does not augment effectiveness and may add to toxicity. Although beneficial and safe in the majority of RA patients, NSAIDS should be used with caution and awareness of possible complications. As with all therapies for RA, these first-line agents should be monitored for effectiveness by the usual parameters. The error often made with NSAID therapy is the prolonged use of these agents alone despite apparent disease progression and the need for more effective treatment.

Corticosteroids

Since their initial use for RA over 40 years ago,[43] corticosteroids (CS) have remained an important adjunct to RA therapy. The original enthusiasm for the beneficial effects of these drugs in RA was modified when trials in the 1950s showed no clear arrest of disease progression.[44] Additionally, the hazards of chronic therapy became increasingly apparent. Questions still remain regarding the remittive nature of CS. Review of the earlier studies suggests that patients treated with prednisone develop fewer erosions than do those treated with aspirin or placebo.[45, 46] The lowest dose required for this effect is unknown and may be higher than that generally accepted for use in RA. As a result, the current application of CS therapy is for symptomatic relief of inflammation. It is considered "bridge therapy" between NSAIDS and second-line drugs and is useful for suppression of acute flares of disease.

Despite considerable clinical and laboratory experience with CS, the mechanisms of their activity are only partially defined. The immunosuppressive and anti-inflammatory action of CS derive from a combination of effects on leukocyte circulatory kinetics, cellular functions, and soluble mediators. CS-induced alterations in vascular permeability, neutrophil surface charge, bone marrow release, and circulatory half-life result in an absolute and relative neutrophilia. Temporary redistribution of lymphocytes (particularly CD4-positive T cells) and monocytes to extravascular sites precipitates a profound lymphopenia and monocytopenia. These changes occur maximally 4 to 6 hours after administration of CS and abate by 24 hours.

CS alter leukocyte function by regulating gene transcription through CS-cell receptor binding. T-cell proliferation, B-cell activation, and the bactericidal and fungicidal action of monocytes are suppressed in this manner. The cellular activity of neutrophils is relatively refractory to CS. CS restrict the production of T-cell and monocyte soluble mediators. In addition, CS block prostaglandin synthesis by induction of lipocortin antiphospholipase proteins, which inhibit arachidonic acid release from cell membranes.

These mechanisms, operating in variable degrees, explain most of the anti-inflammatory actions of CS.

The toxicities of CS therapy are myriad (Table 4). Side effects are usually dependent upon the dose and duration of therapy. Risk of infection increases with doses greater than 20 mg of prednisone per day or after a cumulative dose greater than 700 mg of prednisone.[47] Low-dose CS therapy (less than 10 mg of prednisone per day given as a single morning dose) diminishes the risk of infection and hypothalamic-pituitary-adrenal axis suppression compared to split doses or single evening doses. Osteoporosis, an important sequela of CS therapy, may occur unpredictably with even low-dose and alternate-day therapy. Although studies of preventive measures for osteoporosis are limited, empiric therapy with supplemental calcium and 25-hydroxy-vitamin D may be warranted during chronic CS treatment. Newer preparations of CS with less osteopenic effect are under current consideration by the Food and Drug Administration.

The goal of CS therapy is to maximize control of underlying disease while minimizing the likelihood of adverse reactions. In this regard, alterna-

TABLE 4.
Side Effects of Corticosteroids*

Cataracts (posterior subcapsular)
Glaucoma
Hypertension
Congestive heart failure in predisposed patients
Peptic ulcer disease
Pancreatitis
Cushingoid appearance (truncal obesity, moon facies)
Hyperglycemia
Secondary adrenal insufficiency
Electrolyte changes (sodium retention, hypokalemia)
Myopathy
Osteoporosis
Aseptic necrosis
Psychosis
Alterations in mood or personality
Pseudotumor cerebri
Thin fragile skin, ecchymoses

*Adapted from Axelrod L: Glucocorticoids, in Kelley WN (ed): *Textbook of Rheumatology*. Philadelphia, WB Saunders Co, 1989, p 852.

tive methods of CS administration have been explored. Although alternate-day therapy is associated with fewer side effects as mentioned, it does not prevent osteoporosis and usually is inadequate for controlling symptoms in RA. Large intermittent intravenous "pulse" doses of CS (1 g methylprednisolone) have gained popularity in a number of rheumatic conditions. Studies in patients with RA have shown a short-lived improvement in symptoms, but no impact on development of erosions.[48] Pulse CS therapy in combination with other agents has yielded mixed results.[49, 50] This mode of CS administration for RA is not without hazard and should be considered experimental at this time.

Intraarticular (IA) CS injections are useful for suppressing symptomatic synovitis. Deleterious effects of IA therapy are infrequent but include tendon rupture, systemic absorption, and rarely, septic arthritis. Since repeated injections may lead to joint damage, no more than four injections yearly at 3-month intervals is recommended.

Generally accepted guidelines for CS use in RA have emerged despite the aforementioned uncertainties. Low dose therapy with 5 to 7.5 mg of prednisone as a single morning dose is the preferred regimen for patients with severe and persistent symptoms in whom NSAIDS have been ineffective. The older, seronegative RA patient may be particularly responsive to CS, and may experience fewer serious side effects with this regimen than with NSAIDS.[51] Upon initiating CS therapy, the duration of therapy, the use of additional agents, and a tapering schedule must be considered. A slow taper, approximately 1-mg decrements every 3 weeks, usually circumvents the acute flares seen with the abrupt cessation of as little as 5 mg per day of prednisone.

Second-Line Therapy

Once the determination is made that therapy with NSAIDS and CS has reached maximum usefulness, more aggressive therapy is usually instituted. The drugs used have been classified under a number of headings that describe their presumed efficacy and action: disease modifying antirheumatic drugs (DMARDS), slow acting antirheumatic drugs (SAARD), remission-inducing drugs, immunosuppressive drugs, and second-line agents. While these agents may have only some of these properties in common, and although their mechanisms of action differ, they do share the feature that they are used as second-line therapy after NSAIDS and CS.

Gold Salts

Gold salts, the oldest of the current second-line drugs, was utilized for RA in the 1930s after the discovery that gold halted the growth of mycobacteria, initially believed to be the causative agent of RA.[52] At that time, a 70% to 80% favorable response was reported for gold-treated patients. Since then, the efficacy of gold has been studied extensively in controlled clinical trials, observational studies, and meta-analyses. Clinical effects (joint count, grip strength, functional capacity, ESR)[53] and radiographic benefits[54] have been documented in a number of these trials. A review of drug therapy effects from 17 studies suggested that gold treatment retards radiographic progression of RA.[55] In a meta-analysis of second-line drug efficacy, gold was determined to be as effective as other drugs and better than placebo.[56]

Recent studies, however, have cast doubt on the effectiveness of gold salts. A study in 1988 showed no significant difference in outcome among gold, sulfasalazine, and placebo.[57] A 5-year observational study of patients on intramuscular (IM) gold showed no change in joint count or functional status.[58] This has led to the opinion by some that gold therapy is at best marginally beneficial,[59, 60] although discarding its use entirely would seem to be unwarranted.

Besides the potential antimicrobial action of gold, a number of additional effects may explain its antiarthritic activity. A reduction in CRP, ESR, RF, and polyclonal immunoglobulins has been associated with its administration. During gold therapy, the complement cascade is partially inactivated, T-lymphocyte and monocyte functions including cytokine production are blocked, and neutrophil chemotaxis, migration, and phagocytosis are inhibited. In addition, reactive oxygen species associated with tissue damage are inhibited by gold.[61] The degree to which the benefits of gold in RA are attributable to these effects is unknown, particularly since many of these studies were only conducted in vitro.

Gold has the highest toxicity and patient dropout rate of the second-line drugs.[56] The important side effects include dermatitis, membranous glomerulonephritis, and bone marrow suppression.[62] Diarrhea and occasionally cholestatic jaundice may develop and usually subside with drug cessation. Parenteral and oral gold differ in their frequency of various adverse reactions: mucocutaneous and hematologic complications arise less commonly with oral gold, whereas gastrointestinal (GI) side effects occur more than twice as frequently with oral gold than with parenteral therapy.[63] Parenteral gold is associated with the nitroid reaction, a vasomotor response manifested by dizziness, flushing, and hypotension in as many as a third of patients after injection. Interestingly, patients who are HLA-DR3 positive may have increased susceptibility to gold toxicity in addition to increased responsiveness to its therapeutic effect.[64]

Injectable gold therapy is initiated in test doses of 10 mg the first week followed by 25 mg the next week. Subsequent doses of 50 mg each week are given until a cumulative dose of 1 g is attained. Higher weekly doses are associated with greater toxicity, but may be necessary for some patients to achieve results. Maintenance therapy is generally 25 to 50 mg every 2 to 4 weeks indefinitely.

Gold compounds are available as three preparations: gold sodium thiomalate (GSTM), gold thioglucose (GSTG), and the only oral form, auranofin. Nitroid reactions are more often associated with GSTM; GSTG, however, is more difficult to administer. While some toxicities are less frequent with auranofin than with injectable gold, auranofin is considered less effective.[56] Regardless of the preparation used, close monitoring with careful history, physical, and laboratories is essential for early recognition of toxicity.

Antimalarials

Quinacrine was the first antimalarial agent reported to show a therapeutic benefit in RA.[65] Chloroquine and subsequently hydroxychloroquine, both 4-aminoquinoline derivatives, have been the antimalarial agents of choice for RA, primarily because of their superior safety profile. Early studies described improvement with antimalarials in such variables as grip strength, joint count, ESR, and overall assessment, but at twice the current recommended dose.[66–68] Although effectiveness may be dose-related,[69] studies utilizing lower doses have demonstrated clinical efficacy[70,71] with decreased side effects.[72–74] However, when radiologic findings were compared, these studies failed to show a statistically significant difference in radiographic progression between those who were treated with antimalarials and those who were not.[55]

Antimalarials have been measured against a number of other second-line drugs with respect to efficacy and toxicity. Compared to gold, antimalarials showed less efficacy in some studies[75,76] and equal benefit in others.[77,78] When both toxicity and efficacy were combined using life table analysis, hydroxychloroquine was superior to gold, penicillamine, and levamisole in one study,[79] but was no different than other second-line drugs in a more recent study.[63] Additional comparisons to penicillamine and sulfasalazine show hydroxychloroquine to be less effective, but better tolerated.[80–83]

The actions of antimalarials are varied. These drugs inhibit the activity of many enzymes, including the release of lysosomal enzymes that cause tissue damage. Neutrophil chemotaxis and phagocytosis are blocked as well. Mitogen-induced lymphocyte proliferation is reduced with chloroquine, as well as macrophage production of interleukin-1 (IL-1). Hydroxychloroquine has been shown to inhibit IL-1 mediated cartilage degradation in vitro.[84]

Ocular side effects have been the major toxicity of concern with antimalarial therapy, although numerous other adverse reactions commonly occur, particularly GI symptoms. Difficulty with accommodation and convergence develops often, manifesting as blurred vision. The symptom of seeing halos around lights may be an indication of corneal deposits of antimalarial salts which develop in 95% and 20% of patients receiving chloroquine and hydroxychloroquine, respectively. These deposits are reversible within days to weeks of stopping the drug and do not cause visual loss.

The incidence of serious retinopathy associated with antimalarial therapy, defined as visual field loss to white objects and prominent macular pigment defects (bull's eye), is very low.[85] Nevertheless, it can result in irreversible loss of vision. Patients may perceive a decrease in visual acuity and central scotoma or peripheral field constriction. Other characteristic retinal changes, such as pigmentary stippling and transient central scotoma to red objects also occur but do not necessarily progress to permanent visual loss, and revert with drug discontinuation.[86]

The daily dose of antimalarial drugs rather than the cumulative dose appears to influence the development of ocular toxicity.[69, 87] The lowest dose for maximum effectiveness and minimum toxicity is 400 mg hydroxychloroquine per day (6.5 mg/kg) and 250 mg chloroquine per day (4 mg/kg).[74, 85] However, ocular complications have been noted rarely despite these low doses. Ophthalmologic examinations should be performed before initiating therapy, and every 6 months thereafter, to screen for the aforementioned lesions. Self-administered tests like the Amsler grid may detect early lesions.[85, 86]

The impact of antimalarial therapy on the associated symptoms and abnormal laboratories of RA is not realized for many weeks to months. The drugs should be continued for 6 months before treatment is considered a failure. Once the patient experiences a favorable response, therapy should be continued at full dose until remission is achieved. Subsequently, the dose may be halved for 6 months and then slowly discontinued. Relapse does occur and is often responsive to reinstitution of antimalarial therapy. NSAIDS and antimalarials may be administered concomitantly. The addition of other second-line therapy may be necessary at some point if the disease process continues.

D-Penicillamine

DPA, discovered as a byproduct of penicillin, was first used for its copper chelating properties in the treatment of Wilson's disease in the 1940s.[88] An additional property that led to its use in RA was the ability of DPA to dissociate IgM RF, thus decreasing its circulating titer.[89] Three chief characteristics of DPA biochemistry that explain its usefulness in a variety of clinical settings are: (1) chelation of various heavy metals (Wilson's disease); (2) thiol-disulfide interchange reaction which dissociates IgM RF as well as renal stone formation in cystinuria; and (3) thiazolidine formation by aldehyde cross-linking of collagen (scleroderma, primary biliary cirrhosis). This last property is the basis of the antivitamin B6 effect of DPA. Postulated anti-inflammatory and immunosuppressive effects of DPA include interference with leukocyte chemotaxis and helper T-cell function.[90]

After DPA was utilized with success in a patient with RA and vasculitis in 1964,[92] uncontrolled trials in the 1970s reported greater than 50% improvement in parameters of disease activity in RA patients treated with DPA.[93–95] The first double-blind placebo controlled trial was conducted over 12 months in 105 patients who had failed conventional therapy.[96] A significant improvement in pain, morning stiffness, grip strength, functional status, and ESR, as well as a fall in RF titer was noted in DPA-treated patients. Premature termination of DPA therapy was due primarily to adverse reactions rather than treatment failure, whereas the opposite was the case for the control group. No change in radiographic progression of disease was noted in either group.

Subsequent double-blind controlled trials have confirmed the efficacy of DPA in RA.[97, 98] DPA has been measured against gold in many trials.[99–103] In general, DPA and IM gold were comparable in efficacy and response pattern. Although the overall incidence of adverse reactions was greater for DPA, withdrawal from therapy for adverse reactions was more frequent for gold.[103] Like gold, DPA exerts a gradual clinical effect; up to 6 months of therapy is required to achieve maximum benefit. DPA is superior to oral gold with regard to efficacy, but withdrawal for side effects is more frequent with DPA than with oral gold.[99]

Life table analyses and meta-analyses have compared DPA to numerous other second-line drugs.[56, 63, 104, 105] Sulfasalazine (SSZ) and DPA were comparable in the incidence of treatment withdrawal for both toxicity and inefficacy.[56, 104] The probability of remaining on long-term DPA therapy is similar to other drugs except methotrexate (MTX).[63]

A number of serious side effects associated with DPA therapy have limited its clinical usefulness.[106] Of the hematologic side effects, thrombocytopenia occurs most commonly and can be managed by reducing the daily dose. Leukopenia and aplastic anemia have also been observed. Considered a later complication of DPA therapy, proteinuria and the nephrotic syndrome can result from immune-complex-mediated membranous nephropathy in a significant number of patients receiving this drug. Therapy may be continued with minor dosage adjustments as long as proteinuria does not exceed 2 g per 24 hours. Renal lesions tend to resolve only gradually after drug discontinuation.

Some of the most frequent side effects associated with DPA are dermatologic, occurring both early and late in therapy. Early rashes include mild pruritus, urticaria, and eczema while those seen later, which usually require drug cessation, include bullous dermatitis, pemphigus foliaceus, and pemphigus vulgaris. Other early side effects include anorexia, nausea, diarrhea, stomatitis, mouth ulcers, and loss of taste. Hypogeusia occurs early but gradually returns to normal by 3 months. Neither dosage changes nor mineral supplementation improve this side effect. Rare complications include polymyositis, myasthenia gravis, and drug fever.

Various dosage regimens have been examined in an attempt to reduce side effects.[97, 107] Based on the results of these reports, DPA therapy is usually started at 125 mg per day with an increase in the daily dose by 125 mg every 4 to 8 weeks, depending on response and side effects, until a maximum of 1000 mg is reached ("go low, go slow"). However, there is great interpatient variability and a wide range of dosages have been utilized.

Sulfasalazine

SSZ is the conjugate of 5-aminosalicylic acid (5-ASA) and sulfapyridine (SP) linked by an azo bond. It was first manufactured for its dual antibacterial and antiinflammatory properties in the 1930s, when an infectious etiology was a suspected cause of RA. Although SSZ produced favorable results in many RA patients in the 1940s, some negative reports and the expanded use of other drugs limited its application. It was then utilized successfully in inflammatory bowel disease (IBD). In 1980, McConkey reexamined SSZ therapy in 74 RA patients in an open trial that confirmed the previously seen clinical benefit.[108]

Open and controlled trials comparing SSZ with placebo and other second-line agents followed McConkey's report.[109–116] In these short-term trials, SSZ performed as well as gold and DPA while inducing clinical responses more rapidly than these other drugs. However, the ability to find statistically significant differences between therapies was limited in some cases because the number of patients analyzed was small. SSZ has shown superiority over placebo in at least two trials,[112, 113] but surprisingly and without explanation, in one comparative study of placebo, gold, and SSZ, neither gold nor SSZ performed better than placebo.[114]

The use of SSZ in early RA after NSAIDS have failed has been examined in a few trials. A 48-week comparison of hydroxychloroquine (HXY) and SSZ in 60 patients failing NSAIDS favored SSZ for improvement of pain scores, grip strength, and immunoglobulin levels. Other parameters such as ESR, CRP, and joint count were similar between the two groups. By 4 weeks of SSZ therapy, grip strength, morning stiffness, and pain scores had improved significantly over baseline, whereas HXY did not exhibit any effect until week 12.[83] Another 48-week, double-blind trial evaluating radiographic progression of disease showed fewer erosions at the end of the study in patients treated with SSZ than those treated with HXY.[82] In a 3-year follow-up to this report the difference was still evident.[117]

Studies of SSZ for 2 years or more are few. A 2-year comparison study of SSZ and DPA therapy demonstrated improvement above baseline of most parameters measured, but no difference between treatments. One life-table analysis of 317 RA patients receiving gold, DPA, or SSZ showed the same risk of treatment termination at 5 years for both toxicity and inefficacy with a trend favoring gold (81% to 92% risk). SSZ therapy was associated with fewer terminations due to adverse reactions, but withdrawal for lack of efficacy was more common with this agent.[104] A subsequent life-table analysis of 596 RA patients found no difference between SSZ and other second-line drugs except MTX in terms of the risk of treatment termination (50% at 5 years).[105] SSZ performed similarly to IM gold, DPA, and MTX in a meta-analysis of second-line agents.[56]

SSZ is partly absorbed before it is cleaved in the intestine by bacterial enzymes into its two components, 5-ASA and SP. The first, 5-ASA, passes through the colon essentially unabsorbed and is the active portion in IBD. On the other hand, more than 90% of SP is absorbed and, along with its parent compound SSZ, is the portion that has demonstrated activity in RA.[118, 119]

The anti-inflammatory actions of SSZ which may account for its activity in RA include inhibition of thromboxane synthetase and lipoxygenase pathways, neutrophil motility, and proteolytic enzyme activity.[120] Also, few immunomodulating effects such as enhancement of lymphocyte mitogen response, inhibition of lymphocyte proliferation, and RF production have been described in vitro.[120] The alteration of bowel flora, the impairment of folate absorption, as well as the inhibition of synovial neovascularization[121] may be additional modes of action of SSZ in RA. However, the role of these mechanisms in RA is only speculative.

Toxicities associated with SSZ use are well-described from the experience in IBD and appear to occur in a similar pattern in RA. While most adverse reactions are not serious, GI intolerance is frequent, accounting for up to 60% of treatment discontinuations despite the use of enteric-coated tablets. Dose reduction may alleviate some of these symptoms. Since SSZ is acetylated in the liver, patients who are "slow-acetylators" may experience increased side effects[122] related to the serum level of SP. Idiosyncratic toxicities such as rash occur and account for up to 15% of drug withdrawals. Other idiosyncratic reactions rarely develop, but include agranulocytosis, aplastic anemia, pneumonitis, and hepatitis. Male patients should also be advised of the reversible effects on sperm (decreased count and motility) that may develop within 2 months of SSZ therapy.

SSZ is usually instituted at a low dose of one 500 mg enteric-coated tablet twice a day to minimize risk of toxicity. This is usually increased weekly in 500-mg increments until a total daily dose of 2 to 3 g daily is achieved. Once a clinical response is achieved, patients generally continue therapy indefinitely at varying doses.

Methotrexate

MTX, a folate antagonist, has emerged as an important second-line agent in the treatment of RA. Like many antirheumatic drugs, MTX was originally developed for use in nonrheumatic diseases. It was not until 1951 that the efficacy of folate antagonists in RA was demonstrated.[123] However, their potential usefulness was largely ignored until the report by Hoffmeister in 1972, in which 25 of 29 patients receiving low dose weekly IM MTX (10 to 15 mg) showed moderate to marked clinical improvement over a 2-year period.[124] A follow-up to this report on 78 patients treated for up to 15 years again showed marked improvement in 45 patients as measured by morning stiffness, pain, joint count, functional capacity, change in prednisone dose, and ESR. Patients withdrew prematurely due to a lack of initial response in 10, toxicity in 7, and increasing disease activity in 4. Complete remission was achieved in 28 patients.[125]

Additional open trials in the 1980s confirmed these findings.[126–130] Patients chosen for these studies were generally refractory to therapy with gold, penicillamine, antimalarials, or azathioprine. Unlike other second-line medications, MTX induced an initial response usually within 4 weeks with a maximal response by 2 to 4 months. Route of administration was both IV,[128] IM, and oral at doses ranging from 7.5 mg to 50 mg weekly. Overall, short-term effectiveness reported in these studies was considerable.

Subsequent short-term, placebo-controlled clinical trials of low-dose weekly MTX, both oral and IM, led to the approval by the FDA of this drug for RA in 1988. Again, patients with disease activity refractory to conventional therapy were selected for study.[131–134] In two crossover trials,[132, 133] disease flare was noted with drug discontinuation. A pooled analysis of these data revealed between 15% and 46% improvement in morning stiffness, joint count and pain, global assessment by patient and physician, and ESR.[135]

Comparison of MTX to other second-line drugs has been conducted in a number of randomized, prospective trials. Both gold and MTX significantly improved a number of standard clinical variables in three short-term, randomized, double-blinded trials, but no difference was found between the two therapies.[136–138] Also, radiologic deterioration occurred with equal frequency in MTX and gold-treated patients.[136, 137] However, in all three studies, MTX was better tolerated. When compared to oral gold, MTX produced an earlier, more pronounced response with fewer side effects.[139]

Two trials comparing MTX to azathioprine (AZA) report conflicting results. In a 24-week, prospective, controlled trial, 42 patients treated with MTX and AZA showed significant improvement from baseline in 9 efficacy variables.[140] Although there was a trend favoring MTX, no statistical difference was detected between treatment groups. Efficacy was maintained for both groups at 52 weeks.

A subsequent 48-week, randomized, double-blind trial showed marked superiority in efficacy and toxicity of MTX over AZA at 24 and 48 weeks in 64 patients studied.[141] Discrepancy between these two studies is ascribed to the number of patients studied and the dropout rate.

The measurement of time to termination of therapy has been utilized to estimate drug efficacy as well. Two such analyses showed that, compared to therapy with IM and oral gold, antimalarials, penicillamine, azathioprine, and sulfasalazine, MTX therapy was of considerably longer duration, and termination of therapy for both inefficacy and toxicity was less likely. One meta-analysis of second-line drugs comparing ESR, joint count, grip strength, and combined effect size showed the greatest improvement in joint count with MTX, but found little difference between drugs for other parameters.[56] The smaller number of MTX-treated patients and the increased disease severity may have influenced these results.

Long-term experience with low dose weekly MTX has been reviewed both prospectively and retrospectively over the last 10 years.[125, 142–150] As in the short-term trials, drug effect was noted early in the course of therapy with greatest response occurring at up to 6 months. A plateau in effect developed from 6 months to 2 years of treatment, with some patients requiring increasing doses of MTX.[144, 145, 147] Other patients were able to reduce their MTX dose.[125] Reduction in mean prednisone dosage was accomplished in a number of patients while on MTX therapy.[144, 147] In addition, the probability of continuing therapy after 1 year, 2 years, and 5 years was approximately 70%, 50% to 65%, and 50%, respectively.

Two open prospective trials updating previous reports of a cohort sampling of patients[143, 151] followed for almost 8 years were recently published. Overall responsiveness was sustained throughout the study period with 46%[148] and 62%[149] of patients remaining on therapy. Toxicity rather than lack of efficacy was cited as the primary reason for drug discontinuation.

An important marker of drug efficacy is radiographic evidence of disease arrest. A recent meta-analysis reviewed the radiologic findings of 11 studies published between 1970 and 1991.[150] MTX and non-MTX treated patients treated with gold salts or AZA were compared for rates of radiologic progression. When compared to AZA, MTX exhibited a slower rate of progression.[140, 152] However, the MTX and gold groups were comparable in their rates of radiologic progression. No overall difference in radiographic progression was detected between MTX and non-MTX treated patients. Other reviews suggest that RA is indeed halted with therapy, but the rate at which this becomes apparent may vary with the disease course, timing of treatment, and timing of radiographs.

Although MTX is effective therapy for RA, the mechanism by which it suppresses disease activity is unclear. MTX binds to dihydrofolate reductase, preventing the formation of tetrahydrofolate and thus producing an intracellular depletion of folate coenzymes. Consequently, DNA and RNA synthesis is interrupted. In addition to its antifolate effects, low dose MTX may also possess anti-inflammatory and immunosuppressive properties through which it controls RA symptoms. MTX has been shown to decrease IgM and IgA RF production,[153] reduce 5-lipoxygenase pathway products,[154] modulate IL-1 activity,[155] inhibit mononuclear cell proliferation,[156] and prevent neovascularization.[91] Whether these mechanisms contribute to MTX effectiveness in RA is still unknown.

The long-term experience with low dose MTX in RA described previously has established that patients are able to tolerate this therapy. The occurrence of common GI side effects (nausea, vomiting, dyspepsia, diarrhea, and anorexia) and stomatitis likely reflect the effect of MTX on cells with high turnover and are usually manageable with dosage adjustment.[157] Anemia, leukopenia, and thrombocytopenia can develop with low-dose MTX. MTX should be used with particular caution in the presence of renal insufficiency and drugs that alter renal clearance of MTX such as aspirin and NSAIDS.[158] Concomitant supplementation with 1 mg folic acid daily can reduce side effects without altering efficacy.[159]

The potential development of serious hepatic and pulmonary toxicity has been of major concern with MTX therapy. Initial reports of MTX in psoriatic patients showed significant liver toxicity associated with daily dosing and high cumulative doses.[160] A poor correlation with elevated transaminases and liver pathology was noted. The experience in RA patients on weekly low dose MTX has not paralleled that of psoriatic patients. Studies evaluating liver biopsies from MTX-treated RA patients have shown a low incidence of hepatic fibrosis (8% to 11%),[161] which is of uncertain clinical significance, and only rare cases of cirrhosis. Furthermore, serial transaminase elevations in most instances correlate with hepatic toxicity as does hypoalbuminemia.[162–164] Significant liver disease did not develop with a cumulative dose of 1.5 g or after 2 years therapy.[164] Risk factors for the development of hepatic toxicity include diabetes mellitus, obe-

TABLE 5.
Recommendations for Liver Biopsy in Patients With Rheumatoid Arthritis Receiving Methotrexate*

I. Baseline biopsy in patients with:
   A. significant alcohol consumption (2 to 3 drinks/day);
   B. a history of hepatitis, jaundice, or liver disease.
II. Initial biopsy to monitor toxicity if:
   A. 6 of 12 monthly determinations of aspartate aminotransferase (AST) are abnormally elevated;
   B. baseline normal serum albumin falls to ≤ 3.3 g/dl;
   C. 3 to 5 of 12 monthly elevations of AST into the abnormal range per year when present for 3 consecutive years.
III. Repeat biopsy for Roenigk Class I, II, IIA (minimal fibrosis) on initial biopsy if circumstances in II (above) apply.

*Adapted from Kremer JM: Liver biopsies in patients with rheumatoid arthritis, receiving methotrexate: Where are we going? *J Rheumatol* 1992; 19:189–191.

sity, and alcohol consumption. Although an HLA-associated predisposition to hepatic toxicity has been conjectured, it has not been confirmed. Given the aforementioned considerations, current recommendations for liver enzyme determinations and liver biopsy are in Table 5.

Pulmonary complications with low-dose MTX therapy have been well described. The most common manifestation is a hypersensitivity pneumonitis presenting with chronic symptoms of nonproductive cough, dyspnea, and malaise, or with acute symptoms of fever, chills, and severe hypoxia. Chest radiographs usually show bilateral interstitial infiltrates. Often the distinction between RA involving the lungs, respiratory infection, and MTX-induced pulmonary toxicity is difficult to determine.

Dosage schedules have been devised to reduce potential toxicities and maintain efficacy. In general, oral MTX therapy is initiated at doses of 5 mg to 7.5 mg as a single weekly dose with increasing doses to up to 10 to 20 mg per week. Splitting the total dose over 24 hours has been advocated in patients who develop GI symptoms, but this may increase other toxicities. Oral and IM MTX have equal bioavailability, but IM therapy may be utilized when higher doses are required or when lack of efficacy or GI side effects occur. A linear relationship between dose efficacy and toxicity has been described.[165] IV therapy has been employed at doses from 10 to 50 mg.[128] Protocols with high-dose IV MTX for refractory RA have shown benefit, but still remain experimental.[166]

Azathioprine

AZA has been used in RA since the early 1960s.[167] This purine analogue is derived from the addition of an imidazole group to 6-mercaptopurine

(6-MP), another purine analogue. In vivo AZA is converted to 6-MP, the active form of the drug. One pathway of 6-MP metabolism is through the enzyme xanthine oxidase. Since allopurinol is a xanthine oxidase inhibitor, its concomitant use with AZA increases AZA toxicity.

AZA possesses a number of immunoregulatory and anti-inflammatory properties which account for its therapeutic effect in RA. By inhibiting nucleic acid synthesis, AZA blocks the proliferation of immunocompetent cells. Therapy with AZA results in both T- and B-cell lymphocytopenia. Primary and secondary antibody responses are suppressed, although lymphocyte blastogenic responses are not significantly affected. Also, established delayed-type cutaneous hypersensitivity remains intact, whereas de novo responses are inhibited. Anti-inflammatory activity results from the inhibition of monocyte precursor cell division, limiting monocyte infiltration at the sites of inflammation. However, cytokine production and release are unaltered by AZA.

Since its initial use in RA, AZA has demonstrated superiority over placebo in various short and long-term double-blind trials.[168–170] These were conducted in patients generally refractory to other second-line therapy who had longstanding disease. Two trials comparing AZA to cyclophosphamide, gold, and chloroquine in patients with disease duration of less than 5 years concluded that AZA was as easy and safe to administer as gold and was at least as effective.[77, 171] AZA has compared favorably to DPA in two trials.[172, 173]

As previously mentioned, comparisons with MTX have been conflicting, but current opinion is that MTX tends to produce a more marked and rapid improvement than AZA. In addition, AZA is no more effective in altering rates of radiologic disease progression than other second-line drugs.[55, 152]

As with other cytotoxic agents, bone marrow suppression is the most worrisome side effect of AZA therapy. Leukocytes are preferentially depleted. However, opportunistic infections develop in the absence of leukopenia, reflecting the important effect of AZA on lymphocytes and monocytes. GI intolerance is the greatest cause of drug discontinuation. Other adverse reactions that occur less frequently include stomatitis, dermatitis, hepatitis, and alopecia. AZA therapy occasionally may result in reversible infertility, but not invariably. Finally, an increased incidence of lymphoreticular malignancies has been reported in renal transplant patients receiving AZA therapy.

Therapy with AZA is usually started at 2 mg per kg per day orally. Clinical effects usually are evident within one month but may take up to 6 months for full effect to be achieved. Dosage adjustments are based on side effects. A recent 12-week trial reported the effectiveness of pulse doses of AZA 300 mg 3 days a week.[174] Additional experience is required before this dosage regimen can be recommended. AZA has been approved by the Food and Drug Administration for use in RA.

Cyclophosphamide

Alkylating agents have been used in the treatment of RA since 1951.[175] As the immunopathogenesis of RA was recognized, interest in these immunoregulating agents expanded.

Cyclophosphamide (CP) has been studied in uncontrolled and controlled trials,[176–178] which have confirmed its effectiveness in intractable RA. A review of radiographs in patients receiving CP in three trials found evidence that therapy halted radiologic disease progression.[55] However, the serious side effects of CP have generally precluded its early or extensive use in RA.

CP and other alkylating agents act by covalently binding to DNA strands. This cross-linking restricts cell division. CP is active during all phases of the cell cycle, including the resting stage, making it a potent cytotoxic immunosuppressant. B cells are selectively suppressed early in the course of CP therapy, but with chronic therapy both B and T cells are depleted equally. Antibody responses and cutaneous delayed hypersensitivity to a new antigen are also suppressed. Other immunosuppressive effects of CP include reduction of elevated immunoglobulin, suppression of monocyte-macrophage function, and inhibition of soluble mediator production.

CP is metabolized in the liver and excreted as active metabolites in the urine. Thus, impaired renal function may increase CP toxicity. Barbiturates and CS alter drug metabolism by inducing hepatic enzymes and increasing the formation of active metabolites. CS also can protect the bone marrow from the neutropenic effects of CP, allowing the use of a higher immunosuppressive dose in some cases.

The major and usually limiting side effect of CP therapy is the dose-dependent bone marrow toxicity that affects leukocytes more than erythrocytes or platelets. Since active metabolites are concentrated in the urine, bladder irritation leading to hemorrhagic cystitis, fibrosis, and malignant transformation can occur. Bladder toxicity can be lessened by encouraging patients to drink large volumes of water and to urinate frequently. Therapy with mesna, which binds the bladder irritant acrolein, may be useful in selected cases. Patients should also be advised that CP therapy can cause irreversible infertility in both men and women. Alopecia with chronic low-dose CP is usually mild. Less common but important side effects include pulmonary fibrosis, hepatotoxicity, and the development of lymphoreticular malignancies. The long-term side effects are usually associated with cumulative dose and duration of therapy.

CP therapy is usually initiated at 50 mg per day orally and increased to a maintenance dose of 1.5 to 2.5 mg per kg per day over the ensuing 4 to 6 weeks. Lower doses have been studied and have failed to show any benefit.[176] A clinical response is usually noted within 2 to 4 weeks. Drug dosage is adjusted based on the leukocyte count in order to maintain a count of 3,000 cells/mm. No correlation between the degree of leukopenia and suppression of synovitis has been found.[176, 178]

Cyclosporine

Cyclosporine (CsA), originally tested as a fungicide, is a potent immunosuppressive agent with activity against both humoral and cell-mediated immune responses. Although its application had been primarily in recipients of solid-organ transplantation to prevent rejection,[179] use has been extended to diseases characterized by exaggerated immune reactivity. The rationale for use in RA stems from the evidence that T cells are critical to the immunopathology of RA. CsA inhibits T-cell activation and proliferation by inhibiting: (1) the generation of T-cell receptors for interleukin-2 (IL-2); (2) the responsiveness of T cells to interleukin-1 (IL-1); and (3) the synthesis of IL-2 and other cytokines. These events are likely calcium dependent and mediated by a recently discovered enzyme, cyclophilin. The effects of CsA on T cells may also result in the suppression of IL-1 synthesis by macrophages, another important cell in the pathology of RA. In addition, CsA suppresses the early stages of B-cell activation directly and indirectly through T-cell inhibition.

Short-term, open, uncontrolled studies of CsA in RA were begun in the late 1970s and continued through the 1980s, followed by placebo-controlled, double-blinded trials. Patients were generally in their sixth decade with longstanding, refractory disease. A number of these earlier trials studied high dose CsA (6 to 10 mg/kg/day as used in transplantation patients).[180–182] Improvement in the number of swollen joints, morning stiffness, and pain scores was evident, but important GI and renal side effects occurred commonly and were the major cause of drug discontinuation. Interestingly, ESR was essentially unaffected, while CRP levels fell dramatically, a phenomenon seen with CsA in the treatment of other autoimmune diseases. Despite short-term benefit, relapse of symptoms occurred within weeks of drug cessation.

In an attempt to reduce side effects, investigators have studied lower starting doses of CsA. An open, uncontrolled trial of 20 patients with advanced RA revealed significant clinical benefit with as low as 2.5 mg to 5 mg/kg/day of CsA. A delay in effect of several weeks was noted at these dosages compared to higher doses.[183] To further define the lowest effective dose of CsA in RA, 10 mg/kg/day was compared to 1 mg/kg/day in a 6-month, randomized, prospective, double-blind trial of 31 patients.[231] Improvement in disease activity was achieved with high-dose CsA as expected, but no statistically significant clinical changes were found in the low dose group. Furthermore, most patients in the low dose group exhibited some degree of significant nephrotoxicity. A subset of patients defined by anergy appeared to have a better response to therapy than those who were not anergic. Subsequent open[184] and double-blinded, placebo-controlled trials[185, 186] of low dose CsA have corroborated that doses of 5 mg/kg/day or less provide the optimal risk/benefit ratio.

Few studies have compared CsA with other second-line agents. In a 6-month open trial of 12 patients, CsA was shown to have superior efficacy compared to AZA. The average dose of CsA was high (6.4 mg/kg/day) and adverse reactions were significant.[187] CsA and D-penicillamine were shown to have comparable efficacy with equal frequency of drug discontinuation.[188] However, therapy was terminated because of toxicity more often in the CsA group than the D-penicillamine group (90% vs. 30%). Studies comparing CsA to MTX are currently underway.

Recently, a preliminary meta-analysis of the efficacy and toxicity reported in five controlled trials of CSA was performed.[189] A composite treatment effect was examined which was similar to one reported in a previous meta-analysis of second-line drugs that consolidated outcome measures.[56] The composite effect in the CsA group was considerably greater than the effect for the placebo group. A comparison with other second-line drugs from the earlier meta-analysis showed that CsA performs as well as conventional therapy, particularly if CRP replaces ESR in the analysis. Toxicity as measured by dropout rates was also comparable to other agents such as oral gold and antimalarials.

Long-term data on safety and efficacy are still scarce. An open study described 16 patients previously responsive to CsA who were continued on therapy for a mean duration of 21 months at an initial dose of 5 mg/kg/day.[190] Efficacy was maintained throughout the study period for the 10 patients still receiving therapy. Two patients discontinued therapy because of disease progression, two because of adverse reactions, and two for other reasons. A predictable rise in serum creatinine during CsA therapy was noted, which was not entirely reversible in all patients after drug discontinuation. A correlation between duration of therapy and decrease in creatinine clearance was not found. Radiographs showed significant progression of disease despite therapy. Another open trial of 20 patients studied over a 16- to 38-month period also showed continued clinical benefit during therapy. Creatinine clearance levels were a median of 19% below pretreatment levels.[232]

A major drawback to therapy with CsA is the nephrotoxicity invariably observed. Glomerular filtration rate and blood flow decrease by 15% to 40%.[191] Animal studies suggest this may be a result of diminished renal blood flow secondary to changes in the renin-angiotensin system and in eicosanoid metabolism, which appears to be a reversible, dose-dependent effect. Chronic irreversible damage has been seen in some patients. Injury to small arterioles, tubular atrophy, and tubulointerstitial fibrosis were observed on biopsies of older patients who were treated with higher doses of CsA and who had higher pretreatment serum creatinine levels than control patients.[192] The clinical relevance of these relatively nonspecific changes is still controversial. Risk factors for CsA nephrotoxicity also include concomitant NSAID use since these drugs alter renal hemodynamics as well.[193]

Other important side effects of CsA therapy include hypertension, hypertrichosis, neurotoxicity, and hepatotoxicity; however, these rarely result in drug withdrawal. The concern of hematologic malignancies associated with CsA therapy has been recently addressed in a review of over 1,000 RA patients receiving CsA.[194] Of the 17 cases of malignancy documented,

TABLE 6.
Safety Guidelines for Cyclosporine Therapy*

1. Use minimum effective dose; ≤ 5 mg/kg/day.
2. Monitor serum creatinine and blood pressure.
3. Decrease dose in 25-mg decrements if serum creatinine rises by >30%.
4. Avoid drugs known to interfere with the bioavailability or action of cyclosporine.
5. Treat sustained hypertension and/or reduce or discontinue cyclosporine.

*Adapted from Tugwell P: Cyclosporine in rheumatoid arthritis: documented efficacy and safety. *Semin Arthritis Rheum* 1992; 3(suppl):30–38.

only 1 was lymphoreticular. The authors concluded that the risk of malignancy was no greater with CsA than with any other second-line therapy. However, because of the potential increased risk of lymphoma observed in transplant patients, CsA-treated patients should be monitored carefully for this possibility.

The role of CsA in RA therapy has yet to be defined, and although many investigations have substantiated its efficacy, CsA therapy for RA is still generally a consideration only after most other second-line agents have failed. When used in RA patients, the guidelines outlined in Table 6 should be followed. Particular attention should be paid to the concomitant use of drugs that alter its metabolism by the liver, such as ketoconazole and erythromycin. The results of ongoing trials will help answer questions regarding the effect of CsA on early RA, on radiographic progression of disease, as well as measures to assure long-term safety.

Immunotherapy

Cytokines.—As the study of cytokines in the pathogenesis of RA has advanced, their role as potential therapy for RA has also been explored. In this regard, interferon-γ (IFN-γ), a lymphokine secreted by activated T cells, has been the most extensively researched of the cytokines. Although IFN-γ has been regarded as an upregulator of the immune system, it possesses a number of properties that led to its initial use in RA. In vitro, IFN-γ inhibits prostanoid production by synovial cells and monocytes. IFN-γ also inhibits production of other proinflammatory cytokines such as interleukin-8 (IL-8) and the bone-resorbing activities of IL-1 and tumor necrosis factor (TNF). Finally, surprisingly low levels of IFN-γ are found in the joints of RA patients.

Early reports of IFN-γ treatment in open, uncontrolled studies noted significant improvement in symptoms after administration.[195–197] The short-term, double-blind, placebo-controlled trials that followed demonstrated only modest improvement in laboratory and clinical parameters of disease activity in RA patients treated with IFN-γ.[198–202] Conclusions from these trials are limited by the fact that patients continued other second-line agents during the study period;[201] patients exhibited a high placebo response;[203] and dosage regimens varied. Side effects were generally minor (fever, chills, nausea, and local reactions at the injection site), but leukopenia[199] and drug-induced lupus[204] have been described.

The biologic activity of cytokines is modulated by naturally occurring inhibitors. Natural IL-1 receptor antagonists recently have been characterized, cloned, and studied in vitro.[205–207] Clinical trials are currently ongoing to assess their anti-inflammatory properties in vivo. Yet another method of targeting T cells for destruction is the use of a genetically engineered fusion protein that combines IL-2 and the toxic component of diphtheria toxin (DAB IL-2). The immunotoxin binds to activated T cells expressing IL-2 receptors and destroys them by delivering the toxin directly to the cells. An open, uncontrolled trial of 13 patients with RA treated with DAB IL-2 reported transient benefit.[208]

Monoclonal Antibodies.—There is now substantial evidence that T cells play a central role in the pathogenesis of RA. Initial trials of immunotherapy directed at T cells included thoracic duct drainage,[209] lymphoid irradiation,[210] and lymphocytopheresis.[211] Although these therapies were cumbersome and clinical improvement was brief, they reinforced the theory that T-cell manipulation was of potential benefit in RA patients. This recognition has led to the development of new therapeutic modalities.

Specific lymphocyte antigens were the targets of the first monoclonal antibodies (mAb) used to treat patients with renal transplant rejection.[212] These mAb were directed against the pan-T-cell antigen CD3, present on all T lymphocytes. Subsequent research has yielded mAb against other pan T-cell antigens including CD5 and CDw52; the activated T-cell antigens CD7 and CD25 (IL-2 receptor); the helper T-cell antigen CD4; and T-cell receptor molecules (Table 7). The cells whose antigens are targeted are destroyed by lympholysis.

Uncontrolled trials of mAb in RA began with anti-CD4 antibody therapy in seven RA patients.[213] Clinical improvement was noted within one week of therapy and sustained for over 3 months in five out of eight patients. However, symptoms were controlled for a relatively short duration. No change in ESR, CRP, or RF was noted. Additionally, CD4+ T cells were depleted from the circulation only temporarily. Subsequent trials of various anti-CD4 mAb have confirmed these initial findings.[214–218]

Antibodies against the pan T-cell antigens CD5 and CDw52 have been under recent investigation. In addition to all mature T cells, CD5 antigen is also present on a subset of B cells which may be involved in autoantibody

TABLE 7.
Monoclonal Antibodies Tested for Use in RA

Monoclonal Antibody	Target	Source	Isotype
RFT2	CD7	Mouse	IgG2a
SDZ CHH-380	CD7	Chimeric (human/mouse)	hIgG1
H 65 RA (CD5+)	CD5	Mouse	IgG1
CAMPATH - 6	CD25 (IL2-R)	Rat	IgG2b
CAMPATH - 1H	CDw52	Humanized rat	hIgG1
V1 T4	CD4	Mouse	IgG2a
M-T151	CD4	Mouse	IgG2a
16H5	CD4	Mouse	IgG1
BL4	CD4	Mouse	IgG2a
B-F5	CD4	Mouse	IgG1
M-T412	CD4	Chimeric (human/mouse)	hIgG1

production. CDw52 is found on both T and B lymphocytes as well as some monocytes. Clinical trials of anti-CD5 in RA have used CD5-plus (CD5 mAb linked to ricin A, a protein synthesis inhibitor). Theoretically, the addition of ricin A enhances effectiveness, but no comparative studies have been done to confirm this. In preliminary reports[219] and phase II trials,[220] half the patients showed a short-term improvement by 50%. Data from these studies also suggests that treatment is more effective when used early in the course of RA. Anti-CDw52 (CAMPATH-1H) is the only humanized mAb currently tested. A recent open trial of CAMPATH-1H reported clinical benefit in seven of eight patients treated, with sustained effect for 8 months in one patient.[221]

T cells express activation antigens after stimulation by a specific antigen. MAb against two T-cell activation antigens have been developed. CAMPATH-6, a rat IgG2b antibody against the IL-2 receptor CD25, was given to three patients with refractory RA.[222] Two of the three patients improved for 3 months. Another mAb against an activation antigen of unclear function, CD7, had no effect in 16 patients studied. Failure of therapy was attributed to an improper isotype or target epitope, or the possibility that CD7 is not relevant to the pathogenesis of RA.[223]

Complications of mAb therapy have been relatively few. Common side effects include fever, chills, malaise, nausea, and headache. In most of the trials using rodent mAb, including humanized and chimeric mAb, treated patients developed antirodent antibodies after either the initial or the second course of treatment. Although this antirodent antibody response has not prevented subsequent retreatments with mAb in some of these patients, a potential risk of adverse reactions as well as a decrease in effectiveness exists.

The results from studies of mAb for the treatment of RA have been encouraging. However, these have been small, uncontrolled trials of patients with advanced, refractory disease. Questions regarding efficacy, toxicity, dosing, duration of therapy, and retreatment must still be answered by future trials. Research is ongoing in creating new mAb against other aspects of the inflammatory process such as cytokines, adhesion molecules, and the HLA-DR molecule.

The specific T cell receptors that form in response to the antigenic stimulus of RA are a potential mAb target. T-cell vaccination has been another intriguing area of research.[224] Intact, inactivated T cells theoretically induce immunity to the pathogenic T-cell clone responsible for disease. The future development of these and other treatments will be directed by a more precise understanding of the immunopathology of RA.

Combination Therapy

Given the probable multifactorial pathogenesis of RA and the lack of precise understanding of how second-line agents work in RA, the use of combinations of drugs has been advocated. Proponents of this approach suggest that the therapy of RA could be similar to that used for malignancies: combinations of drugs with presumably different mechanisms of action given concomitantly will be more effective than any agent used alone.

A number of trials of combination therapies have been published, although many were not rigorously controlled. Boers and Ramsden reviewed seven prospective trials (1956–1989), but found only three which they believed were evaluable.[225] Of these, two showed benefit, but one of these combinations had increased toxicity. The third trial showed only additional adverse reactions. The remaining four studies included data which revealed extra effectiveness but also additional problems with untoward effects. Therefore, these authors suggested that, up until 1989, combination therapy could not be advocated based on these trials.

Paulus contradicted this report in a 1990 review of combination chemotherapy.[236] In this retrospective review, he found multidrug treatment to be advantageous when these protocols utilized methotrexate or cyclophosphamide. Nonetheless, Paulus stated that: "There is as yet no evidence that the efficacy of combinations of DMARDS is synergistic, and there is very little suggestion that it is additive."[226]

Many rheumatologists already employ combination therapy, although these protocols generally have added a cytotoxic drug or gold to preexisting antimalarials which are relatively nontoxic drugs. Under these circumstances, additive toxicity is unlikely, although clear advantages have not been demonstrated.

Two recent multicenter trials deserve review. Williams and co-investigators evaluated auranofin and/or MTX in a 48-week trial involving over 300 patients.[227] Combination therapy only proved advantageous over single drug therapy because of a decreased withdrawal rate due to lack of efficacy compared to either drug alone. Wilkens and co-workers compared AZA and/or MTX in a 24-week trial and found MTX alone and combination treatment more effective than AZ alone, but these regimens did alter outcome.[233]

Although appealing in concept, evidence in support of improved efficacy and avoidance of additive toxicity with second-line combination therapy is lacking. Unfortunately, most of the data in the literature are not derived from rigorously controlled trials, a prerequisite for addressing this issue. However, as rheumatologists become increasingly convinced that early and aggressive therapy of RA is warranted, it is probable that the advantages of a multidrug regimen will be tested. At the present time, however, combination treatment cannot be recommended for RA.

Inverting the Pyramid

As noted earlier in this chapter, the traditional approach to the treatment of RA has been based on the pyramid model. This step-wise protocol includes a broad base consisting initially of patient education, physical and occupational therapy, salicylates, and NSAIDS. If this regimen proves ineffective, increasingly aggressive forms of therapy (e.g., remittive drugs) are added sequentially from least toxic (antimalarial drugs, gold) to more toxic (cytotoxic agents), and finally to experimental procedures and agents. Wilske and Healey have recently challenged this model, suggesting that this slow and conservative method permits major joint destruction to occur since the disease is not aggressively treated early in the course of the process when much of the damage is incurred.[229]

These authors have suggested inversion of the pyramid in which aggressive forms of therapy are used early and, as the disease process is contained, more potent agents are removed and less potent and slower onset drugs are continued. Therefore, they propose initiating therapy with low-dose prednisone for one month following the diagnosis. Should this anti-inflammatory approach fail, they consider the patient "at risk" for joint destruction and a "step-down bridge" approach is instituted.[230] Thus, methotrexate, oral gold, IM gold, and anti-malarial drugs are added to prednisone. In this order, it is anticipated that the most potent and most rapidly acting medications (methotrexate and IM gold) will contain the inflammatory process initially thus permitting time for the slower acting agents (oral gold and antimalarial drugs) to become effective. As the disease remits, drugs are sequentially dropped (methotrexate first, then IM gold, and so forth) until the smallest combination of medications is needed.

Unfortunately, this experience is anecdotal and few data in support of this approach exist. Nonetheless, the concept is provocative and supports the combination chemotherapy protocols which have also been suggested.

A related proposal has been advocated by Fries, which he refers to as the "saw tooth" strategy. This approach utilizes many of the concepts outlined by Wilske and Healey and follows six guiding principles: (1) remittive drugs are employed early in the course of the disease prior to irreversible joint destruction; (2) one or more than one of these agents are used continuously; (3) markers of disease activity and disability are charted to monitor outcome; (4) a threshold is determined at which level therapy is altered; (5) remittive drugs are sequentially changed to more potent agents at each of these thresholds; and (6) pain relievers and anti-inflammatory agents are employed for improvement of symptoms.[231] Like the previously described "inverted pyramid," this protocol represents a conceptual approach to the treatment of RA, but data are still lacking. It is anticipated, however, that such novel protocols will be employed with increasing frequency in attempts to modify disease activity early in the course of RA prior to the advent of irrevocable joint destruction. Clearly, such approaches should be based on well-controlled studies, given the lack of existing data in support of these approaches and the concerns of added toxicities with combinations of medications.

Summary

RA remains a therapeutic challenge. Despite substantial data from therapeutic trials, the precise therapy of this often debilitating disease remains controversial. A variety of agents are available to the clinician for the treatment of this disease, yet the precise timing of their use and the determination of situations in which efficacy is most likely to be observed is still unclear. However, it is obvious that earlier intervention and more aggressive forms of therapy are currently advocated by most rheumatologists. Given the rapidity with which this disease can induce substantial morbidity, the use of second-line agents early in the course of this process is warranted. Whether or not combination therapy provides any benefit is still unproved. As our understanding of the pathogenic mechanisms involved in the development of RA evolve, and with the development of newer immunomodulatory agents, it is likely that more specific forms of therapy can be developed. It is hoped that these protocols will permit more precise treatment of the abnormalities leading to this disease without global suppression of the immune system or other unacceptable side effects.

References

1. Gay S, Koopman WJ: Immunopathology of rheumatoid arthritis. *Curr Opin Rheumatol* 1989; 1:8–14.
2. Venables PJW: Infection and rheumatoid arthritis. *Curr Opin Rheumatol* 1989; 1:15–20.
3. Harris ED, Jr: Rheumatoid Arthritis: Pathophysiology and implications for Therapy. *N Engl J Med* 1990; 322:1277–1289.
4. Mannik M: Rheumatoid factors in the pathogenesis of rheumatoid arthritis. *J Rheumatol* 1992; 19(suppl):46–49.
5. Harris ED, Jr: Excitement in the synovium: The rapid evolution of under-

standing of rheumatoid arthritis and expectations for therapy. *J Rheumatol* 1992; 19(suppl 32):3–5.
6. Wortmann RL: Pathogenesis of rheumatoid arthritis: Basis for future therapies. *Semin Arthritis Rheum* 1991; 21:35–39.
7. Roudier J, Rhodes G, Vaughn JH, et al: The Epstein-Barr virus glycoprotein gp110, a molecular link between HLA DR4, HLA DR1, and rheumatoid arthritis. *Scand J Rheumatol* 1988; 27:367–371.
8. Zwillich SH, Lipsky PE: Molecular mimicry in the pathogenesis of rheumatic diseases. *Rheum Dis Clin North Am* 1987; 13:339–352.
9. Vaughn JH, Kouri T, Petersen J, et al: On the etiology of rheumatoid arthritis. *Scand J Rheumatol* 1988; 74:(suppl)19–28.
10. Gregersen PK: HLA associations with rheumatoid arthritis: A piece of the puzzle. *J Rheumatol* 1992; 19 32:(suppl)7–11.
11. Grennan DM: The immunogenetic basis of rheumatoid arthritis. *Curr Opin Rheumatol* 1989; 1:5–7.
12. Firestein GS: The immunpathogenesis of rheumatoid arthritis. *Curr Opin Rheumatol* 1991; 3:398–406.
13. Panayi GS, Lanchbury JS, Kingsley GH: The importance of the T-cell in initiating and maintaining the chronic synovitis of rheumatoid arthritis. *Arthritis Rheum* 1992; 35:729–735.
14. Arnett FC, Edworthy SM, Bloch DA, et al: The american rheumatism association 1988 revised criteria for the classification of rheumatoid arthritis. *Arthritis Rheum* 1988; 31:315–324.
15. Mitchell DM, Spitz PW, Young DY, et al: Survival, prognosis and causes of death in rheumatoid arthritis. *Arthritis Rheum* 1986; 29:706–713.
16. Eggelmaijer F, Otten HG, De Rooy HH, et al: Significance of rheumatoid factor isotypes in seronegative rheumatoid arthritis. *Rheumatol Int* 1990; 10:43–46.
17. Wolfe F, Cathey MA: The assessment and prediction of functional disability in rheumatoid arthritis. *J Rheumatol* 1991; 18:1298–1306.
18. Bacon PA, Farr M: Assessment of rheumatoid arthritis. *Curr Opin Rheumatol* 1991; 3:421–428.
19. Olsen NJ: Assessment of disease activity in rheumatoid arthritis. *Curr Opin Rheumatol* 1989; 1:21–28.
20. Anderson JJ, Felson DT, Meenan RF, et al: Which traditional measures should be used in rheumatoid arthritis clinical trials? *Arthritis Rheum* 1989; 32:1093–1099.
21. Wolfe F, Kleinheksel SM, Cathey MA, et al: The clinical value of the Stanford Health Assessment Questionnaire Functional Disability Index in patients with rheumatoid arthritis. *J Rheumatol* 1988; 15:1480–1488.
22. Anderson JJ, Firschein HE, Meenan RF: Sensitivity of a health status measure to short-term clinical changes in arthritis. *Arthritis Rheum* 1989; 32:844–850.
23. Ochi T, Iwase R, Yonemasu K, et al: Natural course of joint destruction and fluctuation of serum C1q levels in patients with rheumatoid arthritis. *Arthritis Rheum* 1988; 31:37–44.
24. Rubin LA, Snow KM, Kurman CC, et al: Serial levels of soluble interleukin 2 receptor in the peripheral blood of patients with rheumatoid arthritis: Correlations with disease activity. *J Rheumatol* 1990; 17:597–602.
25. Olsen NJ, Callahan LF, Brooks RH, et al: Associations of HLA-DR4 with rheumatoid factor and radiographic severity in rheumatoid arthritis. *Am J Med* 1988; 84:257–264.

26. Sharp JT: Radiologic assessment as an outcome measure in rheumatoid arthritis. *Arthritis Rheum* 1989; 32:221–229.
27. Leigh JP, Fries JF: Mortality predictors among 263 patients with rheumatoid arthritis. *J Rheumatol* 1991; 18:1307–1312.
28. Willkens RF: Prognostic staging for therapy of rheumatoid arthritis. *Semin Arthritis Rheum* 1991; 21(suppl)1:40–43.
29. Pincus T, Callahan LF: Taking mortality in rheumatoid arthritis seriously - Predictive markers, socioeconomic status and comorbidity. *J Rheumatol* 1986; 13:841–845.
30. Markenson JA: Worldwide trends in the socioeconomic impact and long-term prognosis of rheumatoid arthritis. *Semin Arthritis Rheum* 1991; 21(suppl)1: 4–12.
31. Pincus T, Callahan LF, Vaughn WK: Questionnaire, walking time and button test measures of functional capacity as predictive markers for mortality in Rheumatoid Arthritis. *J Rheumatol* 1987; 14:240–243.
32. Kazis LE, Anderson JJ, Meenan RF: Health status as a predictor of mortality in rheumatoid arthritis: A five year study. *J Rheumatol* 1990; 17:609–613.
33. Darlington LG: Dietary therapy for arthritis. *Rheum Dis Clin North Am* 1991; 17:273–285.
34. Williams HJ: Future prospects for the treatment of rheumatoid arthritis. *Curr Opin Rheumatol* 1989; 1:52–58.
35. Kremer JM, Jubiz W, Michalek A, et al: Fish-oil fatty acid supplementation in active rheumatoid arthritis. A double-blinded, controlled, crossover study. *Ann Intern Med* 1987; 106:497.
36. Gerber LH: Rehabilitation of patients with rheumatic diseases, in Kelley WN (ed): *Textbook of Rheumatology*. Philadelphia, WB Saunders, 1989, pp 1904–1918.
37. Schlegel SI, Paulus HE: Update on NSAID use in rheumatic diseases. *Bull Rheum Dis* 1986; 36:1–8.
38. Cush JJ, Lipsky PE, Postlethwaite AE, et al: Correlation of serologic indicators of inflammation with effectiveness of nonsteroidal antiinflammatory drug therapy in rheumatoid arthritis. *Arthritis Rheum* 1990; 33:19–28.
39. Schlegel SI: *Drugs for Rheumatic Disease*. New York, Churchill Livingstone, 1987, p 203.
40. Fenner H: Nonsteroidal antiinflammatory drugs: benefit/risk evaluation in rheumatic diseases. *J Rheumatol* 1992; 19(suppl)32:98–99.
41. Fries JF, Williams CA, Bloch DA, et al: Nonsteroidal anti-inflammatory drug-associated gastropathy: Incidence and risk factor models. *Am J Med* 1991; 91:213–221.
42. Stewart CF, Evans WE: Drug-drug Interactions with antirheumatic agents: Review of selected clinically important interactions. *J Rheumatol* 1990; 17(suppl)22:16–23.
43. Hench PS, Kendall EC, Slocumb CH, et al: The effect of a hormone of the adrenal cortex (17-hydroxy-11-dehydrocorticosterone: compound E) and of pituitary adrenocorticotropic hormone on rheumatoid arthritis: Preliminary report. *Mayo Clin Proc* 1949; 24:181–197.
44. Empire Rheumatism Council: Multi-centre controlled trial comparing cortisone acetate and acetyl salicylic acid in the long-term treatment of rheumatoid arthritis. *Ann Rheum Dis* 1955; 14:353–367.
45. Joint Committee of the Medical Research Council and Nuffield Foundation: A comparison of prednisolone with aspirin or other analgesics in the treatment of rheumatoid arthritis. *Ann Rheum Dis* 1960; 19:331–337.

46. Harris ED, Jr, Emkey RD, Nichols JE: Low dose prednisone therapy in rheumatoid arthritis: a double-blind study. *J Rheumatol* 1983; 10:713–721.
47. Stuck AE, Minder CE, Frey FJ: Risk of infectious complications in patients taking glucocorticoids. *Rev Infectious Dis* 1989; 2:954–963.
48. Leibling MR, Leib E, McLaughlin K, et al: Pulse methylprednisolone in rheumatoid arthritis. *Ann Intern Med* 1981; 94:21–26.
49. Hansen TM, Kryger P, Elling H, et al: Double blind placebo controlled trial of pulse treatment with methylprednisolone combined with disease modifying drugs in rheumatoid arthritis. *Br Med J* 1990; 301:268–270.
50. Wong CS, Champion G, Smith MD, et al: Does steroid pulsing influence the efficacy and toxicity of chrysotherapy? A double blind, placebo controlled study. *Ann Rheum Dis* 1990; 49:370–372.
51. Lockie LM, Gomez E, Smith DM, et al: Low dose adrenocorticosteroids in the management of elderly patients with rheumatoid arthritis: Selected examples and summary of efficacy in the long-term treatment of 97 patients. *Semin Arthritis Rheum* 1983; 8:373–381.
52. Forestier J: Rheumatoid arthritis and its treatment by gold salts. *J Lab Clin Med* 1935; 20:827.
53. Empire Rheumatism Council: Gold therapy in rheumatoid arthritis: Final report of a multicentre controlled trial. *Ann Rheum Dis* 1961; 20:315.
54. Sigler JW, Bluhm GB, Duncan H: Gold salts in the treatment of rheumatoid arthritis: A double-blind study. *Ann Intern Med* 1974; 80:21–26.
55. Iannuzzi L, Dawson N, Zein N, et al: Does drug therapy slow radiographic deterioration in rheumatoid arthritis? *N Engl J Med* 1983; 309:1023–1028.
56. Felson DT, Anderson JJ, Meenan RF: The comparative efficacy and toxicity of second-line drugs in rheumatoid arthritis: Results of two meta-analyses. *Arthritis Rheum* 1989; 33:1449–1461.
57. Williams HJ, Ward JR, Dahl SL, et al: A controlled trial comparing sulfasalazine, gold sodium thiomalate, and placebo in rheumatoid arthritis. *Arthritis Rheum* 1988; 31:702–713.
58. Epstein WV, Henke CJ, Yelin EH, et al: Effect of parenterally administered gold therapy on the course of adult rheumatoid arthritis. *Ann Intern Med* 1991; 114:437–444.
59. Epstein WV: Parenteral gold therapy for rheumatoid arthritis: A treatment whose time has gone. *J Rheumatol* 1989; 16:1291–1294.
60. Hoffman GS: Rheumatoid Arthritis, in Lichtenstein LM, Fauci AS (eds): *Current Therapy in Allergy, Immunology, and Rheumatology.* St Louis, Mosby-Year Book, 1992, p 161.
61. Harth M: Mechanisms of action of disease modifying antirheumatic drugs. *J Rheumatol* 1992; 19(suppl)32:100–103.
62. Yan A, Davis P: Gold induced marrow suppression: A review of 10 cases. *J Rheumatol* 1990; 17:47–51.
63. Wolfe F, Hawley DJ, Cathey MA: Termination of slow acting antirheumatic therapy in rheumatoid arthritis: A 14-year prospective evaluation of 1017 consecutive starts. *J Rheumatol* 1990; 17:994–1001.
64. Bensen WG, Moore N, Tugwell P, et al: HLA antigens and toxic reactions to sodium aurothiomalate in patients with rheumatoid arthritis. *J Rheumatol* 1984; 11:358–360.
65. Page F: Treatment of lupus erythematosus with mepacrine. *Lancet* 1951; 2:755.
66. Mainland D, Sutcliffe MI: Hydroxychloroquine sulfate in rheumatoid arthritis, a six month double-blind trial. *Bull Rheum Dis* 1957; 13:287–290.

67. Hamilton EBD, Scott JT: Hydroxychloroquine sulfate (Plaquenil) in the treatment of rheumatoid arthritis. *Arthritis Rheum* 1962; 5:502–512.
68. Freedman A, Steinberg VL: Chloroquine in rheumatoid arthritis: A double blindfold trial of treatment for one year. *Ann Rheum Dis* 1960; 19:243–250.
69. Kersley GD, Palin AG: Amodiaquine and hydroxychloroquine in rheumatoid arthritis. *Lancet* 1959; 2:886–888.
70. Popert AJ, Meijers KAE, Sharp J, et al: Chloroquine diphosphate in rheumatoid arthritis: A controlled trial. *Ann Rheum Dis* 1961; 20:18–35.
71. Adams EM, Yocum DE, Bell CL: Hydroxychloroquine in the treatment of rheumatoid arthritis. *Am J Med* 1983; 75:321–326.
72. Scherbel AL, Harrison JW, Atdjian M: Further observation on the use of 4-aminoquinoline compounds in patients with rheumatoid arthritis or related diseases. *Cleveland Clin Q* 1958; 25:95–111.
73. Easterbrook M: Dose relationships in patients with early chloroquine retinopathy. *J Rheumatol* 1987; 14:472.
74. Mackenzie AH: Dose refinements in long-term therapy of rheumatoid arthritis with antimalarials. *Am J Med* 1983; 75:40–45.
75. Dixon JS, Pickup ME, Bird HA, et al: Biochemical indices of responses to hydroxychloroquine and sodium aurothiomalate in rheumatoid arthritis. *Ann Rheum Dis* 1981; 40:480–488.
76. Richter JA, Runge LA, Pinals RS: Analysis of treatment terminations with gold and antimalarial compounds in rheumatoid arthritis. *J Rheumatol* 1980; 7:153–159.
77. Dwosh IL, Stein HB, Urowitz MB, et al: Azathioprine in early rheumatoid arthritis: Comparison with gold and chloroquine. *Arthritis Rheum* 1977; 20:685–692.
78. Bird HA, Le Gallez P, Dixon JS, et al: A single-blind comparative study of auranofin and hydroxychloroquine in patients with rheumatoid arthritis. *Clin Rheumatol* 1984; 3(suppl)1:57–66.
79. Husain Z, Runge LA: Treatment complications of rheumatoid arthritis with gold, hydroxychloroquine, D-penicillamine, and levamisole. *J Rheumatol* 1980; 7:825–830.
80. Bunch TW, O'Duffy JD, Tompkins RB, et al: Controlled trial of hydroxychloroquine and D-penicillamine singly and in combination in the treatment of rheumatoid arthritis. *Arthritis Rheum* 1984; 27:267–276.
81. van Riel PLCM, Nuver-Zwart I, Gribnau FWJ, et al: A double-blind comparative study of sulfasalazine and hydroxychloroquine in patients with rheumatoid arthritis (RA). *Arthritis Rheum* 1988; 31(suppl)4:30.
82. van der Heijde DM, van Riel PLCM, Nuver-Zwart I, et al: Effects of hydroxychloroquine and sulphasalazine on progression of joint damage in rheumatoid arthritis. *Lancet* 1989; 1036–1038.
83. Nuver-Zwart I, van Riel PLCM, van de Putte LBA, et al: A double blind comparative study of sulphasalazine and hydroxychloroquine in rheumatoid arthritis: Evidence of an earlier effect of sulphasalazine. *Ann Rheum Dis* 1989; 48:389–395.
84. Rainsford KD: Effects of anti-inflammatory drugs on catabalin-induced cartilage destruction in vitro. *Int J Tissue React* 1985; 7:123.
85. Easterbrook M: Ocular effects and safety of antimalarial agents. *Am J Med* 1988; 85(suppl)4A:23–29.
86. Bernstein HN: Ocular safety of hydroxychloroquine. *Ann Ophthalmol* 1991; 23:292–296.

87. Rynes RI, Krohel G, Falbo A, et al: Ophthalmologic safety of long-term hydroxychloroquine treatment. *Arthritis Rheum* 1979; 22:832–836.
88. Walshe JM: Penicillamine: New oral therapy for Wilson's disease. *Am J Med* 1956; 21:487–491.
89. Deutsch HF, Morton JI: Dissociation of human serum macroglobulins. *Science* 1957; 125:600.
90. Lipsky PE, Ziff M: Inhibition of human helper T-cell function in vitro by D-penicillamine and CuSo4. *J Clin Invest* 1980; 65:1069–1076.
91. Hirata S, Matsubara T, Saura R, et al: Inhibition of in vitro vascular endothelial cell proliferation and in vivo neovascularization by low-dose methotrexate. *Arthritis Rheum* 1989; 32:1065–1073.
92. Jaffe IA: Rheumatoid arthritis with arteritis: Report of a case treated with penicillamine. *Ann Intern Med* 1964; 61:556–560.
93. Jaffe IA: The treatment of rheumatoid arthritis and necrotizing vasculitis with penicillamine. *Arthritis Rheum* 1970; 13:436–440.
94. Zuckner J, Ramsey RH, Dorner RW, et al: D-Penicillamine in rheumatoid arthritis. *Arthritis Rheum* 1970; 13:131–135.
95. Huskisson EC, Hart FD: Penicillamine in the treatment of rheumatoid arthritis. *Ann Rheum Dis* 1972; 31:402–404.
96. Multicentre Trial Group: Controlled trial of D-penicillamine in severe rheumatoid arthritis. *Lancet* 1973; 1:275.
97. Williams HJ, Ward JR, Reading JC, et al: Low-dose D-penicillamine therapy in rheumatoid arthritis: A controlled, double-blind clinical trial. *Arthritis Rheum* 1983; 26:581–592.
98. Shiokawa Y, Horiuchi Y, Homma M, et al: Clinical evaluation of D-penicillamine by a multicenter double-blind comparative study in chronic rheumatoid arthritis. *Arthritis Rheum* 1977; 20:1464–1472.
99. Hochberg MC: Auranofin or D-penicillamine in the treatment of rheumatoid arthritis. *Ann Intern Med* 1986; 105:528–535.
100. Makisara P, Nissila M, Kajander A, et al: Comparison of penicillamine and gold treatment in early rheumatoid arthritis. *Scand J Rheumatol* 1978; 7:166–169.
101. Barraclough D, Brook A, Brooks P, et al: A comparative study of auranofin, gold sodium thiomalate and D-penicillamine in rheumatoid arthritis: A progress report. *J Rheumatol* 1982; 8(suppl):197–200.
102. Franchimont P, Hauwaert C, Vanschoubroek K, et al: Auranofin and D-penicillamine: A one year comparative study of safety and efficacy in patients with rheumatoid arthritis followed by a two year open assessment. *Clin Rheumatol* 1984; 3(suppl)1:75–82.
103. Huskisson EC, Gibson TJ, Balme HW, et al: Trial comparing D-penicillamine and gold in rheumatoid arthritis: Preliminary report. *Ann Rheum Dis* 1974; 33:532–535.
104. Situnayake RD, Grindulis KA, McConkey B: Long-term treatment of rheumatoid arthritis with sulphasalazine, gold, or penicillamine: A comparison using life-table methods. *Ann Rheum Dis* 1987; 46:177–183.
105. Morand EF, McCloud PI, Littlejohn GO: Life table analysis of 879 treatment episodes with slow acting antirheumatic drugs in community rheumatology practice. *J Rheumatol* 1992; 19:704–708.
106. Cooperative Systematic Studies of Rheumatic Disease Group: Toxicity of long-term low dose D-penicillamine therapy in rheumatoid arthritis. *J Rheumatol* 1987; 14:67–73.
107. Dixon AJ, Davies J, Dormandy TL, et al: Synthetic D-penicillamine in rheu-

matoid arthritis: Double-blind controlled study of a high and low dose regimen. *Ann Rheum Dis* 1975; 34:416–421.
108. McConkey B, Amos RS, Durham S, et al: Sulphasalazine in rheumatoid arthritis. *Br Med J* 1980; 280:442–444.
109. Bird HA, Dixon JS, Pickup ME, et al: A biochemical assessment of sulphasalazine in rheumatoid arthritis. *J Rheumatol* 1982; 9:36–45.
110. Neumann VC, Grindulis KA, Huball S, et al: Comparison between penicillamine and sulphasalazine in rheumatoid arthritis. *Br Med J* 1983; 287:1099–1102.
111. Chalmers IM, Sitar DS, Hunter T: A one-year, open, prospective study of sulfasalazine in the treatment of rheumatoid arthritis: Adverse reactions and clinical response in relation to laboratory variables, drug and metabolite serum levels, and acetylator status. *J Rheumatol* 1990; 17:764–770.
112. Pullar T, Hunter JA, Capell HA: Sulphasalazine in rheumatoid arthritis: A double-blind comparison of sulphasalazine with placebo and sodium aurothiomalate. *Br Med J* 1983; 287:1102–1104.
113. Pinals RS, Kaplan SB, Lawson JG, et al: Sulfasalazine in rheumatoid arthritis. A double-blind, placebo-controlled trial. *Arthritis Rheum* 1986; 29:1427–1434.
114. Williams H, Ward JR, Dahl SL, et al: A controlled trial comparing sulphasalazine, gold sodium thiomalate, and placebo in rheumatoid arthritis. *Arthritis Rheum* 1988; 31:702–713.
115. Porter D, Hunter JA, Capell HA: Prospective trial comparing the use of sulphasalazine and auranofin as second-line drugs in patients with rheumatoid arthritis. *Ann Rheum Dis* 1992; 51:461–464.
116. Bax DE, Amos RS: Sulphasalazine: A safe, effective agent for prolonged control of rheumatoid arthritis: A comparison with sodium aurothiomalate. *Ann Rheum Dis* 1985; 44:194–198.
117. van der Heijde DM, van Riel PLCM, Nuver-Zwart I, et al: Sulphasalazine versus hydroxychloroquine in rheumatoid arthritis: 3-year follow-up. *Lancet* 1992; 335:539.
118. Pullar T, Hunter JA, Capell HA: Which component of sulphasalazine is active in rheumatoid arthritis? *Br Med J* 1985; 290:1535–1538.
119. Neumann VC, Taggart AJ, LeGallez P, et al: A study to determine the active moiety of sulphasalazine in rheumatoid arthritis. *J Rheumatol* 1986; 13:285–287.
120. Pinals RS: Sulfasalazine in the rheumatic disease. *Semin Arthritis Rheum* 1988; 17:246–259.
121. Madhok R, Wijelath E, Smith J, et al: Is the beneficial effect of sulfasalazine due to inhibition of synovial neovascularization? *J Rheumatol* 1991; 18:199–202.
122. Pullar T, Hunter JA, Capell HA: Effect of acetylator phenotype on efficacy and toxicity of sulphasalazine. *Ann Rheum Dis* 1985; 44:831–837.
123. Gubner R, August S, Grusberg V: Therapeutic suppression of tissue reactivity. II. Effect of aminopterin in rheumatoid arthritis and psoriasis. *Am J Med Sci* 1951; 221:176–182.
124. Hoffmeister RT: Methotrexate in rheumatoid arthritis (abstract). *Arthritis Rheum* 1972; 15:114.
125. Hoffmeister RT: Methotrexate therapy in rheumatoid arthritis: 15 years experience. *Am J Med* 1983; 12(suppl):69–73.
126. Wilke WS, Calabrese IH, Scherbel AL: Methotrexate in the treatment of rheumatoid arthritis. *Clev Clin* 1980; 47:305–309.

127. Willkens RF, Watson MA, Paxson CS: Low dose pulse methotrexate therapy in rheumatoid arthritis. *J Rheumatol* 1980; 7:501–505.
128. Michaels RM, Nashel DJ, Leonard A: Weekly intravenous methotrexate in the treatment of rheumatoid arthritis. *Arthritis Rheum* 1982; 25:339–341.
129. Steinsson K, Weinstein A, Korn J, et al: Low dose methotrexate in rheumatoid arthritis. *J Rheumatol* 1982; 9:860–866.
130. Groff GD, Shenberger KN, Wilke WS, et al: Low dose oral methotrexate in rheumatoid arthritis: An uncontrolled trial and review of the literature. *Semin Arthritis Rheum* 1983; 12:333–347.
131. Williams H, Willkens RF, Samuelson CO, Jr., et al: Comparison of low dose oral pulse methotrexate and placebo in the treatment of rheumatoid arthritis: A controlled clinical trial. *Arthritis Rheum* 1985; 28:721–730.
132. Weinblatt ME, Coblyn JS, Fox DA, et al: Efficacy of low dose methotrexate in rheumatoid arthritis. *N Engl J Med* 1985; 312:818–822.
133. Andersen PA, West SG, O'dell JR, et al: Weekly pulse methotrexate in rheumatoid arthritis: Clinical and immunologic effects in a randomized double blind study. *Ann Intern Med* 1985; 103:489–496.
134. Thompson RN, Watts C, Edelman J, et al: A controlled two center trial of parenteral methotrexate therapy for refractory rheumatoid arthritis. *J Rheumatol* 1984; 11:760–763.
135. Tugwell P, Bennett K, Gent M: Methotrexate in rheumatoid arthritis: Indications, contraindications, efficacy, and safety. *Ann Intern Med* 1987; 197:358–366.
136. Rau R, Herborn G, Karger T, et al: A double-blind randomized parallel trial of intramuscular methotrexate and gold sodium thiomalate in early erosive rheumatoid arthritis. *J Rheumatol* 1991; 18:328–338.
137. Rau R, Herborn G, Karger T, et al: A double-blind comparison of parenteral methotrexate and parenteral gold in the treatment of early erosive rheumatoid arthritis: An interim report on 102 patients after 12 months. *Semin Arthritis Rheum* 1991; 21(suppl 1):13–20.
138. Morassut P, Goldstein R, Cyr M, et al: Gold sodium thiomalate compared to low dose methotrexate in the treatment of rheumatoid arthritis: A randomized, double blind 26 week trial. *J Rheumatol* 1989; 16:302–306.
139. Weinblatt ME, Kaplan H, Germain BF, et al: Low dose methotrexate compared with auranofin in adult rheumatoid arthritis. *Arthritis Rheum* 1990; 33:330–338.
140. Hamdy HH, McKendry RJR, Mierins E, et al: Low dose methotrexate compared with azathioprine in the treatment of rheumatoid arthritis. *Arthritis Rheum* 1987; 30:361–368.
141. Jeurissen MEC, Boerbooms, AM, van de Putte LBA, et al: Methotrexate versus azathioprine in the treatment of rheumatoid arthritis. *Arthritis Rheum* 1991; 34:8:961–972.
142. Kremer JM: Long-term methotrexate therapy in rheumatoid arthritis: A review. *J Rheumatol* 1985; 12(suppl):25–28.
143. Kremer JM, Lee JK: A long-term prospective study of the use of methotrexate in rheumatoid arthritis: update after a mean of fifty-three months. *Arthritis Rheum* 1988; 31:577–584.
144. Kremer JM, Lee JK: The safety and efficacy of the use of methotrexate in long-term therapy for rheumatoid arthritis. *Arthritis Rheum* 1986; 29:822–831.
145. Fehlauer CS, Carson CW, Cannon GW, et al: Methotrexate therapy in rheu-

matoid arthritis: 2-year retrospective followup study. *J Rheumatol* 1989; 16:307–312.
146. Weinblatt ME, Maier AL: Long-term experience with low dose weekly methotrexate in rheumatoid arthritis. *J Rheumatol* 1990; 17:33–38.
147. Sany J, Anaya JM, Lussiez V, et al: Treatment of rheumatoid arthritis with methotrexate: A prospective open long-term study of 191 cases (abstract). *J Rheumatol* 1991; 18:1323–1327.
148. Weinblatt ME, Weissman BN, Holdsworth DE, et al: Long-term prospective study of methotrexate in the treatment of rheumatoid arthritis: 84-Month Update. *Arthritis Rheum* 1992; 35:129–137.
149. Kremer JM, Phelps CT: Long-term prospective study of the use of methotrexate in the treatment of rheumatoid arthritis: Update after a mean of 90 months. *Arthritis Rheum* 1992; 35:138–145.
150. Alarcon GS, Lopez-Mendez A, Walter J, et al: Radiographic evidence of disease progression in methotrexate treated and nonmethotrexate disease modifying antirheumatic drug treated rheumatoid arthritis patients: A meta-analysis. *J Rheumatol* 1992; 19:1868–1873.
151. Weinblatt ME, Trentham DE, Fraser PA, et al: Long-term prospective trial of low dose methotrexate in rheumatoid arthritis. *Arthritis Rheum* 1988; 31:167–175.
152. Jeurissen MEC, Boerbooms AM, van de Putte LBA, et al: Influence of methotrexate and azathiorpine on radiologic progression in rheumatoid arthritis. *Ann Intern Med* 1991; 114:999–1004.
153. Alarcon GS, Schrohenloher RE, Bartolucci AA, et al: Suppression of rheumatoid factor production by methotrexate in patients with rheumatoid arthritis: Evidence for differential influences of therapy and clinical status on IgM and IgA rheumatoid factor expression. *Arthritis Rheum* 1990; 33:1156–1161.
154. Sperling RI, Coblyn JS, Larkin JK: Inhibition of leukotriene B4 synthesis in neutrophils from patients with rheumatoid arthritis by a single oral dose of methotrexate. *Arthritis Rheum* 1990; 33:1149–1155.
155. Segal R, Mozes E, Yaron M, et al: The effects of methotrexate on the production and activity of interleukin-1. *Arthritis Rheum* 1989; 32:370–377.
156. Olsen NJ, Murray LM: Antiproliferative effects of methotrexate on peripheral blood mononuclear cells. *Arthritis Rheum* 1989; 32:378–385.
157. Furst DE, Kremer JM: Methotrexate in rheumatoid arthritis. *Arthritis Rheum* 1988; 31:305–314.
158. Stewart CF, Fleming RA, Germain BF, et al: Aspirin alters methotrexate disposition in rheumatoid arthritis patients. *Arthritis Rheum* 1991; 34:14514–1520.
159. Morgan SL, Baggott JE, Vaughn WH, et al: The effect of folic acid supplementation on the toxicity of low-dose methotrexate in patient with rheumatoid arthritis. *Arthritis Rheum* 1990; 33:1:9–18.
160. Roenigk HH, Maibach HI, Weinstein GP: Methotrexate therapy for psoriasis. Guideline revisions. *Arch Dermatol* 1973; 108:35.
161. Brick JE, Moreland LW, Al-Kawas F, et al: Prospective analysis of liver biopsies before and after methotrexate therapy in rheumatoid patients. *Semin Arthritis Rheum* 1989; 19:31–44.
162. Kremer JM, Koff R: A Debate: Should patients with rheumatoid arthritis on methotrexate undergo liver biopsies? *Semin Arthritis Rheum* 1992; 21:376–386.
163. Kremer JM: Liver biopsies in patients with rheumatoid arthritis receiving methotrexate: Where are we going? (editorial). *J Rheum* 1992; 19:2:189–191.

164. Tolman KG, Clegg DO, Lee RG, et al: Methotrexate and the liver. *J Rheumatol* 1985; 12(suppl):29–34.
165. Furst DE, Koehnke RE, Burmeister LF, et al: Increasing methotrexate effect with increasing dose in the treatment of resistant rheumatoid arthritis. *J Rheumatol* 1989; 16:313–320.
166. Shiroky JB: Complications of immunosuppression associated with weekly low dose methotrexate (abstract). *J Rheumatol* 1991; 18:1172–1175.
167. Galens GJ, Bull FE, Bartholomew LE: The treatment of rheumatoid arthritis with G-mercaptopurine and azathioprine. *Arthritis Rheum* 1964; 7:735–737.
168. Urowitz MB, Gordon DA, Smythe HA, et al: Azathioprine in rheumatoid arthritis: A double blind cross over study. *Arthritis Rheum* 1973; 16:411–419.
169. De Silva M, Hazleman BL: Long-term azathioprine in rheumatoid arthritis: A double-blind study. *Ann Rheum Dis* 1981; 40:560–563.
170. Woodland J, Chaput DeSaintonge DM, Evans SJW, et al: Azathioprine in rheumatoid arthritis: Double-blind study of full versus half doses versus placebo. *Ann Rheum Dis* 1981; 40:359–368.
171. Currey HLF, Harris J, Mason RM, et al: Comparison of azathioprine, cyclophosphamide, and gold in treatment of rheumatoid arthritis. *Br J Rheumatol* 1974; 3:763–766.
172. Paulus HE, Williams HJ, Ward JR, et al: Azathioprine versus D-penicillamine in rheumatoid arthritis patients who have been treated unsuccessfully with gold. *Arthritis Rheum* 1984; 27:721–728.
173. Halberg P, Bentzon MW, Crohn O, et al: Double blind trial of levamisole, penicillamine, azathioprine in rheumatoid arthritis. *Dan Med Bull* 1984; 31:403–409.
174. Cseuz R, Zimmerman J, Panayi GS: Daily and alternate-day azathioprine treatment in rheumatoid arthritis: A twelve-week controlled clinical trial (letter). *Br J Rheum* 1992; 31:501–504.
175. Diaz CJ, Garcia EL, Merchante A, et al: Treatment of rheumatoid arthritis with nitrogen mustard: A preliminary report. *JAMA* 1951; 147:1418–1419.
176. Cooperating Clinics Committee of the American Rheumatism Association: A controlled trial of cyclophosphamide in rheumatoid arthritis. *N Engl J Med* 1970; 283:883–889.
177. Townes AS, Sawa JM, Shulman LE: Controlled trial of cyclophosphamide therapy in rheumatoid arthritis. *Arthritis Rheum* 1976; 19:563–573.
178. Fosdick WM, Parsons JL, Hill DF: Long-term cyclophosphamide therapy in rheumatoid arthritis. *Arthritis Rheum* 1968; 11:151–161.
179. White DJG, Calne RY: The use of cyclosporin A immunosuppression in organ grafting. *Immunol Rev* 1982; 65:115–118.
180. Weinblatt ME, Coblyn JS, Fraser PA: Cyclosporin: A treatment of refractory rheumatoid arthritis. *Arthritis Rheum* 1987; 30:11–17.
181. Bowles CA: Long-term treatment of rheumatoid arthritis with cyclosporin (CsA). *Arthritis Rheum* 1987; 32:S61.
182. van Rijthoven AWAM, Dijkmans BAC, Goei The HS, et al: Cyclosporine treatment for rheumatoid arthritis: A placebo-controlled double-blind multicentre study. *Ann Rheum Dis* 1986; 45:726–731.
183. Tugwell P, Bombardier C, Gent M, et al: Low dose cyclosporine in rheumatoid arthritis: A pilot study. *J Rheumatol* 1987; 14:1108–1114.
184. Dougados M, Duchesne L, Awada H, et al: Assessment of efficacy and acceptability of low dose cyclosporine in patients with rheumatoid arthritis. *Ann Rheum Dis* 1989; 48:550–556.
185. Dougados M, Amor B, Awada H: Cyclosporine in rheumatoid arthritis: A

double-blind, placebo controlled study in 52 patients. *Ann Rheum Dis* 1988; 47:127–133.
186. Tugwell P, Bombardier C, Gent M, et al: Low-dose cyclosporin versus placebo in patients with rheumatoid arthritis. *Lancet* 1990; 335:1051–1055.
187. Forre O, Bjerkhoel F, Salvesen CF, et al: An open, controlled, randomized comparison of cyclosporin and azathioprine in the treatment of rheumatoid arthritis: A preliminary report. *Arthritis Rheum* 1987; 30:88–92.
188. van Rijthoven AWAM, Dijkmans BAC, Goei The HS, et al: Comparison of cyclosporine and D-penicillamine for rheumatoid arthritis: A randomized, double blind, multicenter study. *J Rheumatol* 1991; 18:815–820.
189. Wells G, Tugwell P: Cyclosporin A in rheumatoid arthritis: Overview of efficacy. *Br J Rheum* 1993; 32(suppl):51–56.
190. van Rijthoven AWAM, Dijkmans BAC, Goei The HS, et al: Long-term cyclosporine therapy in rheumatoid arthritis. *J Rheumatol* 1990; 18:19–23.
191. Ludwin D, Alexopoulou I: Cyclosporin A nephropathy in patients with rheumatoid arthritis. *Br J Rheumatol* 1993; 32(suppl 1):60–64.
192. Feutren G: Renal morphology after cyclosporin A therapy in rheumatoid arthritis patients. *Br J Rheumatol* 1993; 1993; 32(suppl 1):65–71.
193. Altman RD, Perez GO, Sfakianakis GN: Interaction of cyclosporine A and nonsteroidal anti-inflammatory drugs on renal function in patients with rheumatoid arthritis. *Am J Med* 1992; 93:396–402.
194. Arellano F, Krupp P: Malignancies in rheumatoid arthritis patients treated with cyclosporin A. *Br J Rheum* 1993; 32(suppl 1):72–75.
195. Veys EM, Mielants H, Verbruggen G: Thymic hormones and interferons in the treatment of rheumatoid arthritis. *Scand J Rheumatol* 1988; 76(suppl): 297–304.
196. Lemmel EM, Franke M, Gaus W, et al: Results of a phase-II clinical trial on treatment of rheumatoid arthritis with recombinant interferon-gamma. *Rheumatol Int* 1987; 7:127–132.
197. Wolfe F, Cathey MA, Hawley DJ, et al: Recombinant gamma-interferon in rheumatoid arthritis. *Arthritis Rheum* 1986; 29(suppl):18.
198. Veys EM, Mielants H, Verbruggen G, et al: Interferon gamma in rheumatoid arthritis: A double blind study comparing human recombinant interferon gamma with placebo. *J Rheumatol* 1988; 15:570–574.
199. Cannon GW, Pincus SH, Emkey RD, et al: Double-blind trial of recombinant gamma interferon versus placebo in the treatment of rheumatoid arthritis (abstract). *Arthritis Rheum* 1989; 32:964–973.
200. Lemmel EM, Brackertz D, Franke M, et al: Results of a multicenter placebo-controlled double-blind randomized phase III clinical study of treatment of rheumatoid arthritis with recombinant interferon-gamma. *Rheumatol Int* 1988; 8:87–93.
201. Cannon GW, Emkey RD, Denes A, et al: Prospective two-year followup of recombinant interferon-gamma in rheumatoid arthritis. *J Rheumatol* 1990; 17:304–310.
202. Machold KP, Neumann K, Smolen JS: Recombinant human interferon gamma in the treatment of rheumatoid arthritis: Double blind placebo controlled study. *Ann Rheum Dis* 1992; 51:1039–1043.
203. Weinblatt ME, Maier AL, Emery P: Substantial placebo response with parenteral therapy in active rheumatoid arthritis. *Arthritis Rheum* 1990; 33(suppl):152.
204. Graninger WB, Hassfeld W, Pesau BB, et al: Induction of systemic lupus ery-

thematosus by interferon-gamma in a patient with rheumatoid arthritis. *J Rheumatol* 1991; 18:1621.
205. Arend WP: Interleukin-1 receptor antagonist. A new member of the interleukin-1 family. *J Clin Invest* 1991; 88:1445.
206. Smith RJ, Chin JE, Sam LM, et al: Biologic effects of an interleukin-1 receptor antagonist protein on interleukin-1-stimulated cartilage erosion and chondrocyte responsiveness. *Arthritis Rheum* 1991; 34:78–83.
207. Carter DB, Deibel MR, Jr, Dunn CJ, et al: Purification, cloning expression and biological characterization of an interleukin-1 receptor protein. *Nature* 1990; 344:633–638.
208. Sewell KL, Trentham DE: Rapid improvement in refractory rheumatoid arthritis by an interleukin 2 receptor targeted immunotherapy (abstract). *Clin Res* 1991; 39:314A.
209. Paulus HE, Machleder HI, Levine S, et al: Lymphocyte involvement in rheumatoid arthritis: Studies during thoracic duct drainage. *Arthritis Rheum* 1990; 20:1249–1262.
210. Kotzin BL, Strober S, Engelman EC: Treatment of intractable rheumatoid arthritis with total lymphoid irradiation. *N Engl J Med* 1981; 305:969–974.
211. Emery P, Smith GN, Panayi GS: Lymphocytapheresis: a feasible treatment for rheumatoid arthritis. *Br J Rheumatol* 1986; 25:40–43.
212. Cosimi AB, Colvin RB, Burton RC, et al: Monoclonal antibodies for immunologic monitoring and treatment in recipients of renal allograft. *N Engl J Med* 1981; 305:303–308.
213. Herzog C, Walker C, Pichler W, et al: Monoclonal anti-CD4 in arthritis. *Lancet* 1987; ii:1461–1462.
214. Herzog C, Walker C, Muller W, et al: Anti-CD4 treatment of patients with rheumatoid arthritis: I. Effect on clinical course and circulating T cells. *J Autoimmun* 1989; 2:627–642.
215. Goldberg D, Morel P, Chatenoud L, et al: Immunological effects of high dose administration of anti-CD4 antibodies in rheumatoid arthritis. *J Autoimmun* 1991; 4:617–630.
216. Wendling D, Wijdenes J, Racadoy E, et al: Therapeutic use of monoclonal anti-CD4 antibody in rheumatoid arthritis. *J Rheumatol* 1991; 18:325–327.
217. Horneff G, Burmeister G, Emmrich F, et al: Treatment of rheumatoid arthritis with an anti-CD4 monoclonal antibody. *Arthritis Rheum* 1991; 34:129–140.
218. Reiter C, Kakavand B, Reiber E, et al: Treatment of rheumatoid arthritis with monoclonal CD4 antibody M-T151. *Arthritis Rheum* 1991; 34:525–536.
219. Strand V, Fishwild D: Xoma rheumatoid arthritis investigation group: Treatment of rheumatoid arthritis with anti-CD5 immunoconjugate: Clinical and immunologic findings and preliminary results of retreatment (abstract). *Arthritis Rheum* 1990; 33:S25.
220. Strand V, Lipsky PE, Cannon G, et al: Treatment of rheumatoid arthritis with an anti-CD5 immunoconjugate final results of phase II studies (abstract). *Arthritis Rheum* 1991; 34:S91.
221. Isaacs JD, Watts RA, Hazleman BL, et al: Humanised monoclonal antibody therapy for rheumatoid arthritis. *Lancet* 1992; 340:748–752.
222. Kyle V, Coughlin RJ, Tighe H, et al: Beneficial effect of monoclonal antibody to the interleukin 2 receptor on activated T cells in rheumatoid arthritis. *Ann Rheum Dis* 1989; 48:428–429.
223. Kirkham B, Thien F, Amlot P, et al: Chimeric (human/mouse) CD7 monoclonal antibody treatment in rheumatoid arthritis (abstract). *Br J Rheumatol* 1991; 30(suppl 2):88.

224. van Laar JM, Miltenburg AMM, Verdonk MJ, et al: T-Cell vaccination in rheumatoid arthritis. *Br J Rheumatol* 1991; 30(suppl 2):28.
225. Boers M, Ramsden M: Longacting drug combinations in rheumatoid arthritis: A formal review. *J Rheumatol* 1991; 18:316–324.
226. Paulus HE: The use of combinations of disease-modifying antirheumatic agents in rheumatoid arthritis. *Arthritis Rheum* 1990; 33:113–120.
227. Williams HJ, Ward JR, Reading JC, et al: Comparison of auranofin, methotrexate, and the combination of both in the treatment of rheumatoid arthritis. *Arthritis* 1992; 35:259–269.
228. Willkens RF, Vrowitz MB, Stablein DM, et al: Comparison of azathioprine, methotrexate, and the combination of both in the treatment of rheumatoid arthritis. *Arthritis Rheum* 1992; 35:849–856.
229. Wilske KR, Healey LA: Remodeling the pyramid: A concept whose time has come. *J Rheumatol* 1989; 16:565–567.
230. Healey LA, Wilske KR: Reforming the pyramid: A plan for treating rheumatoid arthritis in the 1990's. *Rheum Dis Clin North Am* 1989; 15:615–619.
231. Fries JF: Reevaluating the therapeutic approach to rheumatoid arthritis: The "sawtooth" strategy. *J Rheumatol* 1990; 17(suppl 22):12–15.
232. Yocum DE, Klipper JH, Wilder RL, et al: Cyclosporin A in severe, treatment-refractory rheumatoid arthritis. *Ann Intern Med* 1988; 109:863–869.
233. Madhok R, Torley HI, Capell HA: A study of the long-term efficacy and toxicity of cyclosporine A in rheumatoid arthritis. *J Rheumatol* 1990; 18:19–23.

Therapy of Acute and Chronic Viral Hepatitis

Jay H. Hoofnagle, M.D.

Director, Division of Digestive Diseases and Nutrition, National Institute of Diabetes and Digestive and Kidney Diseases, National Institutes of Health, Bethesda, Maryland

Viral hepatitis comprises at least five different diseases caused by five different viruses: (1) Hepatitis A or infectious hepatitis is caused by the hepatitis A virus (HAV). (2) Hepatitis B or classical serum hepatitis is caused by the hepatitis B virus (HBV). (3) Hepatitis C, formerly known as classical, parenterally transmitted non-A, non-B hepatitis, is caused by the hepatitis C virus (HCV). (4) Hepatitis D or delta hepatitis is caused by the hepatitis delta virus (HDV). (5) Hepatitis E, or epidemic non-A, non-B hepatitis, is caused by the hepatitis E virus (HEV).[1, 2] All five viruses can cause acute hepatitis; types B, C, and D can also cause persistent infection and chronic hepatitis. Acute viral hepatitis is the probably the most common cause of jaundice and acute liver failure worldwide. Similarly, chronic viral hepatitis is probably the most common cause of cirrhosis and hepatocellular carcinoma.

Therapy of acute and chronic viral hepatitis has recently been advanced by breakthroughs in the understanding of the hepatitis viruses and by development of several safe and potent antiviral substances. Chief among the antiviral agents that have been evaluated is alpha interferon, which now has been approved for use in chronic hepatitis B and C in most countries of the world. Newer antivirals have shown promise but are presently experimental and not generally available. This review will focus largely on alpha interferon with a few comments relating to other antiviral and immunomodulatory agents that have been found promising in early studies and that may warrant use in the future.

Acute Viral Hepatitis

All five forms of viral hepatitis can cause an acute, icteric illness. The clinical symptoms, signs, and biochemical laboratory tests of acute viral hepatitis are generally of little help in separating the five different forms of the disease. Specific diagnosis can be suggested by epidemiologic features and by incubation period, but can only be made with confidence by serologic testing (Table 1).[1] Any approach to therapy of acute viral hepatitis must

TABLE 1.
Five Forms of Viral Hepatitis*

Feature	Hepatitis A	Hepatitis B	Hepatitis C	Hepatitis D	Hepatitis E
Virus	HAV	HBV	HCV	HDV	HEV
	27 nm	42 nm	30–60 nm	35–40 nm	27–34 nm
	Picornavirus	Hepadnavirus	Flavivirus	Satellite	Calicivirus
Genome	ssRNA(+)	dsDNA	ssRNA(+)	ssRNA(−)	ssRNA(+)
	7.5 kb	3.2 kb	9.4 kb	1.7 kb	7.5 kg
Antigens	HA Ag	HBsAg†	HCV Ag	HDV Ag	HEV Ag
		HBcAg			
		HBeAg†			
Antibodies	Anti-HAV†	Anti-HBs†	Anti-HCV†	Anti-HDV†	Anti-HEV
	IgM†	Anti-HBc† (IgM)†			
		Anti-HBe†			
Incubation period	25 days	75 days	50 days	35 days	42 days
	(15–40)	(30–150)	(20–120)	(15–150)	(15–70)
Acute mortality	0.2%	0.2%	0.2%	2–20%	0.2%‡
Chronicity	0%	5–10%	50–70%	5–10%	0%
Spread	Fecal oral	Parenteral	Parenteral	Parenteral	Fecal oral
		Sexual	Sexual ?	Sexual	
		Vertical	Vertical ?		

*From Baron S, Coppenhaver D, Dianzani F, et al (eds): *Interferon: Principles and Medical Applications.* Galveston, Tex, University of Texas Medical Branch at Galveston, Department of Microbiology Press, 1992. Used by permission.
†Commercial assays available
‡Mortality 10% in pregnant women

take into consideration the specific virologic diagnosis, in that the different forms of viral hepatitis may respond differently to therapy.

At present, there is no specific therapy for acute viral hepatitis of proven benefit. Indeed, specific therapy of acute viral hepatitis must be approached with caution. For the most part, acute viral hepatitis is a self-limited disease, and complete recovery with full restoration of liver function and clearance of virus occurs in most patients. The hepatic dysfunction accompanying acute hepatitis alters drug metabolism so that medications are often poorly tolerated. Finally, viral replication is usually decreasing and may have actually ceased by the onset of jaundice and symptoms in acute viral hepatitis.[1] For these reasons, antiviral agents require rigorous proof of efficacy and safety before they can be recommended for patients with acute hepatitis.

There are features of acute viral hepatitis, however, that make antiviral therapy an attractive option. First, even though self-limited, acute viral hepatitis can be severe and convalescence can be prolonged. Therapy to shorten the course of disease, ameliorate symptoms, and speed recovery would be welcomed by most patients and physicians. Second, a percentage of patients with acute hepatitis develop fulminant hepatic failure. Each year in the United States, approximately 2000 persons die and 200 undergo liver transplantation for fulminant hepatitis.[3] Third, a proportion of patients with acute hepatitis B, C, and D develop chronic hepatitis, which ultimately can lead to cirrhosis and hepatocellular carcinoma. The chronicity rate is highest for hepatitis C, where more than half of patients develop chronic infection and at least a quarter of these ultimately develop cirrhosis.[4] To date, two major antiviral agents have been evaluated extensively for their antiviral and beneficial effects in acute viral hepatitis: ribavirin and alpha interferon.

Ribavirin (1-beta-D-ribofuranosyl-1H-1,2,4-triazole-3-carboxamide: virazole; Viratek, San Rafael, Calif) is a guanosine-like nucleoside analogue first synthesized in 1972. Ribavirin was found to have broad activity against several DNA and RNA viruses in vitro and to have clinical efficacy in humans against influenza A and B, respiratory syncytial virus, and Lassa fever.[5] Ribavirin was also found to be safe; its only significant side effect being a dose-related and reversible hemolysis.

There have been several randomized controlled trials of ribavirin in symptomatic acute viral hepatitis reported from Brazil,[6] India,[7] and Mexico.[8] Patients received ribavirin in doses of 400 to 800 mg daily for 10 to 14 days. In all studies, serum bilirubin, alanine aminotransferase (ALT), and aspartate aminotransferase levels decreased more rapidly on ribavirin than with placebo therapy. However, the differences were somewhat modest, and there was no mortality or significant morbidity even in the control patients. Finally, in none of the studies was the diagnosis of the type of hepatitis clear. Although the investigators assumed that the patients treated had viral hepatitis due to hepatitis A, it is equally possible that most were due to hepatitis E and that some were due to hepatitis B and C. These controlled trials were very promising, but hardly conclusive. In view of the demonstrated effects of ribavirin against HAV in vitro[9] and against HBV[10] and HCV[11, 12] in vivo, further evaluation of this agent is needed, but only in the context of controlled studies in which virologic markers are carefully evaluated. The correct dose and regimen of ribavirin in viral hepatitis also needs to be evaluated. At present, however, ribavirin is not available and should not be used in cases of acute viral hepatitis outside of controlled trials.

Alpha interferon is a host protein made by several cell types (macrophages and B cells) in response to viral infection and other antigenic stimuli.[13] Alpha interferon acting through cell surface receptors induces a set of intracellular enzymes that inhibit viral replication and make the cells resistant to viral infection. Alpha interferon is closely related to beta interferon which differs antigenically but which has similar biologic actions and acts through the same receptor. Endogenously produced alpha interferon probably plays a major role in response to viral challenge and recovery from viral infection. During the course of viral hepatitis, levels of alpha interferon are minimally elevated, and some evidence suggests that the interferon response is blunted in hepatitis virus infections. Alpha interferon has been shown to have in vitro activity against HAV and HBV in cell culture.[14, 15] When given parenterally to humans with chronic hepatitis B, C, and D, alpha interferon has been found to lower virus titers in both serum and liver and to induce long-term remissions in a proportion of patients with chronic hepatitis B, C, and D.[16] On the basis of these findings, small studies of alpha (and beta) interferon have been carried out in selected patients with acute viral hepatitis.

Interferon Therapy of Acute Hepatitis B.—The success of alpha interferon in treating chronic hepatitis B led to several pilot studies of this agent in acute disease. These small studies suggested that alpha interferon might be beneficial, especially in fulminant[17] and protracted cases.[18] Subsequently, a large prospective randomized controlled trial of alpha interferon was carried out in Greece among 100 patients with acute icteric hepatitis B.[19] Patients were randomized to receive either 1 or 3 million units (mu) of alpha interferon or placebo three times weekly for 6 weeks. Preliminary analysis failed to demonstrate any advantage of interferon therapy over placebo in time to resolution of symptoms, fall of serum aminotransferases to normal, or loss of HBsAg and HBeAg from serum. Indeed, all 100 patients ultimately recovered; there were no deaths from fulminant hepatitis and no patient developed chronic hepatitis. In a separate uncontrolled trial among 12 patients from Spain with fulminant hepatitis, alpha interferon failed to demonstrate any evidence of benefit of therapy; the mortality rate was 83% which was similar to historical controls.[20] Thus at present, there is no evidence of benefit of alpha interferon therapy in either typical or fulminant acute hepatitis B.

Interferon Therapy of Acute Hepatitis D.—There have been no controlled trials of alpha interferon in acute delta hepatitis, this disease being somewhat rare and quite difficult to diagnose during the acute phase.[1] Nevertheless, isolated case reports and small uncontrolled series suggest that alpha interferon has little effect on the course of acute delta hepatitis. In a pilot study of alpha interferon from Spain, 9 of 12 patients with fulminant hepatitis had either acute co-infection or super-infection with HDV; 7 (78%) of these patients died and 1 of the 2 survivors developed chronic delta hepatitis and cirrhosis.[20]

Interferon Therapy of Acute Hepatitis C.—The evidence for benefit of alpha interferon in acute hepatitis C is stronger than in acute hepatitis B or D. There have been four prospective controlled trials of alpha interferon therapy of acute hepatitis C (Table 2).[21–24] All four trials were conducted on patients who were being followed prospectively after blood transfusion as a part of epidemiologic studies on posttransfusion hepatitis and the efficacy of blood donor screening. All four studies were relatively small, and several were discontinued early because of a dwindling number of cases of posttransfusion hepatitis C after the introduction of blood donor screening for anti-HCV. All four trials demonstrated a rapid improvement in serum aminotransferases and a decrease in the incidence of chronic hepatitis C among the interferon-treated patients. While these results were promising, it should be pointed out that cases of chronic hepatitis C still occurred despite treatment. It is unclear whether therapy during the acute phase offered additional benefit over delayed therapy during the chronic phase. Further follow-up on the treated patients and detailed analysis of the effects of therapy on HCV RNA are needed to fully address the advisability of treatment of acute hepatitis C.

Recommendations for Antiviral Therapy in Acute Viral Hepatitis.—Currently, antiviral therapy for acute viral hepatitis must be considered experimental and treatments should only be given as a part of controlled trials. There is little evidence to suggest that alpha interferon is effective in acute hepatitis B and D. In acute hepatitis C, alpha interferon may have an effect in speeding the time to recovery and decreasing the

TABLE 2.
Alpha Interferon Therapy of Acute Hepatitis C: Four Trials*

		Normal ALT at 12 mo.	
Authors	**No. Treated**	**Interferon**	**Placebo**
Omata et al.[21]	20	64%	11%
Alberti et al.[22]	22	57%	37%
Viladomiu et al.[23]	28	57%	31%
Rumi et al.[24]	45	61%	42%

*From Baron S, Coppenhaver D, Dianzani F, et al (eds): *Interferon: Principles and Medical Applications.* Galveston, Tex, University of Texas Medical Branch at Galveston, Department of Microbiology Press, 1992. Used by permission.

rate of chronicity. However, it is important to stress that 50% of patients with acute hepatitis C recover spontaneously and that the improvement in the chronicity rate with alpha interferon therapy has been modest. For these reasons, it is prudent to reserve interferon therapy for those cases of acute hepatitis C in which it is clear that chronic infection is developing. As a general guideline, initiation of alpha interferon would be appropriate in patients with acute hepatitis C whose serum aminotransferases remained elevated (or HCV RNA persists) for more than 2 months after onset of illness. Alpha interferon is generally well tolerated during acute hepatitis (see sections below on side effects and monitoring recommendations) and is reported to result in prompt improvement in serum aminotransferases. The optimal dose and duration of therapy with alpha interferon is not known; it is reasonable to use the same regimen recommended for chronic hepatitis C, i.e., 3 mu given subcutaneously three times weekly for 24 weeks.

Chronic Viral Hepatitis

Chronic viral hepatitis can be caused by persistent infection with the hepatitis B, C, or D viruses. The three forms of chronic viral hepatitis are similar in clinical, serum biochemical, and histologic features and can only be distinguished reliably by serologic testing.[1] The natural history of the three forms of chronic viral hepatitis are also quite similar in that all three can lead to cirrhosis and all three have been associated with the development of hepatocellular carcinoma.

Chronic hepatitis C is the most common form of chronic viral hepatitis in the United States accounting for 60% to 70% of cases.[2,4] The disease tends to be insidious and silent and, after years to decades, leads to cirrhosis in about 25% of cases.[25] Hepatitis C is most often seen in parenteral drug abusers and in blood transfusion or blood product recipients. Approximately 0.4% of volunteer blood donors in the United States are chronically infected with HCV.

Chronic hepatitis B accounts for 20% to 30% of chronic viral hepatitis and leads to cirrhosis in 30% to 40% of cases. Hepatitis B is most often seen in parenteral drug abusers, recipients of blood products, medical care workers, and sexually promiscuous persons including male homosexuals. Hepatitis B is also common among immigrants from areas of the world where this disease is endemic such as Africa and Asia. Between 0.1% and 0.2% of American volunteer blood donors are chronic carriers of hepatitis B.

Chronic delta hepatitis is the most uncommon form of chronic viral hepatitis, probably accounting for less than 5% of cases. Delta hepatitis, however, is the most severe form of viral hepatitis and leads to cirrhosis in up to 70% of cases, often within a few years of onset of disease.[26] Delta hepatitis occurs only in persons who are infected with hepatitis B and are HBsAg positive. Delta hepatitis is found most commonly among parenteral drug abusers and recipients of multiple blood products.

In recent years there have been several important advances made in the therapy of chronic viral hepatitis. The rationale for treatment has been to alter the natural history of disease, to prevent development of cirrhosis, end-stage liver disease, and hepatocellular carcinoma. These are long-term objectives that are difficult to document in clinical trials, largely because cirrhosis develops in only 20% to 30% of patients and usually takes years to decades to appear. For these reasons, most studies on antiviral therapy have relied upon more short-term criteria for improvement, such as disappearance of symptoms, decrease in hepatitis disease activity (as assessed by serum aminotransferase activities and by liver histology), and decrease in infectivity (as assessed by serum and hepatic levels of viral genome or antigens). Studies of the natural history of all forms of chronic viral hepatitis support use of these short-term outcomes as predictive of eventual improvement in the natural history of these diseases.[25–27] Nevertheless, it needs to be stressed that recommendations for therapy of chronic viral hepatitis are based upon evidence on short-term outcomes.

At present only alpha interferon has been shown to be beneficial in treating chronic viral hepatitis. Several other newer antiviral agents have demonstrated great promise, especially in chronic hepatitis B. However, the margin of long-term benefit and the level of toxicity of these newer agents remain incompletely characterized.

Chronic Hepatitis B

Diagnosis and Course of Chronic Hepatitis B.—Chronic hepatitis B is diagnosed by the finding of elevations in aminotransferases and HBsAg in serum for at least 6 months.[1] Chronic hepatitis B should be differentiated from the chronic "inactive" HBsAg carrier state in which HBsAg is present in serum, but there is little or no disease activity. Serologic testing can help to make this separation, in that patients with chronic hepatitis B will have evidence of HBV replication, as shown by the presence of HBV DNA or HBeAg in addition to HBsAg in serum. In contrast, inactive HBsAg carriers have normal serum aminotransferases and no HBeAg or HBV DNA in serum. In some unusual cases of chronic hepatitis B, HBsAg and HBV DNA without HBeAg are detected in serum.[28, 29] These individuals are infected with a strain of HBV with a mutation in the precore region of viral genome that allows for replication, but prevents synthesis and secretion of HBeAg. This HBeAg-negative mutant form of HBV is rare in the United States, but is common in Mediterranean countries and Asia.

Liver biopsy is helpful, both in the diagnosis and staging of chronic hepatitis B. Histology generally reveals variable degrees of portal, periportal, and parenchymal inflammation and necrosis, and fibrosis. Immunostaining will reveal HBcAg in the nuclei and occasionally in the cytoplasm of hepatocytes. Testing for HBV DNA demonstrates the presence of full-length as well as shorter, replicative intermediate forms of the viral genome.[27]

Trials of Alpha Interferon in Chronic Hepatitis B.—Multiple prospective randomized controlled trials have shown that a 4- to 6-month course of alpha interferon is effective in inducing a remission in 25% to 40% of patients with chronic hepatitis B.[30–43] The largest such trial from the United States included 169 patients and was the result of a collaborative group of investigators from 12 different institutions.[30] In that study, a 4-month course of alpha interferon given subcutaneously in doses of 5 mu daily induced sustained remissions in disease in 37% (15 of 41) of treated patients, an outcome noted in only 7% (3 of 43) of control subjects. A lower dose of interferon (1 mu daily) was less effective, yielding a remission rate of only 17% (7 of 41 patients). Finally, pretreatment of patients with a short course of prednisone did not increase the response rate to interferon alone (16 of 44 patients: 36%). Several other controlled trials from the United States,[31, 32] South America,[33] Europe,[34–40] Africa,[41] Australia,[42] and Asia[43] have yielded similar results using both recombinant and lymphoblastoid alpha interferons in doses of 4 to 5 mu daily or 9 to 10 mu thrice weekly for 3 to 6 months. Long-term follow-up on patients treated in the initial studies has shown that the remissions in disease were generally sustained, symptoms and signs of chronic liver disease resolved in all patients, complications of cirrhosis after remission in disease were rare, and the majority of patients ultimately became HBsAg as well as HBeAg and HBV DNA negative.[44]

Current Recommendations for Therapy of Chronic Hepatitis B.—Alpha interferon is currently recommended for patients with well-compensated chronic hepatitis B with HBsAg, HBeAg, and HBV DNA in serum. Patients should have elevations in serum aminotransferase activities but no evidence of advanced ("decompensated") liver disease, such as severe wasting, ascites, variceal hemorrhage, or hepatic encephalopathy. Liver biopsy is recommended before treatment to verify the diagnosis and stage the activity and severity of the disease. In patients with contraindications to liver biopsy, this procedure need not be performed, and recommendations for therapy can be made entirely on the basis of clinical and serum biochemical features.

The recommended regimen of alpha interferon is 4.5 to 5 mu daily or 9 to 10 mu thrice weekly given either subcutaneously or intramuscularly for 16 weeks. Patients should be fully informed of the side effects of alpha interferon and the expected results of treatment before starting interferon. The first several doses of interferon should be given under close supervision, as side effects are maximal with the initial injections and can be severe. Patients should be carefully taught to measure out and administer the interferon, as well as how to dispose of the used needles and syringes.

Side Effects of Alpha Interferon.—Side effects are greatest with the initial dose of alpha interferon.[45] When given in doses of 1 mu or greater, alpha interferon usually induces an "influenza-like" syndrome approximately 4 to 8 hours after the injection. Typical symptoms are fever, chills, fatigue, muscle aches, headaches, backaches, nausea, and poor appetite. Some patients develop diarrhea or vomiting. With very high doses (>10 mu), confusion, delirium, coma, hypotension, cyanosis, and even vascular collapse can occur.[45–48] These initial symptoms generally last for 4 to 12 hours and are much reduced with the second and third injections. Typically, after the first week of treatment, the only symptoms induced with each injection are a mild feverishness and muscle aches. Acetaminophen given at the time of the injection can help to blunt these initial side effects.

With prolonged therapy, the late side effects of alpha interferon occur (Table 3). The most common side effects are fatigue and muscle aches. These can be severe and dose-limiting. Some patients also develop nausea, poor appetite, weight loss, indigestion, and diarrhea. Approximately 15% of patients develop psychological side effects, typically anxiety, depression, irritability, and moodiness.[48, 49] These psychological side effects are the major reason for having to discontinue interferon early. Patients should be warned that they may become irritable, anxious, and moody, as these symptoms are often not considered to be caused by the therapy, and they may result in serious disruptions in the family or workplace. Therapy for these side effects is difficult; the irritability may respond to counseling

TABLE 3.
Side Effects of Alpha Interferon*

Systemic
Fatigue, myalgias, fever, headache, backache, anorexia, weight loss, nausea, vomiting, diarrhea, abdominal cramps, hair loss.

Neurologic
Difficulty concentrating, lack of motivation, sleep disturbance, delirium, disorientation, coma, seizures, electroencephalographic changes.

Psychological
Anxiety, irritability, depression, social withdrawal, decreased libido, paranoid or suicidal ideation, return of craving for alcohol or drugs.

Hematologic
Decrease in platelets, white blood cells, and hematocrit.

Infectious
Increased susceptibility to bacterial infections, especially bronchitis, sinusitis, furuncles, urinary tract infections. In rare instances, pneumonia, lung abscess, brain abscess, septicemia, bacterial peritonitis.

Autoimmune
Development of autoantibodies, anti-interferon antibodies, hyperthyroidism, hypothyroidism, other autoimmune diseases.

Other
In rare instances, proteinuria, interstitial nephritis, nephrotic syndrome, cardiac arrhythmias, congestive heart failure, acute exacerbation of liver disease.

*From Baron S, Coppenhaver D, Dianzani F, et al (eds): *Interferon: Principles and Medical Applications.* Galveston, Tex, University of Texas Medical Branch at Galveston, Department of Microbiology Press, 1992. Used by permission.

and encouragement, but usually requires a modification in interferon dosage. In some cases, methylphenidate (15 to 30 mg once to twice daily) may be helpful.[45] Severe psychological side effects such as acute psychosis, delirium, paranoia, suicide attempts, and coma have also been described with interferon therapy, especially in patients with preexisting CNS disorders.[47–49] These side effects should lead to discontinuation of interferon.

Alpha interferon also induces some degree of bone marrow depression, and a decrease of the white blood cell and platelet counts by 25% to 50% is not uncommon.[45, 46] Patients with a predisposition to bacterial infections will often develop an infection during interferon therapy. In patients with an established cirrhosis, bacterial infections during treatment are common and can be severe and even life-threatening.[50] Other severe side effects of alpha interferon include seizures,[51] nephrotic syndrome or acute interstitial nephritis,[52] cardiac arrhythmias and acute congestive heart failure,[53] and acute exacerbation of the liver disease.[50] These are rare and are generally reversible.

Alpha interferon therapy can induce autoimmune phenomena and cause autoimmune conditions. More than 50% of patients treated for 4 months with alpha interferon develop autoantibodies, the most common being antinuclear, anti–smooth muscle, and antithyroid antibodies.[54] Approximately 2% of patients with chronic viral hepatitis treated with alpha interferon for 4 to 6 months will develop an autoimmune condition, the most common being thyroiditis with either hypothyroidism or hyperthyroidism.[55] Other autoimmune conditions linked to interferon therapy include thrombocytopenia purpura, hemolytic anemia, rheumatoid arthritis, lupus erythematosus-like syndromes, and type I diabetes.[56–58] The autoantibodies generally decrease in titer and disappear, and most (but not all) of the autoimmune conditions resolve when therapy is stopped.[54]

Finally, antibodies to alpha interferon can develop during therapy, especially when using recombinant interferons. These antibodies are generally transient and low in titer and rarely affect the response to treatment.[30, 31]

Monitoring of Patients on Therapy.—Patients with chronic hepatitis B should be seen, questioned regarding side effects, examined, and have blood taken for serum aminotransferases and blood counts every 1 to 4 weeks while on interferon therapy. The frequency of visits should be dictated by the severity of the hepatitis and the occurrence of side effects. Liver biochemical tests and tests for HBV markers should be obtained at the beginning and end of therapy and again 4 to 12 months afterwards to assess whether a sustained response has occurred. Tests of thyroid function (TSH) at the start and end of therapy are also appropriate, as autoimmune thyroid disease develops in 2% to 3% of patients treated with alpha interferon.[55]

Side effects of interferon can limit therapy in chronic hepatitis B.[45] The recommended doses of interferon are high, and 10% to 40% of patients will require a dose reduction because of intolerable side effects,[30] such as severe fatigue, depression, irritability, or bone marrow suppression. In these situations, the dose should be decreased by one-fourth to one-half. Side effects that can lead to early discontinuation of therapy include severe exacerbation of disease, acute bacterial infections, marked depression or anxiety, psychosis, seizures, congestive heart failure, and acute renal failure. Bone marrow suppression is common with interferon therapy, but rarely requires dose adjustment or stopping treatment.

Definition of Response.—A response to therapy in chronic hepatitis B is defined as a sustained loss of HBV DNA from serum, accompanied or followed by a loss of HBeAg, and fall of aminotransferases into the normal range (Fig 1).[30–32] HBV DNA levels generally decrease by 50% to 70% when interferon is started,[46] but this marker of viral replication remains detectable until several months into treatment when it falls to undetectable levels in patients with a sustained response.

While the loss of HBV DNA during treatment is suggestive that a beneficial response has occurred, proof requires further follow-up and demonstration of loss of HBeAg, which may not occur for several months after treatment is stopped. For these reasons, a long-term beneficial response cannot be claimed to have occurred until 6 to 12 months after treatment. Subsequent relapse with reappearance of HBV DNA, HBeAg, and disease activity occurs in 10% to 15% of patients who lose HBV DNA on treat-

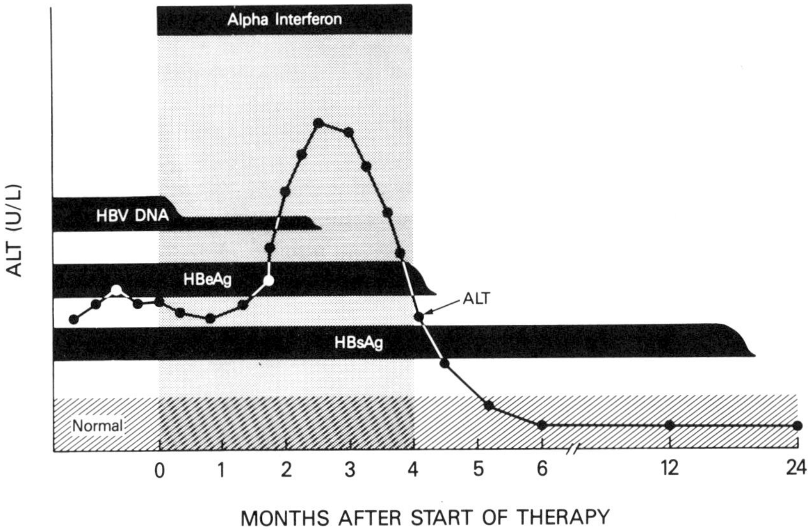

FIG 1.
Course of patient with chronic hepatitis B treated with alpha interferon who responded to treatment with clearance of hepatitis B virus *(HBV)* DNA, hepatitis B e antigen *(HBeAg)*, improvement in serum alanine aminotransferase *(ALT)*, and ultimately a loss of hepatitis B surface antigen *(HBsAg)*. (From Baron S, Coppenhaver D, Dianzani F, et al (eds): *Interferon: Principles and Medical Applications.* Galveston, Tex, University of Texas Medical Branch at Galveston, Department of Microbiology Press, 1992. Used by permission.)

ment, usually during the 6- to 12-month follow-up period. Relapse is most frequent among patients who have unusual serologic features,[29] who are immunosuppressed,[59] or who have advanced liver disease.[50]

Serum aminotransferase activities are fairly reliable indicators of the degree of hepatic inflammation and necrosis in chronic viral hepatitis and are the best means of monitoring the hepatitis disease activity, short of liver biopsy. With a sustained response to interferon therapy, aminotransferases should fall into the normal range. However, this response may be delayed for 1 to 6 months after the loss of HBV DNA and HBeAg. Furthermore, the aminotransferases may paradoxically increase early in therapy. Indeed, a flare of hepatitis during therapy in chronic hepatitis B is a favorable sign indicating activation of the immune system, immune lysis of infected heptocytes, and thus a beneficial response to treatment (Fig. 1).[30]

Some patients lose HBsAg in addition to HBeAg and HBV DNA after interferon therapy, thus indicating a complete response and eradication of the viral infection. In early studies, loss of HBsAg was said to be uncommon[34] and larger controlled trials suggested that this occurred in 10% to 20% of responders. However, in long-term follow-up studies, up to 65% of persons who became HBeAg negative with treatment ultimately became HBsAg negative.[44] The loss of HBsAg usually occurred 1 to 5 years after treatment and was followed by appearance of anti-HBs in most patients.

Increasing the Response Rate in Chronic Hepatitis B.—Alpha interferon therapy leads to a beneficial response in 25% to 40% of patients. Attempts to increase this response rate by combination with other antiviral drugs, immunomodulating agents, and multiple courses of treatment have not yielded higher response rates.[60–62]

A commonly used approach to increasing the response rate to interferon has been to pretreat patients with a short course of prednisone.[63] The withdrawal of prednisone induces an acute flare of the hepatitis which should make the patient more susceptible to interferon treatment. However, prospective studies have failed to show a consistent benefit of pretreatment with prednisone above that with interferon alone.[30, 40, 43] Furthermore, prednisone treatment can worsen the course of chronic hepatitis B[64] and can induce severe and even life-threatening exacerbations of disease.[30] Thus, at present, corticosteroids should not be used for the treatment of chronic hepatitis B.

Predictors of a Response to Alpha Interferon in Chronic Hepatitis B.—The average response rate to interferon can be increased by selecting patients who are most likely to respond. Retrospective analyses have identified several features that help predict a response to treatment in chronic hepatitis B (Table 4).[30–43, 59] The features that have most commonly been associated with a response are high initial levels of aminotransferases and low initial titers of HBV DNA. In some studies, female gender, a history of acute hepatitis, and a short, known duration of disease were associated with a favorable treatment outcome. In contrast, Asian ethnicity and infection in childhood predisposed to a lack of response to treatment.[43, 65] Finally, response to interferon appeared to depend upon

TABLE 4.
Alpha Interferon Therapy of Chronic Hepatitis B: Predictors of a Response

High serum aminotransferases (>100 U/L)
Low serum HBV DNA (<100 pg/mL)
Short duration of disease
History of acute hepatitis
Female sex
Non-Asian ethnicity
No other serious illness (renal failure, immunosuppression, AIDS)

an intact immune system; thus patients with renal failure, HIV infection, or immunosuppressive therapy were unlikely to respond.[59] Overall, the height of the serum aminotransferases is probably the most convenient and useful means of predicting a response.[31]

Patients with Atypical Forms of Chronic Hepatitis B.—The current recommendations for interferon therapy in chronic hepatitis B are for patients with typical, well-compensated disease. These criteria eliminate many patients who are deserving of some form of therapy, including patients with minimal elevations in serum aminotransferases, children, Asian patients, patients with atypical serological results, patients with decompensated liver disease, and those who are immunosuppressed.

Normal Aminotransferases.—Patients with chronic hepatitis B or the HBsAg carrier state with normal aminotransferases generally should not receive interferon. Such patients rarely have significant underlying liver disease. Furthermore, the response rate to interferon is low in patients with inactive disease and aminotransferases that are minimally elevated.[30, 31, 43] An exception to this is the patient with extrahepatic manifestations of hepatitis B such as glomerulonephritis who has been found to have a high rate of response.[66]

Children.—Children with chronic hepatitis B typically have mild disease and serum aminotransferases may be normal or near normal. Trials of interferon in children with minimal aminotransferase elevations have yielded poor response rates.[65] However, in pilot studies of children with moderate to severe chronic hepatitis B, the response rates have been similar to those in adults.[67, 68] Children in general tolerate alpha interferon well, the major side effects being hair loss and occasionally personality change. Alpha interferon has not been approved for use in children with chronic hepatitis B, and large multicenter controlled trials in children with chronic hepatitis B are currently underway in the United States and Europe. These trials are evaluating alpha interferon in doses of 5 to 6 mu/m^2

given three times weekly for 16 to 24 weeks. The criteria for treatment are the same as in adults: aminotransferase elevations and HBeAg and/or HBV DNA in serum.

Asians.—Several studies of chronic hepatitis B conducted in the Far East have reported low response rates to alpha interferon among Asian patients.[43, 65, 69] Even in studies from Western countries, Asian patients have had a low response rate in comparison to Western patients.[35, 59] Yet, many of the Asian patients entered into these studies with chronic hepatitis B had minimal or no elevations in aminotransferase activities, despite the presence of HBV DNA and HBeAg in serum. Subsequent trials of alpha interferon among Asians with high aminotransferases have demonstrated response rates similar to those in Europeans.[43] At present, interferon therapy is recommended for Asian patients with chronic hepatitis B, but they should be informed of the generally low rate of response if aminotransferases are minimally elevated.

Atypical Serologic Patterns.—Most but not all patients with chronic hepatitis B have HBsAg, HBeAg, and HBV DNA in serum. Some patients, however, harbor an HBV mutant with a nucleotide substitution in the precore region of the genome which creates an early "stop" codon and blocks the synthesis of HBeAg. These patients have HBsAg and HBV DNA without HBeAg in serum.[28, 29] This HBeAg-negative mutation is common in Italy, Greece, and parts of Asia, but is rare in the United States and Northern European countries. Despite the lack of HBeAg, these patients often deserve therapy. There have been three controlled trials of alpha interferon therapy in patients with the HBeAg-negative mutant, all three of which showed benefit for therapy.[29, 70, 71] However, one study suggested that the response rate in patients with the HBeAg-negative mutant was lower than that in HBeAg-positive patients and that these patients were particularly prone to relapse or reactivation of disease, weeks to months after treatment.[29] An additional problem was that without HBeAg, it was difficult to assess whether a response to therapy had occurred. In the controlled trials of alpha interferon, the presence of normal aminotransferases and absence of HBV DNA 12 months after therapy were used as an indication of a sustained beneficial response. Liver biopsy results were also helpful in that HBcAg was detected in hepatocytes if the disease and viral replication were still active, but was absent once a sustained treatment response occurred. Thus, alpha interferon therapy can be recommended for patients with chronic hepatitis B who lack HBeAg, but monitoring with HBV DNA and careful follow up is needed to document a response to treatment and to determine whether it is sustained. Some investigators have recommended longer courses of therapy (24 instead of 16 weeks) and retreatment if relapse occurs.[29]

Decompensated Liver Disease.—Perhaps the most challenging treatment group of patients with chronic hepatitis B are those with advanced or decompensated liver disease. This group is defined by the presence or history of ascites, hepatic encephalopathy, variceal hemorrhage, persistent jaundice (bilirubin greater than 4 mg/dl), or wasting. Dramatic beneficial responses have been noted in approximately 35% of these patients.[50, 72, 73] However, a sustained response is unlikely if the disease is far advanced (Child's Class C) and if the patient has intractable ascites, marked wasting, or presence of hepatic encephalopathy. In addition, patients with cirrhosis often have an exacerbation of disease within the first few weeks of starting interferon, and this exacerbation of disease can be severe and life-threatening. For these reasons, patients with clinically apparent cirrhosis should be treated only by physicians with experience in using interferon and in caring for patients with hepatic failure. Patients with cirrhosis often do not tolerate the doses used in patients with well compensated disease. Therapy should be started at doses of 1 to 2 mu three times weekly and increased based upon tolerance. Patients need to be monitored carefully for side effects, especially bacterial infections, psychiatric complications, and worsening of the liver disease.

Immunosuppressed Patients.—Chronic hepatitis B is common among immunosuppressed individuals, such as oncology patients, renal dialysis patients, patients with solid organ transplants, and patients with human immunodeficiency virus (HIV) infection. Unfortunately, these individuals rarely have a beneficial response to interferon therapy. After solid-organ transplantation, for instance, the high doses of prednisone and cyclosporine appear to block the antiviral effects of interferon, and long-term responses to treatment are rare.[74] Patients with established acquired immunodeficiency syndrome (AIDS) and severe immune deficiency also do not usually respond to interferon therapy with loss of HBV DNA or HBeAg.[75] On the other hand, patients with HIV infection with normal immune parameters are able to respond to treatment and should be considered candidates for therapy if they fulfill other criteria.[31, 35] Thus, alpha interferon therapy is not recommended in individuals with major immune deficiencies. Patients with chronic hepatitis B who are on renal dialysis or who have a solid organ transplant should not be treated with alpha interferon outside of controlled trials.

Nonresponders.—A common and difficult problem in chronic hepatitis B is the management of patients who fail to respond to an adequate course of alpha interferon treatment. In the "nonresponder" patient, serum HBV DNA levels decrease with treatment but remain present, as do HBeAg and HBsAg (Fig 2). Interestingly, aminotransferases often improve slightly during the last months of therapy, but this improvement is not generally sustained. When therapy is stopped, serum HBV DNA levels and aminotransferases usually return to pretreatment values. These nonresponder patients rarely benefit from retreatment and should be followed without therapy, unless serum levels of HBV DNA decrease or serum aminotransferases increase, in which case a second course of therapy might be appropriate.

Other Therapies of Chronic Hepatitis B.—Because alpha interferon induces remissions in only 25% to 40% of patients, other approaches to therapy are being actively investigated. Other antiviral and immunomodulatory agents currently under evaluation include thymosin,[76] le-

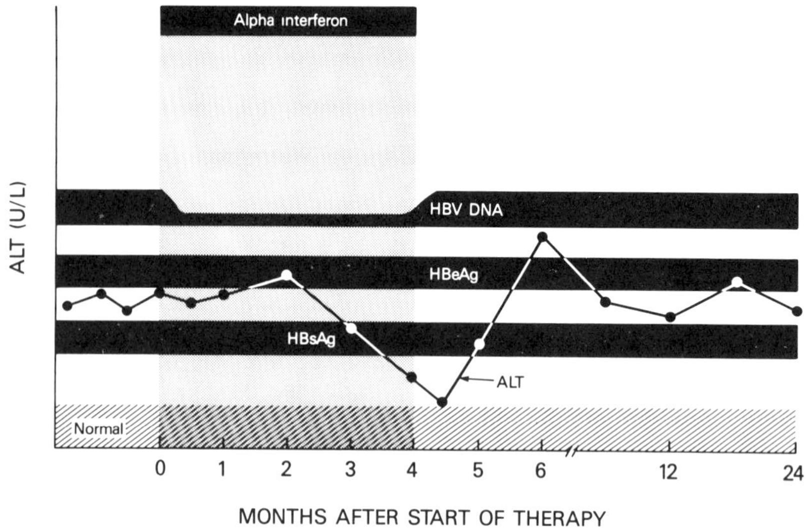

FIG 2.
Course of patient with chronic hepatitis B treated with alpha interferon who had a transient inhibition of HBV DNA, but who did not have an improvement in ALT or loss of HBeAg or HBsAg. (From Baron S, Coppenhaver D, Dianzani F, et al (eds): *Interferon: Principles and Medical Applications*. Galveston, Tex, University of Texas Medical Branch at Galveston, Department of Microbiology Press, 1992. Used by permission.)

vamisole,[62] interleukin-2,[77] gamma interferon,[61, 78] granulocyte-macrophage colony-stimulating factor,[79] acyclovir,[80, 81] gancyclovir,[82] suramin,[83] foscarnet,[84] dideoxyinosine,[85, 86] ribavirin,[10] and other nucleoside analogues.[87, 91] Many of these agents have been promising, but none has been proven effective in inducing long-term remissions in chronic hepatitis B at a rate higher than that which occurs spontaneously. In studies of combinations of antiviral agents with alpha interferon, the response rate has actually been *lower* than with interferon alone,[60–62] perhaps because many of these agents are immunosuppressive.

Among the agents tried in pilot studies as therapy for chronic hepatitis B, the most promising have been thymosin, famciclovir, and 3-thiacytidine (3TC). *Thymosin* is a general term for cytokines isolated from the thymus which have differentiation or growth effects on immunocytes.[92] The first biologically active polypeptide isolated from thymosin extracts was thymosin alpha-1, which has been cloned and synthesized. In a small pilot study, a 6-month course of thymosin alpha-1 led to remissions in chronic hepatitis B in a high proportion of patients.[76] The mechanism of action of thymosin alpha-1 is unclear. The protein induces T-cell maturation and improves CD4/CD8 ratios when administered in vivo. The intracellular actions of thymosin are not yet characterized. Thymosin is given in parenteral form as a subcutaneous injection usually two to three times weekly. There have been no side effects reported in patients who receive thymosin. Thymosin is currently being evaluated as therapy of chronic hepatitis B in a large, multicenter, randomized, double-blind trial of 6 months of therapy with alpha thymosin vs. placebo. The results of that trial are eagerly awaited.

Famciclovir and 3-TC are substituted nucleoside analogues which have recently been shown to have activity against HBV in vitro and in vivo.[87, 88] Both agents are relatively nontoxic and can be taken by mouth. In pilot studies of different doses of these agents, a 4-week course of therapy led to 70% to 90% inhibition of serum HBV DNA levels, but long-term remissions in disease (loss of HBV DNA and HBeAg) were uncommon.[87] Preliminary studies of more prolonged courses of therapy of FIAU and 3-TC are now being designed.

In light of the many recent breakthroughs in the understanding of hepatitis B, the future of therapy of this disease is promising. The development of animal models of chronic HBV infection[91, 93, 94] and cell culture systems for studying HBV replication[89, 90, 95–97] have provided the tools to screen large numbers of antiviral substances for activity against HBV. In addition, the recent worldwide search for antiviral therapy for HIV infection will no doubt uncover many important agents that might also be effective in chronic viral hepatitis. Finally, other technological advances have provided potentially valuable, innovative approaches to therapy of chronic hepatitis B. For instance, preliminary in vitro and in vivo studies have suggested that use of antisense oligonucleotides,[96] ribozymes directed against HBV RNA,[97] monoclonal antibodies to HBsAg,[98] and HBV antigen-specific T cells[99] may be helpful in eradicating HBV infection. These advances indicate that a rational, safe, and effective therapy for chronic hepatitis B may soon be available.

Chronic Delta Hepatitis

Diagnosis and Clinical Course.—The diagnosis of chronic delta hepatitis can be made in a patient with HBsAg and high titers of anti-HDV in serum. Confirmation can be made by demonstrating histologic evidence of chronic hepatitis with HDV antigen in hepatocytes or by finding HDV RNA in serum. Chronic delta hepatitis tends to be severe and progressive, up to 70% of patients eventually develop cirrhosis.[26] Conventional therapies and corticosteroids are ineffective in chronic delta hepatitis.

Trials of Alpha Interferon.—Several pilot studies suggested that alpha interferon lowered serum levels of HDV RNA and resulted in improvements in serum aminotransferases and liver histology in approximately 50% of patients.[100–102] Subsequent controlled trials of interferon, however, showed that the improvement in the disease activity was rarely sustained. Although serum aminotransferase activities and liver biopsy histology often improved during treatment, relapse of disease was almost universal when therapy was stopped.[103–106] These trials, however, used rather short courses and low doses of interferon. In a recent controlled trial from Italy, higher doses of alpha interferon (9 mu three times weekly) given for up to 1 year resulted in sustained improvements in liver disease in 45% of the patients.[107] Indeed, a percentage of patients with delta hepatitis, after prolonged treatment periods, have become HBsAg negative and subsequently lost all evidence of active HDV infection and chronic hepatitis.

Recommendations for Therapy of Chronic Delta Hepatitis.—At present, alpha interferon is not approved for use against chronic delta hepatitis in the United States. Because of the severity and progressive nature of chronic delta hepatitis, however, therapy is often recommended even though the optimal regimen for treatment with alpha interferon has not been established. The indications for treatment are the presence of raised serum aminotransferases, HBsAg and anti-HDV in serum, chronic hepatitis disease activity by liver biopsy, and HDV antigen in liver.

An appropriate dose of alpha interferon for chronic delta hepatitis is 4 to 5 mu daily or 9 to 10 mu three times weekly.[100, 107] The optimal duration of therapy is unknown. If serum aminotransferases do not fall by at least 50% (and to within 1.5 times the upper limit of the normal range) within 3 months, treatment should be stopped. If aminotransferases improve, interferon should be continued at the highest dose that can be tolerated. Unfortunately, side effects are common with this dose of interferon and modification of the dose may be necessary. Therapy should be continued for at least 1 year. If HBsAg becomes undetectable, therapy can be stopped early, as relapse is unlikely (Fig 3). However, if HBsAg remains present,

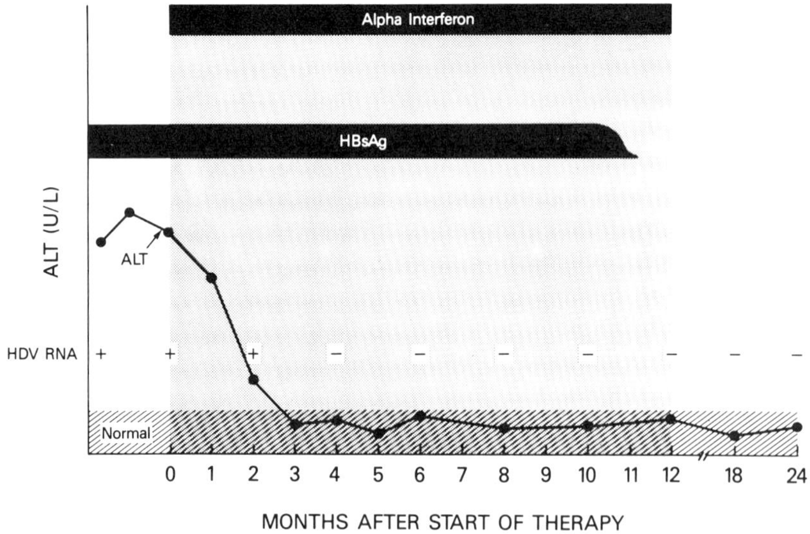

FIG 3.
Course of patient with chronic delta hepatitis treated with alpha interferon who had a sustained response with improvements in serum ALT and eventually loss of HBsAg. (From Baron S, Coppenhaver D, Dianzani F, et al (eds): *Interferon: Principles and Medical Applications.* Galveston, Tex, University of Texas Medical Branch at Galveston, Department of Microbiology Press, 1992. Used by permission.)

relapse can occur even after prolonged therapy (Fig 4). Nevertheless, it is appropriate to stop treatment at 1-year intervals and assess whether relapse occurs. In the even of a relapse, patients can be treated again if their tolerance of interferon was acceptable. Other recommendations regarding evaluation, monitoring and follow-up are identical to those described for treatment of chronic hepatitis B.

The role of alpha interferon therapy in chronic delta hepatitis is also not established for special groups of patients such as children, immunosuppressed patients, and those who have decompensated liver disease. Small trials of alpha interferon in children with chronic delta hepatitis suggest that they respond to treatment in a manner and at a rate similar to adults.[108] In addition, in small studies, patients with chronic delta hepatitis and HIV infection have responded to alpha interferon therapy at rates similar to patients without HIV infection.[109] Too few patients with advanced liver disease due to delta hepatitis have been treated with alpha interferon to recommend therapy generally. At present, liver transplantation is recommended for patients with advanced chronic delta hepatitis with decompensated liver disease.[110]

Other Therapies of Chronic Delta Hepatitis.—The HDV is a defective RNA virus that requires the presence of HBsAg to induce active infection and liver disease.[100] Both animal model and tissue culture systems[111, 112] have been developed for evaluation of HDV replication, its interactions with HBV, and the effects of antiviral substances. Using in vitro

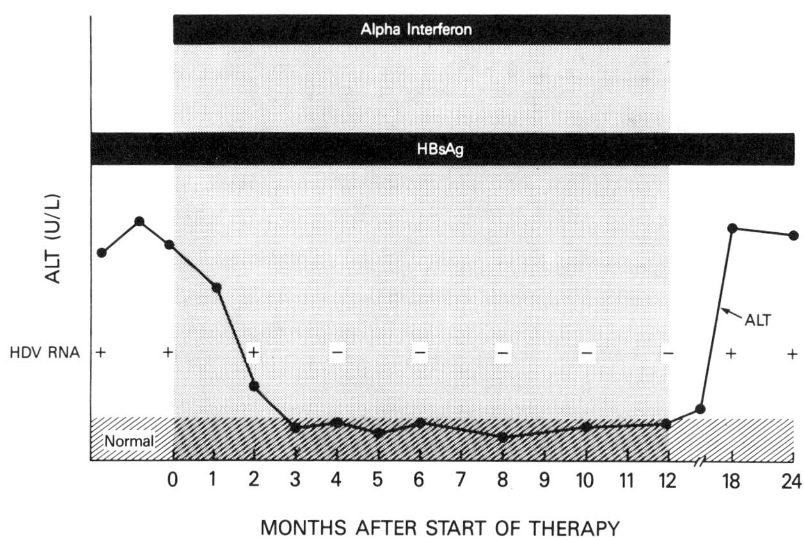

FIG 4.
Course of patient with chronic delta hepatitis treated with alpha interferon who had a transient response during therapy but relapsed when interferon was stopped. (From Baron S, Coppenhaver D, Dianzani F, et al (eds): *Interferon: Principles and Medical Applications.* Galveston, Tex, University of Texas Medical Branch at Galveston, Department of Microbiology Press, 1992. Used by permission.)

systems, several antiviral agents have been found to have activity against HDV replication. However, appropriate studies in humans have not been done, nor is it clear whether antiviral treatment should be directed against HDV or HBV replication. Thus, agents developed to treat chronic hepatitis B should probably also be tried against chronic hepatitis D. Furthermore, the serious nature of chronic delta hepatitis and its unique virus challenge both the basic and clinical researcher to develop innovative approaches to treat this disease.

Chronic Hepatitis C

Diagnosis and Clinical Course.—Chronic hepatitis C is diagnosed by finding elevations of serum aminotransferases for at least 6 months along with anti-HCV in serum and liver histology compatible with chronic hepatitis.[1] Diagnosis is problematical for several reasons. First, 5% to 15% of patients with chronic hepatitis C do not have anti-HCV detectable using current immunoassays (false-negative results).[4] Second, a proportion of patients with other forms of liver disease without HCV infection test positive for anti-HCV (false-positive results). Finally, some patients have both chronic hepatitis C and another form of liver disease, and deciding which disease is causing the hepatic injury (and thus should be treated) is difficult. With future improvements in assays for detection of antibodies, antigens, and genomic sequences of HCV, these problems should lessen. At present, reliance upon anti-HCV testing alone to make the diagnosis of hepatitis C is not completely reliable, and confirmatory testing is often needed. Confirmation of hepatitis C can be made based upon a compatible history (blood transfusion, drug abuse, exposure to blood or blood products), or by confirmatory antibody tests (immunoblot assays or neutralization),[4, 113] or by detection of HCV antigens in liver (by immunofluorescence microscopy),[114] or by assaying HCV RNA in serum or liver (by reverse-transcription followed by polymerase chain reaction [RT-PCR]).[4, 115]

Chronic hepatitis C tends to be a silent but insidious disease. Long-term natural history studies suggest that 25% to 30% of patients with chronic HCV infection ultimately develop cirrhosis, and a large proportion of these patients develop complications of cirrhosis, portal hypertension, or liver failure.[4, 25] Chronic hepatitis C also appears to be an important cause of hepatocellular carcinoma.[116] Thus, the major rationale for therapy of chronic hepatitis C is to arrest disease activity, decrease symptoms if present, and prevent cirrhosis and possibly liver cancer. Most trials of antiviral therapy, however, have focused upon short-term outcomes, such as decreases in serum aminotransferases, loss of HCV RNA from serum or liver, and improvements in liver histology.

Trials of Alpha Interferon.—Pilot studies of alpha interferon were started before the identification of HCV, but nevertheless demonstrated that therapy was followed by marked improvements in serum aminotransferases in 70% to 80% of patients.[117] Subsequently, multiple randomized controlled trials documented that a 6-month course of alpha interferon in doses of 2 to 5 mu thrice weekly was followed by a fall of serum aminotransferases into the normal range and improvement in liver histology in approximately 50% of patients.[118–129] Retrospective analyses demonstrated that the decrease in aminotransferases was accompanied by a fall in HCV RNA levels in blood and that most patients who developed normal aminotransferases on therapy became HCV RNA negative.[130] Subsequent studies have shown that the decrease in serum HCV RNA reflects a decrease or disappearance of liver HCV RNA as well as HCV antigen.[131, 132]

Unfortunately, most studies of alpha interferon therapy of chronic hepatitis C also reported a high relapse rate once therapy was stopped. Relapses were marked by a return of serum HCV RNA and biochemical evidence of liver injury. Thus, in most studies the rate of sustained, long-term responses to alpha interferon has been only 25% to 30%.[118–129] More prolonged courses of therapy with higher doses of alpha interferon are now being evaluated in prospective studies.

Current Recommendations for Therapy of Chronic Hepatitis C.—Alpha interferon is currently recommended for patients with well-compensated chronic hepatitis C with persistently raised serum aminotransferases, chronic hepatitis disease activity by liver biopsy, and serologic or epidemiologic evidence of HCV infection (anti-HCV or a history of exposure to blood or blood products before the onset of hepatitis).

The recommended regimen of alpha interferon for chronic hepatitis C is 3 mu given 3 times weekly either subcutaneously or intramuscularly for 6 months (24 weeks). Actually the optimal dose and duration of therapy are controversial, with some investigators recommending higher doses (5 mu three times weekly) for more prolonged periods (12 months or 48 weeks).[16] The initial evaluation and initiation of therapy should follow the general recommendations given for chronic hepatitis B. A liver biopsy to document the severity of disease, the activity of the inflammation and necrosis, and degree of fibrosis is advisable but not mandatory, if there are serious contraindications to liver biopsy. Patients should be fully apprised of the expected results and side effects.

Monitoring of Patients on Therapy.—Patients with chronic hepatitis C should be seen, questioned about side effects, and have blood tested for aminotransferases and blood counts every 1 to 4 weeks while on therapy. The frequency of visits should be dictated by the severity of the liver disease and the degree of side effects. Evaluation should continue for at least 6 months after stopping therapy to assess whether the response is sustained. Follow-up liver biopsies are not needed unless retreatment is considered.

In cases of hepatitis C, aminotransferases usually decrease during interferon therapy, the degree of decrease varying from patient to patient. Worsening of aminotransferases (doubling of the pretreatment levels) during therapy of chronic hepatitis C is a reason for concern and should lead to early discontinuation of therapy. Several cases of acute exacerbation of hepatitis C with alpha interferon therapy have been reported, and some of these exacerbations have been severe and even life-threatening.[133, 134] The cause of the exacerbation is unclear; some patients are found to have autoimmune hepatitis rather than hepatitis C as initially suspected.

Definition of Response.—Several patterns of change in aminotransferases can occur with interferon therapy of chronic hepatitis C (Fig 5). Approximately 25% of patients have a *sustained beneficial response* (see Fig 5,A).[16, 117, 118] In these patients, aminotransferases begin to fall within the first months of treatment and are often normal by 2 to 3 months. Simultaneous testing for HCV RNA in serum reveals that the fall in aminotransferases is accompanied by a loss of this marker of viremia.[130] Aminotransferases remain normal and HCV RNA undetectable even after therapy is stopped. Another 25% of patients have a complete response while on interferon but promptly *relapse* when treatment is stopped (see Fig. 5,B). These patients may become negative for HCV RNA on treatment, but redevelop this viral marker when interferon is stopped and aminotransferases rise. A third group consists of about 25% of the patients

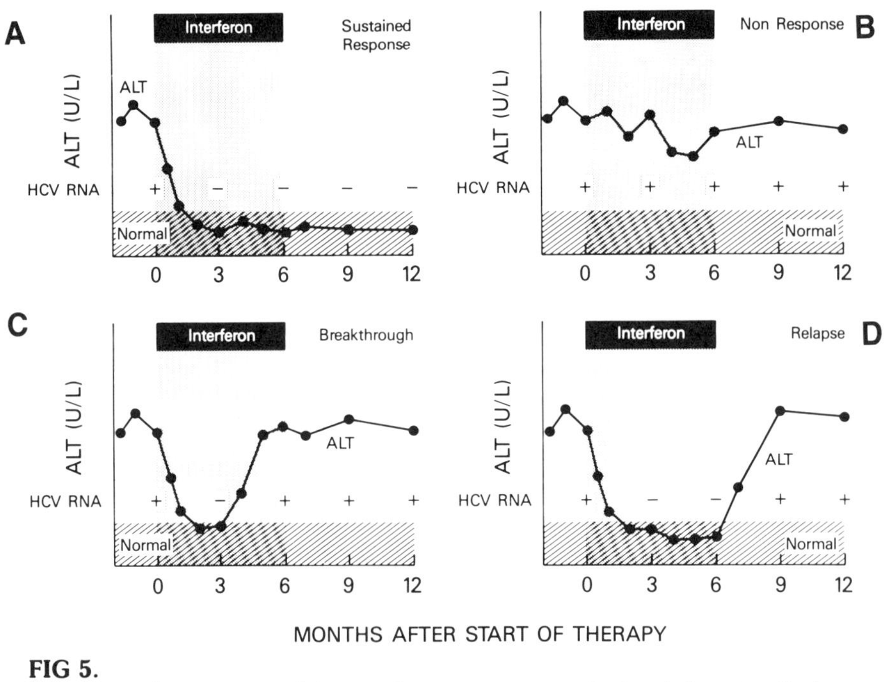

FIG 5.
Four types of response to alpha interferon in patients with chronic hepatitis C. *A*, a sustained complete response. *B*, no response to treatment. *C*, a partial and transient response with breakthrough during therapy. *D*, a transient complete response with relapse when therapy was stopped. (From Baron S, Coppenhaver D, Dianzani F, et al (eds): *Interferon: Principles and Medical Applications.* Galveston, Tex, University of Texas Medical Branch at Galveston, Department of Microbiology Press, 1992. Used by permission.)

who have a *partial or transient response* only (see Fig. 5,C); in these patients, serum aminotransferases decrease but do not become normal or become normal only transiently *(breakthrough)* and then rise despite continuation of interferon. Such patients may manifest a fall of aminotransferases into the normal range if the dose of alpha interferon is increased, but not all patients will be able to tolerate the increased side effects that accompany the higher dose. A final 25% of patients have *no response* to interferon (see Fig 5,D). In these patients, serum aminotransferase activities remain elevated and serum HCV RNA present throughout interferon treatment.

A long-term response to alpha interferon is usually defined as persistence of normal aminotransferases for at least 1 year after therapy. Longer follow-up on patients treated with alpha interferon is available on very few patients. In one study, 2- to 7-year follow-up demonstrated that responses were sustained and patients continued to be asymptomatic of liver disease, to have normal serum aminotransferases, and to have no HCV RNA in serum.[135] In a second study, late relapses were described and not all patients with a sustained response based upon aminotransferase levels continued to be HCV RNA negative.[136] Long-term follow-up is, of course, important in ultimately defining the optimal dose and duration of interferon therapy for chronic hepatitis C.

Predictors of Response.—There are no completely reliable features that help to predict which patient is likely to respond to treatment.[137] Responses to interferon usually occur within 2 to 3 months of starting therapy; thus, if aminotransferases have not improved after 12 weeks of treatment, interferon should be stopped early.[118] Nonresponders need not be treated for the full 24 weeks.

Retrospective analyses have indicated a few clinical features that weakly predict whether the patient will have a response to therapy and whether the response will be long-term. In multivariate analyses of large numbers of patients, the two features that best predict a response are the absence of cirrhosis and a short, known duration of aminotransferase elevations.[138] Thus, a long-term response is most likely to occur in the patient with chronic hepatitis C who has had disease for less than 5 years and is not shown to have cirrhosis upon liver biopsy. These predictive factors are quite different from those that predict a response in chronic hepatitis B and point again to the many dissimilarities between these two diseases which clinically are often indistinguishable.

Increasing the Response Rate in Chronic Hepatitis C.—Most attempts to increase the response rate in chronic hepatitis C have focused on using longer periods of treatment. Unfortunately, the findings from these studies have been contradictory; a 12-month course yielded a higher long-term response rate in one large randomized controlled study from Italy[139] but not in another.[140] Indeed, high response rates have been reported in a study from Japan using a 2-month course of treatment alone.[141] At present a 24-week course is recommended, but the high relapse rate with such therapy makes a 48-week course appealing.

There is little information regarding the efficacy of retreatment or use of higher doses of alpha interferon. Retreatment should be advised only for those patients who had a beneficial response to an initial course of therapy with few side effects, but who subsequently relapsed. In this situation, use of a more prolonged course and perhaps higher doses of interferon is advisable.[16]

Patients with Atypical Forms of Chronic Hepatitis C.—Current recommendations for alpha interferon therapy in chronic hepatitis C are for patients with typical, well-compensated disease. The criteria for selecting patients eliminate some who may deserve treatment, such as those with normal aminotransferases, children, patients with atypical serologic results, those with advanced liver disease, and those who are immunosuppressed.

Normal Aminotransferases.—Patients with chronic HCV infection have various degrees of liver injury. Many patients with this infection will have no elevations in serum aminotransferases. Some of these may have a degree of chronic hepatitis by liver biopsy.[142] These patients are often detected when they donate blood and are found to be anti-HCV positive. At present, one would not recommend treatment of patients with chronic hepatitis C who have normal or near-normal aminotransferases. Chronic HCV infection can be benign and not associated with progressive liver injury.[25] These patients should be followed and treated only if biochemical evidence of disease becomes manifest.

Children.—Preliminary reports on alpha interferon therapy of chronic hepatitis C in children indicate that the response rates in children are similar to those in adults.[143] There is no evidence that children are either more or less susceptible to the effects of interferon, and treatment is recommended in doses of 3 mu/m^2 three times weekly for 24 weeks. The criteria for treatment and procedures for monitoring therapy should be the same as those for adults.

Atypical Serologic Patterns.—Some patients with chronic hepatitis C test negative for anti-HCV by currently available immunoassays. These patients can be said to have cryptogenic hepatitis. Important diagnoses to exclude in this situation are autoimmune hepatitis, drug-induced liver injury, sclerosing cholangitis, Wilson's disease, and alpha-1-antitrypsin deficiency. In some cases the diagnosis of chronic hepatitis C can be established by research assays for HCV RNA in serum or HCV antigen in liver. In other cases, however, the diagnosis remains elusive and the severity of disease warrants some form of treatment. There is a need for caution in using alpha interferon in this situation, because patients with autoimmune hepatitis can exhibit a severe worsening of the hepatitis with treatment.[133] For this reason, it is appropriate to try a course of corticosteroids before trying alpha interferon in patients with cryptogenic hepatitis in whom a specific diagnosis cannot be made. If there is no response to corticosteroids, a trial of interferon is warranted.

Decompensated Liver Disease.—Patients with advanced chronic hepatitis C and clinically apparent cirrhosis can respond to interferon treatment.[144] These patients, however, have troublesome side effects from interferon such as severe fatigue, weight loss, anorexia, bacterial infections, and psychological changes. As in chronic hepatitis B, only patients with early or mildly decompensated cirrhosis should be treated. For advanced cases, liver transplantation offers the only possibility for a sustained improvement in health.

Immunosuppressed Patients.—Patients with immune deficiencies or those receiving immunosuppressive medications are frequently infected with HCV and represent a difficult group of patients to manage.[144] Chronic hepatitis C is common among oncology patients, renal dialysis patients, patients with HIV infection, and patients who have received a solid organ transplant.[145–147] Furthermore, the immunosuppression itself may worsen the underlying liver disease. There have been no prospective, controlled trials of therapy of chronic hepatitis C in immunosuppressed patients. Small pilot studies have suggested that patients with a combination of HCV and HIV infection can respond to alpha interferon therapy.[148] Furthermore, preliminary reports of therapy of patients with recurrent hepatitis C after liver transplantation suggest that alpha interferon can suppress viral replication and improve serum aminotransferases even in the face of large doses of immunosuppressive medications.[74, 149] The safety and relative benefit of interferon therapy in these situations are still unclear and warrant further study. At the present time, immunosuppressed patients should probably not receive alpha interferon outside of prospective controlled trials.

Nonresponders.—There is currently little information to suggest that nonresponder patients benefit from a repeat course of interferon. These patients are excellent candidates for future trials of other antiviral agents. Patients who have no response to alpha interferon should also be carefully evaluated for the possibility of having another form of liver disease, perhaps unrelated to their HCV infection such as autoimmune or alcoholic hepatitis.

Patients who respond to alpha interferon initially but relapse when therapy is stopped can occasionally benefit from higher doses of interferon given for a more prolonged period.[130] Other patients may benefit from long-term therapy aimed at suppressing the disease activity rather than inducing a long-term remission. However, these uses of alpha interferon must be considered experimental and only used if the response to treatment is clear cut, the underlying disease severe, and the interferon well tolerated.

Other Therapies of Chronic Hepatitis C.—Pilot studies of other antiviral agents that might be used alone or in combination with interferon in chronic hepatitis C have recently been initiated. The most promising such antiviral agent is ribavirin. In two pilot studies, a 6-month course of ribavirin therapy was found to lead to a decrease in aminotransferases in the majority of patients with chronic hepatitis C.[11, 12] The decrease in aminotransferases was similar to that seen with alpha interferon therapy in chronic hepatitis C. Unfortunately, the improvements in aminotransferases were not accompanied by improvements in liver histology or HCV RNA levels. The possible role of long-term therapy with ribavirin or combinations of this drug with alpha interferon awaits further investigations.

Few other antiviral agents have been evaluated in patients with chronic hepatitis C. A preliminary study from Spain indicated that gamma interferon had little effect on serum aminotransferases in patients with chronic hepatitis C.[150] Future advances in therapy of chronic hepatitis C would be benefitted most by development of reliable tissue culture systems for evaluating HCV replication and the effect of antiviral agents.[151]

Summary

Viral hepatitis comprises five different diseases caused by five different viral agents: hepatitis A, B, C, D, and E virus. All five forms can cause acute hepatitis, only hepatitis B, C and D can cause chronic hepatitis. Alpha interferon has been shown to be effective in inducing sustained remissions in all three forms of chronic viral hepatitis. Its efficacy in acute viral hepatitis has not been documented, although preliminary results suggest that interferon may decrease the chronicity rate of acute hepatitis C.

In *chronic hepatitis B,* alpha interferon therapy with 5 mu daily or 10 mu three time weekly for 16 weeks will induce a long-term remission in disease with loss of HBV DNA and HBeAg from serum in 25% to 40% of patients and ultimately, a loss of HBsAg in approximately half of the responders. Patients likely to respond are those with high initial serum aminotransferases and low levels of HBV DNA.

In *chronic hepatitis C,* therapy with 3 to 5 mu of alpha interferon 3 times weekly for 24 to 48 weeks will induce a temporary remission in disease with loss of HCV RNA from serum, fall of aminotransferases into the normal range and improvement in liver histology in 50% of patients and a sustained remission persisting after therapy is stopped in 25% of patients. Patients with a short duration of disease and without cirrhosis are the most likely to respond. Unfortunately, there are no completely reliable means of predicting which patients are likely to respond to interferon and which of these will have a lasting response.

In *chronic hepatitis D,* a prolonged course of alpha interferon given in doses of 3 to 5 mu daily or 9 to 10 mu three times weekly results in remission in disease as marked by loss of HDV RNA from blood and fall of aminotransferases into the normal range in up to 50% of patients. Unfortunately, this response is rarely sustained after treatment unless HBsAg becomes negative, which occurs in only a small number of patients.

Despite the benefits of alpha interferon therapy in many patients with chronic viral hepatitis, several shortcomings of this therapy are evident: less than 50% of patients respond, side effects can be problematical, and some patients are not appropriate for therapy. Thus, interferon is not indicated for patients with advanced cirrhosis or for those who are severely immunosuppressed. Alpha interferon is an important first step in therapy for chronic viral hepatitis, but further approaches are needed to increase its efficacy and safety.

References

1. Hoofnagle JH, Di Bisceglie AM: Serologic diagnosis of acute and chronic viral hepatitis. *Semin Liver Dis* 1992; 11:73–83.
2. McQuillan GM, Alter M, Everhart JE: Viral hepatitis, in Everhart JE (ed): *Digestive Diseases in the United States: Epidemiology and Impact.* Washington DC, Government Printing Office, in press, 1993.
3. Annual Report of the U.S. Scientific Registry for Organ Transplantation and the Organ Procurement and Transplantation Network 1990. Richmond, Va, UNOS; Bethesda, Md, Division of Organ Transplantation, Health Resources and Services Administration.
4. Alter HJ: Descartes before the horse: I clone, therefore I am. The hepatitis C virus in current perspective. *Ann Intern Med* 1991; 115:644–649.
5. Gilbert DE, Knight V: Biochemistry and clinical applications of ribavirin. *Antimicro Agents Chemo* 1986; 30:201–205.
6. Sanchez FS, Sosa IRG, Vargas GM: Treatment of type A hepatitis with ribavirin, in Smith RA, Knight V, Smith JAD (eds): *Clinical Applications of Ribavirin.* New York, Academic Press, Inc, 1984, pp 193–201.
7. Ayrosa-Galvao PA, Castro IO: The effect of 1-beta-D-ribofuranosyl-1,2,4-triazole-3-carboxamide on acute viral hepatitis. *Ann NY Acad Sci* 1977; 284:278–283.
8. Patki SA, Gupta P: Evaluation of ribavirin in the treatment of acute hepatitis. *Chemotherapy* 1982; 28:298–303.
9. Widell A, Hansson BG, Oberg B, et al: Influence of twenty potentially antiviral substances on in vitro multiplication of hepatitis A virus. *Antiviral Res* 1986; 6:103–112.
10. Fried MW, Fong T-L, Swain, MG, et al: Hepatitis B virus (HBV) DNA suppression during long-term therapy with ribavirin. *Gastroenterology* 1992; 102:A808.
11. Reichard O, Andersson J, Schvarcz R, et al: Ribavirin treatment for chronic hepatitis C. *Lancet* 1991; 337:1058–1061.
12. Di Bisceglie AM, Shindo M, Fong T-L, et al: A pilot study of ribavirin therapy for chronic hepatitis C. *Hepatology* 1992; 16:649–654.
13. Peters M: Mechanisms of action of interferon. *Semin Liver Dis* 1989; 4:235–239.
14. Vallbracht A, Flehmig B: Elimination of a persistent hepatitis A infection in cell cultures by interferon, in Kirchner H, Schellekens H (eds): *The Biology of the Interferon System.* New York, Elsevier, pp 339–345, 1985.
15. Tur-Kaspa R, Teicher L, Laub O, et al: Alpha interferon suppresses hepatitis B virus enhancer activity and reduces viral gene transcription. *J Virol* 1990; 64:1821–1824.
16. Hoofnagle JH, Di Bisceglie AM: Antiviral therapy of viral hepatitis, in Galasso GJ, Whitley RJ, Merigan TC (eds): *Antiviral Agents and Viral Diseases of Man,* ed 3. New York, Raven Press, pp 415–459, 1990.
17. Levin S, Hahn T: Interferon system in acute viral hepatitis. *Lancet* 1982; 1:592–595.
18. Iwarson S, Norkrans G, Nordenfelt E, et al: Interferon treatment in acute

hepatitis B infection with prolonged course. *Scand J Infect Dis* 1980; 12:233–234.
19. Tassapoulos NC, Hadziyannis SJ, Wright GE: Recombinant human interferon alfa-2b in the management of acute type B hepatitis (abstract). *Hepatology* 1989; 10:576.
20. Sanchez-Tapias JM, Mas A, Bruguera M, et al: Recombinant alpha-2c interferon therapy in fulminant viral hepatitis. *J Hepatology* 1987; 5:205–210.
21. Omata M, Yokosuka O, Takano S, et al: Resolution of acute hepatitis C after therapy with natural beta interferon. *Lancet* 1991; 338:914–915.
22. Alberti A, Chemello L, Benvegnu L, et al: Pilot study of interferon alpha-2a therapy in preventing chronic evolution of acute hepatitis C, in Hollinger RB, Lemon S, Margolis H (eds): *Viral Hepatitis and Liver Disease,* Baltimore, Williams and Wilkins, pp 656–658, 1991.
23. Viladomiu L, Gonzalez A, Lopez-Talavera JC, et al: A randomized controlled trial of alpha-interferon in acute posttransfusion C hepatitis (abstract). *J Hepatology* 1990; 11:S64.
24. Rumi MG, Lampertico P, Soffredini R, et al: Serum HCV-RNA in patients with acute hepatitis C treated with recombinant interferon alfa (abstract). *Hepatology* 1992; 16:72A.
25. Di Bisceglie AM, Goodman ZD, Ishak KG, et al: Long-term clinical and histopathological follow-up of chronic posttransfusion hepatitis. *Hepatology* 1991; 14:969–974.
26. Rizzetto M, Verme G, Recchia S, et al: Chronic hepatitis in carriers of hepatitis B surface antigen, with intrahepatic expression of the delta antigen: An active and progressive disease unresponsive to immunosuppressive treatment. *Ann Intern Med* 1983; 98:437–441.
27. Di Bisceglie AM, Waggoner JG, Hoofnagle JH: Hepatitis B virus deoxyribonucleic acid in liver of chronic carriers. Correlation with serum markers and changes associated with loss of hepatitis B e antigen after antiviral therapy. *Gastroenterology* 1987; 93:1236–1241.
28. Carman WF, Jacyna MR, Hadziyannis S, et al: Mutation preventing formation of hepatitis B e antigen in patients with chronic hepatitis B infection. *Lancet* 1989; ii:588–591.
29. Brunetto MR, Oliveri F, Rocca G, et al: Natural course and response to interferon of chronic hepatitis B accompanied by antibody to hepatitis e antigen. *Hepatology* 1989; 10:198–202.
30. Perrillo RP, Schiff ER, Davis GL, et al: A randomized controlled trial of interferon alfa-2b alone and after prednisone withdrawal for the treatment of chronic hepatitis B. *N Engl J Med* 1990; 323:295–301.
31. Hoofnagle JH, Peters MG, Mullen KD, et al: Randomized controlled trial of a four-month course of recombinant human alpha interferon in chronic type B hepatitis. *Gastroenterology* 1988; 95:1318–1325.
32. Di Bisceglie AM, Bergasa N, Fong T-L, et al: A randomized controlled trial of recombinant alpha interferon therapy for chronic hepatitis B (abstract). *Hepatology* 1991; 14:70A.
33. Perez V, Tanno H, Gay O, Barclay CA: Treatment of chronic active hepatitis B with recombinant interferon alpha A, in Hollinger FB, Lemon SM, Margolis HS (ed): *Viral Hepatitis and Liver Disease,* Baltimore, Williams and Wilkins, pp 851–854, 1991.
34. Alexander GJM, Brahm J, Fagan EA, et al: Loss of HBsAg with interferon therapy in chronic hepatitis B virus infection. *Lancet* 1987; i:66–69.
35. Thomas HC, Dusheiko GM, Lok ASF, et al: Comparative study of three

doses of interferon alpha-2a in chronic active hepatitis B, in Hollinger FB, Lemon SM, Margolis HS (eds): *Viral Hepatitis and Liver Disease.* Baltimore, Williams and Wilkins, pp 641–642, 1991.

36. Realdi G, Gattovich G, Pastore G, et al: Problems in the management of chronic hepatitis B with interferon: Experience in a randomized multicenter study. *J Hepatology* 1990; 11:S129–S132.
37. Sarraco G, Mazzella G, Rosina F, et al: A controlled trial of human lymphoblastoid interferon in chronic hepatitis B in Italy. *Hepatology* 1989; 10:336–341.
38. Carreno V, Porres JC, Mora I, et al. A controlled study of treatment with recombinant interferon alpha in chronic hepatitis B virus infection: Induction and maintenance schedules. *Antiviral Research* 1989; 8:125–137.
39. Muller R, Baumgarten R, Markus R, et al: Treatment of chronic hepatitis B with alpha-2b. *J Hepatology* 1990; 11:S137–S140.
40. Fevery J, Elewant A, Michielsen P, et al: Efficacy of interferon alfa-2b with or without prednisone withdrawal in the treatment of chronic viral hepatitis B. A prospective double-blind Belgian-Dutch study. *J Hepatology* 1990; 11:S108–S112.
41. Dusheiko GM, Paterson AC, Pitcher L, et al: Recombinant leucocyte interferon treatment of chronic hepatitis B: An analysis of two therapeutic trials. *J Hepatology* 1986; 3:S199–S207.
42. Williams SJ, Craig PI, Cooksley WGE, et al: Randomized, controlled trial of recombinant human interferon-alphaA for chronic active hepatitis B. *Aust NZ J Med* 1990; 20:9–19.
43. Lok ASF, Wu P-C, Lai C-L, et al: A controlled trial of interferon with or without prednisone priming for chronic hepatitis B. *Gastroenterology* 1992; 102:2091–2097.
44. Korenman J, Baker B, Waggoner J, et al: Long-term remission in chronic hepatitis B after alpha-interferon therapy. *Ann Intern Med* 1991; 114:629–634.
45. Renault PF, Hoofnagle JH: Side effects of alpha interferon. *Sem Liver Dis* 1989; 9:273–277.
46. Dooley JS, Davis GL, Peters M, et al: Pilot study of recombinant human alpha interferon for chronic type B hepatitis. *Gastroenterology* 1986; 90:150–157.
47. Smedley H, Katrak M, Sikora K, et al: Neurological effects of recombinant human interferon. *Br Med J* 1983; 286:262–264.
48. Renault PF, Hoofnagle JH, Park Y, et al: Psychiatric complications of long-term interferon alpha therapy. *Arch Intern Med* 1987; 147:1577–1580.
49. McDonald EM, Mann AH, Thomas HC: Interferons as mediators of psychiatric morbidity: An investigation in a trial of recombinant alpha-interferon in hepatitis-B carriers. *Lancet* 1987; 2:1175–1178.
50. Kassianides C, Di Bisceglie AM, Hoofnagle JH, et al: Alpha interferon therapy in patients with decompensated chronic type B hepatitis, in Zuckerman AJ (ed): *Viral Hepatitis and Liver Disease.* New York, Alan R Liss, 1988, pp 840–843.
51. Janssen HLA, Berk L, Vermeulen M, et al: Seizures associated with low-dose alpha-interferon (letter) *Lancet* 1990; 336:1580.
52. Averbuch, SD, Austin HA, Sherwin SA, et al: Acute interstitial neprhritis with the nephrotic syndrome following recombinant leukocyte interferon therapy for mycosis fungoides. *N Engl J Med* 1984; 310:32–35.
53. Deyton LR, Walker RE, Kovacs JA, et al: Reversible cardiac dysfunction as-

sociated with interferon alfa therapy in AIDS patients with Kaposi's sarcoma. *N Engl J Med* 1989; 321:1246–1249.
54. Mayet W-J, Hess G, Gerken G, et al: Treatment of chronic type B hepatitis with recombinant alpha-interferon induces autoantibodies not specific for autoimmune chronic hepatitis. *Hepatology* 1989; 10:24–28.
55. Lisker-Melman M, Di Bisceglie AM, Usala SJ, et al: Development of thyroid disease during therapy of chronic viral hepatitis with alpha interferon. *Gastroenterology* 1992; 102:2155–2160.
56. McLaughlin P, Talpaz M, Quesada JR: Immune thrombocytopenia following alpha interferon therapy in patients with cancer. *JAMA* 1985; 254:1353–1354.
57. Akard LP, Hoffman R, Elias L, et al: Alpha interferon and immune hemolytic anemia (letter). *Ann Intern Med* 1986; 105:306.
58. Chazerain P, Meyer O, Kahn MR. Rheumatoid arthritis-like disease after alpha-interferon therapy (letter). *Ann Intern Med* 1992; 116:427.
59. Brook MG, Karayiannis P, Thomas HC: Which patients with chronic hepatitis B virus infection will respond to alpha interferon therapy? A statistical analysis of predictive factors. *Hepatology* 1989; 10:761–763.
60. Garcia G, Smith CI, Weissberg JI, et al: Adenine arabinoside monophosphate in combination with human leukocyte interferon in the treatment of chronic hepatitis B: A randomized, double-blind, placebo-controlled trial. *Ann Intern Med* 1987; 107:278–285.
61. Di Bisceglie AM, Rustgi VK, Kassianides C, et al: Therapy of chronic hepatitis B with recombinant alpha and gamma interferon. *Hepatology* 1990; 11:266–270.
62. Fattovich G, Giustina G, Brollo L, et al: Therapy for chronic hepatitis B with lymphoblastoid interferon-alpha and levaminsole. *Hepatology* 1992; 16:1115–1119.
63. Perrillo R, Regenstein F, Peters M, et al: Prednisone withdrawal followed by recombinant alpha interferon in the treatment of chronic type B hepatitis: A randomized controlled trial. *Ann Intern Med* 1988; 109:95–100.
64. Hoofnagle JH, Davis GL, Pappas SC, et al: A short course of prednisolone in chronic type B hepatitis: Report of a randomized, double-blind, placebo-controlled trial. *Ann Intern Med* 1986; 104:12–17.
65. Lai CL, Lok ASF, Lin HS, et al: Placebo-controlled trial of recombinant alpha-interferon in Chinese HBsAg-carrier children. *Lancet* 1987; 2:877–880.
66. Lisker-Melman M, Webb D, Di Bisceglie AM, et al: Glomerulonephritis caused by chronic hepatitis B virus infection: Treatment with recombinant human alpha-interferon. *Ann Intern Med* 1989; 111:479–483.
67. Ruiz-Moreno M, Rua MJ, Molina J, et al: Prospective, randomized controlled trial of interferon-alpha in children with chronic hepatitis B. *Hepatology* 1991; 13:1035–1039.
68. Utili R, Sagnelli E, Galanti B, et al: Prolonged treatment of children with chronic hepatitis B with recombinant alpha 2a-interferon: A controlled, randomized study. *Amer J Gastro* 1991; 86:327–330.
69. Lok ASF, Lai CL, Wu PC, et al: Long-term follow-up in a randomised controlled trial of recombinant alpha-2 interferon in Chinese patients with chronic hepatitis B infection. *Lancet* 1988; 2:298–302.
70. Hadziyannis S, Bramou T, Makris A, et al: Interferon alfa-2b treatment of HBeAg negative/serum HBV DNA positive chronic active hepatitis type B. *J Hepatology* 1990; 11:S133–S136.
71. Fattovich G, Farci P, Brollo L, et al: A randomized controlled trial of lympho-

blastoid interferon-alpha in patients with chronic hepatitis B lacking HBeAg. *Hepatology* 1992; 15:584–589.
72. Hoofnagle JH, Di Bisceglie AM, Waggoner JG, et al: Alpha interferon for patients with clinically apparent cirrhosis due to chronic hepatitis B. *Gastroenterology* 1993; 104:1116–1121.
73. Perrillo R, Tamburro C, Regenstein F, et al: Treatment of decompensated chronic hepatitis B (CHC) with a titratable, low dose regimen of recombinant interferon alfa-2b (rIFN a-2b) (abstract). *Hepatology* 1992; 16:126A.
74. Wright HI, Gavaler JS, Van Thiel DH: Preliminary experience with alpha-2b interferon therapy of viral hepatitis in liver allograft recipients. *Transplantation* 1992; 53:121–124.
75. Thomas HC, Karayiannis P, Brook G: Treatment of hepatitis B virus infection: Factors predicting response to interferon. *J Hepatology* 1991; 13:S4–S7.
76. Mutchnick MG, Appelman HD, Chung HT, et al: Thymosin treatment of chronic hepatitis B: A placebo controlled pilot trial. *Hepatology* 1991; 14:409–415.
77. Nishioka M, Kagawa H, Shirai M, et al: Effects of human recombinant interleukin 2 in patients with chronic hepatitis B: A preliminary report. *Am J Gastroenterol* 1987; 82:438–442.
78. Lau JYN, Lai CL, Wu PC, et al: A randomised controlled trial of recombinant interferon-gamma in Chinese patients with chronic hepatitis B virus infection. *J Med Virol* 1991; 34:184–187.
79. Martin J, Bosch O, Quiroga JA, et al: Recombinant human granulocyte-macrophage colony stimulating factor (rhGM-CSF) in the treatment of chronic hepatitis B (abstract). *Hepatology* 1992; 16:67A.
80. Alexander GJM, Fagan EA, Hegarty JE, et al: Controlled clinical trial of acyclovir in chronic hepatitis B virus infection. *J Med Virol* 1987; 21:87–87.
81. Berk L, Schalm SW, de Man RA, et al: Failure of acyclovir to enhance the antiviral effect of alpha lymphoblastoid interferon on HBe seroconversion in chronic hepatitis B: A multi-centre randomized controlled trial. *J Hepatol* 1992; 14:305–309.
82. Locarnini SA, Guo K, Lucas CR et al: Inhibition of HBV DNA replication by ganciclovir in patients with AIDS. *Lancet* 1989; 2:1225–1226.
83. Loke RHT, Anderson MG, Coleman JC, et al: Suramin treatment for chronic active hepatitis B—toxic and ineffective. *J Med Virol* 1987; 21:97–99.
84. Bain VG, Daniels HM, Chanas A, et al: Foscarnet therapy in chronic hepatitis B virus e antigen carrier. *J Med Virol* 1989; 29:152–155.
85. Fried MW, Korenman JC, Di Bisceglie AM, et al: A pilot study of 2′,3′ dideoxyinosine for the treatment of chronic hepatitis B. *Hepatology* 1992; 16:861–864.
86. Catterall AP, Moyle G, Hopes EA, et al: Dideoxyinosine for chronic hepatitis B infection. *J Med Virol* 1992; 37:307–309.
87. Thursz M, Thomas H: Future therapy for B virus chronic hepatitis, in Miguet JP, Dhumeaux D (eds): *Progress in Hepatology 93*. Paris, John Libbey Eurotext, 1993, pp 99–107.
88. Doong SL, Tsai CH, Schinazi RF, et al: Inhibition of the replication of hepatitis B virus in vitro by 2′,3′-dideoxy-3′-thiapyrimidine and related analogues. *Proc Natl Acad Sci USA* 1991; 88:8495–8499.
89. Price PM, Banergee R, Acs G. Inhibition of the replication of hepatitis B virus by the carbocyclic analogue of 2′deoxyguanosine. *Proc Natl Acad Sci USA* 1989; 86:8541–8544.

90. Suzuki S, Lee B, Luo W, et al: Inhibition of duck hepatitis B virus replication by purine 2′,3′dideoxynucleosides. *Biochem Biophy Res Commun* 1988; 156:1144–1151.
91. Ponzetto A, Forzani B, Busi C, et al: Adenine arabinoside monophosphate and acyclovir monophosphate coupled to lactosaminated albumin inhibit woodchuck hepatitis virus replication at low doses. *Hepatology* 1991; 14:16–23.
92. Goldstein AL, Low TLK, Thurman GB, et al: Current status of thymosin and other hormones of the thymus gland. *Recent Prog Hormone Res* 1981; 37:369–415.
93. Tsiquaye KN, Collins P, Zuckerman AJ: Screening of antiviral drugs for treatment of hepatitis B. *J Hepatol* 1986; 2:S45–48.
94. Korba BE, Cote PJ, Tennant BC, et al: Woodchuck hepatitis virus infection as a model for the development of antiviral therapies against HBV, in Hollinger FB, Lemon SM, Margolis HS (eds): *Viral Hepatitis and Liver Disease.* Baltimore, Williams and Wilkins; 1991, pp 641–642.
95. Korba BE, Gerin JL: Use of a standardized cell culture assay to assess activities of nucleoside analogs against hepatitis B replication. *Antiviral Res* 1992; 17:1–16.
96. Wu GY, Wu CH: Specific inhibition of hepatitis B viral gene expression in vitro by targeted antisense oligonucleotides. *J Biol Chem* 1992; 267:12436–12439.
97. Weizsaecker FV, Blum HE, Wands JG: Ribozyme mediated cleavage of hepatitis B and duck hepatitis B virus RNA (abstract). *Hepatology* 1992; 16:88A.
98. Lever AML, Waters J, Brook MG, et al: Monoclonal antibody to HBsAg for chronic hepatitis B virus infection with hypogammaglobulinaemia (letter). *Lancet* 1990:335:1529.
99. Lok ASF, Liang RHS, Chung H-T: Recovery from chronic hepatitis B (letter). *Ann Intern Med* 1982; 116:957.
100. Hoofnagle JH: Type D (delta) hepatitis. *JAMA* 1989; 261:1321–1325.
101. Thomas HC, Farci P, Shein R, et al: Inhibition of hepatitis delta virus replication by lymphoblastoid human alpha interferon. *Prog Clin Biol Res* 1987; 234:277–290.
102. Di Bisceglie AM, Martin P, Lisker-Melman M, et al: Therapy of chronic delta hepatitis with interferon alfa-2b. *J Hepatology* 1990; 11:S151–S154.
103. Hadziyannis SJ: Use of alpha-interferon in the treatment of chronic delta hepatitis. *J Hepatology* 1991; 13:S21–S26.
104. Porres JC, Carreno V, Bartholome J, et al: Treatment of chronic delta infection with recombinant human interferon alpha 2c at high doses. *J Hepatology* 1989; 9:338–350.
105. Rosina F, Rizzetto M: Treatment of chronic type D (delta) hepatitis with alpha interferon. *Sem Liver Dis* 1989; 9:264–266.
106. Rosina F, Pintus C, Meschievitz C, et al: A randomized controlled trial of a 12-month course of recombinant human interferon-alpha in chronic delta (type D) hepatitis: A multicenter Italian study. *Hepatology* 1991; 13:1052–1056.
107. Farci P, Mandas A, Lai CE, et al: Randomized controlled trial of high and low doses of interferon (IFN) alpha-2a (Roferon-A) in chronic HDV hepatitis: An interim report, in Hollinger FB, Lemon SM, Margolis H (eds): *Viral Hepatitis and Liver Disease,* Baltimore, Williams and Wilkins, 1991, pp 672–673.

108. Craxi A, Di Marco V, Volpes R, et al: Treatment with interferon alfa-2b of chronic HDV hepatitis in children (abstract). *J Hepatology* 1990; 11:S175.
109. Buti M, Esteban R, Roget M, et al: Longterm treatment with recombinant alfa-2 interferon in patients with chronic delta hepatitis and human immunodeficiency antibodies (abstract). *J Hepatology* 1989; 9:S131.
110. Rizzetto M, Chiaberge E, Negro F, et al: Liver transplantation in hepatitis delta virus disease. *Lancet* 1987; 2:469–471.
111. Petcu DJ, Aldrich CE, Coates L, et al: Suramin inhibits in vitro infection by duck hepatitis B virus, Rous sarcoma virus, and hepatitis delta virus. *Virology* 1988; 167:385–392.
112. Mason WS, Taylor JM: Experimental systems for the study of hepadnavirus and hepatitis delta virus infections. *Hepatology* 1989; 9:635–645.
113. Van der Poel CL, Cuypers HTM, Reesink HW, et al: Confirmation of hepatitis C virus infection by new four antigen recombinant immunoblot assay. *Lancet* 1991; 337:317–319.
114. Krawczynski K, Beach MJ, Bradley DW, et al: Hepatitis C virus antigen in hepatocytes: Immunomorphologic detection and identification. *Gastroenterology* 1992; 103:622–629.
115. Farci P, Alter HJ, Wong D, et al: A long-term study of hepatitis C virus replication in non-A, non-B hepatitis. *N Engl J Med* 1991; 325:98–104.
116. Kiyosawa K, Sodeyama T, Tanaka E, et al: Interrelationship of blood transfusion, non-A, non-B hepatitis and hepatocellular carcinoma: Analysis by detection of antibody to hepatitis C virus. *Hepatology* 1990; 12:671–675.
117. Hoofnagle JH, Mullen KD, Jones DB, et al: Treatment of chronic non-A, non-B hepatitis with recombinant human alpha interferon: A preliminary report. *N Engl J Med* 1987; 315:1575–1578.
118. Davis GL, Balart LA, Schiff ER, et al: Treatment of chronic hepatitis C with recombinant interferon alfa: A multicenter randomized, controlled trial. *N Engl J Med* 1989; 321:1501–1505.
119. Di Bisceglie AM, Martin P, Kassianides C, et al: Recombinant interferon alfa therapy for chronic hepatitis C: A randomized, double-blind, placebo-controlled trial. *N Engl J Med* 1989; 321:1506–1510.
120. Jacyna MR, Brooks MG, Loke RHT, et al: Randomised controlled trial of interferon alfa (lymphoblastoid interferon) in chronic non-A, non-B hepatitis. *Br Med J* 1989; 298:80–82.
121. Marcellin P, Boyer N, Giostra E, et al: Recombinant human alpha-interferon in patients with chronic non-A, non-B hepatitis: A multicenter randomized controlled trial from France. *Hepatology* 1991; 13:393–397.
122. Saracco G, Rosina F, Torrani Cerenzia MR, et al: A randomized controlled trial of interferon alfa-2b as therapy for chronic non-A, non-B hepatitis. *J Hepatology* 1990; 11:S43–S49.
123. Ferenci P, Vogel W, Pristautz H, et al: One-year treatment of chronic non-A, non-B hepatitis with interferon alfa-2b. *J Hepatology* 1990; 11:S50–S56.
124. Weiland O, Schvarcz R, Wejstal R, et al: Therapy of chronic post-transfusion non-A, non-B hepatitis with interferon alfa-2b: Swedish experience. *J Hepatology* 1990; 11:S57–S62.
125. Gomez-Rubio M, Porres JC, Castillo I, et al: Prolonged treatment (18 months) of chronic hepatitis C with recombinant alpha-interferon in comparison with a control group. *J Hepatology* 1990; 11:S63–S67.
126. Realdi G, Diodata G, Bonetti P, et al: Recombinant human interferon alfa-2a in community-acquired non-A, non-B chronic active hepatitis: preliminary results of a randomized, controlled trial. *J Hepatology* 1990; 11:S68–S71.

127. Causse X, Godinot H, Chevallier M, et al: Comparison of 1 or 3 MU of interferon alfa-2b and placebo in patients with chronic non-A non-B hepatitis. *Gastroenterology* 1991; 101:497–502.
128. Lin R, Schoeman MN, Craig PI, et al: Can the response to interferon treatment be predicted in patients with chronic active hepatitis C? *Aust NZ J Med* 1991; 21:387–392.
129. Makris M, Preston FE, Triger DR, et al: A randomized controlled trial of recombinant interferon-alpha in chronic hepatitis C in hemophiliacs. *Blood* 1991; 78:1672–1677.
130. Shindo M, Di Bisceglie AM, Cheung L, et al: Decrease in serum hepatitis C viral RNA during alpha-interferon therapy for chronic hepatitis C. *Ann Intern Med* 1991; 115:700–704.
131. Fong T-L, Shindo M, Feinstone S, et al: Detection of replicative intermediates of hepatitis C viral RNA in liver and serum of patients with chronic hepatitis C. J Clin Invest 1991; 88:1058–1060.
132. Di Bisceglie AM, Krawczynski K, Brazzeal D, et al: Hepatitis C viral antigen (HCVAg) in liver: Effect of antiviral therapy (abstract). *Hepatology* 1992; 16:131A.
133. Papo T, Marcellin P, Bernuau J, et al: Autoimmune chronic hepatitis exacerbated by alpha-interferon. *Ann Intern Med* 1992; 116:51–53.
134. Shindo M, Di Bisceglie AM, Hoofnagle JH: Acute exacerbation of liver disease during interferon alfa therapy for chronic hepatitis C. *Gastroenterology* 1992; 102:1406–1408.
135. Shindo M, Di Bisceglie AM, Hoofnagle JH: Long-term follow-up of patients with chronic hepatitis C treated with alpha interferon. *Hepatology* 1992; 15:1013–1016.
136. Marcellin P, Boyer N, Martinot-Peignoux M, et al: Detection of serum HCV RNA by polymerase chain reaction (PCR) in patients with chronic hepatitis C with sustained response to recombinant alpha interferon (abstract). *J Hepatology* 1992; 16:S8.
137. Lindsay KL, Davis GL, Bodenheimer HC, et al: Predictors of relapse and response to re-treatment in patients with an initial response to recombinant alpha interferon (rIFN) therapy for chronic hepatitis C (abstract). *Hepatology* 1990; 12:847.
138. Camma C, Craxi A, Tine F, et al: Predictors of response to alpha-interferon (IFN) in chronic hepatitis C: a multivariate analysis on 361 treated patients (abstract). *Hepatology* 1992; 16:131A.
139. Alberti A, Chemello L, Diodati G, et al. Treatment of chronic hepatitis C with different regimens of interferon alpha-2a (IFN-2A) (abstract). *Hepatology* 1992; 16:75A.
140. Craxi A, Di Marco V, Lo Iacono O, et al: Lymphoblastoid alpha-interferon for post-transfusion chronic hepatitis C: A randomized trial of 6 vs. 12 months treatment (abstract). *J Hepatology* 1992; 16:S8.
141. Omata M, Ito Y, Yokosuka O, et al: Randomized, double-blind placebo-controlled trial of eight-week course of recombinant alpha-interferon for chronic non-A, non-B hepatitis. *Digest Dis Sci* 1991; 36:1217–1222.
142. Alberti A, Morsica G, Chemello L, et al: Hepatitis C viraemia and liver disease in symptom-free individuals with anti-HCV. *Lancet* 1992; 340:697–698.
143. Ruiz-Moreno M, Rua MJ, Castillo I, et al: Treatment of children with chronic hepatitis C with recombinant interferon-alpha: A pilot study. *Hepatology* 1992; 16:882–885.

144. Martin P, Di Bisceglie AM, Kassianides C, et al: Rapidly progressive non-A, non-B hepatitis in patients with human immunodeficiency virus infection. *Gastroenterology* 1989; 97:1559–1561.
145. Martin P, Munoz SJ, Di Bisceglie AM, et al: Recurrence of hepatitis C infection following orthotopic liver transplantation. *Hepatology* 1991; 13:719–721.
146. Pereira BJG, Milford EL, Kirkman RL, et al: Transmission of hepatitis C virus by organ transplantation. *N Engl J Med* 1991; 325:454–460.
147. Ferrell LD, Wright TL, Roberts J, et al: Hepatitis C viral infection in liver transplant recipients. *Hepatology* 1992; 16:865–876.
148. Boyer N, Marcellin P, Degott C, et al: Recombinant interferon-alpha for chronic hepatitis C in patients positive for antibody to human immunodeficiency virus. *J Infect Dis* 1992; 165:723–724.
149. Wright TL, Ferrell L, Lake J, et al: Hepatitis C viral RNA in patients on interferon (IFN)-alpha for post-liver transplant (OLTx) hepatitis (abstract). *Gastroenterology* 1992; 102:A910.
150. Saez-Royuela F, Porres JC, Moreno A, et al: High doses of recombinant alpha-interferon or gamma-interferon for chronic hepatitis C: A randomized, controlled trial. *Hepatology* 1991; 13:327–331.
151. Shimizu YK, Iwamoto A, Hijikata M, et al: Evidence for in vitro replication of hepatitis C virus genome in a human T-cell line. *Proc Natl Acad Sci USA* 1992; 89:5477–5481.

Emerging Concepts in the Management of Vasculitic Diseases

Gary S. Hoffman, M.D.

Head, Vasculitis and Related Diseases Section, Laboratory of Immunoregulation, National Institute of Allergy and Infectious Diseases, National Institutes of Health, Bethesda, Maryland; Chairman, Department of Rheumatic and Immunologic Diseases, Cleveland Clinic Foundation, Cleveland, Ohio

Anthony S. Fauci, M.D.

Chief, Laboratory of Immunoregulation and Director, National Institute of Allergy and Infectious Diseases, National Institutes of Health, Bethesda, Maryland

The Treatment of Systemic Vasculitis

The cornerstone for successful treatment of any potentially serious illness is making an accurate diagnosis as quickly as possible, recognizing prognosis, and anticipating the effects of disease and treatment on other concurrent illnesses.[1] Meeting these goals is often a difficult task in patients with systemic vasculitides, for which clinical manifestations may mimic infection malignancy, endocrinopathy, coagulopathy, multifocal emboli, drug toxicity, or poisoning. Many of these competing diagnoses may be ruled out by a thorough history and physical examination, and some others can be assessed within hours by appropriate laboratory studies. Suspicion of systemic vasculitis should be especially heightened when combinations of the following features are present: rash with palpable purpura, glomerulonephritis, peripheral neuropathy, preexisting features of autoimmunity (e.g., systemic lupus erythematosus, rheumatoid arthritis), and evidence of regional ischemia. Still, situations may arise when one cannot be certain whether fever, rash, a heart murmur and/or pulmonary infiltrates are due to infection (e.g., endocarditis), multifocal emboli, or vasculitis. Under some circumstances there may be a need to provide therapies that address more than one contingency pending definitive diagnosis. Sometimes this approach may seem counterproductive, such as simultaneously prescribing broad-spectrum antibiotics and immunosuppressive medications. Definitive studies, including biopsy of abnormal sites and/or angiography, will minimize the risk of prolonged inappropriate treatment for other suspected diseases.

It is important to recognize that the systemic vasculitides are uncommon, and that even major referral centers may encounter no more than 5 to 10 newly diagnosed patients with any one type of systemic vasculitis per year. Consequently, almost all studies of treatment have been uncontrolled. In addition, patients with different presentations and prognoses have not been stratified to assess the benefit of varying intensity of therapy in proportion to disease severity. Nonetheless, in those instances where a consensus of opinion exists, this will be stated. In other cases, the authors will indicate what they believe is the most reasonable approach.

Regardless of the specific vasculitic diagnosis (Table 1),[2] the severity of disease, anatomic distribution of involvement, rate of progression, and preexisting conditions should determine the aggressiveness of immunosuppressive therapy. For example, if manifestations of hypersensitivity vasculitis were limited to the skin and joints, and appeared to be associated with a

TABLE 1.
Vasculitis Syndromes*

Systemic Necrotizing Vasculitis
Polyarteritis nodosa
Wegener's granulomatosis
Allergic angiitis and granulomatosis of Churg-Strauss
Polyangiitis overlap syndrome
Hypersensitivity Vasculitis
Henoch-Schönlein purpura
Drug-induced vasculitis
Vasculitis associated with infectious disease
Vasculitis associated with neoplasms
Vasculitis associated with autoimmune disease
Giant Cell Arteritis
Temporal arteritis
Takayasu's disease
Kawasaki's Disease
Behçet's Disease
Cogan's Syndrome
Buerger's Disease

*From Hoffman GS, Kerr GS: Recognition of systemic vasculitis in the acutely ill patient, in Mandell BF (ed): *Management of Critically Ill Patients With Rheumatologic and Immunologic Diseases.* New York, Marcel Dekker, Inc, in press, 1994. Used by permission.

self-limiting respiratory infection or use of a new medication, then symptomatic treatment and medication withdrawal may be adequate therapy. However, if severe systemic disease occurred, and included major visceral organs, then treatment should begin with high-dose glucocorticoids (GC), such as prednisone (1 mg/kg/day). Whether GC should be given as a single morning dose, in 2 or 3 split doses, or as a large intravenous "pulse" or "bolus" (e.g., methylprednisolone 1 g), or whether a cytotoxic agent should be used at the onset will require individualization based on diagnosis and disease severity. For example, most patients with giant cell arteritis will dramatically improve after GC therapy alone,[3] whereas most patients with generalized Wegener's granulomatosis (WG), including glomerulonephritis, will progress to renal failure and death if not treated with GC plus a cytotoxic agent (e.g., cyclophosphamide).[4–8] Acute Kawasaki syndrome, which should be treated with salicylates and high dose intravenous immunoglobulin, is an exception to the GC/cytotoxic drug therapy guidelines provided for other systemic vasculitides.

While physicians may continue to debate the proper use of immunosuppressive agents, all would agree that successful treatment of these patients may be extremely complex and that their care requires frequent scrutiny of disease activity and attention to complications of therapy. Involvement of special organ systems will often require a multidisciplinary team approach: Behçet's disease (BD)—internal medicine, ophthalmology, neurology, and surgery; WG—internal medicine, nephrology, otolaryngology, ophthalmology, and surgery; Takayasu's arteritis (TA)—internal medicine, invasive radiology, and vascular surgery.

Initial Therapeutic Interventions

Polyarteritis Nodosa.—Untreated polyarteritis nodosa (PAN) has been estimated to have a 5-year mortality rate in excess of 85% (Table 2).[9, 10] Treatment with high dose GC has decreased this figure to about 30% to 45%.[10–14] When GC have been used in conjunction with an immunosuppressive/cytotoxic agent (usually cyclophosphamide and less often azathioprine, about 2 mg/kg/day), the 5-year mortality was reported to be 20% to 25%,[10, 12] and relapses were less frequent[14] than noted with GC therapy only. Clinical features that have most adversely affected survival include intestinal ischemia, cardiac involvement, and renal insufficiency. A reasonable approach to treatment in PAN, in the setting of normal renal function and in the absence of critical organ ischemia, would be to initiate therapy with GC only. If improvement did not follow within days, if deterioration occurred, or if renal, cardiac, intestinal, or central nervous system disease became apparent, daily therapy with a cytotoxic agent should be added.

About one third of patients with PAN have serologic markers of hepatitis B virus (HBV) infection. These patients usually have circulating immune complexes that contain HBV surface antigen and antibodies. Biopsies of

TABLE 2.
Polyarteritis Nodosa: Clinical Profile*

Abnormality†	Frequency, %
Fever	40–75
Musculoskeletal	50–80
Skin	30–50
Neurological (PNS‡ > CNS)	55–75
Renal	60–75
Hypertension	30–55
Cardiac	10–60
Pulmonary	occasional–50
Gastrointestinal	14–60

*From Hoffman GS, Kerr GS: Recognition of systemic vasculitis in the acutely ill patient, in Mandell BF (ed): *Management of Critically Ill Patients With Rheumatologic and Immunologic Diseases.* New York, Marcel Dekker, Inc, in press, 1994. Used by permission.

†In "classical" PAN the lungs are not involved. Some reported series of patients do not conform to these classification guidelines and include patients that are PAN-like, who might be considered by others as having an overlap syndrome.

‡PNS = peripheral nervous system; CNS = central nervous system.

involved blood vessels have revealed deposition of immune complexes. These observations have led to trials of plasmapheresis to remove immune complexes from the circulation and antiviral treatment with vidarabine to limit viral replication.[12–14] Patients in these studies received GC therapy for only 2 weeks and were not treated with cytotoxic agents. Of the patients studied, 72% recovered, and viral antigen was cleared from the circulation in most others. These preliminary results are encouraging and will, it is hoped, be confirmed by others.

Churg-Strauss Syndrome.—Churg-Strauss Syndrome (CSS; allergic angiitis and granulomatosis) is much less common than PAN and consequently information about its therapy is even more anecdotal. CSS appears to be more responsive to GC than PAN. The same principles noted for PAN would apply for adding a cytotoxic agent, but the need is less frequent (Table 3).

Wegener's Granulomatosis.—Untreated or inadequately treated

TABLE 3.
Churg-Strauss Syndrome (Allergic Angiitis and Granulomatosis): Clinical Profile*

Abnormality	Frequency, %
Eosinophilia	100
Asthma	100
Allergic rhinitis	70
Fever	85
Musculoskeletal	20–50
Skin	30–75
Neurological (PNS† > CNS)	63–70
Renal	30–40
Hypertension	30–54
Cardiac abnormalities	40–85
Pulmonary (chest radiograph)	72–96
Gastrointestinal	17–92

*From Hoffman GS, Kerr GS: Recognition of systemic vasculitis in the acutely ill patient, in Mandell BF (ed): *Management of Critically Ill Patients With Rheumatologic and Immunologic Diseases*. New York, Marcel Dekker, Inc, in press, 1994. Used by permission.
†PNS = peripheral nervous system; CNS = central nervous system.

Wegener's granulomatosis (Table 4) is associated with a mean survival time of 5 months.[7] Treatment with GC alone increases mean survival time to about 12 months.[8] These sobering statistics have been dramatically altered by (1) aggressive combination therapy with prednisone and daily cyclophosphamide, as well as (2) recognizing milder more indolent forms of disease without renal involvement (about 20% of WG). In a recent review from the National Institutes of Health (NIH), 158 patients were evaluated and treated for up to 24 years, the mean followup period being 8 years. Mortality from WG or complications of treatment occurred in 13%.[6] Although combined drug therapy has been life-saving for many patients, it has become clear that for limited indolent disease such treatment may have excessive risk. Palliation of limited disease may be achieved with only GC therapy, but disease progression and relapses occur frequently. A total of 45 patients with generalized WG were referred to the NIH, having been treated with only GC. Of these, 20 (44%) had improved initially, but eventually all 45 patients failed GC therapy. An additional 12 patients with lim-

TABLE 4.
Wegener's Granulomatosis: Clinical Profile*

Abnormality	Frequency, %
Otolaryngic†	92
Pulmonary	85
Sinusitis	85
Glomerulonephritis	77
Nasal or nasopharyngeal inflammation	68
Nasal deformity ("saddle nose")	28
Musculoskeletal	67
Eye	52
Fever	50
Skin	46
Otitis media	42
Hearing loss	35
Neurological (PNS‡ > CNS)	23
Subglottic stenosis	16
Weight loss (>10% usual body weight)	15
Pericarditis	6
Myocarditis	<2
Gastrointestinal	uncommon

*Adapted from Hoffman GS, Kerr GS, Leavitt RY, et al: Wegener's granulomatosis: Prospective clinical and therapeutic experience with 85 patients for 21 years. *Ann Intern Med* 1992; 116:488–498.
†Combines all ENT manifestations. Most patients have multiple ENT abnormalities.
‡PNS = peripheral nervous system; CNS = central nervous system.

ited WG (no renal involvement) were treated initially with only GC; 8 improved, including 2 (17%) who achieved long-term remission, and 6 who later worsened. Overall, of 57 patients receiving single drug GC therapy, 96% failed to achieve remission (Hoffman and Fauci, unpublished observations, 1993). Attempts to identify less toxic therapies for mild disease include trials of daily trimethaprim-sulfamethoxazole.[15–17] This experience has been anecdotal[6, 18] and only occasionally convincing. Further prospective controlled studies with this agent are required before it can be considered clearly effective.

In the setting of severe life-threatening disease, most would agree that GC and daily low dose cyclophosphamide (2 mg/kg and in extreme situations up to 4 mg/kg for several days) remain the treatment of choice[6, 19–21] (Fig 1). However, even in this setting, toxicity is distressing and has led to trials of high dose intravenous ("pulse") cyclophosphamide and studies of other cytotoxic agents such as methotrexate. Preliminary results indicate that pulse cyclophosphamide and GC may provide substantial initial improvement, but is not as effective as daily low dose cyclophosphamide therapy in maintaining improvement.[19, 20]

In a study of 35 patients, weekly methotrexate therapy (0.15–0.30 mg/kg, oral or intramuscular) has been relatively well tolerated and has resulted in a 75% remission rate, which included the discontinuation of GC medication (Hoffman and Fauci, unpublished observations, 1993) (Fig 2). The mean followup period for this study is 1½ years. Thus, although promising, these results should be considered preliminary, pending further experience.

Of all the systemic vasculitides, WG is an excellent example of the necessity for a multidisciplinary team approach to achieve the best possible outcome. Chronic otitis media may require tympanotomy and drainage tubes. Hearing loss may progress to require hearing aids. Nasal and sinus disease may be complicated by chronic crusting, mucopurulent discharge, and secondary infection, which may require daily irrigation and occasionally débridement or surgery. Subglottic stenosis may require dilatation, resection, tracheostomy or even extensive reconstructive sur-

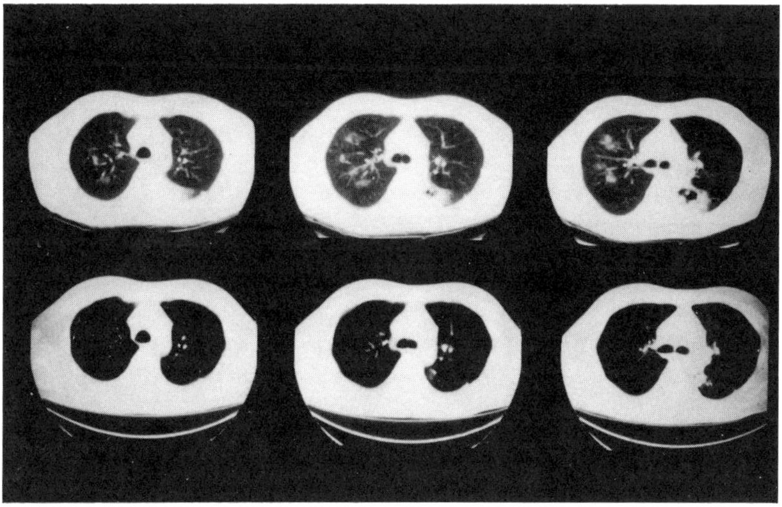

FIG 1.
Wegener's granulomatosis. Exacerbation of pulmonary disease was associated with multiple infiltrates, nodules, and cavitating nodules *(upper three images)*. Marked improvement followed after 1 month of prednisone and cyclophosphamide therapy *(lower 3 images)*.

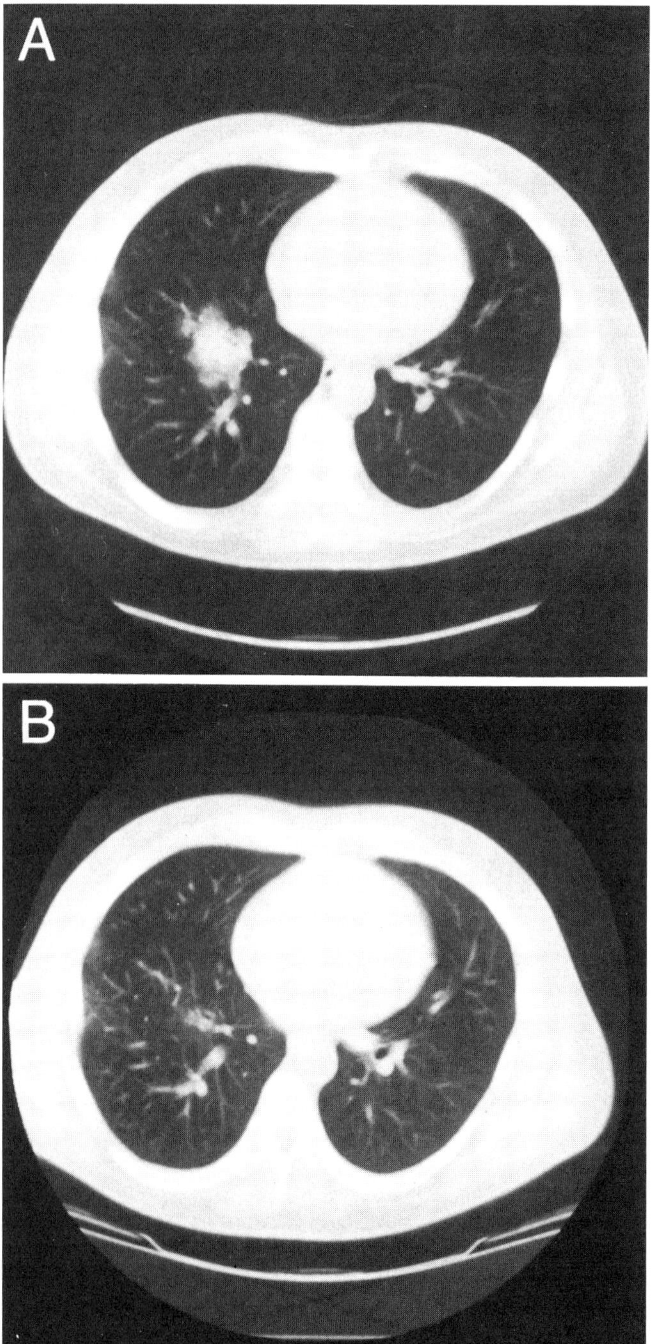
A
B

gery. Retroorbital pseudotumor and lacrimal duct obstruction may require ophthalmic surgery as well as medical treatment. Immunosuppressive therapy may lead to infectious complications that may require diagnostic bronchoscopy and biopsies, whereas toxic complications such as cyclophosphamide-cystitis or malignancy may require urological studies and treatment.

Hypersensitivity Vasculitides.—Hypersensitivity vasculitides (HV) are a heterogeneous group of disorders linked by the clinical impression of a certain sensitizing antigenic exposure being responsible for acute inflammation and injury to small blood vessels (e.g., arterioles, capillaries and venules). The skin is the principal organ affected and "crops" of lesions tend to occur and evolve within the same time frame. The skin may or may not be a representative "window" to similar lesions in other organ systems. In only a minority of cases is the offending antigen identified with certainty. Because visceral involvement is less common and less severe and since the prognosis is better than for PAN, WG, or CSS, a more cautious therapeutic approach is advised. If illness is mild and a drug reaction is suspect, the likely causative medication should be discontinued. If the precipitant may have been a self-limiting or treatable infection, cautious followup and antibiotics may be adequate. However, in the setting of visceral ischemia or glomerulonephritis, it would be prudent to treat with daily GC. Persistent resolution of abnormalities should lead to a slow taper and discontinuation of GC over 4 to 8 weeks.[1]

Henoch-Schönlein Purpura.—Henoch-Schönlein purpura (HSP) is a subset of HV that occurs principally in children and rarely in adults (Table 5). Most patients have a self-limiting monophasic illness of less than 4 weeks' duration. Up to 40% may have recurrences that follow a period of well-being. Guidelines for treatment are the same as those applied to HV in general. Although gastrointestinal involvement may occur in up to 70%, a minority of patients may have the serious gastrointestinal complications of hemorrhage, intussusception, infarction, perforation, or obstruction.[1, 22–24] About 40% of patients develop renal abnormalities, and one half of these have elevation of serum creatinine and urea nitrogen. Progressive renal failure is uncommon. Whether GC therapy affects the eventual outcome of HSP has been debated. Well-controlled studies have not been performed. Until such are available,

---

FIG 2.
Wegener's granulomatosis. After a disease-free period of 5 years, this patient presented with increasing sinusitis and polyarthritis. Evaluation revealed asymptomatic nodular pulmonary lesions on CT scan **(A)** and glomerulonephritis. Following 1 month of daily prednisone and weekly methotrexate therapy, pulmonary lesions markedly diminished **(B)**, and remission was later achieved. Treatment with cyclophosphamide was relatively contraindicated because of previous cyclophosphamide-induced hemorrhagic cystitis.

TABLE 5.
Henoch-Schönlein Purpura: Clinical Profile*†

Abnormality	Frequency, %
Rash	100
Fever	75
Joints	68
Preceding infection	66
Abdominal pain	53
Guaiac positive stools	49
Extremity edema	46
Melena	38
Hematuria	38
Scalp edema	24
Hematemesis	11

*From Hoffman GS, Kerr GS: Recognition of systemic vasculitis in the acutely ill patient, in Mandell BF (ed): *Management of Critically Ill Patients With Rheumatologic and Immunologic Diseases,* New York, Marcel Dekker, Inc, in press, 1994. Used by permission.
†Pediatric series

we would advocate GC therapy for serious abdominal-intestinal findings and renal impairment. The role, if any, of cytotoxic therapy in HSP is even less clear.

Behçet's Disease.—Spontaneous relapsing and remitting features of BD make evaluation of treatment in any single patient complex and confusing (Table 6). Most investigators feel that GC therapy is usually palliative for acute inflammatory features of BD. However, numerous reports document the failure of some patients to sustain improvement. Controlled studies of the efficacy of daily colchicine therapy have yielded conflicting results.[25, 26] Visual complications may affect up to 85% of patients and lead to blindness in 25%, making expert ophthalmology consultation essential. Because ocular manifestations of BD have been more carefully studied than most other causes of morbidity, it is useful to review those results. Severe ocular disease that is not responsive to topical and/or systemic GC has been treated with variable success with the addition of chlorambucil, cyclophosphamide, azathioprine, or cyclosporine.[27–33] Recent double-blind, controlled studies of cyclosporine and azathioprine have convincingly demonstrated that each of these agents does provide palliation beyond that achieved with prior GC[30] or colchicine therapy.[33] Concurrent with ocular improvement, most patients

TABLE 6.
Behçet's Disease: Clinical Profile*

Abnormality	Frequency, %
Aphthous oral ulcers	100
Aphthous genital ulcers	67–74
Uveitis	50–80
Cutaneous vasculitis	56–84
Arthritis	30–50
Meningoencephalitis	10–30
Gastrointestinal	50

*From Hoffman GS, Kerr GS: Recognition of systemic vasculitis in the acutely ill patient, in Mandell BF (ed): *Management of Critically Ill Patients With Rheumatologic and Immunologic Diseases*, New York, Marcel Dekker, Inc, in press, 1994. Used by permission.

also experienced improvement in extraocular features such as mucosal ulcers and skin lesions.

Takayasu's Arteritis.—Approximately two thirds of all patients with TA will have symptoms and signs of disease that indicate active inflammation (Table 7). About half of these individuals will respond to GC therapy and will be successfully tapered off medicine without disease relapse. However, about half of TA patients with clinically active disease will be GC-resistant or will not be able to stop treatment without relapse. Those individuals may improve and require less GC, when daily cyclophosphamide[34] or weekly methotrexate therapy is initiated (Fig 3) (see discussion of WG).[35, 36] The most difficult management problems in TA occur in those patients who have clinically silent, progressive disease, which may include a normal erythrocyte sedimentation rate (as many as 20%). Active disease in asymptomatic individuals has been recognized by periodic arteriographic studies that have revealed new sites of stenosis or aneurysm formation. Still other individuals, who are clinically "silent," but require bypass surgery for old critically stenotic lesions, may provide histopathologic evidence of unsuspected active disease from tissue obtained at the origin and insertion of the surgical graft[37] (personal observations). In one vascular surgery study of 33 patients, preoperative signs of active inflammation were "rarely" found, but 22% of 41 vascular specimens had evidence of acute inflammation and 20% had signs of chronic inflammation, which was of less clear significance.[37] These observations emphasize the importance of

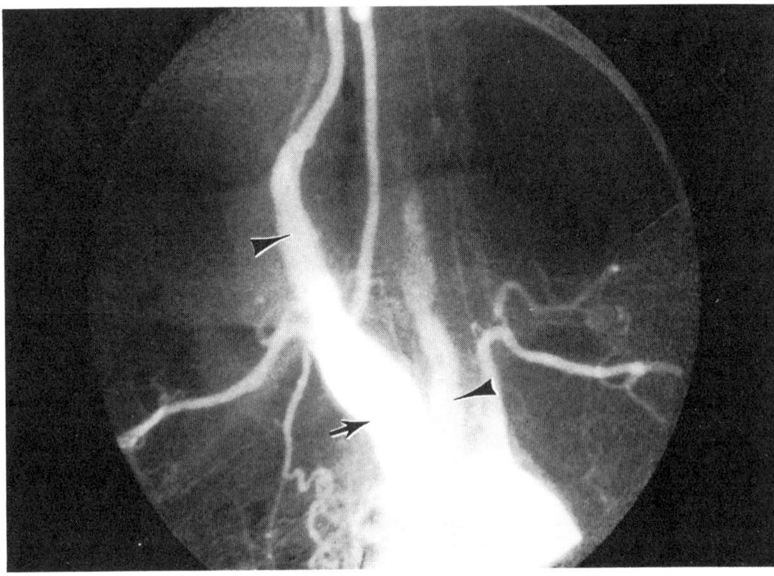

FIG 3.
Takayasu's arteritis. Inflammatory vascular disease in this 35-year-old woman led to aneurysms of the innominate *(arrow)* and common carotid *(arrowheads)* arteries. The left common carotid artery also has a more distal stenotic segment. The left vertebral artery has been reduced to a threadlike remnant. Dilatation of the aortic root caused severe aortic regurgitation, congestive heart failure, and led to successful aortic valve replacement. Right renal artery stenosis (not shown) was treated by angioplasty. Remission was not achieved with prolonged glucocorticoid therapy. The addition of methotrexate was followed by remission and the ability to decrease prednisone to 5 mg every other day.

intraoperative biopsies in all TA vascular surgery patients. The finding of unsuspected active disease obligates immediate GC therapy. It has been assumed, although not proved, that the likelihood of sustained graft patency would be enhanced by decreasing inflammation. Similar reasoning has been applied to recommendations to suppress any suspicious signs of disease activity before surgery.[38] These therapeutic goals are frustrated by tests for inflammatory markers such as clinical features, the erythrocyte sedimentation rate (ESR), or serum concentrations of the von Willebrand factor antigen[39] not being sufficiently sensitive or specific to identify all patients with active disease.

The most common causes of death from TA are due to hypertensive or primary cardiac, renal, and central nervous system disease.[40, 41] In some patients stenosis and/or occlusion of all extremity large vessels may make monitoring blood pressure unreliable. One may only learn of severe central hypertension in such patients during angiography with pressure recordings.

TABLE 7.
Takayasu's Arteritis: Clinical Profile*

Abnormality	Frequency, %
Dizziness	20–50
Syncope	13–25
Stroke	14–20
Headache	28–57
Congestive heart failure	28–31
Palpitations	33–43
Precordial pain	13–25
Visual disturbances	8–30
Hypertension	21–59
Dyspnea	11–72
Myalgias and/or arthralgias	30–56
Vascular bruits	86–96
Pulse deficit	50–96
Claudication	29–40
Fever	8–44
Erythema nodosum	0–16

*From Hoffman GS, Kerr GS: Recognition of systemic vasculitis in the acutely ill patient, in Mandell BF (ed): *Management of Critically Ill Patients With Rheumatologic and Immunologic Diseases,* New York, Marcel Dekker, Inc, in press, 1994. Used by permission.

The ideal goal of medical therapy, to prevent permanent vascular morphologic changes, is often not achieved. Vascular bypass procedures have been successful in diminishing morbidity and mortality in carefully selected patients with stenoses of cerebral, coronary, peripheral, or renal arteries.[37, 38, 42, 43] Less often, dilatation of the aortic root may lead to severe aortic regurgitation, requiring an aortic graft and aortic valve replacement.[43] The usual limitations of vascular surgery are further complicated by the possibility of active TA leading to graft occlusion at the origin or insertion. As many as 20% to 33% of bypass procedures will require revision at a later time.[38, 42] There are a number of unanswered questions affecting vascular surgery in TA: (1) Do the limitations in detecting active disease justify preoperative and postoperative GC therapy for all patients? (2) Should patients with anatomically severe, but asymptomatic lesions have prophylactic surgery (e.g., bilateral common carotid occlusion), or should one temporize until ischemic symptoms occur? (3) Is there a difference in long-term graft patency comparing use of autologous vein or artery to synthetic materials? (4) Does chronic anticoagulation with antiplatelet agents or coumadin affect graft patency? (5) Does transluminal angioplasty have comparable success to bypass surgery for certain lesions?

Temporal Arteritis (giant cell arteritis of the elderly).—GC continues to be the most effective therapy for a giant cell arteritis (GCA) (Table 8). Prednisone (1 mg/kg/day) will reduce symptoms within 1 to 2 days and often eliminate symptoms within a week. One month after clinical and laboratory (ESR) parameters have normalized, GC tapering can begin. Occasional patients may neither achieve complete remission, nor be able to be tapered off GC. Cytotoxic/immunosuppressive agents have been recommended for such individuals by some authors, but the utility of these agents as demonstrated in controlled comparative trials has not been addressed.[3]

Whether polymyalgia rheumatica (PMR) is usually a feature of GCA or a separate, distinct process has significant implications for initial treatment (i.e., high doses [1 mg/kg/day] or low doses [0.2–0.3 mg/kg/day] of prednisone). Therapy hinges on whether one accepts or rejects the notion that PMR, in the absence of symptoms of cranial or systemic vasculitis, may be

TABLE 8.
Temporal Arteritis: Clinical Profile*

Abnormality	Frequency, %
Headache	60–90
Fever	21–48
Polymyalgia rheumatica	47
Visual signs/symptoms	36–40
Claudication	
Extremity	5–8
Jaw	36–67
Vertigo	12
Tenderness of temporal artery	55–69
Absent temporal artery pulse	40–51

*From Hoffman GS, Kerr GS: Recognition of systemic vasculitis in the acutely ill patient, in Mandell BF (ed): *Management of Critically Ill Patients With Rheumatologic and Immunologic Diseases*, New York, Marcel Dekker, Inc, in press, 1994. Used by permission.

associated with temporal artery biopsies that reveal GCA in as many as 30% to 40% of cases.[44, 45] Because vasculitis may be characterized in part by "skip lesions" or nonuniform vascular involvement, a negative biopsy does not rule out GCA. In addition, it is not uncommon for patients who are initially diagnosed as having PMR to later "develop" temporal arteritis.[46, 47] Further confounding this problem is the recognition that symptoms of PMR may be the first indication of other inflammatory conditions such as rheumatoid arthritis.[48]

If one accepts that symptoms of PMR alone are inadequate to rule out a diagnosis of GCA, the certainty that high dose GC is appropriate therapy can be enhanced, if a temporal artery biopsy revealed vasculitis. In the setting of a negative biopsy, if PMR is still assumed to be a reflection of GCA, then one risks the possibility of overtreating, if in fact PMR is a mild disease, truly distinct from GCA. The pitfalls in the understanding and treatment of PMR obligate careful followup.

Polyangiitis Overlap Syndromes.—The term polyangiitis overlap syndrome[49] has been applied to patients who have had typical features of vasculitis common to more than one diagnostic entity. An example would be a patient with arteriographic features of both PAN and TA. Some patients who fail to be easily classified may be best served with the tentative diagnosis of undifferentiated systemic vasculitis. These individuals may with time evolve to have a more clearly defined syndrome. The heterogeneity of this group does not allow for dogmatic recommendations regarding treatment. Assessment of disease severity, anatomic distribution, rate of progression, and comorbid conditions should determine aggressiveness of therapy.

Chronic Therapy

Because most systemic vasculitides are not definitively cured, realistic goals include diminishing morbidity from disease and treatment, while hoping that the underlying process will go into an extended treatment-induced remission or becoming self-limiting (Tables 9–11). Examples of vasculitides that may be monophasic are HV, HSP, PAN, and TA. However, many individuals with PAN, TA, WG, CSS, BD, and GCA achieve remission and then subsequently relapse. Patients who relapse do not possess any clinical or serological markers that predict risk of recurrence. Thus, regardless of how well a patient with these disorders has fared over time, the physician is obligated to maintain careful followup. This is especially true for those processes that involve the kidney as a target organ. Renal recurrences may not be apparent until advanced renal injury has occurred.

Embarking on GC therapy should alert the clinician to consider acute and subacute effects on intravascular volume, blood pressure, glucose metabolism, electrolyte balance, wound healing, and opportunistic infections. This is especially important in the elderly and in patients with preexisting hypertension, cardiac disease, and diabetes mellitus. When treatment is in-

TABLE 9.
Monitoring Glucocorticoid Therapy*

Acute and Chronic Effects
Fluid balance
Blood pressure
Cardiac function
Glucose metabolism
Electrolyte balance
Wound healing
Infection
Alterations in mental status
Chronic Effects
Cataracts
Myopathy
Aseptic necrosis
Osteoporosis/fractures

*Risks are directly proportional to dose, frequency (e.g. split daily, daily alternate day doses), and duration of therapy.

dicated for systemic vasculitis, high doses should be maintained until all manifestations of *active* disease have abated. Tapering prednisone should follow after about one month. The literature does not provide a consensus opinion about the subsequent strategy for tapering GC. Our preference is to reduce prednisone on an alternate-day basis so that within another 2 to 3 months, in the absence of relapse or exacerbations, a dose of about 1 mg/kg every other day is achieved. During the ensuing 2 to 3 months, tapering of the alternate-day schedule continues until GC therapy is discontinued. Waxing and waning of disease may force alterations in these guidelines. The rationale for this approach is well established[5, 50, 51] and has been recently reviewed.[6, 52] The immunologic defects induced by GC are dependent on dose, frequency, and duration of treatment. As each factor increases, the incidence of opportunistic infections and other side effects increases. In addition to those toxicities that may occur within several months of starting GC therapy, chronic treatment increases the risks of cataracts, myopathy, aseptic necrosis, osteoporosis, and pathologic fractures. The use of alternate-day prednisone (single A.M. dose) is associated with less toxicity than daily treatment. Nonetheless, toxicity is still greater than when patients are not receiving GC at all.[6]

Pneumonia is the most common life-threatening infection in the immunocompromised host. It is a complication likely to confuse the clinician when it occurs in the setting of a vasculitic disease that includes the lungs

TABLE 10.
Monitoring Chronic Therapy With Commonly Used Cytotoxic Agents*

Risks of Therapy	Cyclophosphamide	Azathioprine	Methotrexate
Infection	+	+	+
Malignancy	+	+	rare
Cystitis	+	−	−
Bone marrow suppression	+	+	+
Infertility	+	−	rare
Teratogenicity	+	+	+
Liver toxicity	−	rare	+
Cirrhosis	−	−	rare
Drug-induced pneumonitis	+	rare	+

*Conventional therapeutic doses for autoimmune diseases: cyclophosphamide, 2 mg/kg/day; azathioprine, 2 mg/kg/day; methotrexate, 10-25 mg once a week. Dose reduction is required when renal impairment is present.

(e.g., WG, CSS, and overlap syndromes). The problem is compounded by an increased frequency of infections due to virulent microorganisms such as gram-negative bacteria. *Staphylococcus aureus, Pneumocystis carinii,* as well as opportunistic fungi or mycobacteria. Because immunosuppressive therapy limits ability to contain infections, sepsis and mortality of up to 40% may result from infectious pneumonitis in immunocompromised patients in general.[52, 53] Thus, pneumonitis in the GC-treated patient is a medical emergency. This caveat is no less true for the patient who does not appear febrile and toxic. GC may blunt fever, malaise, and anorexia. Infections may progress in relative clinical silence, even to abscess formation.

The indications for adding a cytotoxic agent have been provided in discussions of initial therapy. However, in some vasculitides that respond to GC, relapses become so common that continuous prednisone therapy may begin to produce more morbidity than the underlying illness. Cytotoxic therapy should be considered in this setting for enhancing the likelihood of remission as well as for GC-sparing effects. Cyclophosphamide has been the most thoroughly studied cytotoxic agent for treatment of vasculitis. In a recent review of its use in WG over a period of 24 years, it was associated with cystitis (43%), bladder cancer (2.8%, 33 × expected rate), lymphoma (1.5%, 11 × expected rate), myelodysplasia (2%), infertility (>57% of women), and an increased frequency of infections, especially when used in conjunction with GC.[6] Although such treatment may be lifesaving, and may be the best known means of achieving remission in se-

TABLE 11.
Treatment of the Systemic Vasculitides

Illness	Usual Immunosuppressive Therapy	Other Therapies	Severe Features	Comment
Hypersensitivity vasculitis, including Henoch-Schonlein purpura	None	Careful followup. Treat infections that may have precipitated vasculitis. Withdraw suspected precipitants (e.g., medications). Glucocorticoids for severe features	Critical visceral ischemia, hemorrhage, renal disease.	Cytotoxic agents: indications for use would be rare life-threatening complications unresponsive to glucocorticoids.
Giant cell (temporal) arteritis	Glucocorticoids	Cytotoxic agents*	Glucocorticoid-resistance. Progressive visual loss, stroke, cardiac ischemia	
Takayasu's arteritis	Glucocorticoids	Cytotoxic agents. Cardiology and vascular surgery evaluation and care. Angioplasty. Anticoagulation.†	Glucocorticoid-resistance. Progressive aortic root dilatation and valvular insufficiency. Cerebral, cardiac and renal ischemia. "Critical" stenosis may be symptomatic or asymptomatic.	Silently progressive disease complicates diagnosis and treatment. About 50% require a second agent. No controlled studies of medical and surgical interventions have been reported.

Polyarteritis nodosa and Churg-Strauss vasculitis	Glucocorticoids	Cytotoxic agents	Progressive renal, neurologic gastrointestinal and cardiac disease.	Role of plasmapheresis, high dose IV immunoglobulin and vidarabine therapy for hepatitis B virus associated PAN are under study.
Wegener's granulomatosis	Glucocorticoids + cyclophosphamide	Otolaryngic, ophthalmic and urologic consultation and care. Methotrexate or azathioprine + glucocorticoids.	Diffuse pulmonary hemorrhage, progressive renal disease.	Glucocorticoids alone may be palliative, but rarely produce lasting remission. Roles of trimethoprim/ sulfamethaxazole and IV immunoglobulin are under study.
Behçet's disease	Glucocorticoids Colchicine‡	Chlorambucil, azathioprine, cyclophosphamide, cyclosporine. Ophthalmic and surgical consultation may be necessary.	Central nervous system vasculitis, multiple gastrointestinal ulcers and perforations.	Role of second agent immunosuppressive therapies have been best defined in studies of progressive ocular disease.
Kawasaki's syndrome	High dose IV immunoglobulin salicylates		Coronary aneurysms and ischemia.	

*Cytotoxic agents have not been critically evaluated in this disease.
†Role of routine anticoagulation has not been defined.
‡Role of colchicine is controversial.

vere systemic vasculitides, it may also cause substantial morbidity and even mortality. Its use requires close vigilance of bladder and bone marrow effects, titration of dose, high oral fluid intake to dilute cyclophosphamide-derived bladder toxins (e.g., acrolein), and urological consultation for any sign of bladder toxicity. The time from initial use of cyclophosphamide to detecting bladder cancer may be as brief as 7 months to as long as 10 to 15 years, even after medication has been discontinued.[6]

Many investigators are currently studying alternative modes of cytotoxic therapy. However, under the best of circumstances the effects of such agents are too broadly immunosuppressive. The most promising opportunities for treatment in the future may be realized through a better understanding of cytokines and immunologically active, cloned human proteins that are being produced by recombinant DNA technology.

Immunotherapy/Biological Agents

Intravenous immunoglobulin (IVIg) is obtained from large normal human plasma pools. It is prepared to minimize the content of Ig molecules other than those of the IgG isotype. The principal use of IVIg has been treatment of patients with hypogammaglobulinemia. The first report of efficacy in the treatment of an autoimmune disease, idiopathic thrombocytopenic purpura (ITP), appeared in 1981. The beneficial effect of IVIg in ITP has since been confirmed.[54] High dose IVIg (2 g/kg) has subsequently been shown to be safe and effective in reducing signs of systemic inflammation and preventing coronary artery aneurysms that are of vasculitic origin in Kawasaki syndrome (KS). When untreated, coronary aneurysms occur in 15% to 22% of children. IVIg-treated patients have 3 to 4.5 times fewer coronary aneurysms than patients treated with just aspirin.[54, 56] Although the mechanisms of immunosuppressive action of IVIg in these illnesses have not been completely elucidated, some reported effects that may be relevant in KS include: (1) diminution of activated, helper T cells, (2) increase in suppressor/cytotoxic T cells, and (3) decrease in spontaneous IgG and IgM production.[58] In ITP, additional important mechanisms might include: (1) blockade of Fc receptors on phagocytic cells of the reticuloendothelial system, resulting in decreased clearance of opsonized platelets, and (2) formation of complexes between antiidiotypic antibodies in IVIg and idiotypic determinants of antiplatelet antibodies. Idiotype-antiidiotype complexes may result in neutralization of autoantibodies, down-regulation of B-cell receptors for antigen (thus causing a decrease in autoantibody production), and/or binding to T-cell receptors to influence their activation and regulatory properties.[54, 59] In other settings IVIg has also been shown to attenuate complement-dependent immune injury[60] and diminish natural killer (NK) cell activity.[61] These reports encouraged an open trial of IVIg in patients with antineutrophil cytoplasmic, antibody-positive, systemic vasculitis. Improvement was noted within 3 weeks in 7 of 7 patients.[62] Other preliminary studies suggest efficacy in rheumatoid arthritis[63] and idiopathic myositis.[64–66] These encouraging results will need to be confirmed by others.

Immunoregulation and Recombinant Proteins

Preliminary studies in patients with several forms of systemic vasculitis have demonstrated the presence of elevated serum levels of proinflammatory cytokines such as interleukin-1 (IL-1), IL-2, and tumor necrosis factor (TNF).[67] Peripheral blood mononuclear cells from systemic vasculitis patients have also manifested increased gene expression for TNF-α.[68] Following GC and/or cytotoxic therapy, these cytokine levels diminished markedly.[67]

Proteins From Recombinant Technology for Therapeutic Purposes.—In recent years, recombinant DNA technology has provided opportunities to produce many different recombinant proteins (Table 12). Most relevant to acute and/or chronic inflammatory conditions has been the cloning of human genes for normal proteins that function as cytokine antagonists or competitors. One example is the recombinant human IL-1 receptor antagonist (rh IL-1ra).[69–71] In vitro studies of IL-1ra activity have shown diminution of IL-1-induced: collagenase production by chondrocytes, prostaglandin E_2 (PGE_2) production by fibroblasts and synovial cells, IL-2 production by T lymphocytes,[72] and endothelial cell activation with

TABLE 12.
Anti-Cytokine Therapy: Potential Application of Products From Recombinant DNA Technology*†

Potential Agents	Selected Actions
rh IL-1ra	Decreases lymphocyte IL-2 production, endothelial cell activation, WBC-endothelial cell interaction and PGE_2 production.
rh IL-1r	Binds circulating IL-1.
rh IL-4	Decreases monocyte production of IL-1, TNF and PGE_2.
rh TGF-β	Decreases monocyte production of IL-1, TNF, and B-lymphocyte proliferation, and Ab, and decreases IL-2r expression.

*Rationale: Patients with systemic vasculitis have increased levels of proinflammatory cytokines in their serum (e.g., IL-1, IL-2, TNF). GC/cytotoxic therapy has been shown to reduce inflammatory cytokine levels, concurrent with clinical improvement.
†rh IL-1ra = recombinant human IL-1 receptor antagonist; WBC = white blood cell; PGE_2 = prostaglandin E_2; TNF = tumor necrosis factor; TGF-β = transforming growth factor β; GC = glucocorticoids.

consequent endothelial cell-leukocyte adhesion.[71] rh IL-1ra has been evaluated in animal models and human disease. Gram-negative, endotoxin-induced shock is associated with high circulating levels of IL-1 and TNF. These cytokines appear to act synergistically in contributing to tissue damage and death. Treatment of rabbits with rh IL-1ra after they received lethal doses of endotoxin has been shown to markedly diminish inflammation and disruption of vascular integrity and to prevent death.[73] Clinical trials of rh IL-1ra in patients with septic shock are now under way. In another human study, rh IL-1ra has been evaluated in a model of chronic inflammation, rheumatoid arthritis. Although, the results are preliminary, daily subcutaneous injections appeared to result in significant palliation within 7 days.[74] Soluble rh IL-1r would be expected to have similar effects to rh IL-1ra.

Interleukin-4, a product of activated T lymphocytes, has both inhibitory and stimulatory effects on a variety of cells. Among these effects are inhibition of monocyte production of IL-1, TNF-α, and PGE_2. In vitro effects of IL-4 on monocytes are similar to those obtained with dexamethasone.[75] Recombinant human IL-4 has been produced and is an attractive candidate for clinical trials in inflammatory diseases.

Transforming Growth Factor-β.—Transforming growth factor-β (TGF-β) has also been shown in vitro to inhibit endotoxin-induced production of IL-1 and TNF in monocytes, T-lymphocyte and thymocyte proliferation, IL-2 receptor expression, B-lymphocyte proliferation and antibody production, and the generation of NK and cytotoxic T cells. Human rTGF-β has also recently been produced.[76]

Monoclonal Antibody Therapy.—Recombinant DNA technology has also provided opportunities to produce monoclonal monospecific antibodies (MAb) from hybridoma cell lines. Thus far, the greatest success in achieving stable fusion of hybridoma partners has occurred with rodent myeloma cells. Unfortunately, such MAb products include components that are rodent-derived and foreign to the human recipient. These MAbs may generate neutralizing immune responses that decrease potential immunomodulatory effects and/or cause serum sickness. Recent advances have allowed for the monospecific hypervariable regions of MAbs to be annealed to the constant and variable regions of human immunoglobulin molecules, thus producing a "humanized" MAb. It is anticipated that such a product would retain specificity and minimize foreign protein antigenicity.[77]

The effectiveness of MAb treatment in autoimmune disease has been demonstrated in murine lupus erythematosus. MAb to L3T4 (helper/inducer) lymphocytes was given to mice with established disease from which 20% of animals had already died. One-year survival among treated animals was greater than four times that of untreated controls. Similar palliation has also been achieved with anti-L3T4 MAb was used to treat experimental autoimmune allergic encephalitis, myasthenia gravis, and collagen-induced arthritis.[78] Preliminary studies with MAb in man have demonstrated significant palliation in one patient with systemic vasculitis[79] and several patients with chronic inflammatory arthritis.[80]

MAb can also be prepared to inhibit the effects of cytokines. In a study of *E. coli*-induced endotoxin shock in baboons, MAb to TNF was given 2 hours before experimental bacteremia and completely protected animals from acute shock, organ failure, and death.[81]

Our enhanced understanding and ability to more precisely manipulate immunoinflammatory events with biological products offers unprecedented opportunities for disease palliation and minimizing GC and other toxic therapies in the future. However these advances change our approach to treatment, they will not provide a cure for systemic vasculitides. That goal will more likely be achieved only after we have learned more about factors that predispose patients to these diseases, as well as the precipitants that trigger abnormal immunoregulation.

References

1. Hoffman GS, Kerr GS: Recognition of systemic vasculitis in the acutely ill patient, in Mandell BF (ed): *Management of Critically Ill Patients with Rheumatologic and Immunologic Diseases.* New York, Marcel Dekker, Inc, in press. 1994.
2. Fauci AS, Haynes BF, Katz P: The spectrum of vasculitis: clinical, pathologic, immunologic and therapeutic considerations. *Ann Intern Med* 1978; 80:660–676.
3. Hunder GG: Giant cell (temporal) arteritis. *Rheum Dis Clin NA* 1990; 16:399–409.
4. Fauci AS, Wolff SM: Wegener's granulomatosis: studies in eighteen patients and a review of the literature. *Medicine* 1973; 52:535–561.
5. Fauci AS, Haynes BF, Katz P, et al: Wegener's granulomatosis: Prospective clinical and therapeutic experience with 85 patients for 21 years. *Ann Intern Med* 1983; 98:76–85.
6. Hoffman GS, Kerr GS, Leavitt RY, et al: Wegener's granulomatosis: An analysis of 158 patients. *Ann Intern Med* 1992; 116:488–498.
7. Walton EW: Giant cell granuloma of the respiratory tract (Wegener's granulomatosis). *Brit Med J* 1958; 2:265–270.
8. Hollander D, Manning RT: The use of alkylating agents in the treatment of Wegener's granulomatosis. *Ann Intern Med* 1967; 67:393–398.
9. Frohnert PP, Sheps SG: Longterm follow-up study of polyarteritis nodosa. *Am J Med* 1967; 43:8–14.
10. Leib ES, Restivo C, Paulus HE: Immunosuppressive and corticosteroid therapy of polyarteritis nodosa. *Am J Med* 1979; 67:941–947.
11. Fauci AS, Katz P, Haynes BF, et al: Cyclophosphamide therapy of severe systemic necrotizing vasculitis. *N Engl J Med* 1979; 301:235–238.
12. Guillevin L, Du LTH, Godeau P, et al: Clinical findings and prognosis of polyarteritis nodosa and Churg-Strauss angiitis: A study of 165 patients. *Brit J Rheumatol* 1988; 27:258–264.
13. Guillevin L, and the Cooperative Study Group for the Study of Polyarteritis Nodosa: Treatment of polyarteritis nodosa and Churg-Strauss angiitis: Indica-

tion of plasma exchange results of three prospective trials in 162 patients. *Apheresis* 1990; 337:309–317.
14. Guillevin L, Jarrousse B, Lok C, et al: Longterm followup after treatment of polyarteritis nodosa and Churg-Strauss angiitis with comparison of steroids, plasma exchange, and cyclophosphamide to steroids and plasma exchange. A prospective randomized trial of 71 patients. *J Rheumatol* 1991; 18:567–574.
15. DeRemee RA, McDonald TJ, Weiland LH: Wegener's granulomatosis: Observations on treatment with antimicrobial agents. *Mayo Clin Proc* 1985; 60:27–32.
16. DeRemee RA: The treatment of Wegener's granulomatosis with trimethoprim/sulfamethoxazole: Illusion or vision? *Arthritis Rheum* 1988; 31:1068–1072.
17. Israle HL: Sulfamethoxazole-trimethoprim therapy for Wegener's granulomatosis. *Arch Intern Med* 1988; 148:2293–95.
18. Leavitt RY, Hoffman GS, Fauci AS: Response: The role of trimethaprim/sulfamethoxazole in the treatment of Wegener's granulomatosis. *Arthritis Rheum* 1988; 31:1073–1074.
19. Hoffman GS, Leavitt RY, Fleisher TA, et al: Treatment of Wegener's granulomatosis with intermittent high-dose intravenous cyclophosphamide. *Am J Med* 1990; 89:403–410.
20. Steppat D, Gross WL: Stage adapted treatment of Wegener's granulomatosis. *Klin Wochenschr* 1989; 67:666–671.
21. Pusey CD, Gaskin G, Rees AJ: Treatment of primary systemic vasculitis. *APMIS Suppl* 1990; 19:48–50.
22. Allen DM, Diamond LK, Howell DA: Anaphylactoid purpura in children (Henoch-Schönlein Syndrome) *AMA J Dis Child* 1960; 99:147–168.
23. Feldt RH, Stickler GB: The gastrointestinal manifestations of anaphylactoid purpura in children. *Mayo Clin Proc* 1962; 37:465–473.
24. Kauffman RH, Herrmann WA, Meyer CJLM, et al: Circulating IgA-immune complexes in Henoch-Schönlein purpura. *Am J Med* 1980; 69:859–866.
25. Aktulga E, Altac M, Muftuoglu A, et al: A double blind study of colchicine in Behçet's disease. *Haematologica.* 1980; 65:399–402.
26. Mizushima Y, Matsumura N, Mori M, et al: Colchicine in the treatment of Behçet's disease. *The Ryumachi* 1978; 18:2–116.
27. O'Duffy JD, Robertson DM, Goldstein NP: Chlorambucil in the treatment of uveitis and meningoencephalitis of Behçet's disease. *Am J Med* 1984; 76:75–84.
28. O'Duffy JD: Vasculitis in Behçet's disease. *Rheum Dis Clin North Am* 1990; 16:423–31.
29. Michelson JB, Friedlaender MH: Behçet's disease. *Int Ophthalmol Clin* 1990; 30:271–278.
30. Yazici H, Pazarli H, Barnes GC, et al: A controlled trial of azathioprine, in Behçet's syndrome. *N Engl J Med* 1990; 322:281–285.
31. Nussenblatt RB, Palestine AG, Chan CC, et al: Effectiveness of cyclosporin therapy for Behçet's disease. *Arthritis Rheum* 1985; 28:671–679.
32. Diz-Llopis M, Cervera M, Menezo JL: Cyclosporin A treatment of Behçet's disease: A long-term study. *Curr Eye Res* 1990; 9:17–23.
33. Masuda K, Urayama A, Kogure M, et al: Double-masked trial of cyclosporin versus colchicine and long-term open study of cyclosporin in Behçet's disease. *Lancet* 1989; 1:1093–1096.
34. Shelhamer JH, Volkman DJ, Parillo JE, et al: Takayasu's arteritis and its therapy. *Ann Intern Med* 1985; 103:121–126.

35. Hoffman GS, Leavitt RY, Kerr GS, et al: Treatment of Takayasu's arteritis with methotrexate. *Arth Rheum* 1991; 34(suppl):S74.
36. Liang GC, Nemickas R, Madayag M: Multiple percutaneous transluminal angioplasties and low dose pulse methotrexate for Takayasu's arteritis. *J Rheumatol* 1989; 16:1370–1373.
37. Lagneau P, Michel JB, Vuong PN: Surgical treatment of Takayasu's disease. *Ann Surg* 1987; 205:157–166.
38. Kieffer E, Piquois A, Bertel A, et al: Reconstructive surgery of the renal arteries in Takayasu's disease. *Ann Vasc Surg* 1990; 4:156–165.
39. Ciompi ML, Marotta G, Pucetti L, et al: Behavior of von Willebrand factor antigen in follow-up of polymyalgia rheumatoid/giant cell arteritis. *Scand J Rheumatol* 1988; 17:491–495.
40. Ishikawa K: Natural history and classification of occlusive thromboaortopathy (Takayasu's disease). *Circulation* 1978; 57:27–35.
41. Ishakawa K: Survival and morbidity after diagnosis of occlusive thromboaortopathy (Takayasu's disease). *Am J Cardiology* 1981; 47:1026–1032.
42. Giordano JM, Leavitt RY, Hoffman GS, et al: Experience with surgical treatment of Takayasu's disease. *Surgery* 1991; 109:252–258.
43. Amano J, Suzuki A: Coronary artery involvement in Takayasu's arteritis. Collective review and guidelines for surgical treatment. *J Thorac Cardiovasc Surg* 1991; 102:554–60.
44. Hamilton CR, Shelley WM, Tumulty PA: Giant cell arteritis: Including temporal arteritis and polymyalgia rheumatica. *Medicine* 1971; 50:1–27.
45. Fauchald P, Rygvold O, Oystase B: Temporal arteritis and polymyalgia rheumatica. Clinical and biopsy findings. *Ann Intern Med* 1972; 77:845–852.
46. Lundberg I, Hedfors E: Restricted dose and duration of corticosteroid treatment in patients with polymyalgia rheumatica and temporal arteritis. *J Rheumatol* 1990; 17:1340–1345.
47. Kyle V, Hazleman BL: Treatment of polymyalgia rheumatic and giant cell arteritis. I. Steroid regimens in the first two months. *Ann Rheum Dis* 1989; 48:658–661.
48. Hoffman GS: Polyarteritis: the differential diagnosis of rheumatoid arthritis. *Sem Arthritis Rheum* 1978; 8:115–141.
49. Leavitt RY, Fauci AS: Polyangiitis overlap syndrome. Classification and prospective clinical experience. *Am J Med* 1986; 81:79–85.
50. Fauci AS, Dale DC, Balow JE: Glucocorticosteroid therapy: mechanisms of action and clinical considerations. *Ann Intern Med* 1976; 84:304–315.
51. Dale DC, Fauci AS, Wolff SM: Alternate-date prednisone. Leukocyte kinetics and susceptibility to infections. *N Engl J Med* 1974; 291:1154–1158.
52. Hoffman GS, Fauci AS: Respiratory disease in patients treated with glucocorticoids, in Shelhamer J et al (eds): *Respiratory Diseases in the Immunosuppressed Host.* New York, JB Lippincott Co, 1991, chapter 43.
53. Mukwaya G: Immunosuppressive effects and infections associated with corticosteroid therapy. *Pediatr Infect Dis J* 1988; 7:499–504.
54. Dwyer JM: Manipulating the immune system with immune globulin. *N Engl J Med* 1992; 326:107–116.
55. Newburger JW, Takahashi M, Burns JC, et al: The treatment of Kawasaki syndrome with intravenous gamma globulin. *N Engl J Med* 1986; 315:341–347.
56. Newberger JW, Takahashi M, Beiser AS, et al: A single intravenous infusion of gamma globulin as compared with four infusions in the treatment of acute Kawasaki syndrome. *N Engl J Med* 1991; 324:1633–1639.

57. Furusho K, Nakano H, Shinomiya K, et al: High-dose intravenous gamma globulin for Kawasaki Disease. *Lancet* 1984; 2:1055–1058.
58. Leung DYM, Burns JC, NewBurger JW, et al: Reversal of lymphocyte activation in vivo in the Kawasaki syndrome by intravenous immunoglobulin. *J Clin Invest* 1987; 79:468–472.
59. Dietrich G, Rossi F, Kazatchkine MD: Modulation of autoimmune responses with normal polyspecific IgG for therapeutic use, in Melechers A (ed): *Progress in Immunology VII* 1989; pp 1221–1227. Proceeding of the 7th International Congress of Immunology, Berlin, 1989.
60. Basta M, Kirshbom P, Frank MM, et al: Mechanism of therapeutic effect of high-dose intravenous immunoglobulin. Attenuation of acute, complement-dependent immune damage in a guinea pig model. *J Clin Invest* 1989; 84:1974–1981.
61. Engelhard D, Waner JL, Kapoor N, et al: Effect of intravenous immune globulin on natural killer cell activity: Possible association with autoimmune neutropenia and idiopathic thrombocytopenia. *J Pediatr* 1986; 108:77–81.
62. Jayne DRW, Davies MJ, Fox CJV, et al: Treatment of systemic vasculitis with pooled intravenous immunoglobulin. *Lancet* 1991; 337:1137–1139.
63. Becker H, Mitropoulou G, Helmke K: Immunomodulating therapy in rheumatoid arthritis by high dose intravenous immunoglobulin. *Klin Wochenschr* 1989; 67:286–290.
64. Cherin P, Herson S, Wechsler B, et al: Efficacy of intravenous gammaglobulin therapy in chronic refractory polymyositis and dermatomyositis: an open study with 20 adult patients. *Am J Med* 1991; 91:162–168.
65. Gelfand EW: The use of intravenous immune globulin in collagen vascular disorders: A potentially new modality of therapy. *J Allergy Clin Immunol* 1989; 84:613–16.
66. Lang BA, Laxer RM, Murphy G, et al: Treatment of dermatomyositis with intravenous gammaglobulin. *Am J Med* 1991; 91:169–172.
67. Grau GE, Roux-Lombard P, Gysler C, et al: Serum cytokine changes in systemic vasculitis. *Immunology* 1989; 68:196–198.
68. Deguchi Y, Shibata N, Kishimoto S: Enhanced expression of the tumour necrosis factor/cachectic gene in peripheral blood mononuclear cells from patients with systemic vasculitis. *Clin Exp Immunol* 1990; 81:311–314.
69. Eisenberg SP, Evans RJ, Arend WP, et al: Primary structure and functional expression from complementary DNA of a human interleukin-1 receptor antagonist. *Nature* 1990; 343:341–346.
70. Hannum CH, Wilcox CJ, Arend WP, et al: Interleukin-1 receptor antagonist activity of a human interleukin-1 inhibitor. *Nature* 1990; 343:336–340.
71. Carter DB, Deibel MR Jr, Dann CJ, et al: Purification, cloning expression and biological characterization of an interleukin-1 receptor antagonist protein. *Nature* 1990; 344:633–638.
72. Arend WP, Joslin FG, Thompson RC, et al: An IL-1 inhibitor from human monocytes. Production and characterization of biologic properties. *J Immunol* 1989; 143:1851–1858.
73. Ohlsson K, Björk P, Bergenfeldt M, et al: Interleukin-1 receptor antagonist reduces mortality from endotoxin shock. *Nature* 1990; 348:550–552.
74. Lebsack ME, Paul CC, Bloedow DC, et al: Subcutaneous IL-1 receptor antagonist in patients with rheumatoid arthritis. *Arthritis Rheum* 1991; 34 (suppl):S45.
75. Hart PH, ViHi GF, Burgass DR, et al: Potential antiinflammatory effects of interleukin 4: Suppression of human monocyte tumor necrosis factor α, interleu-

kin 1, and prostaglandin E2. *Proc Natl Acad Sci USA* 1989; 86:3803–3807.

76. Chantry D, Turner J, Abney E, et al: Modulation of cytokine production by transforming growth factor-β. *J Immunol* 1989; 142:4295–4300.
77. Mayforth RD, Quintans J: Designer and catalytic antibodies. *N Engl J Med* 1990; 323:173–178.
78. Wofsy D, Seaman WE: Reversal of advanced immune lupus in NZB/NZW F1 mice by treatment with monoclonal antibody to L3T4. *J Immunol* 1987; 138:3247–53.
79. Mathieson PW, Cobbold SP, Hale G, et al: Monoclonal-antibody therapy in systemic vasculitis. *N Engl J Med* 1990; 323:250–254.
80. Herzog C, Wallur C, Pichler W, et al: Monoclonal anti-CD4 in arthritis. *Lancet* 1987; 2:1461–1462.
81. Tracey KJ, Fong Y, Hesse DG, et al: Anti-cachectin/TNF monoclonal antibodies prevent septic shock during lethal bacteremia. *Nature* 1987; 330:662–664.

Human Immunodeficiency Virus and Acquired Immunodeficiency Syndrome: An Update

Steven M. Schnittman, M.D.

Chief, Medical Branch, Division of AIDS, National Institute of Allergy and Infectious Diseases, National Institutes of Health, Bethesda, Maryland

Anthony S. Fauci, M.D.

Chief, Laboratory of Immunoregulation, Director, National Institute of Allergy and Infectious Diseases, National Institutes of Health, Bethesda, Maryland

The decade of the 1980s witnessed the emergence of a new pandemic, the acquired immunodeficiency syndrome (AIDS). The impact that human immunodeficiency virus (HIV) and AIDS have had on the world is unparalleled in modern times. Within the United States, over 250,000 persons have developed AIDS, and over 1 million Americans are believed to be infected with HIV.[1] The pandemic is particularly devastating in sub-Saharan Africa, and early reports of a rapid expansion of this epidemic throughout Southeast Asia and India are sobering indeed, for it is here that over one third of the world's population resides. Even if the rate of new infections in the Western world reaches a plateau, it will be overshadowed by this explosion of new infections in the Third World and the extraordinary public health, social, and political upheavals in its wake.

The purpose of this update is to review some of the important scientific and clinical advances that have occurred in HIV/AIDS over the past year. These advances will be summarized in the following major categories: (1) Scope of the Epidemic and Epidemiology; (2) Virology/Pathogenesis; (3) Therapeutics; (4) Vaccines; and (5) Special Topics.

Scope of the Epidemic and Epidemiology

AIDS was first recognized in mid-1981 when unusual clusters of *Pneumocystis carinii* pneumonia (PCP) and Kaposi's sarcoma were reported in young, previously healthy homosexual men in New York City, Los Angeles, and San Francisco. Soon after these initial reports in the United States, AIDS was identified in Europe, the Caribbean, and Africa. Today, AIDS is a global pandemic, and the World Health Organization (WHO) estimates that at least 10 million people are infected worldwide.[2] It is projected that between 40 and 100 million individuals may be infected with HIV by the year 2000 (Fig 1). The problem of HIV infection has been particularly devastating to equatorial Africa where infection has been observed in 28% of women attending prenatal clinics in Kampala, Uganda,[3] 32% of pregnant women in Kigali, Rwanda,[4] and 35% of women attending sexually transmitted disease (STD) clinics in Kinshasha, Zaire.[5] Recent studies determining the seroprevalence of HIV-1 in Thailand (10.9% in young males in Chiang Mai)[6] and India (4.9% in STD clinic patients, 30% of prostitutes of Bombay and Pune [R. Bollinger and T. Quinn, personal communication, 1992]) project a gloomy forecast for Asia as we enter the next century.

It is estimated that 40,000 adults are newly infected with HIV in the United States every year.[7] The principal modes of HIV transmission continue to include sexual contact, parenteral exposure to blood (predominantly by intravenous drug users who share needles and other paraphernalia), and mother to child during the perinatal period. In the United States, sexual transmission of HIV infection continues to predominate (61%), with the majority of infections occurring as a result of homosexual contact. However, the frequency of heterosexual transmission of HIV continues to rise slowly. Of new AIDS cases reported to the Centers for Disease Control (CDC) during a 12-month period, 3.1% of all cases in men and 34.8% of all cases in women were classified as heterosexually transmitted.[8] For adolescents and young adults (13 to 24 years of age), 13.4% of cases reported from 1989 to 1991 resulted from heterosexual contact, compared with 8.4% of cases reported prior to 1989. A recent analysis of expected trends of AIDS cases in the United States has predicted that the infection rate among non–drug-using heterosexuals will increase over the next 5 years, leading to a doubling of heterosexual AIDS cases by 1995, in contrast to trends in other risk categories.[9]

There has been an extraordinary increase in cases of HIV/AIDS in the inner cities. Unlike the plateau projected for the nation, the incidence of AIDS for the District of Columbia was projected to increase by 34% between 1990 and 1994.[10] This second wave of the epidemic is occurring in injection drug users and heterosexuals. It was estimated that among District of Columbia residents aged 20 to 64 years, 0.3% of white women, 2.9% of white men, 1.6% of black women, and 4.9% of black men were living with HIV infection as of January 1, 1991.

A recent study[11] was conducted among heterosexual couples identified at HIV counseling and testing sites in California. The overall risk of HIV infection for long-term female partners of infected men was 20%, while for long-term male partners of women it was 1.4% (a single case). The explanation for this lopsided odds ratio of infection remains unclear but may be associated with confounding variables or more likely may merely reflect the fact that as with certain other sexually transmitted diseases, it is considerably easier for a woman to be infected by a man than it is for a man to

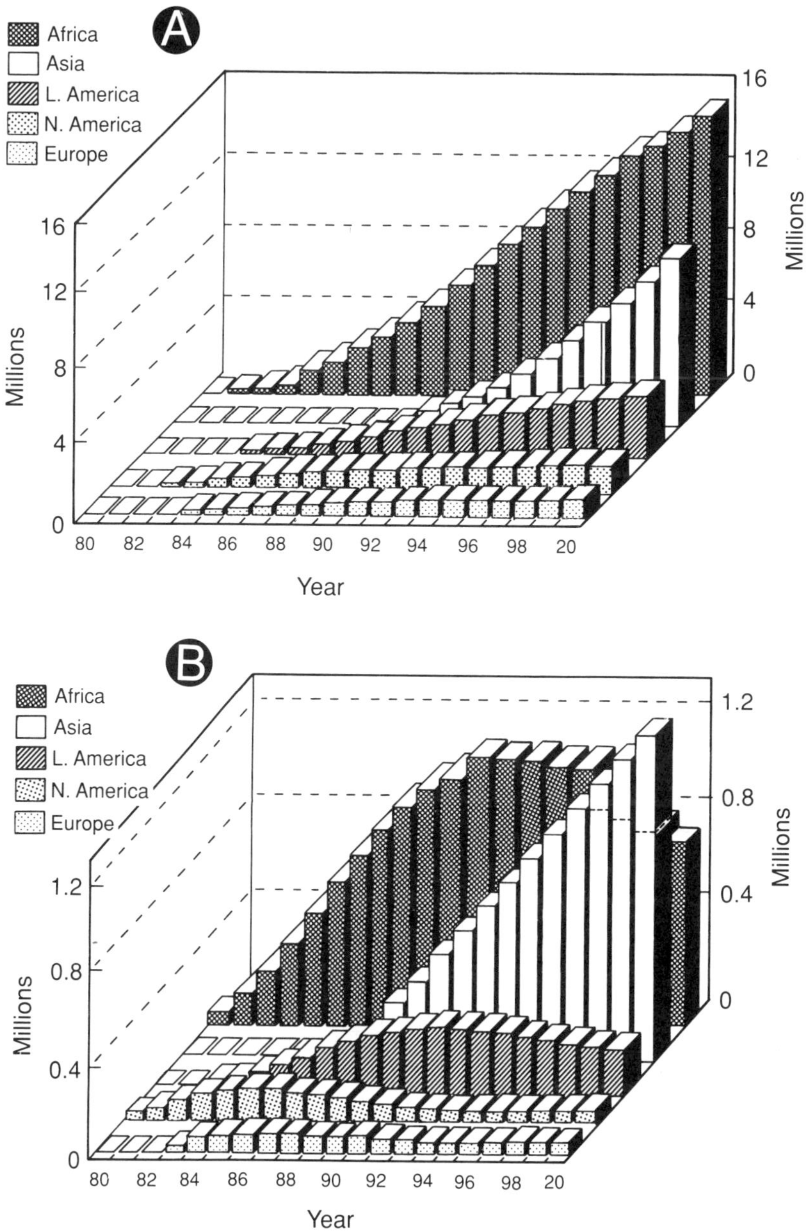

FIG 1.
A, estimated/projected cumulative adult HIV infections, 1980–2000. **B,** estimated/projected annual adult HIV infections, 1980 to 2000. Graphs depict estimated cumulative HIV-1 infections **(A)** and estimated annual HIV-1 infections **(B)** in Europe, North America, Latin America, Asia, and Africa, from 1990 to the present with projections to the year 2000. (Data from World Health Organization statistics.)

be infected by a woman. In this regard, studies of prostitutes in Nairobi have demonstrated a threefold to fivefold increased risk of transmitting HIV-1 when a sexually transmitted disease, in particular, genital ulcerative disease, is present.[12]

Parenteral exposure to blood and blood products represents a mode of transmission of HIV in the United States that has changed markedly in frequency. New infections from contaminated blood transfusions or clotting factor concentrates are extraordinarily rare. In contrast, 24% of all new infections over the past 12 months are parenteral transmissions resulting from the sharing of needles or other drug-related paraphernalia among intravenous (IV) drug users (S. Vermund, personal communication, 1992). Infection rates among the IV drug–using population is expected to continue to grow over the next few years. As a consequence, given the fact that women of childbearing age may be IV drug users themselves or the heterosexual partners of IV drug users, the number of new cases of pediatric HIV infections is also expected to continue to climb. This trend will be particularly apparent among minority (African-American and Hispanic) populations in inner cities where there is a high incidence of IV drug use.

Although maternal-fetal transmission of HIV is well documented, many questions remain unanswered concerning the timing of transmission in relationship to birth, the rate of transmission, and the risk factors for transmission. During 1991, it is estimated that 1,500 to 1,800 children were born infected with HIV-1 in the United States based on 25% to 30% transmission rates.[13] In the European Collaborative Study[14] of mother-to-infant transmission of HIV from predominantly asymptomatic mothers, the frequency of infected infants was less than 15%. Other studies of women with more advanced HIV disease suggest higher rates of transmission approaching 30% to 40%. Several recent studies have addressed the timing of transmission and suggest that infection is more likely to occur as a peripartum event (e.g., studies of twins that demonstrated greater likelihood of transmission to first-born compared to second-born).[15] Two studies have suggested that the titer of maternal immunoglobulin G (IgG) against the neutralizing V3 loop in the envelope (env) protein is inversely correlated with transmission of HIV to the fetus, but this remains to be confirmed.[16, 17]

One study[18] examined the association between the stage of HIV-1 infection in the mother and perinatal transmission. The Mothers and Infants Cohort Study identified 74 infants, infected and uninfected, born to HIV-1 seropositive mothers. Mothers whose lowest prepartum $CD4^+$ T-cell level was less than 20% were found to be at greater risk of transmitting the infection to their child: 10 of 24 transmitters vs. 9 of 50 nontransmitters had less than 20% $CD4^+$ T cells (relative risk 2.07). The association was even stronger when the analysis was limited to $CD4^+$ T-cell levels obtained during the third trimester. The study strongly supports the concept of increased risk of perinatal transmission of HIV-1 infection in mothers with advanced disease, i.e., low prepartum $CD4^+$ T-cell levels.

Parenteral exposure to blood has also resulted in a small but definite occupational risk of HIV-1 infection for health care workers. In a recent collaborative study,[19] the risk of seroconversion following a documented parenteral exposure to the blood of an HIV-infected patient was determined to be less than 0.3%. Because of this very low incidence of seroconversion, studies to determine the value of post-exposure antiretroviral prophylaxis in the health care setting are impractical.

The risk of transmission of HIV-1 from an infected health care worker to the patient has recently received considerable attention following the documented transmission of HIV-1 from an infected dentist to several of his patients.[20] Despite the many questions raised by this isolated incident, including the level of sterilization practices employed, it is evident from a number of "look back" studies of patients who had invasive procedures performed by an HIV-positive surgeon or dentist that the risk of such an occurrence is extremely small.

Virology/Pathogenesis

HIV-1 is a member of the lentivirus subfamily of human retroviruses and is the etiologic agent of AIDS in the vast majority of cases throughout the world. HIV-2 is another human retrovirus that causes AIDS and is endemic in parts of West Africa; it is closely related to simian immunodeficiency virus (SIV) and may be less pathogenic than HIV-1. Human T-cell leukemia-lymphoma virus (HTLV-I) is associated with adult T-cell malignancies. It was isolated only a few years before the first cases of AIDS were described. HTLV-I and HTLV-II are also found with increased frequency in HIV-1 infected populations, particularly injection drug users. According to currently available information, HTLV-II does not cause disease.

Viral Life Cycle

HIV-1 displays a tropism for $CD4^+$ T lymphocytes.[21–24] The CD4 molecule, expressed on the helper/inducer subpopulation of human T cells, is the receptor for HIV-1. The external env glycoprotein of HIV-1, gp120, binds with high affinity to the CD4 molecule. After the binding of viral gp120 to CD4 on the surface of the T cell, HIV-1 enters the cell by direct fusion of the env glycoprotein with the cell membrane. The fusion process is believed to involve fusion of the cell membrane with an env gp41 glycoprotein which is noncovalently attached to gp120. Like other retroviruses, upon entry of the viron into the cell, the env particle is converted into an enzymatically active nucleoprotein complex. The virion-associated reverse transcriptase (RT) transcribes the genomic RNA into unintegrated double-stranded DNA. Although resting cells can be infected with HIV, activation of the cell is required for efficient and complete reverse transcription of genomic RNA. The virally-encoded integrase enables the viral DNA to integrate into the host cell's chromosomal DNA. In HIV infection, a substantial amount of HIV DNA may exist as unintegrated DNA, which may contribute to cytopathicity.

Once the provirus has been integrated, both cellular and viral factors are necessary to initiate expression of viral genes.[25, 26] The cellular factors may be either constitutively produced or may be induced by a variety of activating signals. After activation of HIV provirus by cellular factors, the first viral genes are expressed which encode nonstructural proteins with regulatory functions (Table 1). The most critical of these proteins is Tat, which is a potent transactivator of HIV gene expression and is essential for HIV replication. It operates by both initiating RNA transcription of HIV and by stimulating production of full-length RNA transcripts.

The full-length RNA transcripts are multiply spliced and transported to the cytoplasm, where they are expressed as regulatory proteins. One of these regulatory proteins, Rev, functions to effect the transport of unspliced and singly spliced mRNA from the nucleus to the cytoplasm. These mRNAs encode the structural and enzymatic proteins of HIV that are essential for assembly of infectious virions at the cell membrane. The virion RNA and core proteins associate with viral envelope proteins that are located at the cell membrane, and the mature virion forms by budding from the cell surface.

There are other, less well understood, regulatory and accessory genes expressed by HIV-1.[25, 26] Nef is a nuclear product that has had both negative and positive regulatory functions ascribed to it. The apparent discrepancy may be related to different viral isolates and/or cell lines used in vitro. The only in vivo study unequivocally demonstrated enhanced cytopathic effect for Nef in the SIV/rhesus model. VPR is a virion-associated product that is a trans-acting protein that accelerates the rate of HIV-1 replication and of virus-induced cytopathic effect. VPR is the only regulatory protein present in the virus particle. VPU is a protein that disrupts intracellular gp160-CD4 complex accumulation in the endoplasmic reticulum, thereby facilitating the processing of gp160 to gp120/gp41. VPU also facilitates assembly and budding of virus particles from infected cells. Vif, or viral infectivity factor, is a nuclear protein that increases the infectivity of free virus particles, perhaps by facilitating gp160 processing.

Viral Expression and Latency

Previous studies have demonstrated that the $CD4^+$ T cell is the principal reservoir of HIV-1 in the peripheral blood of infected individuals.[29] There is evidence that only a small fraction of virally infected cells actually express virus. A unique feature of the HIV-1 life cycle is the ability of the provirus to persist in a quiescent state without production of viral mRNA or proteins.[27, 28] Cellular factors play an important role in HIV expression from latently infected cells. One cellular factor, NF-κB, binds to a specific segment of certain cellular genes and initiates transcription of host cell DNA (e.g., promoter region of interleukin-2). In the case of HIV-infected cells, NF-κB proteins induced by various cytokines bind to consensus sequences located in the long-terminal repeat (LTR) region of HIV proviral DNA. This binding results in the stimulation of HIV RNA transcription and the eventual production of virions. The HIV LTR also contains other se-

TABLE 1.
HIV Regulatory and Accessory Genes Primer

Gene	Gene Product	Location	Function
tat	Tat (Trans-activator)	Nucleus	Positive transcriptional trans-activator of all viral genes
rev	Rev (Regulator of HIV structural proteins)	Nucleus	Responsible for the accumulation and nuclear transport of viral structural mRNAs
nef	Nef (Negative factor)	Nucleus	Both negative and positive regulatory functions are ascribed to Nef in vitro by different groups. The apparent discrepancy may be related to different viral isolates and/or cell lines
			The only in vivo study (SIV/rhesus monkey) unequivocally demonstrated a cytopathic effect enhancement property for Nef in this animal model
vpr	VPR	Virion	Trans-acting protein accelerating the rate of HIV-1 replication, and of virus-induced cytopathic effect; the only regulatory protein present in the virus particle
vpu	VPU	Cytoplasm	Disrupts intracellular gp160-CD4 complex accumulation in endoplasmic reticulum, thereby facilitating the processing of gp160 to gp120/gp41
			Facilitates assembly and budding of virus particles from infected cells
vif	VIF (Viral infectivity factor)	Nucleus	Increases the infectivity of free virus particles, perhaps by facilitating gp160 processing

quences that bind cellular transcription factors. These sites (Sp1 binding site, TATA box) as well as NF-κB binding sites are involved in HIV activation following exposure to heterologous viral genes, including herpes simplex virus (HSV), cytomegalovirus (CMV), Epstein-Barr virus (EBV), adenovirus, hepatitis B virus, human HSV-6, and HTLV-I. Experiments suggest that these viruses can act as cofactors in HIV infection by influencing the rate of HIV replication. However, the true role of these viruses as cofactors in vivo remains to be determined.

Recent studies[30] examining the peripheral blood of asymptomatic individuals have shown that HIV-1 is harbored predominantly as full-length, unintegrated complementary DNA. The demonstration that a large fraction of HIV-1 DNA can exist in an extrachromosomal state in infected individuals is in agreement with other reports. However, the results presented in this study attribute the extrachromosomal DNA pool in HIV-1-infected individuals to infection of quiescent T cells, restricted integration, and establishment of a latent and inducible HIV-1 reservoir. These quiescent T cells from infected patients, upon activation in vitro, demonstrated integration of the extrachromosomal unintegrated DNA. Because T-cell activation is a prerequisite for viral DNA integration, the contribution of factors affecting T-cell activation (mitogenic agents, opportunistic infection) to the reactivation of unintegrated HIV-1 DNA forms becomes apparent. Therefore, quiescent T cells may be a major and inducible HIV-1 reservoir in infected individuals.

Cytokines, which are important constituents of immune cell activation that act as physiologic inductive signals in the regulation of immune responses, also play a role in the regulation of HIV expression.[31] Tumor necrosis factor-alpha (TNF-α) has been shown to upregulate HIV expression in chronically infected T- and monocytic-cell lines, whereas two other cytokines, IL-6 and granulocyte macrophage-colony stimulating factor (GM-CSF), induce virus expression in monocyte lineage cells only. In addition, TNF-α acts synergistically with either IL-6 or GM-CSF. These cytokines also induce HIV expression in primary monocyte/macrophage cultures (Fig 2). Other studies have shown that both TNF-α and IL-6 function in an autocrine/paracrine fashion in the induction of HIV expression.[32, 33] Interestingly, it has been shown that TNF-α triggers virus expression by induction of transcription activating factors which bind to the NF-κB binding site in the HIV LTR. In contrast, IL-6 and GM-CSF induce HIV expression predominantly by postranscriptional mechanisms. IFN-γ alone induces HIV expression from chronically infected monocytic cells and in combination with phorbol esters redirects virion formation from the plasma membrane to intracytoplasmic vacuoles.[34]

It has also been shown that certain cytokines possess the ability to inhibit HIV expression. INF-α decreases HIV expression in both acutely and chronically infected cells by inhibiting viral budding.[35] Transforming growth factor-beta (TGF-β), another cytokine, down-regulates constitutive as well as induced expression of HIV by both transcriptional and posttranscriptional mechanisms.[36] However, TGF-β is bifunctional in its regulation

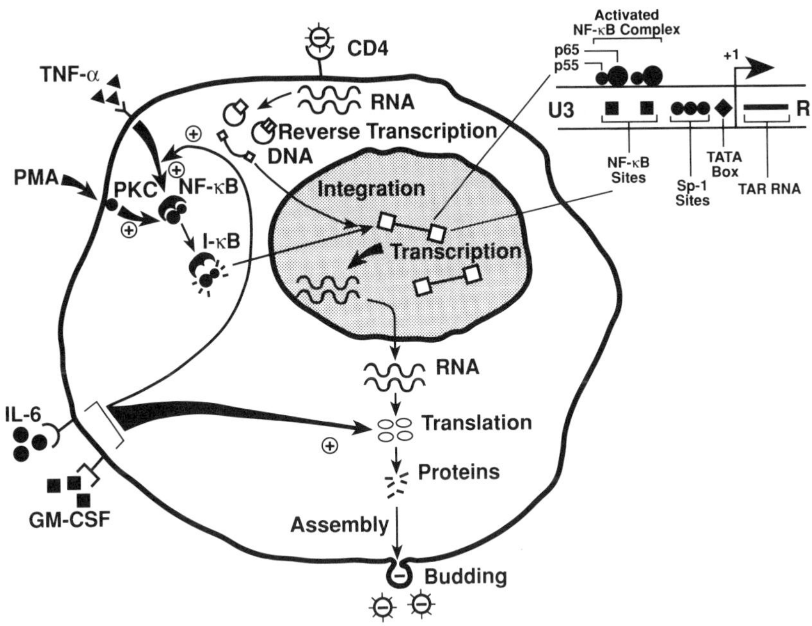

FIG 2.
Mechanisms of cytokine-mediated induction of HIV expression in monocytes/macrophages.

of HIV expression since under certain circumstances in vitro it can actually enhance HIV replication.

CD4 Positive T-Cell Depletion and Dysfunction

A direct relationship between HIV burden and CD4$^+$ T-cell depletion has been established by several groups.[37–43] However, the precise mechanisms by which HIV causes a loss in CD4$^+$ T cells remains poorly understood. A number of different mechanisms have been considered in an attempt to explain this important area of pathogenesis (Table 2).

It has been postulated that HIV can exert its deleterious effects both directly and indirectly. One direct mechanism of cell killing may be the formation of holes in the cell membrane as a consequence of viral budding. In addition, insertion of viral env proteins into the cell membrane can cause ion fluxes and loss of cell viability. Another possible mechanism which has been observed in other retroviral systems is accumulation of unintegrated viral DNA in the cell cytoplasm. It has also been suggested that binding of HIV env proteins to intracellular CD4 molecules may result in cell death. In some experiments, the intracellular CD4-gp160 complexes were noted to have filled the nuclear pores, potentially disrupting the nuclear-cytoplasmic transport pathways.

The low frequency of infected circulating CD4$^+$ T cells and the low level

TABLE 2.
Potential Mechanisms of Depletion of $CD4^+$ T Cells in HIV Infection

1. Direct cytopathic effect on HIV
2. Infection by HIV of a $CD4^+$ T-cell precursor or stem cell
3. Selective depletion of a subset of $CD4^+$ T cells or nonlymphoid $CD4^+$ cells that are trophic for $CD4^+$ T cells and thus critical for the propagation of the entire $CD4^+$ T-cell pool
4. Induction of secretion of soluble substances toxic to $CD4^+$ T cells by HIV-infected $CD4^+$ T cells and/or monocytes
5. Syncytia formation between uninfected and infected $CD4^+$ T cells
6. Autoimmune phenomena
7. Superantigen effects with nonrandom activation of $CD4^+$ T cells expressing particular Vβ T-cell receptors, enhancing their susceptibility to infection with HIV
8. Apoptosis or programmed cell death of stimulated $CD4^+$ T cells

of viremia seen in the early stages of HIV infection does not correlate with the progressive depletion of $CD4^+$ T cells and immune dysfunction seen even with early stage disease. Pantaleo et al.[44] have studied patients with early HIV-1 infection and compared the viral burden in $CD4^+$ T cells in peripheral blood to that in lymphoid organs utilizing quantitative DNA polymerase chain reaction (PCR). They demonstrated that the frequency of HIV-1 infected $CD4^+$ T cells is substantially higher (from ½ to 1 log) in the lymphoid tissue compared to the peripheral blood. Furthermore, high levels of HIV-specific mRNA were detected by in situ hybridization and RNA PCR in lymphoid tissue but not in cell suspensions of peripheral blood mononuclear cells (PBMC, PBL). These findings indicate that a heavy viral load resides in the lymphoid organs of patients with early stage disease, suggesting that these tissues may function as major reservoirs for HIV. In addition, the finding of a heavy viral load as well as active virus replication in the lymphoid organs of patients in early disease may explain the progressive depletion of $CD4^+$ T cells and the immune dysfunction associated with the early stages of HIV infection when peripheral blood viral burden and replication is very low.

In a related study by Aoki-Sei et al.,[45] quantitative assays of HIV-1 DNA and mRNA in various tissues of 10 HIV-1 infected patients with AIDS or AIDS-related complex (ARC) were performed. The number of HIV-1 DNA copies obtained in tissues were much higher than those obtained in PBMCs from the same patients; furthermore, RNA PCR identified the lymph node and spleen as the primary compartments of actively HIV-producing cells. These studies support the concept that lymphoid tissue is the site for active replication of HIV-1 in patients throughout the course of infection and that the combination of a quantitative RNA PCR with concurrent DNA PCR may provide the means for assessing the dynamics of viral load in patients with HIV-1 infection.

Several indirect mechanisms of $CD4^+$ T-cell depletion have been implicated in HIV pathogenesis. The destruction of bystander $CD4^+$ T cells by autoimmune phenomena may occur. It is also possible that antibodies directed against certain viral epitopes may crossreact with the usual ligand for CD4. This model[46] suggests that gp120/41 mimics a conserved domain of major histocompatibility complex (MHC) class II and class I determinants. Further work is needed to define whether this process occurs in vivo.

Another indirect mechanism to explain CD4 depletion is that uninfected $CD4^+$ T cells may bind free gp120 molecules and become targets for lysis by antibody-dependent cellular cytotoxicity involving anti-gp120 antibodies. Furthermore, $CD4^+$ T cells may process soluble gp120 and, following antigen presentation, again become targets for cytolysis.

One puzzling aspect of HIV infection is the lack of $CD4^+$ T-cell regeneration, either early in the course of disease, or following antiretroviral therapy. One possible explanation for the inability of the $CD4^+$ T-cell pool to regenerate itself may be infection of CD4 positive T-cell precursors. This has been recently demonstrated for both bone marrow and intrathymic T-cell precursors.[47, 48]

While long-term infection with HIV is characterized by reduction in the number of $CD4^+$ T cells, functional abnormalities in these cells have been noted at all stages of HIV infection.[21] Abnormal T-cell responses to soluble antigen are observed early in the course of HIV infection. Defective T-cell cloning efficiency is another measure of functional impairment of $CD4^+$ T cells. In addition to HIV-induced suppression of $CD4^+$ T-cell responses that result from infection of the cells, it has also been shown that in vitro exposure of these cells to specific HIV proteins (gp120, gp41, p24) in the absence of infection of the cell is sufficient to inhibit antigen-specific responses. HIV env protein may block the interaction between CD4 and MHC molecules that occurs during antigen presentation. Furthermore, binding of gp120 to CD4 may disrupt the normal cellular postreceptor signal transduction pathway.

The hypothesis that superantigens may be involved in the immunopathogenesis of HIV infection resulted from the report of a protein that functions as a superantigen in immunodeficient mice infected with a retrovirus.[49] The virally encoded superantigen in mice was shown to stimulate proliferation and expansion of cells expressing specific T-cell receptor (TCR) β-chain variable (Vβ) regions, an effect seen with superantigens in general. In humans, superantigens have been invoked to explain $CD4^+$ T-cell depletion in HIV-infected individuals, particularly by investigators who have noted Vβ perturbations in such individuals.[46, 50] However, it is much more likely that superantigens function as selective activators of specific Vβ subsets of T cells, leading to T-cell anergy or increased susceptibility to HIV infection. It has been reported that the level of HIV replication in human

T-cell lines expressing specific Vβs was up to 100-fold higher; this suggests that in vivo cells expressing these same Vβs could support enhanced viral replication.[51] Of note, AIDS patients did not exhibit a depletion in the Vβ clones with the highest level of HIV replication implying that in vivo, other mechanisms of T-cell depletion may be active.

Another hypothesis that may explain T-cell depletion in HIV-infected individuals involves the mechanisms of apoptosis of $CD4^+$ T cells.[52] Apoptosis is the process of programmed cell death that occurs among immature thymocytes, whereby the T-cell repertoire is negatively selected, leading to clonal deletion of autoreactive T cells and the establishment of selftolerance. Apoptosis has also been observed in mature murine $CD4^+$ T cells whose CD3 receptors have been crosslinked. In HIV-infected individuals, crosslinking of CD4 may occur as a result of binding of either gp120 or gp120-anti-gp120 complexes to CD4, which may then prepare the cell for apoptosis following antigenic stimulation of the TCR. Several recent studies support the role of apoptosis in $CD4^+$ T-cell depletion.[46, 53] It has been shown that apoptosis occurs following acute HIV infection of lymphoblastoid cells and activated PBL in vitro. In addition, it has recently been reported that $CD4^+$ T cells from asymptomatic HIV-infected individuals undergo apoptosis following in vitro exposure to MHC class II-dependent superantigens or PWM. Spontaneous apoptosis in cultured $CD4^+$ and $CD8^+$ T cells from asymptomatic HIV-infected individuals has also been observed. While this mechanism of cell death remains speculative and further work in this area is needed, apoptosis may explain at least in part the progressive diminution of $CD4^+$ T cells in HIV infection.

Role of Monocyte/Macrophages

Monocytes and macrophages also express the CD4 receptor on their surface and are readily infected by HIV-1.[21] HIV has been detected in monocyte/macrophages from the blood, lung, and brain of HIV-infected individuals. Unlike the significant cell death or syncytial formation that occurs after infection of $CD4^+$ T cells, HIV infection of monocyte/macrophages appears to be persistent and poorly cytopathic with virus particles found predominantly in cytoplasmic vacuoles. This location may shelter the virus from being recognized by the immune system.

Some investigators have reported that certain isolates of HIV display a specific tropism for either monocyte/macrophages or $CD4^+$ T cells but not both. There is some evidence that this tropism may be driven by the amino acid sequence in the V3 loop region of the env glycoprotein. There is also some suggestion that HIV isolates obtained from infected individuals early in the course of infection, which typically are nonsyncytial-inducing, are predominantly monocyte-tropic, whereas the later, more aggressive isolates which are syncytial-inducing are predominantly T-cell-tropic.[54, 55]

The role of circulating monocytes in HIV infection is presently unknown. However, the detection of HIV in macrophages from the lung and brain suggests that tissue-specific macrophages may be a significant target for

HIV in vivo. Sequestration of HIV-1 within tissue macrophages implies that these cells may function as a reservoir of virus infection in the body, as seen in certain lentivirus infections in animals. In this manner, HIV-infected macrophages may spread HIV to susceptible CD4$^+$ T cells during normal antigen presentation.

Because the monocyte/macrophage lineage cell (microglial cell) is most frequently found to be infected in the brain, it is thought that this cell plays an instrumental role in the neuropathogenesis of HIV infection.[27, 56] It is postulated that there is release of cytokines or other factors from the microglial cell that are directly toxic to neurons or lead to inflammation. On the other hand, TNF-α may function as an autocrine inducer of HIV expression in infected microglial cells which could lead to damage of nearby cells. It has recently been shown that damage to rat and human brain cultures occurs after exposure to a variety of factors secreted by HIV-infected mononuclear phagocytes.[57]

Role of B Lymphocytes

In addition to the depletion of CD4$^+$ T cells, HIV-infected individuals exhibit abnormalities in the B-cell limb of the immune response, some of which are secondary to T-cell deficiency, while others are T-cell independent.[21] B-cell function in HIV-infected individuals is severely impaired. The majority of AIDS patients exhibit polyclonal B-cell activation with spontaneous B-cell proliferation, increased Ig secretion, and hypergammaglobulinemia, suggesting chronic activation. A substantial proportion of these activated B cells are specific for HIV epitopes. In addition to spontaneous B-cell hyperactivity, B cells from infected patients exhibit an intrinsic defect in antigen- and mitogen-induced responses at all stages of infection.

IL-6 is a critical factor in the terminal differentiation of activated B cells. It has been shown that exposure of normal PBL to HIV whole-virus preparation induces IL-6 production in vitro, predominantly by monocytes.[58] It has also been shown that IL-6 induces HIV expression in infected monocytes, in synergy with other cytokines.[33] Oyaizu et al.[59] exposed normal PBL to the gp120 and gp160 env glycoproteins in vitro and demonstrated that these env proteins have the ability to induce IL-6 mRNA and biologically active IL-6 protein secretion from the PBL. These findings suggest that monocytes and T cells contribute to the secretion of IL-6, which plays an important role in the pathogenesis of B-cell activation in HIV infection.

B cells themselves secrete TNF-α and IL-6 when activated. It has recently been shown that spontaneously activated B cells from HIV-infected individuals secrete TNF-α and IL-6, which can induce HIV expression in chronically infected monocyte lines.[60]

The high frequency of B-cell lymphomas in patients with AIDS is another manifestation of B-cell disregulation. Work by MacMahon et al.[61] has conclusively shown that EBV plays a major role in primary central nervous system (CNS) lymphoma in AIDS. These workers utilized an RNA in situ hybridization technique on formalin-fixed paraffin-embedded tissues. In each of 21 cases of primary CNS lymphoma, they detected the abundant nuclear expression of short nonprotein-coding EBV transcripts, called EBERs, which are present in all known forms of EBV latency. This was not true of systemic lymphoma in AIDS patients in which only 3 of 7 cases were EBV-EBER in situ positive. Furthermore, primary CNS lymphoma in other immunodeficiency states was rarely associated (2 of 14) with EBV. Therefore, the pathogenic role for EBV as an effector for EBV-associated lymphomagenesis is strongly supported.

Role of Bone Marrow-Derived Dendritic Cells

Immune responses in resting T cells are initiated by the very potent presentation of antigen by bone marrow-derived dendritic cells (DC). While it has been reported that DC can be infected with HIV-1 in vitro,[62] it appears that productive or latent HIV-1 infection of DC in vivo is rare, certainly no greater than in T cells.[63] Furthermore, DC from HIV-infected individuals are capable of expanding $CD4^+$ T cells efficiently. It is postulated that DC may carry HIV-1 into proximity with uninfected T cells and thereby amplify the cytopathic effects of small amounts of virus.[64] After exposure to HIV in vitro, DC continue to present antigens, forming clusters with T cells that are driven to replicate. In this setting, DC infection cannot be detected; however, the clustered T cells form syncytia, release virions, and die. Therefore, the carrier action of HIV-1 by DC may facilitate the lysis and loss of antigen-specific $CD4^+$ T cells in HIV-infected individuals.

Role of Follicular Dendritic Cells in Lymphoid Organ HIV Pathogenesis

As discussed earlier, the lymph node is the principal reservoir for HIV-1-infected $CD4^+$ T cells in the infected individual. Recent work has examined lymph nodes from infected patients utilizing in situ hybridization in combination with immunohistologic labeling techniques and has demonstrated that follicular dendritic cells (FDC) may be infected with HIV-1.[65–67] Alternatively, FDC in their role as filters of the lymph node, can trap HIV virions and present them to uninfected T cells. This would lead to increasing infection of T helper/memory cells within germinal centers and ultimately, immunodeficiency. Indeed, a high level of free and antibody-bound virus has been demonstrated to be attached to FDC in the lymph nodes of HIV-infected individuals during the stage of follicular hyperplasia[68]; this is followed by a gradual loss of FDC and virus with gradual loss of germinal centers and progression to the stages of follicular atrophy and depletion.

Therapeutics

Antiretroviral Therapy

The therapeutic approach to an HIV-infected person in 1993 represents the efforts of nearly a decade of clinical trials based on our increasing understanding of the biology of the virus and the immune response in the infected host. Since many of the clinical manifestations of HIV infection are a direct consequence of the effects of the virus on the immune system, the most logical therapeutic strategy against AIDS is to treat the underlying retroviral disease.

Until late 1991, zidovudine (AZT, ZDV), a dideoxynucleoside reverse transcriptase inhibitor, was the only drug among the antiretroviral agents that had been demonstrated to provide clinical benefit to HIV-infected patients.[69] Over the past 2 years, however, two additional dideoxynucleoside RT inhibitors have been licensed for use, either as a single agent (ddI, Videx), or in combination with ZDV (ddC, Zalcitabine) (Table 3). At the present time, it is recommended that all individuals with CD4 cell counts of 500/mm^3 or less have therapy initiated with ZDV at a dose of 100 mg given 5 or 6 times daily. Such individuals can be expected to have a transient (<6 months) elevation of their CD4 cell counts associated with clinical benefit, the duration of which will vary from individual to individual. In addition, ZDV therapy has a measurable effect on HIV activity as one can see reductions in serum p24 antigen levels, plasma viremia, quantitative cell microcultures, and plasma viral RNA. The toxicities of ZDV are well known, although they are less frequent at the lower doses currently being employed. These toxicities include anemia, leukopenia, thrombocytopenia, myalgias/myositis, nausea, and headache.

For patients who become intolerant of ZDV therapy or clinically progress despite ZDV, recent studies from the AIDS Clinical Trials Group (ACTG) of the National Institute of Allergy and Infectious Diseases provide the rationale for some alternatives. Analysis of one clinical study[70] has demonstrated that in patients with at least 16 weeks of ZDV therapy, ddI appears to be more efficacious than ZDV in delaying time to first new AIDS-defining event or death in patients with ARC or symptomatic disease. In this double-blinded phase III trial, patients with AIDS or ARC and CD4 cell counts <300/mm^3 or asymptomatic HIV infection and CD4 cell counts <200/mm^3 who had been receiving ZDV for at least 16 weeks were randomized to receive either ZDV 100 mg every 4 hrs, ddI 250 mg every 12 hrs, or ddI 375 mg every 12 hrs. Patients randomized to ddI 500 mg/day (but not 750 mg/day) experienced a statistically significant delay in time to first new AIDS-defining event or death compared to those randomized to ZDV (1 year rates 28% vs. 40%, respectively; log rank $P = 0.08$). Toxicities related to ddI use included hyperamylasemia and pancreatitis; however, there were no differences in the cumulative 1 year incidence of peripheral neuropathy (15%) among the treatment arms. CD4 cells were higher in the 2 ddI arms compared to ZDV over the first year on study, with a difference of about 10 cells/mm^3. The fact that initiation of ddI therapy is more efficacious (in delaying new AIDS-defining events) than remaining on ZDV therapy beyond 16 weeks may be a result of the development of resistance to ZDV, without crossresistance (at least initially) to ddI. However, the clinical ramifications of the development of in vitro resistance to nucleoside analogues remains to be defined.

Despite the clear utility of ZDV therapy in patients with AIDS, progres-

TABLE 3.
Approved Therapies for HIV-1 Infection

Agent	Dose	Approved Indications	Common Adverse Effects
Zidovudine (AZT)	100 mg every 4 hr, 5 times daily	CD4 count <500/μl, AIDS, HIV-associated thrombocytopenia	Neutropenia, anemia, nausea, headache, myopathy
Didanosine (ddl)	2 × 100 mg tablets every 12 hr 2 × 75 mg tablets every 12 hr <50 kg	Patients "failing or intolerant" of zidovudine ? switch if <200 CD4 and >4 mo of zidovudine	Diarrhea, nausea, pancreatitis, neuropathy
Zalcitabine (ddC)	2 × 0.375 mg tablets every 8 hr	CD4 <300 only in combination with zidovudine 200 mg every 8 hr and only after zidovudine alone has been tried	Neuropathy, stomatitis, rash, plus those of zidovudine

sion of HIV disease continues to occur in treated patients, with falling CD4 counts, onset of new opportunistic infections, and the emergence of virus isolates with reduced in vitro susceptibility to ZDV. The combination of ZDV and ddC has additive and possibly synergistic activity against HIV-1 in vitro, including isolates resistant to ZDV alone. These observations led to a phase I/II study of concurrently administered ZDV and ddC in patients with advanced HIV disease.[71] In this study, the safety and efficacy of six different combinations of ZDV and ddC were evaluated. Of patients receiving combinations containing 300 or 600 mg of ZDV daily, 69% had an increase of 50 CD4 cells or greater. Regimens containing 600 mg of ZDV daily were more likely to result in persistent increases in CD4 counts above pretreatment values than were the two lowest dose regimens ($P = 0.003$). In addition, rapid and sustained declines in p24 antigenemia were seen in all treatment regimens except for ZDV alone at 150 mg daily.

While the data from this study suggest that combination therapy with ZDV and ddC were well tolerated and appear to lead to enhanced antiviral activity in patients, it must be stressed that this was a small, pilot study with an average of eight patients per arm. It is, therefore, too premature to yield firm conclusions regarding toxicity or recommendation for treatment with any of the combination regimens. Of note, the Food and Drug Administration (FDA) has "conditionally approved" ddC in combination with ZDV for patients with advanced HIV disease on the basis of the CD4 cell rise as a surrogate marker. Final FDA approval as well as more definitive answers to these critical questions awaits the conclusion of the larger phase II/III trials now under way.

Phase I clinical trials are now under way to determine the safety and preliminary antiviral activity of protease inhibitors and a tat inhibitor. Protease inhibitors are targeted at the enzyme that cleaves the gag-pol polyprotein, preventing the formation of infectious virions. The exact mechanisms of action of the tat inhibition are unclear; however, it does prevent transactivation of HIV-1 in vitro. None of these agents focused at new viral targets is expected to eradicate HIV-1 infection. However if these agents demonstrate antiviral activity in vivo, the rapid evaluation of these compounds in combination with nucleoside RT inhibitors will be essential.

Microbial Resistance to Antiretrovirals

Despite the progress made in the development of single-agent therapy for HIV-1 infection, monotherapy with any agent has been associated with the ultimate failure of that therapy, i.e., progression of HIV disease. HIV isolates obtained from individuals during prolonged treatment with ZDV can show decreased sensitivity to ZDV in vitro.[72–75] The development of clinical resistance to antiviral therapy in general occurs in the setting of an immunocompromised host with a chronic or recurrent infection. Factors that contribute to the development of resistance to antiviral drugs include the magnitude and duration of viral replication, the dosing regimen and pharmacokinetic parameters of the antiviral drug, and effects of mutations that confer drug resistance.

Studies comparing small groups of patients demonstrate that partially resistant isolates appear earlier in patients with late-stage HIV infection than in those with early-stage infection.[74, 76] In general, isolates of HIV that are highly resistant to ZDV have been derived from treated individuals in the very late stages of disease. Genotypic analyses of clinical isolates have demonstrated that ZDV resistance is due to specific mutations in the viral RT gene resulting in amino acid substitutions in at least five residues.[72, 77] Highly resistant isolates had substitutions in RT at four residues (Asp67 to Asn, Lys70 to Arg, Thr215 to Phe or Tyr, and Lys219 to Gln) or occasionally in just the first three. Isolates with a partially resistant phenotype had subsets of these substitutions, often with a single substitution at codon 70 or 215.

It has been recently shown that in patients with AIDS who are switched from ZDV to ddI, a decrease in the in vitro sensitivity to ddI and an increase in sensitivity to ZDV emerges. Analysis of the RT coding region reveals a mutation (Leu74 to Val) associated with reduced sensitivity to ddI.[78] The clinical implications of this remain to be defined. In patients receiving therapy with nonnucleoside RT inhibitors (e.g., nevaripine, TIBO, L-compounds, bisheteroarylpiperazines [BHAPs]), there is rapid development of high level phenotypic resistance that is associated with a mutation in the RT (Tyr 181 to Cys).[79] There is some preliminary evidence that the combination of ZDV with a nonnucleoside inhibitor can delay the development of resistance to ZDV.

The clinical implications of in vitro HIV resistance to antiretroviral therapies remains to be elucidated. In a recent study of 23 children with symptoms of HIV-1 disease during extended monotherapy with ZDV, there was a highly significant correlation between decreased in vitro ZDV sensitivity and poor clinical outcome ($P < 0.001$). Age-adjusted CD4 cell counts were lower at the start of treatment and at the time of sampling in children whose viral isolates manifested an increased resistance to ZDV.[80] Studies can only suggest an association but not a cause-and-effect relationship between development of drug-resistance and clinical deterioration. If one accepts the likelihood of the clinical importance of the development of drug resistance, then strategies to prevent or delay the emergence of resistance assume paramount importance. The use of combination antiretroviral therapy is the most logical approach to delaying the onset of resistance. This approach is being actively studied in multiple clinical trials in the United States and abroad, and it is expected that preliminary information from these studies will be available in 1993.

ZDV Therapy in Minorities With HIV

The frequency of HIV infection among black and Hispanic populations is expected to continue to rise because of the growing rate of infection among injecting drug users, a group that is overrepresented within these minorities. The question of whether ZDV is effective in these groups has been raised.[81] Two recent studies on the efficacy of ZDV in minority and female subpopulations have now shed light on this question and should be reassuring to clinicians. While the two studies used different methodologies and both are weakened by the fact that they constitute analyses of subgroups of a larger study (neither being designed to specifically do cross-race or cross-sex comparisons), they both reached the same conclusion—that ZDV appears to be equally efficacious in minorities and whites.

A study by Lagakos et al.[82] combined the data from the two largest clinical trials of ZDV, ACTG studies 016 and 019. The rates of progression to AIDS in subjects receiving ZDV were significantly lower than in subjects receiving placebo among blacks, whites, Hispanics, non-Hispanics, and non–IV drug users. The benefit of ZDV use over placebo was less apparent for women and IV drug users, most likely related to a problem in health care delivery—such populations have been noted to reach health care providers at a later stage in their disease.

In the study by Easterbrook et al.,[83] patients with AIDS or advanced ARC were examined. The study determined that Hispanic and particularly black patients had more advanced disease than white patients, and it was therefore not surprising that such populations had poorer outcomes with respect to survival and development of opportunistic infection. After adjusting for more advanced disease, black race was no longer a significant independent predictor of a lower survival. Most of the excess risk of the development of *Pneumocystis carinii* pneumonia (PCP) in black patients compared with white patients with AIDS was accounted for by differences in the use of PCP prophylaxis. Thus, there were no significant differences among the measured effectiveness of ZDV across different racial groups.

Therapeutic Vaccines

In general, actual infection with a given virus leads to the broadest and most long-lasting immunity in a host. There is preliminary evidence that this may not be the case with HIV-1 infection. The critical hypothesis that is now under intense investigation is whether a more effective immune response can be generated against HIV-1 by postinfection vaccination with HIV-specific antigens.

The concept of therapeutic vaccination for infectious diseases originated in the mid-1800s in Paris with Auzias-Turenne's vaccination of syphilis patients with extracts of syphilitic chancres.[84] In the late 1800s, Pasteur developed the successful concept of postexposure vaccination for rabies. In the 1800s in Berlin, Koch supported the inoculation of tuberculin into patients with tuberculosis (TB) to induce inflammatory responses. Finally, Wright in London in the early 1900s measured serum "opsonizing" activity in response to therapeutic inoculation with microbe-derived vaccines. Except for rabies, these approaches were never demonstrated to be efficacious, and with the advent of antibiotics in the mid-1900s, therapeutic vaccination was essentially abandoned.

Redfield et al. reported on the results of a phase I study of recombinant gp160 in patients with early HIV-1 infection.[85] Thirty patients with Walter Reed stage 1 or 2 ($CD4^+$ T cell count of >400/mm^3) disease received either three or six injections of the HIV env protein. Nineteen of 30 patients demonstrated increased humoral and cellular immune responses to HIV env proteins, including seroconversion to selected env epitopes, and new T-cell proliferative responses to gp160. Response rate was associated with the $CD4^+$ T-cell count prior to vaccination (13/16 with $CD4^+$ T cells >600, 6/14 with $CD4^+$ T cells <600) and with the number of injections. There were no significant adverse effects. At 10 months follow up, mean $CD4^+$ T-cell counts were stable in the 19 responders, but decreased 7.3% in 11 nonresponders. Preliminary studies suggest that responders have decreases in expression of HIV-1 specific mRNA. This remains to be confirmed. This study has now been followed by a 600-patient, randomized, blinded control study of gp160 vaccine vs. placebo in HIV-infected individuals with $CD4^+$ T-cell counts >400/mm^3. Results of this trial may be available in 1993 or 1994.

Results from a double-blind placebo controlled trial involving 52 patients with HIV infection and $CD4^+$ T-cell counts >400 have recently been reported.[86] Forty patients received baculovirus-expressed gp160 while 12 control patients received hepatitis B vaccine. Preliminary analysis shows promising results in terms of novel lymphocyte proliferative responses, development of new or enhanced cytotoxic T-cell responses, and the appearance of new antibody responses to both vaccine and nonvaccine viral antigens. The latter suggests that vaccination has broadened the immune response with enhanced recognition of viral antigens not present in the vaccine preparation. Tsoukas et al.[87] have also studied this same vaccine in an open-labeled phase II study of 21 patients and have detected mean $CD4^+$ T-cell rises of about 85/mm^3. Of note is the fact that no studies reported to date demonstrate clinical efficacy of therapeutic vaccination.

One can identify several critical issues in therapeutic vaccination that remain unanswered. These include the following: What is the evidence that broadening of the immune response to HIV-1 with vaccine leads to reductions in viral expression/viral burden? What are the immunologic parameters (humoral and cellular) that are enhanced with vaccine and do they correlate with clinical outcome? Should HIV-1–infected patients be vaccinated with antigen derived from a viral strain that is antigenically similar or dissimilar to the infecting strain? What role does the glycosylation of env products and choice of adjuvant play in the response to vaccine? How does one best define clinical efficacy? Which patient populations should be targeted for vaccine? How well will individuals respond to vaccine with CD4 counts <500/mm^3? Will combination of vaccine with antiretroviral therapy enhance the vaccine immunogenicity? It is hoped that answers to these questions will be forthcoming as the concept of therapeutic vaccination is intensely investigated over the next few years.

Opportunistic Infections

The currently accepted approaches to the treatment and prevention of opportunistic infections in HIV disease are summarized in Table 4. The benefits in terms of morbidity and mortality of initiation of therapy to prevent development of PCP for individuals with a prior episode of PCP (secondary prophylaxis) as well as for all HIV-infected patients with CD4 cell counts of 200 cells/mm^3 or less (primary prophylaxis) is well documented. New insights into prophylactic therapy were gained as a result of a recently completed study.[88] The study was a phase II comparison of the efficacy of ZDV combined with either trimethoprim-sulfamethoxazole (TMP-SMX), one double-strength tablet daily, or aerosolized pentamidine (AP), 300 mg every 4 weeks by nebulizer, for preventing PCP. The target population included patients who had recovered from an initial episode of PCP and who had no known treatment-limiting adverse reactions to any of the trial therapies. There were 50 recurrences of PCP during the study: 14 among those assigned to TMP-SMX and 36 among those assigned to AP. Participants randomized to TMP-SMX experienced a significant delay in the time to recurrent PCP compared to those randomized to AP (stratified logrank, $P = 0.0002$). The 1-year PCP recurrence rate was estimated to be 4.5% for the TMP-SMX arm and 18.5% for the AP arm. There were no significant differences in survival or toxicity between the arms. The results of this trial provide conclusive evidence of the superior efficacy of TMP-SMX in preventing or delaying recurrent PCP in HIV-infected individuals. However, the results may not apply to patients with less severe immunosuppression, intolerance to one or more of the study medications, or with no prior episode of PCP. Information regarding the best approaches to primary prophylaxis of PCP will be available sometime in 1993.

Cytomegalovirus (CMV) is a common opportunistic infection in patients with AIDS; it is a relatively late manifestation, generally occurring in patients with fewer than 100 CD4$^+$ T cells/mm^3. It causes substantial morbidity and presents in various clinical forms including retinitis, colitis, pneumonitis, esophagitis, and encephalitis. Visual impairment due to CMV retinitis occurs in 7% to 20% of patients with AIDS.

The first agent approved for therapy of CMV retinitis (June 1989) was ganciclovir (DHPG, Cytovene). Ganciclovir is effective in delaying progression of retinitis compared to placebo[89]; however, retinitis eventually progresses despite daily maintenance therapy (median progression time 15 weeks). Ganciclovir also causes profound neutropenia that precludes concomitant ZDV therapy.

Trisodium phosphonoformate (foscarnet) was the second agent approved for therapy of CMV retinitis (September 1991). In patients who were studied with AIDS and CMV retinitis with peripheral retinal disease, the time to progression of retinitis was 3.2 weeks in the control group compared with 13.3 weeks in the group receiving thrice daily foscarnet at 60 mg/kg intravenously for 3 weeks followed by 90 mg/kg daily mainte-

TABLE 4.
Therapy of Opportunistic Infections in AIDS

Pathogen or Disease	Drug	Usual Dose and Route in Adults	Duration	Adverse Effects	Prophylaxis
Pneumocystis carinii pneumonia	1. TMP-SMX 2. Pentamidine isethionate 3. TMP-dapsone	1. 20 mg TMP/100 mg SMX/kg/day IV or po divided every 6 hr 2. 4 mg/kg/day IV 3. 20 mg/kg/day po TMP, 100 mg/day po dapsone	1. 21 days 2. 21 days 3. 21 days	1. Rash, fever, GI symptoms, leukopenia, thrombocytopenia 2. Nephrotoxicity, hepatotoxicity, hypoglycemia, hypotension leukopenia, thrombocytopenia	1. 160–800 mg 3 times a week or po daily 2. Inhalation 300 mg every 4 wk (rule out pulmonary TB) 3. Dapsone 25 mg three times a week or po daily
T. gondii brain abscess	Pyrimethamine + sulfadiazine + folinic acid	75 mg/day po 1.0–1.5 g every 6 hr po 10 mg/day po	6 weeks	Leukopenia, thrombocytopenia, rash, nephrotoxicity, hepatotoxicity	Primary: TMP-SMX (as for PCP) maintenance: pyrimethamine 25 mg/day po + sulfadiazine 2 g/day po
Cryptococcus neoformans meningitis	Amphotericin B	0.5 mg/kg/day IV	6 weeks	Fever, anemia, nephrotoxicity, pancytopenia, hepatotoxicity	Acute therapy followed by lifelong maintenance with fluconazole 100 mg/day po
Candida esophagitis	1. Ketoconazole 2. Fluconazole	1. 400 mg/day po 2. 200–400 mg/day po	1. 21 days 2. 21 days	1. Hepatitis, altered steroid metabolism,	No routine prophylaxis

	3. Amphotericin B	3. 20–25 mg/day (if severe, unresponsive)	3. 10 days	drug interactions 2. GI symptoms, rash, hepatitis 3. See *C. neoformans*	
Oral thrush	1. Clotrimazole oral troche 2. Ketoconazole 3. Fluconazole	1. 6 troches/day po 2. 200 mg/day po 3. 100 mg/day po	1. 21 days 2. 21 days 3. 21 days	1. GI symptoms 2. See candida esophagitis 3. See candida esophagitis	No routine prophylaxis
Herpes simplex mucocutaneous	Acyclovir	200–800 mg 5 times daily po or 10 mg/kg IV every 8 hr	10 days	Pancytopenia, hepatotoxicity	(If recurrent): 200 mg 5 times daily po
Cytomegalovirus retinitis	1. Ganciclovir	1. 5.0 mg/kg every 12 hr IV	1. 21 days	1. Neutropenia, thrombocytopenia, hepatitis	1. Acute therapy followed by lifelong maintenance 6 mg/kg/day IV
	2. Foscarnet		2. 21 days	2. Nephrotoxicity	2. Acute therapy followed by lifelong maintenance 90 mg/kg/day IV
M. avium-complex disseminated	Combination therapy: rifampin (or rifabutin) + ethambutol +clofazamine + clarithromycin ± amikacin	 600 mg/day po 15 mg/kg/day po 100 mg/day po 500 mg twice daily po 7.5 mg/kg every 12 hr IV	Indefinite	Hepatotoxicity Optic neuritis Skin discoloration GI symptoms Nephrotoxicity, ototoxicity	Rifabutin 300 mg po daily for CD4 > 100
Isospora belli enteritis	TMP-SMX	160 mg/800 mg po every 6 hr	10 days	See PCP	No routine prophylaxis
Cryptosporidiosis, Microsporidiosis	No specific therapy identified; supportive care				

nance.[90] The principal adverse effects of foscarnet were seizures, hypomagnesemia, hypocalcemia, and elevations in serum creatinine.

The recently reported Foscarnet-Ganciclovir CMV Retinitis Trial was designed to evaluate the relative safety and efficacy of foscarnet versus ganciclovir for the initial treatment and maintenance of CMV retinitis in patients with AIDS.[91] The study demonstrated that foscarnet and ganciclovir were equally effective in halting the progression of CMV retinitis and preserving vision in patients who are newly diagnosed with the disease. However, results from the trial demonstrated that those patients who received the antiviral drug foscarnet lived longer (median of 12 months) than those who received ganciclovir (median of 8 months). The difference in mortality between patients treated with foscarnet and those treated with ganciclovir could not be fully explained by the differential use of ZDV or other antiretroviral agents by patients in these treatment groups, nor could the difference in survival be explained by variations in disease severity between the two patient groups at the time they entered the study. It is possible that the improved survival seen in patients taking foscarnet could be due to an additive or synergistic antiretroviral effect of combined foscarnet with ZDV. It is clear that further studies are needed to better define the role of foscarnet in patients with advanced AIDS.

Cryptococcal meningitis is the most common life-threatening fungal infection seen in persons with AIDS, occurring in 5% to 8% of patients. Current therapy for treating the acute episode of cryptococcal meningitis includes the administration of amphotericin B combined with flucytosine over a period of 4 to 6 weeks, with success rates in non-AIDS patients of 75% to 85%; however, in AIDS patients this regimen is only 40% to 50% successful. In addition, these drugs are highly toxic. It is clear that more optimal therapy for AIDS-related acute cryptococcal meningitis is needed.

It was recently reported that fluconazole is an effective alternative to amphotericin B as primary treatment of cryptococcal meningitis in patients with AIDS.[92] Fluconazole is a triazole antifungal compound which has high activity against *Cryptococcus neoformans* and has good oral bioavailability, is renally excreted, and has excellent penetration of the central nervous system (CNS). In this study, treatment was successful in 40% of those receiving amphotericin B and in 34% of those receiving fluconazole ($P = 0.40$). No significant differences in mortality were seen between the treatment groups, although there was a higher mortality seen in the first 2 weeks of therapy in the fluconazole treated group. Pretreatment factors predictive of early death included an abnormal mental status, a cerebral spinal fluid (CSF) cryptococcal antigen titer of more than 1:1024, and a positive blood culture for *C. neoformans.* The question remains concerning optimal therapy for patients classified as being high risk. However, this study does show that fluconazole is an effective alternative to amphotericin B for treatment of acute cryptococcal meningitis in patients with AIDS, particularly in patients at low risk for treatment failure.

Relapse of cryptococcal infection in patients with AIDS is a common problem. Studies have demonstrated relapse rates of 50% to 60% and a shorter life expectancy for patients who did not receive some form of chronic suppressive/maintenance therapy. Relapse most likely represents failure of the acute therapy to eradicate infection. One possibility is that acute therapy may sterilize the CSF, but not eradicate infection from extrameningeal studies, such as the urinary tract, which can serve as a focus for relapse. A recent randomized clinical trial that compared fluconazole (200 mg/day orally) with amphotericin B (1 mg/kg/week intravenously) in patients with AIDS who had completed primary therapy for cryptococcal meningitis with amphotericin B demonstrated that fluconazole is superior to weekly amphotericin B in preventing relapse of AIDS-associated cryptococcal meningitis.[93] In this study, 14 of 78 patients receiving amphotericin B (18%) and 2 of 111 patients receiving fluconazole (2%) had relapses of symptomatic disease. In addition, adverse events were reported much less frequently in the fluconazole group (38%) compared with the amphotericin B group (67%). This study strongly suggests that all patients with AIDS who complete primary therapy for cryptococcal meningitis should receive suppressive therapy with fluconazole at a dose of 200 mg/day.

Toxoplasma gondii causes multiple brain abscesses in patients with AIDS, usually those with CD4 cells $<100/mm^3$, and typically presents as a space-occupying cerebral lesion. Headaches and focal neurologic deficits in this population should prompt a computed tomography or magnetic resonance imaging of the brain. The lack of serum IgG antibodies to *T. gondii* makes the diagnosis unlikely; however, IgM serology is not helpful in confirming the diagnosis. Biopsy demonstrates the tachyzoites in brain tissue; however, it is justified in clinically suggestive cases to start empiric treatment and to perform a brain biopsy only if the patient does not respond to therapy within 2 weeks. Therapy consists of pyrimethamine (75 mg orally daily) and sulfadiazine (1–1.5 g orally every 6 hr), together with folinic acid (10 mg daily) with excellent initial response rates. Clindamycin (600 mg orally every 6 hr) can replace sulfadiazine in intolerant patients. After 6 weeks of therapy, patients should be placed on indefinite maintenance therapy with lower doses of pyrimethamine (25 mg orally weekly) and sulfadiazine (500 mg orally weekly) to prevent relapse. While there is no currently approved prophylaxis to prevent initial *T. gondii* abscess formation (in *Toxoplasma*-seropositive patients), several studies have suggested that patients who receive TMP-SMX for PCP prophylaxis have a significantly reduced incidence of toxoplasmosis than those receiving aerosolized pentamidine. Conclusive clinical trials to address *T. gondii* prophylaxis questions are under way.

Candida albicans is a common pathogen in AIDS patients, which primarily causes infection of the upper gastrointestinal tract (oral thrush, esophagitis) or vulvovaginal tract. It is frequently the first clinically recognized manifestation of HIV-1 infection. It can be diagnosed macroscopically (direct observation or endoscopy) and by Gram's stain or histology. Mild disease will respond to topical therapy (nystatin or clotrimazole). Fluconazole (100–200 mg daily) is a highly effective therapy that can eradicate moderate to severe infections. Ketoconazole (200 mg orally every 12 hr) is equally effective and less expensive. Therapy with amphotericin B is reserved for recalcitrant infections of the esophagus. Recurrences of *C. albicans* mucosal infections are common after successful therapy; however, the benign course of these infections makes routine prophylaxis unnecessary.

Mycobacterium tuberculosis (MTB) and *Mycobacterium-avium-complex* (MAC) are common pathogens in HIV-infected patients. MTB often presents as the first opportunistic infection, typically with CD4 positive T-cell counts > 200/mm^3. The impact of MTB and the problem of multidrug-resistant TB are discussed later under Special Topics. In contrast, MAC is typically isolated from patients with far advanced HIV-1 disease (CD4 positive T cells <50 mm^3), and recent studies have indicated that it does contribute to morbidity (fever, weight loss, wasting, diarrhea) and mortality in AIDS patients.[94] By the time the organism is cultured from the blood, the patient may have greater than 10^{10} organisms present per gram of tissue (lymph node, spleen, liver). A variety of antimicrobial agents have some activity against MAC, including rifabutin, clofazamine, clarithromycin, various quinolones, amikacin, and ethambutol; however, the optimal drug regimen that will produce either eradication of MAC or substantial lowering of the MAC burden remains to be defined. Trials to better define the optimal MAC treatment regimens as well as to define the utility of prophylaxis of MAC infection are currently under way. Recently, the FDA approved rifabutin for prophylaxis of MAC infection after two placebo controlled trials demonstrated its efficacy in delaying bacteremia.

The enteric pathogens *Cryptosporidia* and Microsporidia are being identified with increasing frequency in patients with very late-stage HIV infection. These organisms cause severe gastrointestinal (intractable diarrhea, wasting) or biliary disease that impinges significantly on the patient's quality of life. Unfortunately, there is no specific therapy that has been demonstrated to be effective in treating these pathogens. Clinical trials evaluating potential therapies (e.g., paramomycin, albendazole, letrazuril) for these enteric pathogens are in progress.

Vaccines

While considerable progress has been made toward the development of a vaccine to prevent infection with HIV, there are many obstacles on this pathway that are unique to HIV. These features of HIV include its ability to mutate rapidly, its ability to spread from cell to cell, its ability to remain latent or silent in an infected cell for years without expressing viral proteins, as well as its specific attack on the immune system itself.

The goal of most vaccines is to develop protective immunity which usually involves the development of humoral and/or cellular responses. These include: B cells which secrete antibodies, cytotoxic T cells that kill virus-infected cells thus preventing spread of virus, and helper T cells that regulate both of these functions. For HIV-1, however, there remain several major unanswered questions. First, we still do not know which of these types of immune responses are necessary for protection against HIV infection or the progression of HIV disease. Part of the problem in answering this question is that it is unlikely that anyone infected with HIV has been able to effectively eliminate the virus by developing protective immunity. Another difficulty is that only the great apes, such as chimpanzees, can be consistently infected with HIV-1, and even chimpanzees do not develop illness; therefore, we are limited in our ability to dissect out viral biology from immune response in these animals.

The most promising results in vaccine development for HIV infection have come from the model of SIV infection in monkeys. Several groups[95–98] have shown that it is possible to protect monkeys against SIV using a whole-virus vaccine. Interestingly, these vaccines were capable of protecting some monkeys against infection, while protecting other monkeys from developing fatal disease. These studies provide some optimism that the immune system might be able to protect against this virus, but they also suggest that it may be easier to protect against development of disease than to prevent infection altogether.

Another problem somewhat peculiar to HIV is that there are several mechanisms by which different types of antibody and cellular responses against certain components of HIV can contribute to the development of immunodeficiency by inhibiting or even destroying other cells of the immune system. Furthermore, there is evidence that certain antibodies directed against the env of HIV actually enhance rather than neutralize the infectivity of the virus.

The principal site on HIV-1 against which neutralizing antibodies are directed is the V3 loop sequence in the gp120 portion of the env protein.[99] Antibodies against this region generally neutralize viral infectivity and block syncytial formation in a type-specific manner. These antibodies do not block binding of HIV-1 to the CD4 molecule, its cellular receptor. Despite the high degree of variability in the V3 loop sequence, there is a central portion of the loop, that is relatively conserved from isolate to isolate. Therefore, it may be possible to construct a vaccine containing several of these loop sequences that together would elicit antibodies capable of neutralizing 85% or more of the known isolates of HIV. Variability of viral isolates is also a problem in that it occurs during the course of infection in a single individual. Escape variants arise during the course of HIV-1 infection, and over time the patient's serum antibodies lose their ability to neutralize the predominant isolate. Interestingly, some of these escape variants appear to have mutations that arise outside of the V3 loop itself, suggesting that mutations outside an antigenic site can affect the conformation of the V3 loop in such a way that it is no longer recognized by preexisting antibodies.

Despite the presence of neutralizing antibodies in infected patients, these antibodies do not prevent progression of disease. Thus, it is unclear whether such neutralizing antibodies are protective in vivo. Studies of passive transfer of antibodies in chimpanzees have been inconclusive. One study[100] found that neutralizing antibody mixed with a challenge-virus can prevent infection of chimpanzees. Another study[101] found that after immunizing chimpanzees with killed whole-virus and other vaccine preparations, boosting with a V3 loop peptide coupled to a carrier induced a higher level of neutralizing antibody, and two animals were subsequently protected from infection with live HIV challenge, while a third animal showed partial protection. Several studies examining the transfer of HIV-1 infection from mother to fetus/newborns in humans have suggested that antibodies to the V3 loop of gp120 can be protective.[17, 102, 103] The latter two studies demonstrated a significant correlation between the presence of V3 loop antibodies in the mother's blood and the failure to transmit the virus to her offspring. Therefore, there is some reason to believe that a high enough titer of neutralizing antibodies to the V3 loop can be protective, at least against the corresponding strain of HIV.

Several groups have recently reported the finding of antibodies from HIV-infected individuals that recognize conformation-dependent (i.e., discontinuous) epitopes in the gp120 env glycoprotein.[104–107] Two classes of neutralizing antibodies were elicited against HIV-1 in infected humans: (1) type-restricted neutralizing antibodies which arise early in infection and are usually directed against the V3 loop of gp120 recognize linear determinants and do not block CD4 binding, but may interfere with post-receptor binding events involved in viral entry and fusion; and (2) broadly neutralizing antibodies which arise later in the course of infection, and interfere with the binding of gp120 and CD4, and are against diverse HIV-1 isolates. This latter category of antibodies appears to recognize conformational or discontinuous epitopes in the gp120. The majority of antibodies elicited by subunit vaccines recognize linear epitopes in V3 and are type-specific. It is suggested that HIV vaccines that present conformation-dependent neutralization epitopes should be more effective than vaccines using only linear determinants. It will be important to determine the prevalence of conformation-dependent antibodies among people with HIV infection and to see how this correlates with clinical outcome.

Since it may be desirable to elicit a memory response when one is exposed to live HIV-1, it may be useful to include in a vaccine antigenic structures of HIV that can elicit T-cell help. Certain investigators[108] have identified regions of HIV that elicit helper T cells both in mice of multiple histocompatibility types and in humans of multiple HLA types. Four of these regions are in conserved portions of the env protein and should be less subject to the variability problem. It is possible that a handful of such antigenic sites may be sufficient to elicit immunity in the majority of the population. Palker et al.[109] have incorporated a helper T-cell epitope coupled to a V3 loop peptide which has elicited neutralizing activity in animals, and plans for studying this in humans are under way.

Cytotoxic T cells (CTL) specific for HIV-1 may be another critical arm of the immune response necessary to eliminate cells that are already infected with HIV-1, in addition to preventing spread of virus from cell to cell. In individuals infected with HIV-1, the frequencies of specific CTL are at a level higher than that seen in other viral infections. In addition, the CTL activity in the peripheral blood of such individuals can be detected without prior priming. Furthermore, CTL activity declines in patients with progressive HIV disease. CTL activity is detected during the period of acute HIV-1 infection in individuals, prior to the development of antibodies. This is associated with a rapid decline in the level of viral expression, with the subsequent entry into the clinically latent phase of HIV-1 disease. This evidence strongly supports the view that HIV-specific CTL are important in controlling disease progression and suggests that they may also be a critical and necessary component of an immune response elicited by a vaccine.

Other studies[110, 111] have identified an immunodominant antigen site seen by CTL of mice specific for HIV envelope and recognized by $CD8^+$ CTL of HIV-infected humans. This site has also been shown to be recognized by $CD8^+$ CTL of human volunteers immunized with a recombinant vaccinia virus expressing the HIV env protein.[112]

Other experiments suggest that vaccine design should take into account the ability of different HIV isolates to broaden CTL activity following an initial priming immunization.[113] In these studies of mice primed with strain IIIB, only the strain MN-specific env CTLs (but not strain IIIB or RF-specific env CTLs) that were generated following MN antigen boosts were capable of eliciting env CTL populations with broad specificity.

Additional CTL sites have been identified on several HIV proteins including RT,[114, 115] nef,[116] and gag.[117] In each case, there appear to be far fewer sites recognized by CTL than by helper T cells, and this limited number of critical antigenic sites may make it easier for the virus to escape CTL. In addition, because HIV has been found to vary its sequence during the course of infection of a single individual, such variation could contribute to escape of HIV from CTL immunity, leading to progression of disease.

During the past year, a great deal more has been learned about protective immune responses in animal models of HIV vaccines. One group of investigators has shown that protective immunity can be elicited in macaques by recombinant subunit vaccines.[118] The approach taken was a combination-immunization regimen that included the use of live recombinant vaccinia virus containing the entire SIV env for priming and a subunit immunogen (gp160) for boosting. All immunized animals showed high-level antibody response against SIV env antigens, with significant serum neutralizing activities against SIV. After challenge with an IV inoculation of SIV, four control animals readily demonstrated infection, while all four immunized macaques remained virus-negative for at lest 1 year after challenge. These findings argue for further testing of this combination-immunization approach in animal models and ultimately in humans.

In another important study, researchers have reported that macaque monkeys vaccinated with inactivated, whole-virus SIV cloned in human cells can resist challenge with free, uncloned SIV with an env that differed by 20% from the vaccine virus.[119] In this study, six animals vaccinated with SIV and four animals vaccinated with HBsAg were intravenously challenged with homologous virus (SIV with 94% env similarity to vaccine virus), while four animals vaccinated with SIV and two animals vaccinated with HBsAg were intravenously challenged with heterologous SIV (SIV with 81% env similarity to vaccine virus). All control monkeys developed SIV after challenge. In contrast, none of the animals given SIV vaccine became infected.

Because of recent studies suggesting that neutralizing antibodies in SIV vaccine experiments are actually anti-cell antibodies directed against the human cells used to propagate the vaccine virus, the authors investigated this in their experiments. They found that plasma samples depleted of anti-cell antibodies retained high-titer neutralizing activity, and that any anti-cell antibodies elicited in response to whole SIV vaccine did not play a major role in in vitro neutralization of SIV. These studies of inactivated whole-SIV vaccines suggest that the development of an efficacious HIV vaccine might be possible.

As described previously, researchers over the last 2 to 3 years have developed vaccines that can protect a chimpanzee or macaque against infection with cell-free HIV or SIV, respectively. Transmission of HIV in humans can occur with either cell-associated and/or cell-free virus. Therefore, any effective vaccine against HIV must protect against both viral forms. The first experiments that demonstrate protection of chimpanzees against challenge with HIV-infected PBMCs have now been reported.[120] These chimpanzees, which had been previously immunized with a variety of HIV antigens and successfully challenged with cell-free HIV-1, were challenged (along with a control chimpanzee) with HIV-1-infected chimp PBMCs. The control chimpanzee was infected while the vaccinated chimpanzees were all protected. However, one chimpanzee was rechallenged with cell-free HIV-1 1 year after the successful cell-associated HIV-1 challenge (and 2 years following the initial cell-free HIV-1 challenge) and was readily infected. Thus, it appeared that the immune response elicited by vaccination did not persist at a level sufficient to protect against this last virus challenge. It is unclear why the vaccine failed at this point. Equally uncertain is the mechanism by which the vaccine worked in the first place. CTL activity has never been detected in PBMCs from immunized chimpanzees. More likely mechanisms of protection include antibody-dependent cellular cytotoxicity and antibody-complement-mediated cytotoxicity, both of which have been detected previously in the serum of immunized animals. This would include antibodies to the V3 loop which inhibit cell fusion. It is probable, however, that both HIV-specific antibodies and cell-mediated activities synergize to effect protection.

Over the past few years, the AIDS Vaccine Evaluation Units in the United States sponsored by the National Institute of Allergy and Infectious Diseases (NIAID) have been studying several candidate HIV-1 env vaccines in healthy HIV-1 seronegative volunteers (Table 5). Some of these candidates have been tested for their safety and immunogenicity. To date, none of these candidate vaccines caused any serious adverse effects and all demonstrated varying degrees of immunogenicity. Humoral and cell-mediated immune responses were dose-dependent and varied by vaccine preparation. Neutralizing antibodies, albeit of generally low titer, were seen with all vaccine products in most volunteers. In terms of cell-mediated immunity, all vaccine candidates were able to elicit lymphoproliferative responses in most volunteers. CTL activity was seen following vaccination in several individuals. Responses to priming with HIVAC-1e and boosting with VaxSyn rpg160 included both humoral and cell-mediated immune responses (in vaccinia-naive volunteers) and were better than those seen with either vaccine alone. Silicano and coworkers detected $CD8^+$ CTL activity after this priming/boosting in 2 of 2 volunteers at 2 weeks following the boost. However, this activity was no longer detectable 1 year following the boost.

There is a compelling need to identify potential vaccine candidates for efficacy trials. For the majority of the developing world, the rapidity of the rise in new infections with HIV-1 portends tragic consequences. In the United States, the NIAID is preparing for field evaluations of HIV vaccine candidates which, it is hoped, can be initiated by 1994 (S. Vermund, personal communication, 1992). To this end, studies are under way to determine feasibility and seroincidence in persons at high risk for HIV-1 infection. Cohorts are being systematically identified and surveyed for their suitability for HIV vaccine trials. Important information to be gathered includes the feasibility of recruiting and retaining cohorts with seroincidence targets of 2% to 5%, behavioral data on incidence after counseling and testing, level of community acceptance, genetic and immunologic features of the virus circulating in the projected communities, as well as vaccine availability. Preliminary evaluations show that injection drug users in certain eastern U.S. cities may have 1% to 4% annual seroincidence rates. Other U.S. populations with sufficiently high seroincidence for preventive vaccine trials may include young gay men and high-risk heterosexuals. It is estimated that between 2,000 and 5,000 volunteers will be needed to evaluate a vaccine in a community with a seroincidence of 2%, assuming 60% efficacy in preventing infection.

The World Health Organization (WHO) has also formulated a comprehensive strategy for AIDS vaccine development. WHO has initiated a number of activities to strengthen potential sites for vaccine evaluation in developing countries and has identified four countries (Brazil, Rwanda, Thailand, and Uganda) as the initial sites that would receive WHO support, with a final goal of testing the efficacy of preventive vaccines. In collaboration with WHO, these countries have developed national plans which include infrastructure strengthening, training, and research in four areas: HIV virology, clinical trials of candidate vaccines, cohort studies on HIV seroincidence, and social and behavioral studies. This will require close collaboration with other national/international AIDS vaccine research programs and with vaccine manufacturers.

TABLE 5.
Vaccine Trials in Seronegative Individuals Worldwide

Source	Vaccine	Cell System	Strain	Adjuvant	Sites
Envelope proteins					
MicroGeneSys	gp160	Baculovirus/insect	LAV	Alum	NIAID*
ImmunoAG	gp160	Monkey kidney/vaccinia	IIIB	Alum + DOC	NIAID
Chiron/Biocine	env2–3	Yeast	SF2	Emulsion ± MTP-PE	Hospital Canton
				MF59 ± MTP-PE	NIAID
Chiron/Biocine	gp120	Chinese hamster ovary	SF2	MF59 ± MTP-PE	Univ of California, San Francisco
					NIAID
Genentech	gp120IIIB	Chinese hamster ovary	IIIB	Alum	NIAID
Genentech	gp120MN	Chinese hamster ovary	MN	Alum	NIAID
Core proteins/peptides					
Viral Technologies	HGP30	Synthetic p17 peptide		Alum	St. Stephens Univ of California, San Francisco
Brit. Biotech. Ltd.	Ty-gag	Portion p17/p24 + yeast transposon product P1		Alum	St. Mary's Hosp, London
Swiss Serum and Vaccine Institute	V3-PPD	Purified Protein Derivative coupled V3 peptide	MN		SSVI/Rubinstein

Recombinant poxvirus					
Bristol-Myers Squibb Oncogen	vac-gp160	Recombinant vaccinia	IIIB		Univ of Wash, Seattle NIAID
Combination studies					
	vac-gp 160+gp160 (baculovirus) vac-gp160+gp160 + infected autologous cells				Univ of Wash, Seattle NIAID Zagury
Pasteur-Merieux-Connaught (Virogenetics)	CP-125	Canarypox-gp160 plus rgp160 boost	MN/LAI		PMSV/ANRS†
Pasteur-Merieux-Connaught (Transgene)	rgp160	Mammalian plus V3 peptide boost	MN/LAI MN	Alum/IFA Alum/IFA	PMSV/ANRS
Yokohama City Univ, Japan	mixed HIV peptides	KLH carrier synthetic	MN, RF IIIB		

*NIAID = Laboratory of Immunoregulation (first MicroGeneSys Trial) and AIDS Vaccine Evaluation Group: Johns Hopkins University, St. Louis University, University of Rochester, University of Washington, Vanderbilt University (former members: Baylor University, University of Maryland), Duke University (Central Immunology Laboratory), The EMMES Corporation.

†PMSV = Pasteur Merieux Serums et Vaccins; ANRS = Agence Nationale de Recherches sur SID.

Special Topics

CDC Revised Classification System for HIV Infection and Disease in Adolescents and Adults

With the rapid growth of knowledge concerning the natural history of HIV infection, the availability of new antiretroviral agents, and the use of CD4 lymphocyte testing to guide medical management of HIV-infected individuals, there has been an increasing need for a simpler, prognostically oriented system that could be used by clinicians and public health workers for categorizing conditions occurring in persons infected with HIV-1. The revised system[121] can be displayed as a matrix of mutually exclusive categories hierarchically arrayed along two axes. The first axis has three clinical categories of conditions attributable to HIV infection (asymptomatic, symptomatic not AIDS, AIDS). The second axis has three laboratory categories indicative of cell-mediated immune status as measured by $CD4^+$ lymphocyte counts ($CD4^+$ T-cell count/mm^3 >500, 201–499, and <200, or CD4% of total lymphocytes of >25%, 11% to 24%, and <10%, respectively). The revised HIV classification system can be used by states currently conducting surveillance for all cases of HIV infection. Since surveillance definition of AIDS only reflects a fraction of the morbidity caused by HIV infection, the revised classification may be particularly useful in determining the impact of the HIV epidemic on the health care system. In addition, since the $CD4^+$ T-lymphocyte levels of 500 and 200 are the recommended mileposts for initiating antiretroviral therapy and prophylaxis against PCP respectively, the collection of this information can be used to guide clinical care of individuals infected with HIV.

Special Problems of HIV Infection in Women

In 1991, the Surgeon General reported that the incidence of AIDS had increased by 29% in women as compared with 18% in men,[122] and women now comprise over 11% of persons with AIDS in the United States. Due to a marked increase in HIV infection among women during the mid-1980s, the male-to-female ratio of HIV infection in patients attending Baltimore STD clinics declined from 16:1 in 1978–1982 to 1:1 in 1988–1989.[123] Globally, over 3 million women are estimated to die from AIDS during the 1990s.

Gender influences the social and biologic consequences of HIV disease.[124] Women are more likely than men to rely on clinic care or to need drug rehabilitation services. The pharmacokinetics of drugs may vary with gender. In addition, a gender effect on survival of AIDS patients has been described, although the contributions of biologic factors and access-to-care differences remain to be determined.

Several studies have focused on the relationship between HIV disease, human papillomavirus (HPV) infection, and cervical neoplasia. While there are preliminary suggestions of an increased incidence of abnormal Pap smears among HIV-infected women, well-controlled studies remain to be done. One study[125] found, among women undergoing both Pap tests and colposcopic-directed biopsy, that while only 3% had Pap tests suggesting cervical intraepithelial neoplasia (CIN), 42% were documented to have histologic evidence of CIN by biopsy. This questions the adequacy of Pap tests as a screening tool in women with HIV infection. Other studies suggest the aggressive nature of CIN in HIV-infected women. In contrast to HIV seronegative women, women with HIV disease present with more advanced cervical neoplasia, CIN recurs more rapidly when advanced disease is found, and these patients have more rapid fatalities due to advanced cervical disease. These findings argue for more frequent and more aggressive evaluation to detect the presence of CIN in addition to more aggressive treatment when CIN is found.

Several gynecologic infections have been reported to have their natural course modified by HIV infection. Pelvic inflammatory disease (PID) has been noted to appear with less leukocytosis, but with more abscesses and a greater need for surgical intervention. Vaginal candidiasis is a common gynecologic infection in HIV-infected women, and it has been commonly noted in those with normal CD4 counts, prior to the appearance of either oral or esophageal candidiasis. Responses of vaginal candidiasis to topical and oral systemic antifungal agents appear to be good. Genital ulcer disease is common in women with HIV infection, and such women may shed virus more frequently than women without genital ulcers. There are also suggestions that herpes simplex virus, chancroid, and syphilis may be more refractory to recommended therapies, and this should be kept in mind when treating these genital ulcerative diseases.

Regarding obstetrical care, no alteration from standard care is needed for asymptomatic, pregnant HIV-seropositive women. It is appropriate to adhere to the same standards as used for nonpregnant women when trying to guide the use of medications in pregnant women. It is recommended that pregnant women with CD4 counts below 200 receive both antiretroviral therapy as well as prophylaxis against PCP. The benefits vs. the risk of antiretroviral therapy in pregnant women with CD4 counts between 200 and 500 cells/mm^3 is uncertain and should be determined on a case by case basis.

Tuberculosis, Multi-drug Resistant Tuberculosis, and HIV

Tuberculosis has always been an important cause of morbidity and death in the United States as well as the rest of the world. At the beginning of this century, TB was a leading cause of death in the United States. Through the efforts of physicians, public health officials, and researchers combined with improvements in living conditions and the introduction of effective drug therapy, the number of TB cases and deaths steadily declined from 1945 to 1985. However, since 1985, these rates have plateaued and are actually now increasing. An estimated 39,000 excess cases of TB have occurred from 1985 to 1991 (Fig 3). One major contributing

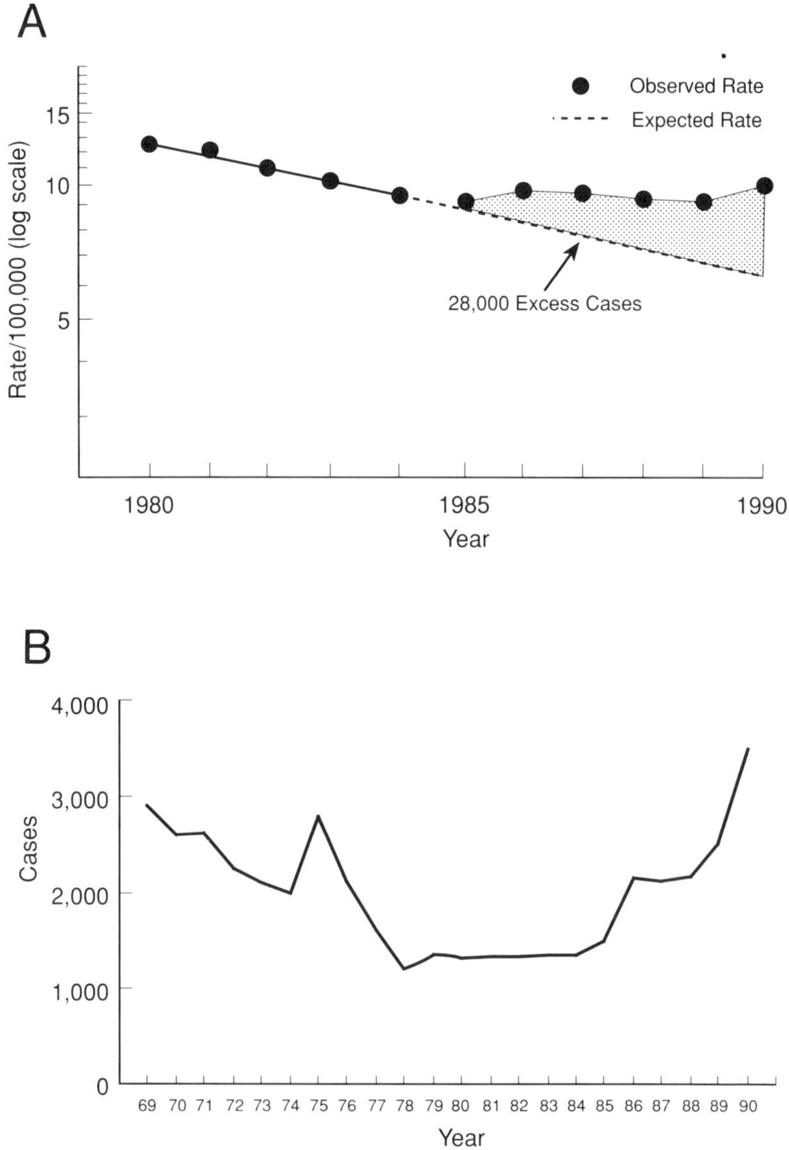

FIG 3.
A, expected and observed U.S. TB cases, 1980 to 1990. (Data from Centers for Disease Control, Atlanta, Georgia. **B,** reported TB cases, New York City, 1969 to 1990. (Data from New York City Department of Health, New York, NY.)

factor to this trend is that individuals infected with HIV are more likely than otherwise healthy persons to reactivate latent TB as well as to develop active disease rapidly when exposed to TB. Other causes include the increased immigration from countries with high TB prevalence, the emergence of drug-resistant strains of TB, and transmission among persons in crowded living environments such as homeless shelters, correctional facilities, and nursing homes. In 1990, nearly 24,000 cases of TB were reported to the CDC, and about 2,000 persons died that year from TB. It is estimated that one third of the world's population is infected with TB, with 10 million new cases developing annually, and 3 million people dying from TB each year. In addition, 10 million individuals in the U.S. are estimated to be infected with TB and are therefore at risk for developing active clinical TB at some point in their lives.

The most serious aspect of the TB problem has been the recent occurrence of outbreaks of multi-drug resistant (MDR) TB, which poses an urgent public health problem.[126–130] The rise in drug-resistant TB and the outbreaks of MDR-TB are a manifestation of serious underlying problems in the health care infrastructure. In a recent survey in New York City, 33% of the patients infected with TB had organisms resistant to at least one drug, and 19% had organisms resistant to both isoniazid (INH) and rifampin, the two most effective drugs available for treating TB. Drug-resistant TB is not limited to New York City. The CDC recently conducted a nationwide survey of drug resistance among all TB cases provisionally reported during the first 3 months of 1991. Overall, 14.9% of patients tested had organisms resistant to at least one antituberculous drug, and 3.3% had organisms resistant to both INH and rifampin. These trends represent a major increase over the last few years.

The CDC,[131] in collaboration with state and local health departments and hospital officials, conducted investigations of six outbreaks of MDR-TB in hospitals, with a total of over 200 cases. In each instance, the epidemiologic evidence of person-to-person nosocomial transmission had been compelling and supported by DNA fingerprinting, i.e., restriction fragment length polymorphism (RFLP). Virtually all of these patients had organisms resistant to both INH and rifampin, and in three hospitals, the outbreak strain was resistant to seven anti-TB drugs. Mortality among patients with MDR-TB has been extraordinarily high (72% to 89%) and is associated with a rapid progression from diagnosis to death on the order of weeks. Over 80% of cases in each outbreak occurred in individuals infected with HIV. These distinctive drug resistance patterns and temporal clustering caused by the extremely rapid progression to active disease in immunocompromised patients with MDR-TB led to the recognition of the outbreaks.[131] At least eight health care workers at the outbreak hospitals have developed active MDR-TB. Four of the eight were HIV seropositive and have died of their TB. These findings support the need of protecting health care workers from infection and disease due to MDR-TB.

In a New York State correctional facility, eight inmates developed MDR-TB in 1991—all of whom were HIV seropositive, and all of whom died. Again, epidemiologic evidence and RFLP analyses suggest transmission within this and other state correctional facilities. In addition, about 50 health care workers at a nearby hospital who were exposed to the inmates had tuberculin skin test conversions.

There are several factors that contribute to outbreaks of MDR-TB in institutional settings. First, TB control programs have difficulty ensuring patient compliance with anti-TB therapy, and poor compliance may lead to the development of drug-resistant organisms, which can be transmitted. Second, there is an increasing incidence of TB in those areas where there is a high seroprevalence of HIV, such as in prisons, homeless shelters, and drug treatment facilities. Therefore, contact between persons with active TB and immunocompromised individuals has risen. Third, institutions may have inadequate infection-control/isolation practices to prevent transmission of TB. In addition, a failure to recognize and diagnose TB, and long delays in laboratory isolation and reporting of species and sensitivity, have contributed to these outbreaks. As a result, initiation of effective anti-TB therapy is delayed, leading to prolonged periods during which patients with MDR-TB are essentially untreated and infectious.

The response to the problem of TB, MDR-TB, and its relation to HIV must be addressed on many levels. First, steps need to be taken to ensure that patients with drug-susceptible TB adhere to the prescribed drug regimen so that drug resistance does not develop (e.g., directly observed therapy). Second, current CDC guidelines to reduce the risk of TB transmission need to be implemented. Third, there need to be epidemiologic studies to better define risk factors for transmission of MDR-TB. Fourth, there must be improved use of currently available tools for diagnosing, treating, and preventing TB. Fifth, research must be intensified to identify more rapid diagnostic techniques, new therapies, and new preventive measures. And finally, education of health workers about MDR-TB and TB infection control must be addressed. A federal TB task force has been established to coordinate these efforts and will require prompt, intense, collaborative action among governmental agencies and the private sector.

Gene Therapy

It has become clear that despite intensive efforts at developing antiretroviral therapies that can arrest HIV viral replication, eradicate infected cell reservoirs, and restore a functional immune system, conventional strategies have thus far failed to achieve these goals. This inability to cure AIDS is contributed to by the unique pathogenic mechanisms of this virus. The development of novel and unorthodox treatment strategies are beginning to receive serious consideration. In its broadest concept, gene therapy is such a novel approach, in that genes that can either be protective of HIV spread or will permit reconstitution of an immune system that is resistant to HIV infection can be used to treat the infected host.

"Intracellular immunization" is a term used to describe a process in which cells are genetically altered to become resistant to pathogens. This process is achieved by stable introduction of a DNA template (i.e., "resistance gene") into cells, whose continuous expression inhibits the expression of an essential viral gene, and hence inhibits viral replication. Since HIV infects hemopoietic cells, insertion of "resistance genes" into such cells could reduce, if not eliminate, the spread of virus in the body. Work by Gilboa's laboratory has developed an intracellular immunization strategy to render cells highly resistant to HIV replication and its cytopathic effects. The salient features of this system are: (1) a novel inhibition strategy utilizing "trans-acting response (TAR) element decoys" to block the function of the tat gene (Fig 4); (2) a tRNA-based expression system required to generate sufficient amounts of TAR RNA; and (3) a novel retroviral design to accommodate tRNA genes, termed double-copy or DC-vector design. The effectiveness of this approach to inhibit HIV replication was demonstrated in cell cultures using an established T-cell line, CEM SS.[132, 133] In brief, since tat must bind to TAR for viral transcription to occur, overexpression of RNA containing TAR is capable of acting as a decoy for tat binding, preventing its binding to the TAR sequence in the viral RNA. This has been demonstrated to inhibit HIV viral replication in the CEM-SS T-cell line. An extension of this inhibition strategy to the rev system (rev responsive element [RRE] decoys) has also been described (T. Lee, personal communication).[134]

Another proposed means of achieving intracellular immunization to HIV is the insertion into bone marrow stem cells of toxin-coding genes linked to the HIV promoter sequence, so-called suicide gene therapy.[135] Such genes would be expressed only at very low levels until they are infected with HIV. Upon infection with HIV, the tat protein would induce high-level expression of the toxin, resulting in the death of the cells harboring the virus. Unfortunately, even the low levels of toxin produced in the absence of HIV could kill normal cells.

A related approach has been suggested by several investigators.[135, 136] This approach would utilize the HSV-1 thymidine kinase (HSV1-TK) which efficiently phosphorylates nucleoside analogs such as acyclovir into monophosphorylated molecules. These are converted into nucleoside triphosphates that are incorporated into elongating DNA by cellular polymerases, causing chain termination and eventually cell death. Thus, high level expression of this gene renders cells sensitive to the cytopathic effects of acyclovir; the drug is harmless to normal human cells, since they do not produce the thymidine kinase needed to activate the drug. This approach has been called "thymidine kinase obliteration." Caruso and Klatzmann recently reported the stable expression of the HSV1-TK gene under the control of the HIV promoter in $CD4^+$ cells.[135] Upon HIV infection these regulatory sequences were transactivated leading to high level expression of HSV1-TK. This led to the death of HIV-infected cells when they were cultured in the presence of acyclovir. The elimination of HIV-infected cells resulted in the halting of HIV spread in the tissue culture. Studies are under way to determine ways to deliver HSV1-TK plasmids into patients with HIV infection. Possible approaches include the use of adenovirus vectors,

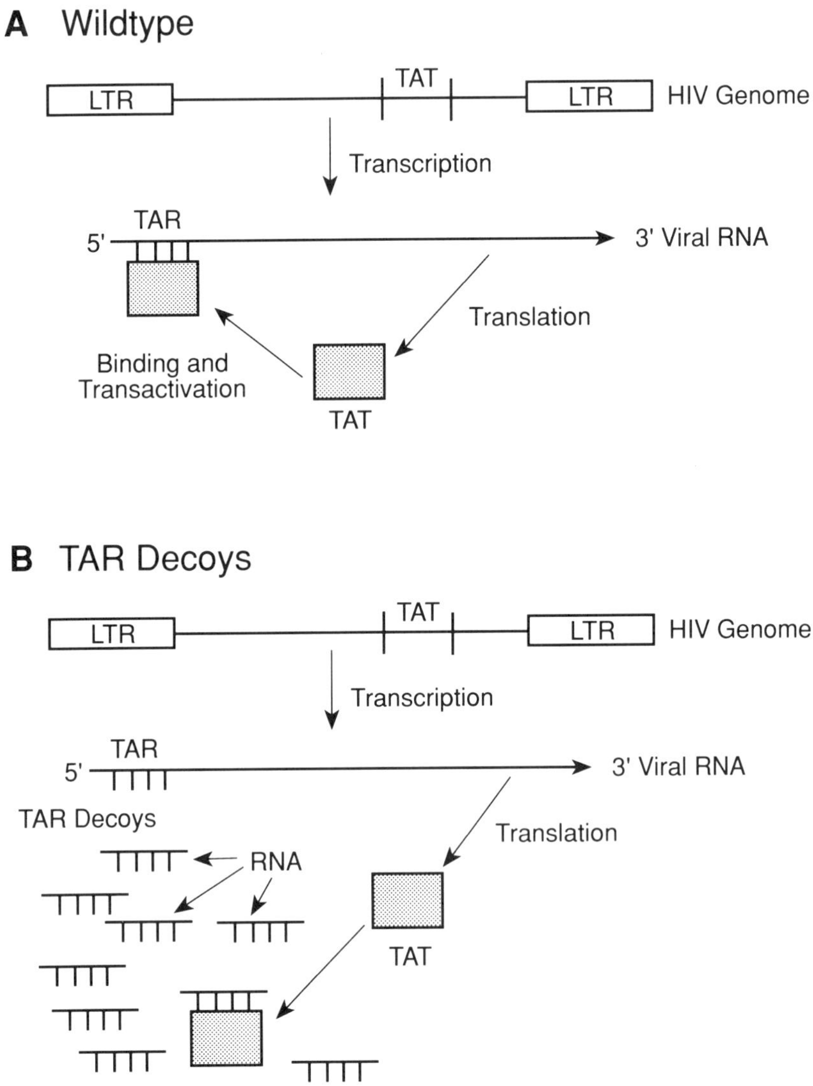

FIG 4.
Gene therapy: HIV replication in the absence **(A)** and presence **(B)** of TAR decoys expressed by a genetically engineered vector. In the wild type infection **(A),** tat protein binds to TAR on expressed HIV viral RNA, leading to transactivation, with production of viral proteins. In the presence of many TAR RNA decoys that have been expressed by a vector, tat protein binds preferentially to the decoys in lieu of the normal binding of tat to viral TAR RNA, thereby inhibiting viral replication.

or murine amphotropic retroviral vectors and packaging cell lines. The aim would be to transfer the genes to stem cells in the bone marrow which would be resistant to HIV infection.

The optimal approach to generating sustained populations of HIV-resistant CD4$^+$ T-cells and monocytes in the HIV infected patient would be via transduction of totipotent hemopoietic stem cells. The insertion of resistance genes into the donor bone marrow-derived stem cell could provide the necessary protection from infection with HIV. The development of effective methods to isolate purified human stem cells and introduce genes into them is still a major hurdle facing the application of intracellular immunization strategies. An alternative approach that is being pursued involves the insertion of the resistance gene directly into CD4$^+$ peripheral T cells. A number of studies have shown that human T cells can be efficiently transduced with retroviral vectors and can persist for over 90 days in the patient. In fact, this approach which targets mature T cells is similar to the first gene therapy protocol for adenosine deaminase deficiency (ADA) deficiency/severe combined immunodeficiency (SCID), which has had some early success. Unfortunately, targeting mature T cells will provide only limited protection from HIV spread in the body, and it is not clear whether this approach will be effective in halting disease progression. Nonetheless, there are plans underway to explore the possibility of transducing viral resistance genes, such as the TAR decoys, into peripheral T cells, in order to determine their survival in HIV-infected individuals.

Summary and Conclusions

Research progress in the understanding of HIV and its effects on the human immune system continues at a rapid pace. Such research is yielding new ideas for chemotherapeutic agents, immunologic stimulators and modifiers, and potential vaccines. Clinical trials to test these approaches are under way. Despite the accomplishments, the epidemic progresses unchecked, resulting in continued suffering and death and enormous demands on the health care system of many nations. Clinicians have had to deal with new and difficult opportunistic infections. Yet advances in the treatment and prevention of these illnesses have benefited many AIDS victims.

In the United States, the AIDS epidemic is now concentrating in the inner cities, involving injection drug users, minorities, heterosexuals, women and their offspring. In the developing world, AIDS continues to be predominantly a heterosexually transmitted disease, where more than one third of prostitutes in central African cities are infected. The major burden of the AIDS epidemic in the remainder of this and the next century will be in India and Southeast Asia, again predominantly via heterosexual spread.

A great deal is now understood concerning the life cycle of HIV. More light has been shed on the interaction of HIV and CD4$^+$ T cells, the cellular and viral factors involved in viral expression vs. latency, the function of the viral regulatory and structural proteins, and the role of cytokines in regulation of HIV expression. Our understanding of the precise mechanisms whereby HIV causes a loss of CD4$^+$ T cells remains incomplete. The direct infection and cell killing of CD4$^+$ T cells is important and is supported by recent evidence demonstrating a high viral burden in these cells in the lymphoid tissue of patients. Over the last 1 to 2 years, there has been new evidence for indirect mechanisms of CD4$^+$ T-cell depletion and/or dysfunction including: autoimmune reactions, perturbations of specific Vβ T-cell receptor populations, infection of T-cell precursors in bone marrow and thymus, immunosuppression and dysregulation by viral proteins, possible superantigen effects, and antigen-induced apoptosis or programmed cell death. New information has come forth in our understanding of B-cell abnormalities in HIV pathogenesis, including the putative role of IL-6 in B-cell activation and the identification of EBV in B-cell lymphomas in the CNS of patients with AIDS. It is expected that these and future discoveries concerning immunopathogenesis of HIV infection will help steer the therapeutic effort.

Major strides continue to be made in the therapeutic arena for HIV infection and its complications. Under the new "accelerated approval" mechanism of the FDA, two nucleoside RT inhibitors have been licensed for late-stage HIV disease, either as a single agent, namely ddI, or in combination with ZDV, namely ddC. In addition, much progress has been made on the molecular level in understanding the development of resistance to antiretroviral therapies. The clinical implications of resistance remain to be defined.

There are early studies under way of newer antiretroviral therapies, including protease inhibitors and tat inhibitors. In addition, newer approaches to treatment of HIV infection have either recently begun or will begin in the very near future. These include therapeutic vaccination with viral proteins in an effort to bolster the immune response and gene therapy which will attempt to insert protective genes into either stem cells or peripheral T cells making such cells resistant to HIV infection or spread (i.e., intracellular immunization).

The results of several important controlled clinical trials have added greatly to the approaches of treatment and prophylaxis of opportunistic infections. The important role of TMP-SMX for the prevention of PCP, the efficacy and effects on survival of ganciclovir and foscarnet for treatment of CMV retinitis, and the utility of fluconazole as an alternative to amphotericin B for treatment and maintenance therapy of cryptococcal meningitis in patients with AIDS have been defined. The new threat from the rising incidence of TB, its interaction with the HIV-infected host, and the development of MDR-TB will clearly be the focus of considerable attention in the coming years.

New progress continues to be made toward the development of a vaccine to prevent HIV infection. The most important epitopes for development of neutralizing antibodies against the various strains of HIV are being defined. In addition, critical immunodominant epitopes needed for development of cytotoxic T-cell responses against HIV-1 are being described, as well as the utility of priming and boosting to broaden the specificity of the response. Some very promising results have come from animal models of vaccine development that have yielded much information about protective immune responses. Successful vaccination-challenge studies in primates provide hope that an effective vaccine will be developed for HIV in humans. To this end, numerous phase I studies of vaccine candidates have been completed and are ongoing in an effort to identify promising vaccines for efficacy trials. A major effort is required to overcome the many obstacles to developing vaccine efficacy trials. While the risks are high, the need to identify an efficacious vaccine for preventing HIV-1 is compelling.

Acknowledgments

The authors would like to thank Dr. Zeda Rosenberg and Dr. Sten Vermund for their scientific contributions and Mary Rust for her editorial assistance.

References

1. Centers for Disease Control: HIV/AIDS surveillance. *CDC* 1992; April:1–18.
2. Mann JM: AIDS—the second decade: A global perspective. *J Infect Dis* 1992; 165:245–250.
3. Hom D, Guay L, Mmiro F, et al: HIV-1 seroprevalence rates in women attending a prenatal clinic in Kampala, Uganda. *VII International Conference on AIDS* 1991; 361. (Abstract)
4. Allen S, Lindan C, Serufilira A, et al: Human immunodeficiency virus infection in urban Rwanda Demographic and behavioral correlates in a representative sample of childbearing women. *JAMA* 1991; 266:1657–1663.
5. Nzila N, Laga M, Thiam MA, et al: HIV and other sexually transmitted diseases among female prostitutes in Kinshasa. *AIDS* 1991; 5:715–721.
6. Theetranont C, Suprasert S, Renyen S, et al: Heterosexually transmitted HIV among young Thai males. *VIII International Conference on AIDS* (abstract). 1992; 226.
7. Estimates of HIV prevalence and projected AIDS cases: Summary of a workshop, October 31-November 1, 1989. *MMWR* 1990; 39:110–2, 117–9.
8. Update: Acquired immunodeficiency syndrome—United States, 1991. *MMWR* 1992; 41:463–468.
9. Brookmeyer R: Reconstruction and future trends of the AIDS epidemic in the United States. *Science* 1991; 253:37–42.
10. Rosenberg PS, Levy ME, Brundage JF, et al: Population-based monitoring of an urban HIV/AIDS epidemic. Magnitude and trends in the District of Columbia. *JAMA* 1992; 268:495–503.
11. Padian NS, Shiboski SC, Jewell NP: Female-to-male transmission of human immunodeficiency virus. *JAMA* 1991; 266:1664–1667.
12. Hook EW, Cannon RO, Nahmias AJ, et al: Herpes simplex virus infection as a risk factor for human immunodeficiency virus infection in heterosexuals. *J Infect Dis* 1992; 165:251–255.
13. Gwinn M, Pappaioanou M, George JR, et al: Prevalence of HIV infection in

childbearing women in the United States. Surveillance using newborn blood samples. *JAMA* 1991; 265:1704–1708.
14. European Collaborative Study: Children born to women with HIV-1 infection: Natural history and risk of transmission. *Lancet* 1991; 337:253–260.
15. Goedert JJ, Duliège AM, Amos CI, et al: High risk of HIV-1 infection for first-born twins. The International Registry of HIV-exposed Twins. *Lancet* 1991; 338:1471–1475.
16. Rossi P, Moschese V, Broliden PA, et al: Presence of maternal antibodies to human immunodeficiency virus I envelope glycoprotein *gp*[120] epitopes correlates with the uninfected status of children born to seropositive mothers. *Proc Natl Acad Sci USA* 1989; 86:8055–8058.
17. Devash Y, Calvelli TA, Wood DG, et al: Vertical transmission of human immunodeficiency virus is correlated with the absence of high-affinity/avidity maternal antibodies to the gp120 principal neutralizing domain. *Proc Natl Acad Sci USA* 1990; 87:3445–349.
18. Burns D, Muenz L, Walsh J, et al: Correlation of perinatal transmission of HIV-1 with mothers lowest prepartum CD4 level. *31st Interscience Conference on Antimicrobials Agents and Chemotherapy* (abstract) 1991; 176.
19. Henderson DK, Fahey BJ, Willy M, et al: Risk for occupational transmission of human immunodeficiency virus type 1 (HIV-1) associated with clinical exposures. A prospective evaluation. *Ann Intern Med* 1990; 113:740–746.
20. Update—transmission of HIV infection during an invasive dental procedure—Florida. *MMWR* 1991; 40:21–7, 33.
21. Rosenberg ZF, Fauci AS: The immunopathogenesis of HIV infection. *Adv Immunol* 1989; 47:377–431.
22. Dalgleish AG, Beverley PC, Clapham PR, et al: The CD4 (T4) antigen is an essential component of the receptor for the AIDS retrovirus. *Nature* 1984; 312:763–767.
23. Klatzmann D, Champagne E, Chamaret S, et al: T-lymphocyte T4 molecule behaves as the receptor for human retrovirus LAV. *Nature* 1984; 312:767–768.
24. McDougal JS, Kennedy MS, Sligh JM, et al: Binding of HTLV-III/LAV to T4+ T cells by a complex of the 110K viral protein and the T4 molecule. *Science* 1986; 231:382–385.
25. Klotman ME, Wong-Staal F: Human immunodeficiency virus (HIV) gene structure and genetic diversity, in Gallo RC, Jay G (eds): *The Human Retroviruses*. San Diego, Academic Press, Inc., 1991, pp 35–68.
26. Haseltine WA: The molecular biology of HIV-1, in DeVita VT Jr., Hellman S, Rosenberg SA (eds): *AIDS: Etiology, Diagnosis, Treatment, and Prevention*. Philadelphia, JB Lippincott Co, 1992, pp 39–59.
27. Fauci AS: The human immunodeficiency virus: infectivity and mechanisms of pathogenesis. *Science* 1988; 239:617–622.
28. Rosenberg ZF, Fauci AS: Immunopathogenic mechanisms of HIV infection: Cytokine induction of HIV expression. *Immunol Today* 1990; 11:176–180.
29. Schnittman SM, Psallidopoulos MC, Lane HC, et al: The reservoir for HIV-1 in human peripheral blood is a T cell that maintains expression of CD4. *Science* 1989; 245:305–308.
30. Bukrinsky MI, Stanwick TL, Dempsey MP, et al: Quiescent T lymphocytes as an inducible virus reservoir in HIV-1 infection. *Science* 1991; 254:423–427.
31. Poli G, Fauci AS: The effect of cytokines and pharmacologic agents on chronic HIV infection. *AIDS Res Hum Retroviruses* 1992; 8:191–197.

32. Poli G, Kinter A, Justement JS, et al: Tumor necrosis factor alpha functions in an autocrine manner in the induction of human immunodeficiency virus expression. *Proc Natl Acad Sci USA* 1990; 87:782–785.
33. Poli G, Bressler P, Kinter A, et al: Interleukin 6 induces human immunodeficiency virus expression in monocytic cells alone and in synergy with tumor necrosis factor alpha by transcriptional and post-transcriptional mechanisms. *J Exp Med* 1990; 172:151–158.
34. Biswas P, Poli G, Kinter AL, et al: Interferon-gamma induces the expression of human immunodeficiency virus in persistently infected promonocytic cells (U1) and redirects the production of virions to intracytoplasmic vacuoles in PMA-differentiated U1 cells. *J Exp Med* 1992; 176:739–750.
35. Poli G, Orenstein JM, Kinter A, et al: Interferon-alpha but not AZT suppresses HIV expression in chronically infected cell lines. *Science* 1989; 244:575–577.
36. Rieckmann P, Poli G, Kehrl JH, et al: Activated B lymphocytes from human immunodeficiency virus-infected individuals induce virus expression in infected T cells and a promonocytic cell line, U1. *J Exp Med* 1991; 173:1–5.
37. Ho DD, Moudgil T, Alam M: Quantitation of human immunodeficiency virus type 1 in the blood of infected persons. *N Engl J Med* 1989; 321:1621–1625.
38. Coombs RW, Collier AC, Allain JP, et al: Plasma viremia in human immunodeficiency virus infection. *N Engl J Med* 1989; 321:1626–1631.
39. Venet A, Lu W, Beldjord K, et al: Correlation between CD4 cell counts and cellular and plasma viral load in HIV-1-seropositive individuals. *AIDS* 1991; 5:283–288.
40. Saag MS, Crain MJ, Decker WD, et al: High-level viremia in adults and children infected with human immunodeficiency virus: Relation to disease stage and CD4+ lymphocyte levels. *J Infect Dis* 1991; 164:72–80.
41. Srugo I, Brunell PA, Chelyapov NV, et al: Virus burden in human immunodeficiency virus type 1–infected children: relationship to disease status and effect of antiviral therapy. *Pediatrics* 1991; 87:921–925.
42. Katzenstein DA, Holodniy M, Israelski DM, et al: Plasma viremia in human immunodeficiency virus infection: relationship to stage of disease and antiviral treatment. *J Acquir Immune Defic Syndr* 1992; 5:107–112.
43. Escaich S, Ritter J, Rougier P, et al: Plasma viraemia as a marker of viral replication in HIV-infected individuals. *AIDS* 1991; 5:1189–1194.
44. Pantaleo G, Graziosi C, Butini L, et al: Lymphoid organs function as major reservoirs for human immunodeficiency virus. *Proc Natl Acad Sci USA* 1991; 88:9838–9842.
45. Aoki S, Yarchoan R, Thomas RV, et al: Quantitative analysis of HIV-1 proviral DNA in peripheral blood mononuclear cells from patients with AIDS or ARC: Decrease of proviral DNA content following treatment with 2′,3′-dideoxyinosine (ddl). *AIDS Res Hum Retroviruses* 1990; 6:1331–1339.
46. Dalgleish AG, Wilson S, Gompels M, et al: T-cell receptor variable gene products and early HIV-1 infection. *Lancet* 1992; 39:824–828.
47. Stanley SK, Kessler SW, Justement JS, et al: CD34+ bone marrow cells are infected with HIV in a subset of seropositive individuals. *J Immunol* 1992; 149:689–697.
48. Schnittman SM, Denning SM, Greenhouse JJ, et al: Evidence for susceptibility of intrathymic T-cell precursors and their progeny carrying T-cell antigen receptor phenotypes TCR alpha beta + and TCR gamma delta + to human

immunodeficiency virus infection: A mechanism for CD4+ (T4) lymphocyte depletion. *Proc Natl Acad Sci USA* 1990; 87:7727–7731.
49. Hugin AW, Vacchio MS, Morse HC,3d: A virus-encoded "superantigen: in a retrovirus-induced immunodeficiency syndrome of mice. *Science* 1991; 252:424–427.
50. Imberti L, Sottini A, Bettinardi A, et al: Selective depletion in HIV infection of T cells that bear specific T cell receptor V beta sequences. *Science* 1991; 254:860–862.
51. Laurence J, Hodtsev AS, Posnett DN: Superantigen implicated in dependence of HIV-1 replication in T cells on TCR VB expression. *Nature* 1992; 358:255–259.
52. Ameisen JC, Capron A: Cell dysfunction and depletion in AIDS: the programmed cell death hypothesis. *Immunol Today* 1991; 12:102–105.
53. Groux H, Torpier G, Montë D, et al: Activation-induced death by apoptosis in CD4+ T cells from human immunodeficiency virus-infected asymptomatic individuals. *J Exp Med* 1992; 175:331–340.
54. Tersmette M, Lange JM, de Goede RE, et al: Association between biological properties of human immunodeficiency virus variants and risk for AIDS and AIDS mortality. *Lancet* 1989; 1:983–985.
55. Tersmette M, Gruters RA, de Wolf F, et al: Evidence for a role of virulent human immunodeficiency virus (HIV) variants in the pathogenesis of acquired immunodeficiency syndrome: Studies on sequential HIV isolates. *J Virol* 1989; 63:2118–2125.
56. Price RW, Brew B, Sidtis J, et al: The brain in AIDS: Central nervous system HIV-1 infection and AIDS dementia complex. *Science* 1988; 239:586–592.
57. Cvetkovich TA, Lazar E, Blumberg BM, et al: Human immunodeficiency virus type 1 infection of neural xenografts. *Proc Natl Acad Sci USA* 1992; 89:5162–5166.
58. Nakajima K, Martinez-Maza O, Hirano T, et al: Induction of IL-6 (B cell stimulatory factor-2/IFN-beta 2) production by HIV. *J Immunol* 1989; 142:531–536.
59. Oyaizu N, Chirmule N, Ohnishi Y, et al: Human immunodeficiency virus type 1 envelope glycoproteins gp120 and gp160 induce interleukin-6 production in CD4+ T-cell clones. *J Virol* 1991; 65:6277–6282.
60. Rieckmann P, Poli G, Kehrl JH, et al: Activated B lymphocytes from human immunodeficiency virus-infected individuals induce virus expression in infected T cells and a promonocytic cell line, U1. *J Exp Med* 1991; 173:1–5.
61. MacMahon EM, Glass JD, Hayward SD, et al: Epstein-Barr virus in AIDS-related primary central nervous system lymphoma. *Lancet* 1991; 338:969–973.
62. Langhoff E, Terwilliger EF, Bos HJ, et al: Replication of human immunodeficiency virus type 1 in primary dendritic cell cultures. *Proc Natl Acad Sci USA* 1991; 88:7998–8002.
63. Cameron PU, Forsum U, Teppler H, et al: During HIV-1 infection most blood dendritic cells are not productively infected and can induce allogeneic CD4+ T cells clonal expansion. *Clin Exp Immunol* 1992; 88:226–236.
64. Cameron PU, Freudenthal PS, Barker JM, et al: Dendritic cells exposed to human immunodeficiency virus type-1 transmit a vigorous cytopathic infection to CD4+ T cells. *Science* 1992; 257:383–387.
65. Spiegel H, Herbst H, Niedobitek G, et al: Follicular dendritic cells are a major reservoir for human immunodeficiency virus type 1 in lymphoid tissues facilitating infection of CD4+ T-helper cells. *Am J Pathol* 1992; 140:15–22.

66. Fox CH, Tenner-R:acz K, R:acz P, et al: Lymphoid germinal centers are reservoirs of human immunodeficiency virus type 1 RNA. *J Infect Dis* 1991; 164:1051–1057.
67. Parmentier HK, van Wichen D, Sie-Go DM, et al: HIV-1 infection and virus production in follicular dendritic cells in lymph nodes. A case report, with analysis of isolated follicular dendritic cells. *Am J Pathol* 1990; 137:247–251.
68. Pantaleo G, Graziosi C, Fauci AS: New concepts in the immunopathogenesis of human immunodeficiency virus (HIV) infection. *N Engl J Med* 1993; 328:327–335.
69. Fischl MA: State of antiretroviral therapy with zidovudine. *AIDS* 1989; 3:S137–43.
70. Kahn JO, Lagakos SW, Richman DD, et al: A controlled trial comparing continued zidovudine with didanosine in human immunodeficiency virus infection. *N Engl J Med* 1992; 327:581–587.
71. Meng TC, Fischl MA, Boota AM, et al: Combination therapy with zidovudine and dideoxycytidine in patients with advanced human immunodeficiency virus infection. A phase I/II study. *Ann Intern Med* 1992; 116:13–20.
72. Larder BA, Kemp SD: Multiple mutations in HIV-1 reverse transcriptase confer high-level resistance to zidovudine (AZT). *Science* 1989; 246: 1155–1158.
73. Land S, Terloar G, McPhee D, et al: Decreased in vitro susceptibility to zidovudine of HIV isolates obtained from patients with AIDS. *J Infect Dis* 1990; 161:326–339.
74. Boucher CA, Tersmette M, Lange JM, et al: Zidovudine sensitivity of human immunodeficiency viruses from high-risk, symptom-free individuals during therapy. *Lancet* 1990; 336:585–590.
75. Rooke R, Tremblay M, Soudeyns H, et al: Isolation of drug-resistant variants of HIV-1 from patients on long-term zidovudine therapy. Canadian Zidovudine Multi-Centre Study Group. *AIDS* 1989; 3:411–5.
76. Richman DD, Grimes JM, Lagakos SW: Effect of stage of disease and drug dose on zidovudine susceptibilities of isolates of human immunodeficiency virus. *J Acquir Immune Defic Syndr* 1990; 3:743–746.
77. Larder BA, Kellam P, Kemp SD: Zidovudine resistance predicted by direct detection of mutations in DNA from HIV-infected lymphocytes. *AIDS* 1991; 5:137–144.
78. St. Clair MH, Martin JL, Tudor-Williams G, et al: Resistance to ddl and sensitivity to AZT induced by a mutation in HIV-1 reverse transcriptase. *Science* 1991; 253:1557–1559.
79. Richman D, Shih C-K, Lowy I, et al: Human immunodeficiency virus type 1 mutants resistant to nonucleoside inhibitors of reverse transcriptase arise in tissue culture. *Proc Natl Acad Sci USA* 1991; 88:11241–11245.
80. Tudor-Williams G, St. Clair MH, McKinney RE, et al: HIV-1 sensitivity to zidovudine and clinical outcome in children. *Lancet* 1992; 339:15–19.
81. Hamilton JD, Hartigan PM, Simberkoff MS, et al: A controlled trial of early versus late treatment with zidovudine in symptomatic human immunodeficiency virus infection. Results of the Veterans Affairs Cooperative Study. *N Engl J Med* 1992; 326:437–443.
82. Lagakos S, Fischl MA, Stein DS, et al: Effects of zidovudine therapy in minority and other subpopulations with early HIV infection. *JAMA* 1991; 266:2709–2712.
83. Easterbrook PJ, Keruly JC, Creagh-Kirk T, et al: Racial and ethnic differences

in outcome in zidovudine-treated patients with advanced HIV disease. *JAMA* 1991; 266:2713–2718.
84. Burke DS: Vaccine therapy for HIV: A historical review of infectious diseases by active specific immunization with microbe-derived antigens. Submitted.
85. Redfield RR, Birx DL, Ketter N, et al: A phase I evaluation of the safety and immunogenicity of vaccination with recombinant gp160 in patients with early human immunodeficiency virus infection. *N Engl J Med* 1991; 324:1677–1684.
86. Valentine F, Katzenstein D, Haslett P, et al: A randomized controlled study of immunogenicity of rgp160 vaccine in HIV infected subjects. *VIII International Conference on AIDS* abstract, 1992.
87. Tsoukas C, Sampeles J, Gold B, et al: Specific active immunotherapy in asymptomatic HIV disease using recombinant gp160. *VIII International Conference on AIDS* (abstract), 1992.
88. Hardy WD, Feinberg J, Finkelstein DM, et al: Trimethoprim-sulfamethoxazole versus aerosolized pentamidine for secondary prophylaxis of Pneumocystis carinii pneumonia in AIDS patients receiving zidovudine: AIDS Clinical Trial Group protocol 021. *N Engl J Med* 1992; 327:1842–1848.
89. Jacobson MA: Ganciclovir therapy for opportunistic cytomegalovirus disease in AIDS. *AIDS Clin Rev* 1990; 149–163.
90. Palestine AG, Polis MA, De Smet MD, et al: A randomized, controlled trial of foscarnet in the treatment of cytomegalovirus retinitis in patients with AIDS. *Ann Intern Med* 1991; 115:665–673.
91. Studies of Ocular Complications of AIDS Research Group, AIDS Clinical Trials Group: Mortality in patients with the acquired immunodeficiency syndrome treated with either foscarnet or ganciclovir for cytomegalovirus retinitis. *N Engl J Med* 1992; 326:213–220.
92. Saag MS, Powderly WG, Cloud GA, et al: Comparison of amphotericin B with fluconazole in the treatment of acute AIDS-associated cryptococcal meningitis. *N Engl J Med* 1992; 326:83–89.
93. Powderly WG, Saag MS, Cloud GA, et al: A controlled trial of fluconazole or amphotericin B to prevent relapse of cryptococcal meningitis in patients with the acquired immunodeficiency syndrome. The NIAID AIDS Clinical Trials Group and Mycoses Study Group. *N Engl J Med* 1992; 326:793–798.
94. Nightingale SD, Byrd LT, Southern PM, et al: Incidence of Mycobacterium avium-intracellulare complex bacteremia in human immunodeficiency virus-positive patients. *J Infect Dis* 1992; 165:1082–1085.
95. Murphey-Corb M, Martin LN, Davison-Fairburn B, et al: A formalin-inactivated whole SIV vaccine confers protection in macaques. *Science* 1989; 246:1293–1297.
96. Desrosiers RC, Wyand MS, Kodama T, et al: Vaccine protection against simian immunodeficiency virus infection. *Proc Natl Acad Sci USA* 1989; 86:6353–6357.
97. Carlson JR, McGraw TP, Keddie E, et al: Vaccine protection of rhesus macaques against simian immunodeficiency virus infection. *AIDS Res Hum Retroviruses* 1990; 6:1239–1246.
98. Sutjipto S, Pedersen NC, Miller CJ, et al: Inactivated simian immunodeficiency virus vaccine failed to protect rhesus macaques from intravenous or genital mucosal infection but prevented disease in intravenously exposed animals. *J Virol* 1990; 64:2290–227.
99. La Rosa GJ, Davide JP, Weinhold K, et al: Conserved sequence and struc-

tural elements in the HIV-1 principal neutralizing determinant. *Science* 1990; 249:932–935.

100. Emini EA, Nara PL, Schleif WA, et al: Antibody-mediated in vitro neutralization of human immunodeficiency type 1 abolishes infectivity for chimpanzees. *J Virol* 1990; 64:3674–3678.
101. Girard M, Kieny MP, Pinter A, et al: Immunization of chimpanzees confers protection against challenge with human immunodeficiency virus. *Proc Natl Acad Sci USA* 1991; 88:542–546.
102. Rossi P, Moschese V, Broliden PA, et al: Presence of maternal antibodies to human immunodeficiency virus 1 envelope glycoprotein gp120 epitopes correlates with the uninfected status of children born to seropositive mothers. *Proc Natl Acad Sci USA* 1989; 86:8055–8058.
103. Goedert JJ, Mendez H, Drummond JE, et al: Mother-to-infant transmission of human immunodeficiency virus type 1: Association with prematurity or low anti-gp120. *Lancet* 1989; 2:1351–1354.
104. Steimer KS, Scandella CJ, Skiles PV, et al: Neutralization of divergent HIV-1 isolates by conformation-dependent human antibodies to Gp120. *Science* 1991; 254:105–108.
105. Ho DD, Fung MS, Cao YZ, et al: Another discontinuous epitope on glycoprotein gp120 that is important in human immunodeficiency virus type 1 neutralization is identified by a monoclonal antibody. *Proc Natl Acad Sci USA* 1991; 88:8949–8952.
106. Thali M, Olshevsky U, Furman C, et al: Characterization of a discontinuous human immunodeficiency virus type 1 gp120 epitope recognized by a broadly reactive neutralizing human monoclonal antibody. *J Virol* 1991; 65:6188–6193.
107. Fung MS, Sun CR, Gordon WL, et al: Identification and characterization of a neutralization site within the second variable region of human immunodeficiency virus type 1 gp120. *J Virol* 1992; 66:848–856.
108. Berzofsky JA: Approaches and issues in the development of vaccines against HIV. *J Acquir Immune Defic Syndr* 1991; 4:451–459.
109. Palker TJ, Matthews TJ, Langlois A, et al: Polyvalent human immunodeficiency virus synthetic immunogen comprised of envelope gp120 T helper cell sites and B cell neutralization epitopes. *J Immunol* 1989; 142:3612–3619.
110. Takahashi H, Cohen J, Hosmalin A, et al: An immunodominant epitope of the human immunodeficiency virus envelope glycoprotein gp160 recognized by class I major histocompatibility complex molecule-restricted murine cytotoxic T lymphocytes. *Proc Natl Acad Sci USA* 1988; 85:3105–3109.
111. Clerici M, Lucey DR, Zajac RA, et al: Detection of cytotoxic T lymphocytes specific for synthetic peptides of gp160 in HIV-seropositive individuals. *J Immunol* 1991; 146:2214–2219.
112. Picard O, Achour A, Bernard J, et al: A 2-year follow-up of an anti-HIV immune reaction in HIV-1 gp160-immunized healthy seronegative humans: Evidence for persistent cell-mediated immunity. *J Acquir Immune Defic Syndr* 1992; 5:539–546.
113. Takahashi H, Nakagawa Y, Pendleton CD, et al: Induction of broadly cross-reactive cytotoxic T cells recognizing an HIV-1 envelope determinant. *Science* 1992; 255:333–336.
114. Hosmalin A, Clerici M, Houghten R, et al: An epitope in human immunodeficiency virus 1 reverse transcriptase recognized by both mouse and human cytotoxic T lymphocytes. *Proc Natl Acad Sci USA* 1990; 87: 2344–2348.

115. Walker BD, Flexner C, Birch-Limberger K, et al: Long-term culture and fine specificity of human cytotoxic T-lymphocyte clones reactive with human immunodeficiency virus type 1. *Proc Natl Acad Sci USA* 1989; 86:9514–9518.
116. Koenig S, Fuerst TR, Wood LV, et al: Mapping the fine specificity of a cytolytic T cell response to HIV-1 nef protein. *J Immunol* 1990; 145:127–135.
117. Nixon DF, Townsend AR, Elvin JG, et al: HIV-1 gag-specific cytotoxic T lymphocytes defined with recombinant vaccinia virus and synthetic peptides. *Nature* 1988; 336:484–487.
118. Hu SL, Abrams K, Barber GN, et al: Protection of macaques against SIV infection by subunit vaccines of SIV envelope glycoprotein gp160. *Science* 1992; 255:456–459.
119. Johnson PR, Montefiori DC, Goldstein S, et al: Inactivated whole-virus vaccine derived from a proviral DNA clone of simian immunodeficiency virus induces high levels of neutralizing antibodies and confers protection against heterologous challenge. *Proc Natl Acad Sci USA* 1992; 89:2175–2179.
120. Fultz PN, Nara P, Barre-Sinoussi F, et al: Vaccine protection of chimpanzees against challenge with HIV-1-infected peripheral blood mononuclear cells. *Science* 1992; 256:1687–1690.
121. Extension of public comment period for revision of HIV infection classification system and expansion of AIDS surveillance case definition. *MMWR* 1992; 40:891.
122. Novello AC: From the Surgeon General, US Public Health Service. *JAMA* 1991; 265:1805.
123. Quinn TC, Groseclose SL, Spence M, et al: Evolution of the human immunodeficiency virus epidemic among patients attending sexually transmitted disease clinics: A decade of experience. *J Infect Dis* 1992; 165:541–544.
124. Minkoff HL, DeHovitz JA: Care of women infected with the human immunodeficiency virus. *JAMA* 1991; 266:2253–2258.
125. Maiman M, Tarricone N, Vieira J, et al: Colposcopic evaluation of human immunodeficiency virus-seropositive women. *Obstet Gynecol* 1991; 78:84–88.
126. Nosocomial transmission of multidrug-resistant tuberculosis to health-care workers and HIV-infected patients in an urban hospital—Florida. *MMWR* 1990; 39:718–722.
127. Centers for Disease Control: Nosocomial transmission of multi-drug resistant tuberculosis among HIV-infected persons—Florida and New York, 1988–1991. *MMWR Rep* 1991; 40:585–591.
128. Edlin BR, Tokars JI, Grieco MH, et al: An outbreak of multidrug-resistant tuberculosis among hospitalized patients with the acquired immunodeficiency syndrome. *N Engl J Med* 1992; 326:1514–1521.
129. Pearson ML, Jereb JA, Frieden TR, et al: Nosocomial transmission of multidrug-resistant Mycobacterium tuberculosis. A risk to patients and health care workers. *Ann Intern Med* 1992; 117:191–196.
130. Fischl MA, Uttamchandani RB, Daikos GL, et al: An outbreak of tuberculosis caused by multiple-drug-resistant tubercle bacilli among patients with HIV infection. *Ann Intern Med* 1992; 117:177–183.
131. Dooley SW, Jarvis WR, Martone WJ, et al: Multidrug-resistant tuberculosis. *Ann Intern Med* 1992; 117:257–259.
132. Sullenger BA, Gallardo HF, Ungers GE, et al: Overexpression of TAR sequences renders cells resistant to human immunodeficiency virus replication. *Cell* 1990; 63:601–608.
133. Sullenger BA, Gallardo HF, Ungers GE, et al: Analysis of trans-acting re-

sponse decoy RNA-mediated inhibition of human immunodeficiency virus type 1 transactivation. *J Virol* 1991; 65:6811–6816.
134. Malim MH, Freimuth WW, Liu J, et al: Stable expression of transdominant rev protein in human T cells inhibits human immunodeficiency virus replication. *J Exp Med* 1992; 176:1197–1201.
135. Caruso M, Klatzmann D: Selective killing of CD4+ cells harboring a human immunodeficiency virus-inducible suicide gene prevents viral spread in an infected cell population. *Proc Natl Acad Sci USA* 1992; 89:182–186.
136. Venkatesh LK, Arens MQ, Subramanian T, et al: Selective induction of toxicity to human cells expressing human immunodeficiency virus type 1 Tat by a conditionally cytotoxic adenovirus vector. *Proc Natl Acad Sci USA* 1990; 87:8746–8750.

Evolving Concepts in the Pathogenesis and Management of Asthma*

E.R. McFadden, Jr., M.D.

Argyl J. Beams Professor of Medicine, Director, Airway Disease Center, Department of Medicine, Case Western Reserve University School of Medicine, Cleveland, Ohio

The word asthma is derived from the Greek αοεμ and is a synonym for "panting" or "breathlessness."[1] For the better part of 4 millennia, asthma has been treated as a nonspecific symptom complex, and periodic attempts at a more precise definition have been unsuccessful. However, within the last 2 decades, the meaning of asthma has been narrowed to describe a distinct medical entity, and over the last 5 years an explosion of studies in airway biology and immunopathology have further sharpened the focus of this illness. Currently, asthma is viewed as a chronic disease of the airways that causes widespread narrowing of the tracheobronchial tree. Asthma is characterized by acute exacerbations of varying degrees of severity that are associated with cough, dyspnea, and wheezing that either resolve spontaneously or with therapy. In unusual circumstances, acute episodes can terminate fatally. Some have characterized asthma in terms of the factors believed to be important in its pathogenesis and pathophysiology, and the concepts of airway inflammation and bronchial hyperresponsiveness have been included in the definition.[2] While there is no doubt that these components are present in asthma, they are not unique to this illness and are found, individually or together, with other forms of airway disease and in patients with atopic rhinitis without lower respiratory problems.[3–6] Hence, the utility of defining asthma using these modifiers is unclear. What appears to be important in asthma is not the mere presence of airway inflammation, but its type and its potential role in producing the bronchial irritability so typical of this illness.

The evolution of the definition of asthma to its current state as a chronic illness with superimposed acute exacerbations is not just an abstract etiologic concept, but rather it has produced profound alterations in therapeutic approaches. Historically, the treatment of asthma has been directed toward symptom relief. Initially, this took the form of using bronchodilators (predominantly oral methylxanthines or nonselective sympathomimetics)

*Supported in part by Specialized Center of Research Grant (SCOR) HL-37117 from NHLBI and General Clinical Research Center Grant MO1 RR 00080 from NCRR.

to treat acute episodes after they developed. With the advent of longer-acting, more conveniently administered drugs, intermittent post hoc use gave rise to scheduled administration to prevent recurrence. As experience with aerosolized β-selective agonists grew in the 1960s and 1970s, they assumed a major role in treatment strategies. Most recently attention has shifted toward controlling the disease by modifying the underlying cellular and biochemical abnormalities believed to be playing a role in pathogenesis. To this end, it has been recommended that drugs with antiinflammatory activities such as cromolyn and inhaled steroids be routinely included in the treatment of patients with recurrent asthma and that β_2-agonists be used as rescue medication rather than on a routine basis.[2] In addition, some have suggested that benefit may be derived in selected patients with asthma from the use of nonspecific antiinflammatory drugs like methotrexate and gold salts. Renewed interest in the development of novel drugs that inhibit mediator synthesis and end-organ effects has also been spurred, and advances in smooth muscle and receptor pharmacology have opened the way to the development of new classes of bronchodilators. The purpose of the present review is to describe the current state of therapy for acute and chronic asthma and to assess the data base underlying it.

Asthma: Magnitude of the Problem

Asthma is a common disease with enormous economic impact. It is estimated that 10 million people are affected in the United States (4%–5% of the population). The overall cost of illness related to asthma in 1990 has been placed at $6.2 billion.[7] An estimated 1.8 million people required emergency room visits in that year and 47.8% of these were children. There were approximately 1.5 and 6.5 million outpatient hospital and physicians' office visits, respectively, and the sum spent on medication approached $713 million. Asthma accounted for 3 million lost work days and more than 10 million days absent from school.

Despite these figures, death rates remain low (4,360 deaths in 1987), but they are rising.[8, 9] Some have suggested that this trend is related to adverse responses to β-agonists (see later), but it is more likely due to improper assessment of the severity of the episodes by the patient and/or physician,[10] inadequate treatment in hospital,[11] and problems of limited availability of health care in certain areas of the country because of socioeconomic constraints.[9] The last issue may be quite significant. In fact, if the death from asthma in the inner city regions of Cook County, Illinois, and New York City are removed from the census, the reported increase for the entire country is barely significant.[12] Obviously, if inroads are to be made into the control of this illness, the application of appropriate therapeutic modalities is mandatory.

Asthma and Airway Reactivity

In asthmatic individuals the responsivity of the airways is markedly increased, and patients with this illness develop bronchial narrowing to a greater extent in response to smaller quantities of physical, chemical, and pharmacologic stimuli than do healthy individuals.[2] As pointed out previously, this phenomenon is the cardinal feature of asthma, and it has been suggested that heightened airway reactivity may be the primary pathogenetic event in the acquisition of the disease. Heightened airway responsiveness also occurs in unaffected first-degree relatives of asthmatic subjects and in some patients with allergic rhinitis, cystic fibrosis, and chronic bronchitis.[3–6] Thus, it is a phenomenon that is familial and also has the capability of being acquired.

The airway reactivity of asthmatics rises with repeated exposure to inciting stimuli and falls with avoidance.[13–15] It also correlates with many clinical features of the illness. When airway reactivity is high, symptoms are more severe and persistent, the acute response to bronchodilator drugs is greater, and the amount of therapy required to control the patient's complaints increases.[16] In addition, the magnitude of diurnal fluctuations in lung function becomes greater and the patient tends to waken at night or in the early morning with breathlessness. Whether the changes in the underlying disease state produce the changes in reactivity or whether the converse occurs has not been established. In any event, the phenomenon of heightened reactivity in asthmatics is an important feature of the illness and can be used in clinical practice not only to diagnose the presence of asthma, but also to help assess its severity and expected treatment requirements.

In both normal and asthmatic subjects, airway reactivity is known to rise following viral respiratory tract infections and exposure to oxidative air pollutants such as ozone and nitrogen dioxide.[17–19] Interestingly, sulfur dioxide does not appear to have this effect.[20] With viruses, airway responsivity can remain elevated for 6 to 8 weeks, while following exposure to ozone reactivity it remains high for only a few days. In asthmatic patients, the inhalation of specific antigen is a potent stimulus to increase reactivity,[13, 14, 21, 22] and exercise, although a common precipitant of acute obstruction, does not have this effect.[23] Recent data indicate that following exposure to immunologic active substances, airway responsiveness will begin to rise within minutes,[22] and can remain elevated for weeks. If the dose of antigen is high enough, acute episodes of obstruction may occur daily for a prolonged period following a single exposure.[16]

One of the most subtle, yet clinically important, manifestations of elevated airway reactivity is an increase in circadian variation in airway tone. In the tracheobronchial tree of humans, airway caliber decreases at night and increases during the day. In normal individuals, the day/night changes are quite small and typically acount for only a 5% to 10% difference in peak flow rates.[24–26] In asthmatics, however, overnight falls and peak flows of 50% or more can occur, and the timing of the decrease tends to correlate with the patient's episodes of nocturnal dyspnea.[24, 26, 27] The more active the underlying illness, the greater the airway lability, and the larger the diurnal fluctuations of lung function. The less active the asthma, the smaller the nocturnal changes.

It is important to appreciate that in the usual course of events, airway function tends to improve during the course of the day following nocturnal problems. Hence, a patient who suffered even a moderately severe to severe episode of asthma in the middle of the night or early morning may come to the office or laboratory the following day and present with a normal physical examination and normal pulmonary mechanics despite the fact that his or her asthma is out of control. If the circadian nature of the airway obstruction is not considered, the significance and seriousness of the patient's complaints may go unrecognized.

Asthma and Airway Inflammation

The cause of the heightened airway reactivity in asthma is unknown, but it is believed to be related to airway inflammation. In autopsy specimens from patients dying in status asthmaticus, exudation of fluid with edema and infiltration of the airway wall with eosinophils, neutrophils, plasma cells, and lymphocytes are found in association with damage to the epithelium, thickening of the basement membrane, goblet-cell hyperplasia, and hyperplasia and hypertrophy of the smooth muscle and capillaries.[28, 29] This, plus the biologic activities of the various cell types found in asthmatic airways, have led to several consensus reports[2, 30] that asthma is an inflammatory disease. While this conclusion will most likely turn out to be correct, currently there is surprisingly little direct information that conclusively links the two. Much of the early support for the inflammatory therapy of the pathogenesis of asthma has been deduced from studying the changes that occur in cell traffic and cell-cell interactions in vivo and in vitro during airway anaphylaxis in animals. Unfortunately, the applicability of this information to humans is far from certain, for no satisfactory animal models of asthma yet exist. With the advent of techniques to lavage and biopsy the tracheobronchial tree of asthmatics, more data in support of the inflammatory hypothesis has been generated, but it is still not possible to translate the cellular changes found in the airway walls of asthmatics into pathophysiologic or clinical events.

The airways of asthmatics can be edematous and infiltrated with eosinophils, plasma cells, and lymphocytes.[31–36] Unlike other forms of inflammation, neutrophils are not prominent, and there is a sparsity of phagocytic cell infiltration and granulation tissue. Aside from the deposition of collagen below the epithelial basement membrane,[37] fibrosis is absent in asthma, and the replacement of the airway with the concentric scarring found in other types of airway inflammation is not a feature of this disease. The factors controlling the extent of the inflammation, its nature, and the tissue reparative response is unknown.

Also unknown is the mechanism by which cellular infiltration produces the abnormalities in airway physiology that are so characteristic of asthma. The latter is a particularly important issue, for the pathologic changes described previously have been reported in asymptomatic patients.[31–34] Thus, the mere presence of inflammation does not necessarily mean active disease. In fact, recent data from our laboratory[38] and others[39] have failed to find any relationship between the intensity of the histologic abnormalities in biopsies from the airways of asthmatics and any index of disease severity.

It is currently hypothesized that the physiologic and clinical features of asthma derive from an interaction among the inflammatory cell types in the airways with the elaboration of chemical mediators whose biochemistry produce an intense local reaction that can be neurally amplified.[40–46] One cell thought to play a pivotal role in this process is the mast cell, but other mediator-releasing cells such as macrophages may also contribute. It has also been suggested that activated T-lymphocytes may also be important in the pathogenesis of asthma.[46a] Lymphocytes secrete signal proteins called cytokines, particularly IL-5, which results in the local accumulation and activation of eosinophils (see later). When stimulated appropriately, mast cells can release histamine and they and macrophages can generate arachidonic acid metabolites such as the leukotrienes and prostaglandins. Platelet-activating factor and bradykinin are also formed. These mediators can cause contraction of bronchial smooth muscles, enhance vascular permeability, produce edema of the airway wall, and elevate mucous production and interfere with its removal.[43, 45, 46] Simultaneously, chemotactic compounds such as neutrophil and eosinophil chemotactic factors of anaphylaxis, leukotriene β_4, platelet activating factor, and hydroxyeicosatetranoic acids attract neutrophils and eosinophils to the site of mediator release and may activate platelets.[43, 45, 46] This second or late phase takes many hours to develop. Once it occurs, however, the cells involved, as well as the resident macrophages, can provide more arachidonic acid metabolites and so enhance both the immediate and delayed phases by initiating a feedback loop. They can also elaborate a family of molecules called histamine-releasing factors[47] which can interact with cells in the mast cell/basophil series and further amplify the inflammatory response. In addition, endothelial and epithelial cells, fibroblasts, lymphocytes, and macrophages also synthesize cytokines whose receptors and biologic functions regulate the response of the other cells in the inflammatory cascade.[48] Cytokines like interleukin-3 (IL-3) and interleukin-5 (IL-5) selectively increase the adherence of basophils and eosinophils, respectively, and IL-3, IL-5, and granulocyte macrophage colony-stimulating factor prolong the survival of eosinophils. Elevated levels of some of these cytokines have been found in airway tissues and fluids in asthmatics.[49–52] This observation is not a uniform feature in all asthmatics, however,[51] and its specificity is open to question since similar phenomena have been observed in atopic patients without asthma.[52] The latter is a theme that recurs with such repetitiveness (see later) that it raises the issue as to whether "inflammation" is more of a general marker of atopy rather than a pathognomonic feature of asthma.

For inflammatory cells to travel from the vascular bed to the site of need, adhesion molecules on their surface must be activated so that the cells can attach to similar molecules on the endothelium and move through the vessel wall. Adhesion molecules are known to be upregulated in asthma,[53] suggesting that inflammatory cells are responding to chemoattractants. This has given rise to the notion that antiadhesion molecule antibodies, by interfering with cell migration, may be beneficial in this disease. Whether such promise will be fulfilled remains to be determined, but the solution is unlikely to be straightforward given that the changes are neither specific nor selective. Adhesion molecule upregulation develops with multiple stimuli including the methods used to obtain the cells from the lungs and occurs with the intraairway installation of antigen in nonasthmatic atopic people.[53]

Perhaps the most important cells in the late reaction are the eosinophils. These cells contain cationic and major basic protein in their granules and are capable of damaging the airway epithelium in animals after prolonged contact, causing it to be shed into the lumen. Major basic protein has been found in the blood and sputum of asthmatics, and its levels fall with therapy.[54] Major basic protein and/or cationic protein have also been detected in endobronchial biopsies and bronchoalveolar lavage fluid of asthmatics,[33–35, 55–57] and it is likely that they contribute to the epithelial damage. Denudation of the epithelium, besides resulting in a loss of barrier and secretory function, can also theoretically expose sensory nerve endings, thereby setting the stage for the activation of neurogenic inflammatory pathways.[44] It has been postulated that mediators released in the vicinity of sensory fibers could result in antidromic conduction down sensory nerves, resulting in retrograde release of neuropeptides like substance P, calcitonin gene-related peptide, and neurokinin A, which augment smooth muscle contraction, enhance vascular permeability, and promote mucus production.[44] This system may be regulated by enzymes like neutral endopeptidases which are bound to the membranes of epithelial cells and cleave and inactivate tachykinins such as substance P.[58] As yet, there are no data in asthmatics defining the role that neurogenic inflammation plays in this condition.

To provide data on the applicability of the inflammatory cascade described above to the pathogenesis of asthma, investigations have turned to bronchial washings and/or endobronchial biopsies. The results of these studies have been presented in depth in two recent reviews[12, 40] and will only be highlighted here. In general, the findings have been supportive, but there is too much variability in the data to draw definitive conclusions. Increased numbers of mast cells, eosinophils, epithelial cells, lymphocytes, and neutrophils have been observed in fluids from bronchoalveolar lavage (BAL) in asthmatics as compared with normal subjects, but the observations are inconsistent with some authors recording one effect and others another. The only consistent theme is an elevated level of eosinophils particularly after immunologic bronchoprovocation.[12] Again, specificity is a problem, for such changes occur in nonasthmatics with rhinitis.[59, 60] Further, although BAL provides cells for study, their origin is unclear and the available data indicate poor correlation between the histologic pattern in airway fluids and endobronchial biopsies taken at the same time.[33, 34, 38, 60, 61]

Comparisons of the number and types of inflammatory cells in the bronchial walls in asthmatics and normals in biopsy studies have not yielded clear cut results either. Using light and/or electron microscopic techniques, some researchers have observed an increase in mast cells[32] and eosinophils,[33, 55] while others have not found any differences.[34] Further, some investigations have recorded an increase in one cell type, but not in others,[32, 33] and one study reported increased numbers of eosinophils in some of the subjects examined, but an absence in others with similar degrees of impairment.[55]

The mere presence of cells in the airways is obviously insufficient to produce heightened airway reactivity or bronchial asthma. Many, such as mast cells and macrophages, are resident there and others are normal transients. Hence, to cause pathological change, the cells must have abnormal secretory or regulatory function, interact negatively with the tissue matrix through which they pass, and/or be exposed to abnormal activating signals. Alternatively, the cells and the signals to which they respond may be normal, or nearly so, and the defect may lie in the factors regulating local host defenses. In any event, to produce airway obstruction and the clinical syndrome of asthma, secondary messengers are required. As indicated earlier, it is believed that the mediators of anaphylaxis fulfill this function.

In atopic asthmatics exposed to an antigen to which they are sensitive, the appearance of inflammatory mediators in blood,[62] urine,[63] or bronchoalveolar lavage fluid[64–70] in conjunction with airway narrowing offers reasonable, although indirect, evidence that these compounds may be involved in the induction of the pathophysiologic changes of the immediate reaction. One agent that has been discussed in depth because of its multiplicity of actions is platelet-activating factor.[71] Several studies have suggested that this compound increases airway reactivity in some normal subjects[72, 73]; hence, its potential role in the pathogenesis of asthma could be quite important. Others have not found this effect.[74]

Mediators, per se, do not explain the whole picture, however, for such compounds have been found in the blood of individuals with mast cell diseases such as cold and cholinergic urticaria[75, 76] and in the airways of atopic nonasthmatics[53, 65–67] who did not have any complaints referable to the lungs. Thus, the mediators of asthma appear to need a unique substrate upon which to exhibit their effects. In this regard, the action of platelet-activating factor is particularly curious. In contrast to other mediators like histamine, prostaglandin $F_2\alpha$ and leukotrienes C and D, asthmatics do not appear to be hyperresponsive to the actions of this compound and there is no consistent effect on airway reactivity in this group.[71, 77] It has been suggested that because asthmatics are chronically exposed to platelet-activating factor, they develop a tachyphylaxis to its exogenous administration that does not occur in normal subjects.[71, 72] Since no such effect is seen with any other of the putative mediators believed to be involved in asthma, this explanation may need to be reexamined.

The situation is even less clear with respect to the importance of the infiltrative phase produced by chemotactic mediator on airway physiology. The current school of thought holds that the influx of cells results in bronchial narrowing 3 to 8 hours after antigen exposure (the so called "late asthmatic response"), and it is this factor that is responsible for elevating airway reactivity.[14] Although this view is widely accepted, there are a number of lines of evidence that do not support it. For example, only about 50% of asthmatics have a late reaction to antigen in the laboratory,[78] yet according to current theory, mast cell degranulation from antigen exposure would produce an infiltrative phase in all patients. Consequently, the two events may not be related as to cause and effect. Moreover, a late reaction is not necessary to increase airway reactivity following immunologic stimuli.[14, 22] It is now appreciated that post-antigen, bronchial responsivity rises shortly after the early response begins.[22] Further, some stimuli, such as exercise, produce late reactions in a small number of subjects[79] yet do not influence airway reactivity,[23] while others like ozone or nitrogen dioxide disease reactivity but do not have a late component.[18, 19]

The role of mediators in producing bronchial hyperresponsiveness or the late reaction is also difficult to understand from a pharmacologic point of view. Cromolyn, when given before antigen, prevents both the early and late responses as well as the subsequent increase in reactivity in asthmatics.[80] The explanation given for this phenomenon is that cromolyn interferes with mediator release in phase one and so aborts the inflammatory cascade of the second phase. Yet, this drug can be given after mediator generation and release occurs, and it will still attenuate the increase in reactivity even though the late reaction is unaffected.[81] Equally perplexing is the fact that β-agonists, which are quite potent mast cell stabilizers,[82] also interfere with mediator release, yet these drugs neither inhibit the late response nor reduce airway reactivity.[80, 83–85] Finally, corticosteroids, which have no direct action on human pulmonary mast cells[86] or the early response to antigen when given acutely,[80] abort the late phase and attenuate the resulting bronchial hyperresponsiveness.[83–85]

It has also been suggested that the epithelial denudation thought to be secondary to the release of proteins from the granules of eosinophils leads to heightened airway responsiveness.[33, 34] In the studies purporting such an effect, the findings were purely association and the correlations incorporated normal subjects as an anchor. Others, using blinded techniques, have not confirmed this hypothesis,[32, 38] and there are data to suggest that the epithelial denudation seen in biopsies from asthmatics may actually be artifactually induced by the biopsy procedures used.[33, 34]

Despite the great strides made, it is apparent that the cellular and biochemical mechanisms involved in the pathogenesis and pathophysiology of asthma are not yet completely understood. There is ample evidence that the airways of asthmatics contain an active inflammatory process, but the factors that control this process and the stimuli that convert a cellular influx into altered physiology remain obscure.

Pharmacology of Asthma

There are five classes of drugs that are routinely used in the treatment of asthma. Three of them, the adrenergic agonists, methylxanthines, and anticholinergics, are bronchodilators and are employed to relieve the symptoms of acute airway obstruction. The other two classes, the glucocorticoids and antiinflammatory agents such as cromones and nedocromil, do not dilate the airways but produce their effects by modulating the various components of acute and subacute inflammation.

Adrenergic Agonists

The adrenergic agonists, or sympathomimetics, are a group of compounds that mimic the effects of the adrenal medullary hormones and neurotransmitters of the sympathetic nervous system, hence their name. They are compounds of simple chemical structure that produce their effects at a biochemical level through the activation of β-receptors on the cell surface and the formation of cyclic adenosine monophosphate (cAMP).[87, 88] The beta effect can be subdivided into two components: β_1 and β_2, and only the latter with its increase in high energy phosphate compounds in respiratory smooth muscle is of major therapeutic use in airway disease. The β_1 effect is cardiac and results in positive inotropism. Hence, the most desirable drug of this type is one with only selective β_2 activity.

β_2 Agonists are the most potent bronchodilators known, and the selective, relatively long-acting compounds that are currently available have made a major impact on the treatment of asthma. These compounds relax airway smooth muscle throughout the tracheobronchial tree in both normal and asthmatic individuals. The inhaled route is the preferred means of administration because of its more rapid onset of action and fewer side effects. β_2 Agonists are functional antagonists and will reverse the effects of all known spasmogens. They also increase chloride flux and water movement in the epithelium,[89] facilitate mucociliary transport,[90] and reduce vascular permeability.[91] In addition they inhibit the release of acetylcholine from postganglionic nerves in the airway.[92] There is very little practical clinical difference between the various agents available in the United States (albuterol, terbutaline, fenoterol, bitolterol, and pirbuterol). Each has an onset of effect within minutes, a duration of action of 3 to 6 hours, similar selectivity for β_2-receptors, and when given in similar doses, produces the same degree of bronchodilatation.[87, 93] Adrenergic agonists are the treatment of choice for active episodes of asthma[94] and are effective therapy for the relief of bronchospasm from any cause. They can also be used prophylactically to prevent exercise-induced asthma. Despite arguments to the contrary, use of β_2-agonists does not lower airway reactivity,[80, 83, 84, 95] although some data show that such therapy can reduce the degree of inflammation in the airways.[96]

Recent advances involving very large substitutions into the catechol structure have produced salmeterol (a chemical analogue of albuterol) and formoterol.[97, 98] These two compounds are potent bronchodilators that have durations of action of 8 to 12 hours. Hence, they may be potentially very useful in preventing obstruction due to repetitive exposure to spasmogens over the day and in controlling nocturnal bronchospasm.[99, 100] With these agents a child could prevent exercise-induced asthma for an entire day by simply inhaling 2 puffs of salmeterol or formoterel before leaving home in the morning. In a large series of patients, salmeterol administered twice-a-day has been found to be as efficacious as albuterol given four times daily.[103] It has also been suggested that salmeterol may prevent the increase in bronchial reactivity that follows the inhalation of antigen;[101] however, this effect may have been due to prolonged bronchodilatation rather than to any alteration of the basic mechanism involved in heightened airway responsiveness.[103] Salmeterol has been shown to inhibit the appearance of various inflammatory mediators in urine after antigen challenge,[102] but this is to be expected based upon the class action of β_2-agonists on mast cell degranulation.

The major side effects of β_2-agonists are tremor, palpitations, and tachyarrhythmia, which are dose dependent.[87] The first appears to be a specific β_2-effect. The others may occur from direct stimulation of β_1-cardiac receptors or reflexly secondary to β_2-mediated vasodilatation. At higher doses, increases in blood glucose, insulin, nonesterified free fatty acids, lactate, pyruvate, and ketones have been reported, as have decreases in serum potassium, phosphate, calcium, and magnesium.[103–106] Typically, these metabolic effects are small and do not produce clinical problems, although ketoacidosis has been reported to develop in patients with diabetes after therapy with albuterol.[106] Hypokalemia occurs more frequently after intravenous administration, and, although usually minor in degree, it can aggravate the potassium loss induced by glucocorticoids or diuretics. Additional problems encountered with the use of the inhaled route of therapy are the inability of some patients to master the proper technique required with metered-dose inhalers and the lack of physician knowledge in instructing them. It has been estimated that perhaps as many as 40% to 50% of patients who use inhalers are not able to coordinate activation of the device and inhalation despite careful teaching,[107–109] and that as many as 60% of general internists may not know how to demonstrate the proper procedures or to detect and correct improper ones.[110, 111]

To overcome the difficulties with coordination and to enhance aerosol deposition in the lower airways, a number of inhalational aids have been added to conventional metered-dose inhalers, and different types of inhalers have been developed. These inhalational aids are collectively known as "spacers" and fall into three categories: tubes without valves, tubes or reservoirs with valves, and collapsible bags. Large volume spacers and tubes with valves are particularly useful. Unfortunately, their bulk frequently makes patients reluctant to carry such devices with them or to use them in public. Other solutions have been the development of breath-activated nonpressurized dry powder aerosols (Spinhaler, Rotahaler, Turbuhaler, and Diskhaler) and a breath-activated, pressurized, metered-dose inhaler.[112] All of these devices are as effective as conventional metered-dose inhalers and obviate the need for spacers while eliminating problems of discoordination.

Controversies Surrounding the Use of β_2-Agonists

Aside from the very rare occurrence of a paradoxical bronchospastic response,[113] β_2-agonists were thought to be free of any adverse pulmonary consequences. In an attempt to explain the increase in asthma death rates that have been reported in some countries,[88, 114] attention has turned toward the possibility of these drugs contributing to the process. Epidemiologic data from New Zealand have indicated that treatment with fenoterol is associated with an increased risk of death from asthma.[115–117] Although these findings were originally challenged on technical grounds, the effect continued to be observed even after the methodological problems in the original studies were corrected.[117] Based upon all of the evidence, the phenomenon appears to be related only to fenoterol, because the control populations in these investigations who were using other β_2-agonists did not have an increased death rate.[115–117] A case control study from Canada on asthma deaths and near deaths also highlights the adverse consequences of the use of fenoterol, but claims that increased use of all selective β-agonists may lead to serious adverse consequences.[118] This has not been the case in the United Kingdom. From 1980 to 1990, the number of prescriptions for metered-dose inhalers of β-agonists tripled while the number of deaths from asthma remained constant.[119] Further, no evidence of a direct association between the use of high doses of β-agonists via a compressor-driven nebulizer and mortality could be found in 271 New Zealand patients dying from asthma.[120] The major difficulty in the investigations claiming positive effects is that causality has not been demonstrated. Escalation of the underlying disease process may cause a need for increased medication and not the converse.

Do β-Agonists Worsen Lung Function or Unfavorably Alter Asthma?

Proponents of this therapy point to the fact that β-agonists produce tachyphylaxis to their bronchodilating activities[121, 122] and increase airway reactivity.[83, 84, 123] It is important to appreciate, however, that not all studies have reported these effects,[95, 124–125] and in those which have, the alterations are small enough that their clinical significance is doubtful. The typical consequences of tachyphylaxis are only a slight reduction in peak bronchodilatation with a shortening of duration of effect.[121, 123] The changes in reactivity are even less impressive, and the magnitude of the reductions reported are actually small enough to be within the error of the measurement itself.[83, 84] Two other potential disadvantages of β-agonists have been postulated: (1) The effect of these compounds in preventing mast cell degranulation may be detrimental and interfere with the antiinflammatory effects of heparin. (2) The bronchodilating effect may unknowingly expose patients to large quantities of inhaled antigen or other immunologically active spasmogens producing magnified delayed effects.[126] There are no data to suggest that either of these events occur. For example, long-acting theophyllines would also produce sustained bronchodilation, yet they are not associated with worsening asthma via increased subliminal exposures. Moreover, it is unclear as to why inhibition of mast cell degranulation by β-agonists should evoke adverse results, when the same situation produced by others (cromolyn or nedocromil) is a sought-after therapeutic effect.

In addition to the aforementioned, it has been suggested that the regular use of β_2-agonists results in poorer control of asthma than when the drugs are taken on an as-needed basis.[127] Fenoterol was the compound employed in this study, but the authors argue that their results apply to all types of β-agonists. Fortunately, this does not appear to be the case. One issue of this study is that the alterations in mechanics are so small that even though statistically significant, it is difficult to assess their physiologic meaning. Futher, others have performed similar studies and have reached different conclusions.[97, 128, 129] In one multicenter investigation involving 234 asthmatics, daily scheduled multiple doses of albuterol produced significantly better control of symptoms and lung function than did an on-demand intermittent regimen,[97] and in another, the regular use of salmeterol was more efficacious than on-demand albuterol.[129] Finally, attempts to directly confirm the aforementioned adverse events by using a similar study design have not been successful.[129a]

To provide definitive answers which confirm or refute the concerns about β_2-agonist therapy for asthma will undoubtedly require large controlled trials. However, given that millions of Americans have used tens of millions of β_2-agonist inhalers per year for more than a decade, the chances of adverse reactions being manifest clinically, if they were occurring, would be quite high. Even a 0% to 5% effect would produce tens to hundreds of thousands of affected individuals in short order, yet asthma deaths are only 4 to 5 thousand per year. Of these, few have been conclusively linked to untoward medication effects. Until definitive data become available to the contrary, β_2-agonists are still the drug of choice for sympatomatic relief. There is nothing to preclude their regularly scheduled use in patients with asthma. This recommendation should not be interpreted as a complacent approach to our therapeutic treatment of this disease. Asthma mortality has increased in the United States, and, until we understand why, constant reassessment of our pharmacologic interventions is required.

Methylxanthines

The methylxanthines consist of caffeine, theophylline, and theobromine. Theophylline is currently the most widely used. The major pharmacologic activity of theophylline in the management of asthma is the relaxation of bronchial smooth muscle. This effect is greatest when the muscles are constricted. Theophylline improves contractility of the diaphragm, rendering it less susceptible to fatigue. It also accelerates mucociliary transport and antagonizes the effects of adenosine on mast cells, reducing mediator release.[130, 131] Finally, theophylline stimulates medullary respiratory centers, promotes diuresis, and induces a positive inotropic cardiac effect.[130, 131]

The bronchodilating activity of theophylline is proportional to the logarithm of the serum concentration over the range of 3 to 25 μg/mL. The degree of improvement in lung function is small at levels less than 10 μg/mL, and serious side effects increase in frequency at levels above 25 μg/mL, and so the therapeutic range is usually taken as 10 to 20 μg/mL. It is important to recognize that these values are arbitrary, and that many patients have excellent control with levels below 10 μg/mL, whereas others need high levels to relieve their symptoms. Thus, one should treat the patient and not the concentration in the blood.

The efficacy of theophylline in controlling the symptoms related to reversible airway obstruction is well documented. This agent abolishes the signs and symptoms of chronic asthma, reduces the need for emergency medications, and permits the withdrawal of oral glucocorticoids.[130–135] The issue of whether methylxanthines interact synergistically with β_2-agonists is controversial.[136] While there may be some positive effect in chronic therapy, there is virtually none in acute situations.[94] Theophylline has no major chronic effect on airway reactivity, although it can provide protection against acute spasmogens.[85] Despite its effectiveness, theophylline is only a medium-potency bronchodilator. In controlled studies dealing with the therapy of acutely ill asthmatic patients, adrenergic agonists have been found to produce more rapid relief and three to four times more bronchodilatation than intravenous aminophylline.[94]

The mechanism responsible for the bronchodilator effect of theophylline is unknown. It was formerly thought that the drug increased the intracellular levels of cAMP by the inhibition of phosphodiesterase. However, this point of view is no longer tenable. Phosphodiesterase activity is not reduced at the concentrations of theophylline achieved with the usual therapeutic doses. Further, other phosphodiesterase inhibitors are not bronchodilators. It has been suggested that theophylline antagonizes adenosine receptors.[131] This may not be conclusive, however, because enprofylline, a closely related drug with greater bronchodilator activity, is not an adenosine antagonist.

For the long-term management of reversible airway obstruction, both rapid and sustained-release formulations of theophylline are available, and the choice of product depends upon the therapeutic goal desired. In the treatment of acute symptoms, a rapidly absorbed compound such as uncoated tablets or liquids can be used. These formulations can rapidly produce therapeutic blood levels, and since there are no important differences in their absorption characteristics, they can be used interchangeably. For long-term prophylaxis, however, serum concentrations may fluctuate widely with these formulations, necessitating unacceptably short dosage intervals. To overcome this problem, a number of sustained-release formulations have been developed. These compounds provide improved time-concentration profiles with little variation between peak and trough serum levels, allowing longer intervals between doses. Presently, agents are available that permit twice daily or once daily dosage. The very long-acting drugs are particularly helpful in the management of nocturnal symptoms.

The modern use of methylxanthines places heavy emphasis on the attainment of stable serum concentrations in the therapeutic range. When sustained-release preparations are to be employed, the dose of medication should be adjusted according to the clinical response and the theophylline blood levels. Since it takes a minimum of three to four half-lives to reach a steady state, theophylline levels should be determined only after 3 to 4 days of therapy and then only with respect to the timing of the dose. With twice-a-day compounds, blood samples should be drawn 4 to 6 hours after a dose to determine the peak level and 10 to 12 hours after administration to obtain the trough level. With once daily formulations, peaks and troughs occur at 12 and 24 hours, respectively. With this information, dosage adjustment is easily accomplished if required. Thereafter, if the patient is doing well, periodic monitoring of the trough level is all that is required.

Theophylline clearance is decreased markedly in neonates and elderly persons, in the presence of acute and chronic hepatic dysfunction, in cardiac decompensation including cor pulmonale, and during febrile illnesses.[130] Clearance is increased in children, cigarette smokers, users of marijuana, and in those ingesting a high-carbohydrate low-protein diet. In each of these circumstances, dosage requirements fall and rise in concert with the changes in clearance. Concurrent medications also influence elimination. Clearance falls with the use of macrolide antibiotics (erythromycin and troleandomycin), allopurinol, cimetidine, and propranolol. It rises with phenobarbital, phenytoin, and other drugs capable of inducing hepatic enzyme formation.

One of the major disadvantages with theophylline is that it has a narrow therapeutic window and the potential for untoward reactions. The side effects of theophylline are nervousness, nausea, vomiting, anorexia, abdominal discomfort, and headache.[137] Theophylline also increases gastric acid secretions. Increasing plasma levels tend to be associated with increasing complaints; however, in one study, approximately 1% of children and 4% of adults were unable to tolerate the drug even at very low levels.[138] The risk of serious toxic effects such as seizures and cardiac arrhythmias increases when the plasma levels exceed 30 μg/mL.[137] Theophylline has been further implicated in learning difficulties and behavioral problems in children.[139] These findings, however, are controversial[140] and this drug is considered safe to use in both children and adults.

Anticholinergics

The anticholinergic drugs consist of atropine sulfate, atropine methylnitrate, and ipratropium bromide. They are among the oldest forms of therapy for airway disease, but can only be administered by inhalation. All of these agents are bronchodilators that override the smooth muscle constrictor and secretory consequences of the liberation of the neurotransmitter of the parasympathetic nervous system. Anticholinergics block reflex bronchoconstriction and can reverse acute airway obstruction,[141] but they offer relatively poor protection against most airway spasmogens and have no effect at all on antigen exposure.[142] They do not alter airway reactivity.[142, 143] It has been suggested that anticholinergic and sympathomimetic drugs interact positively and produce greater bronchodilator activity together than either does alone.[144] While some studies have shown this effect, the majority have not.[145] Further, in those that report a positive response,[144] the bronchodilatation seen with the sympathomimetics is generally much less than that recorded in other investigations conducted in similar circumstances.[94] Thus, the synergism appears to be due to a suboptimal adrenergic effect. Many studies, however, do show a prolonged duration of bronchodilatation when anticholinergics and β-adrenergics are used simultaneously.[145]

The major disadvantages of the anticholinergics are that they have a slow onset of action, and peak bronchodilator activity may not be reached for 30 to 60 minutes. Consequently, their use has been superseded by more rapidly acting agents. Further, atropine sulfate is rapidly absorbed from respiratory mucosal sites, and its systemic effects can present a number of unwanted symptoms in the smooth muscle or neurologic paths of multiple organ systems. In addition, in high doses, atropine sulfate can interfere with mucociliary transport by increasing sputum viscosity and decreasing ciliary motility.[141] The new quaternary compounds (atropine methylnitrate and the ipratropium bromides) are devoid of these side effects.[141] Hence, they represent a major advance in this form of treatment.

The anticholinergics are medium potency bronchodilators, and their role as a single first-line therapy for asthma is open to question. Because of their relatively slow rate of onset, most clinicians would tend to use other agents in emergency situations. There are, however, a group of patients who respond quite favorably to the antimuscarinics. Unfortunately, in our current state of knowledge, there is no good way of prospectively determining who they are without a clinical trial. Consequently, in treating acute obstruction, many authorities would recommend employing anticholinergics as second-line therapy in patients who are severely ill and unresponsive to β-agonists and methylxanthines. In nonacute situations, anticholinergic agents frequently can be of great help in the treatment of the paroxysmal cough associated with irritated airways. They can also be quite useful on occasion in reducing sputum volume in patients with bronchorrhea.

Glucocorticoids

Corticosteroids are among the most effective forms of treatment available for asthma. They are also the only class of drugs routinely used for this disease that are associated with major systemic side effects. Thus, they have been typically employed as a last resort in controlling symptoms when bronchodilators and other agents have failed. With the advent of potent inhaled compounds, this trend has changed and many now consider aerosol glucocorticoids as a first-line treatment. Steroids have been used for the treatment of asthma for over 40 years, and all agree as to their effectiveness. Given this long experience, one would think that the dose-response relationships of these compounds would be well established. Unfortunately, as with other aspects of asthma therapy, this is not the case. Basic issues, such as when steroids should be employed, the optimum dose required to induce a remission in acute or chronic situations, and the schedule of administration, are all still a matter of considerable uncertainty.

Virtually every available glucocorticoid has been used systemically in the treatment of acute and chronic asthma, yet there is little to suggest that one compound provides major therapeutic advantage over another at comparable doses. There are, however, differences in side effects and cost. Of the two injectable corticosteroids (methylprednisone and hydrocortisone), the former has greater antiinflammatory potency, lower mineralocorticoid activity, and a lower cost. Thus, methylprednisone should be the drug of choice for intravenous therapy. In North America, prednisone is the most popular oral agent, while in other parts of the world, the use of prednisolone predominates. Drugs such as cortisone and prednisone need to be hydroxolated before they become active, but in the absence of liver disease, there is nothing to indicate that these agents are any less effective than prednisolone or methylprednisolone which do not require hydroxalation. Further, there are no apparent differences in the manner in which steroid-dependent asthmatics, asthmatics naive to steroids, and normal subjects bind, distribute, or metabolize glucocorticoids. Consequently, these factors are not important issues in determining dosage.

The mechanisms by which steroids improve asthma are unknown. Those that are potentially important are a diminution in the numbers of circulating inflammatory cells, especially eosinophils, vasoconstriction of small vessels, and a reduction in the metabolism of arachidonic acid via the inhibition of phospholipase A_2.[146, 147] Improving β-adrenergic function is often cited as a major activity, but only contradictory and insufficient data are available in humans to support this position.[148–150]

Glucocorticoids are not bronchodilators. Several studies involving a few patients have suggested that glucocorticoids, in and of themselves, can acutely improve lung function over the course of several hours,[151, 152] but neither of these effects have been confirmed in series with larger numbers.[149, 153–162] Rather, the weight of evidence demonstrates that in exacerbations of asthma, steroids augment the action of bronchodilators and require a minimum of 6 to 12 hours to initiate significant increments in pulmonary mechanics in symptomatic patients.[149, 154–158, 161, 162] This time delay fits nicely with the concept that the beneficial activities of glucocorticoids develop via the manufacture of specific new proteins through gene induction. Hence, when steroids are employed in the treatment of acute asthma, one cannot slacken the other forms of therapy, but must continue to use bronchodilators aggressively until the steroids take effect. The use of corticosteroids as a single agent for the treatment of acute asthma is unacceptable.

Of the many dosage schedules that have been proposed, few have been objectively tested. Those that are in use currently have been empirically determined. To treat acute exacerbations, doses of steroids ranging between 10 and 15 mg/kg/24 hours of hydrocortisone or the equivalent appears to be required.[163] A clinical response can be expected within 24 to 36 hours. In chronic asthma, 0.5 mg/kg/day of prednisolone or 1.0 mg/kg/day of prednisone is usually adequate to bring about a remission.[163] In this situation, improvement is usually apparent within 3 to 4 days of beginning treatment, but it may be delayed for a week or more in unusual cases. With the availability of topically effective steroid aerosols, the issue of how long to continue oral steroids has been muted. With these formulations, less reliance can be placed on oral steroids as maintenance therapy, and in many cases exacerbations can be treated by increasing the frequency of aerosol use. Thus, the need for daily or even alternate day treatment plans can be greatly reduced or obviated.

Beclomethasone dipropionate, triamcinolone acetonide, flunisolide, and budesonide (not yet available in the United States) are potent, topically active glucocorticoids that are characterized by a considerable degree of regional first-pass metabolism. Thus, these agents can be directly delivered to the airways to achieve high local concentrations without producing systemic side effects. Inhaled steroids were originally used to replace oral agents in people with moderately severe and severe asthma.[164–167] These formulations reduce the frequency of acute episodes of asthma and the need for concurrent medications, lessen the requirements for oral steroids, and lower airway reactivity.[164–168] The majority of clinicians have seen patients who have improved greatly on inhaled steroids; therefore, the perceptions of the effectiveness of these agents is very positive. Surprisingly, however, there are not any studies that show that inhaled glucocorticoids either induce remissions in patients with moderate to severe disease or improve asthma intensity even one clinical unit (i.e., from severe to moderate disease). One investigation reported large increases in pulmonary function in patients with very compromised pulmonary mechanics,[168a] but this study selected the participants for inclusion based upon their response to oral steroids. In general, there is an inverse relationship between the intensity of the patient's illness and the effectiveness of inhaled glucocorticoids. The more severe the obstruction, the less effective aerosol steroids become in producing objective remissions.[169]

As experience with these compounds has grown, the idea has been advanced that inhaled steroids should be first-line therapy in any patient with chronic symptoms irrespective of severity, rather than something to try when all else has failed. In support of this claim, recent investigations have shown that inhaled steroids in recommended doses provide better symptom control than methylxanthines[168] and β_2-agonists[95] in individuals with mild disease. Steroid aerosols reduce the symptomatic manifestations of asthma and the severity of bronchial hyperresponsiveness over a period of weeks.[83–85, 95, 170–172] Airway reactivity falls as a function of duration of therapy[171, 172] and rises again when the drugs are stopped.[171] Not all studies have found inhaled glucocorticoids to improve bronchoreactivity, however,[173, 174] and this effect has been only inconsistently observed with oral glucocorticoids despite being specifically sought.[175, 176, 176a]

The mechanism by which reactivity is lowered is unknown and may or may not relate to a change in the extent of inflammation in the airways. Three recent studies have examined the effects of inhaled steroids on airway inflammation through the use of serial biopsies.[94, 174, 176] Each found that treatment reduced cellularity as assessed by light microscopy. In one study this reduction was associated with a decrease in airway reactivity, but no change in the extent of mast-cell degranulation was observed on electron microscopic examination.[176] In another there was a diminution in the frequency of free eosinophilic granules seen on electron microscopic examination, but neither these nor the other cellular changes were associated with any alterations in airway responsiveness.[174] The final investigation complicated this picture further by showing that both steroids and terbutaline reduced inflammation, but that only the former lowered reactivity.[96] Steroids had no effect on the degree of basement-membrane thickening.[174]

Although reduction of bronchial hyperresponsiveness by the use of steroid aerosols has received a great deal of attention, the changes reported are typically very minor, on the order of one-half log or less.[83–85, 170–172, 175, 177–182] Therefore, their clinical and physiologic relevance is uncertain. Their size precludes them from being the sole cause of the improvements seen in the clinical state. This matter is complicated further by the fact that the majority of the studies that have examined this issue involved virtually asymptomatic patients with normal lung function.* Only a few studies have examined patients with more severe disease, and the results could actually have derived from improvements in airway geometry without a change in the underlying state of responsivity.[80, 175, 179] Moreover, there is some indication that even though airway reactivity is reduced by steroids in the laboratory, these agents may not provide any protection against specific precipitants of asthma.[81, 177]

*References 83, 84, 95, 170–172, 177, 178, 180–182.

The effects of steroids are dose-dependent. In many areas, high-dose aerosolized steroids (doses that are two or more times the conventionally recommended quantities) are commonly used to control unstable asthma.[183–185] Although this approach diminishes the need for oral glucocorticoids, it carries a risk of increasing side effects and, in fact, all of the untoward consequences of oral steroids have now been reported with aerosols. In addition to causing thrush and dysphonia, which are specific problems with the inhaled route,[186, 187] large quantities of aerosolized steroids, because of their increased availability for systemic absorption, lead to suppression of adrenal function in adults and children,[188, 189] cataract formation,[190] interference with bone metabolism,[191] decreased linear growth in children,[192] and purpura and thinning of the skin.[193]

Antiinflammatory Agents

Cromolyn.—Cromolyn is an agent that is employed in the treatment of asthma to attenuate the bronchial narrowing that follows exposure to a variety of acute provocations and to reduce airway reactivity on a chronic basis. Cromolyn is extremely safe and its low incidence of side effects and broad range of activities suggest that it can be effectively employed in individuals with recurrent symptoms, particularly if there is an allergic diathesis. This drug has no bronchodilatory activity, and its chief mechanism of action is believed to be related to its ability to stabilize mast cells and ameliorate airway inflammation on an acute and chronic basis. Although there is no direct proof of this assumption in humans, cromolyn has been found to be associated with a decrease in BAL eosinophil levels in asthmatics.[194] Since other drugs with more potent mast cell stabilizing properties have not worked in asthma,[195] only part of cromolyn's activity can be attributed to this factor. The composite data on cromolyn in the literature indicates that this drug improves lung function and reduces airway reactivity, but it does not typically promote a diminution of steroid dosage.[196–198] Cromolyn blocks the immediate and late response to antigen and inhibits the subsegment increases in bronchial reactivity that follow such exposures.[80]

In addition to its presumed antiinflammatory actions in chronic situations, cromolyn also can be used prophylactically. As with antigen, a single dose of cromolyn given 15 to 20 minutes before exercise,[199] exposure to cold air,[200] sulfur dioxide,[201] or industrial chemicals like diisocyanate[202] will prevent acute airway obstruction from developing. From a clinical standpoint, this means that a patient who has intermittent exposure to either immunologic or nonimmunologic stimuli that provoke acute episodes of asthma, but who is otherwise well, need not use this drug on a continuous basis. Rather, such individuals can readily be protected by taking cromolyn only before contact with the precipitant. With a stimulus such as exercise, cromolyn will interact positively with β-adrenergic agonists to produce a greater protective effect than either drug alone.[203]

The effect of cromolyn on bronchial reactivity is variable and not all patients respond. This matter has been reviewed recently and approximately

80% of studies show a diminution in reactivity, while the remainder do not show any benefit.[198] The reasons for this dichotomy are unknown. In the positive studies, patients have more symptom-free days and require less concomitant medication. It is of interest that this result occurs even though the changes in bronchial responsiveness that develop are quite small, again, suggesting an as yet undefined mechanism of action.

Cromolyn is most efficacious in atopic patients with seasonal disease or in those who are experiencing perennial stimulation of their airways.[197, 198] It also works in some nonatopics,[204] but since there is no prospective way of determining who will benefit, a therapeutic trial should be undertaken. If the goal is to reduce airway inflammation and promote long range healing, the drug needs to be administered on a regular 4-times-daily basis for at least a month.

Nedocromil.—Nedocromil is a new antiinflammatory agent that is chemically and pharmacologically distinct from glucocorticoids and cromolyn sodium and has recently been released for sale in the United States. Nedocromil has a spectrum of activity similar to cromolyn and controlled trials have shown it to reduce symptoms, improve lung function, and decrease bronchial hyperresponsiveness.[205, 206] Nedocromil blocks both the early and late reactions to antigen and provides protection in asthmatics against challenges with metabisulfite, adenosine, exercise, inflammatory mediators, and sensory neuropeptides.[205] In some studies, nedocromil was found to provide significant benefit to patients who were not adequately controlled by inhaled steroids.[206, 207] It does not, however, appear to have a steroid-sparing effect in those who require maintenance oral glucocorticoids.[208] Like cromolyn, nedocromil is extremely well tolerated and the most commonly reported problem is a bitter taste. Headache, nausea, and vomiting occur occasionally. The mechanism of action is unknown and presumed to be related to mast cell stabilization.

Ancillary Antiinflammatory Therapy

Methotrexate.—To date there have been five controlled[209–212a] and two open studies[213, 214] that have examined the effects of methotrexate as a steroid-sparing agent in asthma. Three of the five double blind investigations found favorable results,[209–211] and two were negative.[212, 212a] The open studies can only be viewed as exploratory because of the lack of controls. Examination of the data in the positive studies demonstrate that the effects, although statistically significant, were uniformly small and of questionable physiologic relevance. In the first paper of this series,[209] the use of methotrexate was associated with an average reduction in prednisone dosage of approximately 9 mg/day. While this seems large, most of the decrease could be accounted for by three subjects who were taking very high doses initially. The remaining two papers reported large-percentage reductions in the dose of prednisone[210] and prednisolone[211] (30% and 50%, respectively) with methotrexate. In absolute terms, however, the doses were reduced by only 3.6 and 6.1 mg/day. There was no effect of methotrexate on lung function or asthma symptoms; thus, even the patients who responded remained steroid-dependent asthmatics. Given the potential serious side effects of methotrexate and its seemingly minor consequence on steroid reduction and asthma severity, more studies need to be performed before this therapy can be recommended for routine clinical use.

Gold.—Because of their antiinflammatory activities in rheumatoid arthritis, gold salts have been used to treat asthma. Uncontrolled studies have suggested a beneficial effect.[215] Controlled trials, however, have not shown any uniform results, and only minor improvements in some of the subjects have occurred.[216, 217] In one such study, the patients were felt to be doing better by their physicians, but there were no differences in pulmonary function or in the number of acute episodes.[216] In another study, some of the patients taking steroids were able to decrease the dose slowly over time, but the effect was minor.[217] Here too, more data are required before firm conclusions regarding efficacy can be reached, and routine clinical use is not recommended.

Mediator Antagonists

Antihistamines.—Histamine is one of the major mediators of immediate hypersensitivity and exhibits a variety of actions that are known to be of relevance to asthma. This compound increases vascular permeability, produces both direct and indirect bronchoconstriction, disrupts the barrier function of the airway epithelium, and may influence both mediator release and immunoregulatory function of inflammatory cells.[43, 45] Consequently, it seems reasonable to attempt to control asthma with antihistamines. In the past, such efforts were not very successful, in part, because of the lack of selectivity of the available agents. With the advent of potent, highly specific H_1-antagonists, this potential form of therapy has been revisited. Although drugs like azelastine, citerizine, terfenadine and astemizole have some intrinsic bronchodilator activity and offer some protection against immunologic and nonimmunologic precipitants of asthma, the effect is small and readily eclipsed by the traditional therapeutic modalities presently in use.[218, 219] Ketotifen, an H_1-antagonist, also inhibits mast cell degranulation and attenuates the response to inhaled antigen in the laboratory.[219] Because of this property and its H_1-antagonism, it has been suggested that ketotifen would be effective in the treatment of asthma. Unfortunately, long-term clinical studies with this drug have not been impressive.[220, 221] In the past, it has been agreed that antihistamines should not be used by asthmatics. Such prohibitions do not appear appropriate and there are no data that demonstrate that asthma is worsened by the administration of an H_1-blocker.

Lipid Mediator Antagonists and Enzyme Inhibition.—Like histamine, the lipid mediators generated from arachidonic acid metabolism (prostaglandins, thromboxane, platelet activating factor, and the leukotrienes) have the potential of producing many of the abnormalities seen in asthma. Consequently, effort is being directed toward the development of specific receptor antagonists and synthesis inhibitors.[222] Studies with various leukotriene D_4 antagonists have produced mixed results in acute challenge studies, but all of the clinical data are not yet in. Similarly, the search for enzyme inhibitors has not been uniformly successful. For example, drugs that inhibit cyclooxygenase, and so the formation of prostaglandins and thromboxane, have no therapeutic value in asthma.

A new compound, zileuton, which inhibits 5-lipoxygenase, shows some promise. This drug interferes with the formation of the leukotrienes and has been found to offer some protection against isocapnic hyperventilation of cold air.[222] Curiously, it does not protect against other bronchoconstrictors.[222] Preliminary clinical trials indicate that it has bronchodilator reactivity, at least in some patients, and that the chronic administration reduces asthma symptoms and improves lung function.[223]

Guidelines for Therapy

Management of Acute Exacerbations.—The goal in treating acute asthma is to eliminate the patient's symptoms and improve lung function as quickly as possible with a minimum of side effects. In the past, first-line therapy consisted mainly of infused aminophylline. However, comparative studies in emergency room settings demonstrated that sympathomimetics produced three times more bronchodilatation then did aminophylline and that aerosol therapy was as effective as the parenterol route and produced less untoward effects.[94] Consequently, β_2-agonists have become the treatment of choice for acute airway obstruction. The means of administering the aerosols does not appear to be important, and studies have shown that both compressor-driven, hand-held nebulizers and multiple doses from a metered-dose inhaler equipped with a spacer will produce the same results.[234, 235] The caveat is that the latter must be given by a health care provider for maximum effectiveness. In the emergency room at our institution, acutely ill asthmatics are treated with 2.5 mg of albuterol by hand-held nebulizer every 20 minutes for 3 doses. Peak flow (PEFR) is recorded before and at the end of the treatment period. The patients are discharged when they become asymptomatic and the PEFR reaches 60% of normal. Those who do not meet both of these criteria at the end of the hour are tested further and reassessed in another 60 minutes. Using this regimen, our experience to date with over 500 patients demonstrates that approximately 80% can be discharged from the emergency room, in 2 hours or less with only a 4% return rate over the next week. Those who remain symptomatic and who have a PEFR less than 60% of expected at 2 hours are admitted (≈20%) of the population). Previous experiments have shown that such individuals need around-the-clock, aggressive care to improve.[158] Our data further indicate that a minimum of 48 hours is required to make these patients asymptomatic and to begin normalizing their PEFR.

It has become fashionable to administer glucocorticoids to all acutely ill asthmatics in the emergency room as first-line treatment in an effort to reduce admissions[226] and to prevent relapse after discharge.[227] While this approach is intuitively appealing, the data base supporting it is not very firm. As indicated previously, the onset of action of glucocorticoids is toc slow[149, 154–158, 161, 162] to have much of a benefit in an acute situation in an emergency room. In fact, of the 20% or so of patients who require admission to the hospital, the evidence is overwhelming that days, not hours, of steroid treatment are necessary to end the attack (see McFadden[163] for an analysis of steroid responses in acute asthma). It is important to note that the one study purporting to show an advantageous effect of steroids on acute asthma morbidity and admissions did not standardize either the quantity or duration of care given in the emergency room and did not find any significant differences in pulmonary function between the steroid and control groups.[226] A subsequent investigation using more rigorous initial therapy could not confirm the original report.[228]

The issue of whether steroids will prevent or minimize acute episodes of asthma from recurring is also not clear. Leaving aside the matter of whether oral glucocorticoids should be employed for such a purpose (i.e., should every acute episode of asthma be treated with steroids?), the database on the aforementioned subject needs to be expanded before firm conclusions can be reached. An early study recommending such an approach was flawed in that no objective assessments of patient improvement or lung function were presented.[229] Others have concluded that steroids worked in this capacity, but again, analysis of objective parameters does not confirm much benefit.[230, 231] Some of these deficits were corrected in a recent report when patients were carefully followed for 2 weeks with serial pulmonary function measurements and symptom diaries.[227] The authors of this report concluded that an 8-day course of prednisone significantly reduced the rate of relapse during the first 10 days following the emergency visit. Analysis of these data, however, show a curious pattern. The differences in relapse rates were most marked between days 4 and 10, and there were no significant differences between groups after this time, or perhaps before it. In our experience, only the recurrence of symptoms within 2 days of an emergency room visit is associated with a relapse from the original attack. Symptomatic episodes beyond this time are difficult to ascribe to a continuation or recrudescence of the original attack. Again, controlled trials that address all relevant variables are needed.

Management of Chronic Asthma

As with the treatment of acute asthma, the chronic management of this disease has evolved substantially over the last decade. Reliance on oral medications, and the heavy emphasis on theophylline, particularly in children, has been replaced by aerosolized β_2-agonists. The most recent recommendations include the early use of antiinflammatory agents.[2] Upon reviewing the literature, one has the sense of a forward movement in therapeutic management, and while this is true, it is important to appreciate that major gaps still exist in our knowledge and that too much of the therapy of asthma remains empirical.

In general terms, the major aim of treatment is to achieve a stable asymptomatic state with the best pulmonary function possible, utilizing whatever medications are necessary to achieve this goal. Once this has been accomplished, the drugs should be systematically withdrawn, beginning with the most toxic, until the lowest quantity of medication necessary to maintain the patient's well being has been reached. A reduction in the dosage and quantity of medications minimizes untoward reactions, forestalls the likelihood of tachyphylaxis, and substantially reduces the cost of treatment. The guidelines devised by the National Institutes of Health for the management of asthma[2] are a good starting point for such a program. They provide algorithms for patient care, including standard doses and sequencing of medications, and deal with education and monitoring. These recommendations are limited, however, by the absence of a critical examination of the efficacy of the various therapeutic strategies and the failures to consider the need for the withdrawal of medication and/or its adjustments.

Patients with infrequent attacks of asthma and those whose disease is predominantly associated with seasonal components can be managed easily on an as-needed basis with inhaled β_2-agent and drugs such as cromolyn or nedocromil. The adrenergic agonists will reverse acute symptomatology and the other drugs, when given prior to the onset of and during seasonal antigen exposure, will prevent and/or ameliorate immunologic increases in airway reactivity. Cromolyn and nedocromil are also quite useful in blocking the symptomatic consequences of acute antigen exposure. Thus, they can be given prophylactically on an as-needed basis in patients who experience intermittent contact to antigens to which they are sensitive. In these circumstances, chronic daily treatment is not required. Inhaled β_2-agonists provide much better prophylaxis against bronchoconstrictors other than antigen than either cromolyn or nedocromil and are the drugs of choice to prevent acute obstruction from nonimmunologic stimuli.

In patients with active disease who have unstable lung function, as indicated by increasing or persistent symptoms, an attempt should be made to reduce the underlying airway irritability by adding cromolyn, inhaled glucocorticoids, or both to the regimen. Since these drugs frequently take weeks to produce the desired effect, one may also wish to use a long-acting theophylline compound or a short, but intense course of oral corticosteroids to speed remission (i.e., 40 to 60 mg of prednisone daily for 4 days, followed by a decrease in the dose every 4 days over a period of 16 to 20 days until the dose reaches zero). In these circumstances, it is essential to monitor the peak expiratory flow rate and to base the adjustments in medication on the patient's symptoms and lung-function measurements. In severely ill patients, the use of oral glucocorticoids, in addition to the other measures listed above, is mandatory. If nocturnal episodes predominate, either a long-acting theophylline compound or a sustained-release oral β_2-agonist can be included to provide sufficient medication to last the night through. The availability of salmeterol and formoterol will also help solve this problem.

Although there is currently great enthusiasm for the use of cromolyn and, particularly, inhaled steroids in the context of the antiinflammatory treatment theory of asthma,[2] it should be remembered that both types of drugs have been used for almost 2 decades, during which time asthma morbidity and mortality have been rising. It may have been that we were using them incorrectly, but that possibility remains to be proved. In general, cromolyn and inhaled steroids work best in patients with the least severe disease, and as severity rises, their effectiveness diminishes.[169, 196]

The choice of whether to use steroids or cromolyn is open to debate. In some investigations, steroids proved more efficacious in controlling asthma than did cromolyn,[178, 179] whereas in others the effects of the drugs were equal.[232] Cromolyn does have the advantage of being able to block acute precipitants of asthma, whereas steroids do not. This latter factor provides some rationale for using both compounds together in patients whose asthma is difficult to manage. Determining which drug to use, when to use it, and how much to give will require major international cooperative trials.

A reduction in the dose of medication on the basis of symptoms and lung function is possible because asthma, unlike other inflammatory airway diseases, does not usually cause progressive structural damage. Tapering should be systematic, guided by close communication between physician and patient, and requires the use of objective measures of disease activity. Oral drugs should be withdrawn first, followed by a diminution in the frequency of aerosols. Some researchers advocate reducing the frequency of β_2-agonist administration from regular use to use only when needed, while maintaining the dose of aerosolized steroids and cromolyn. When this is accomplished, the doses of the antiinflammatory agents are lowered. Others reduce the dose of antiinflammatory agents to a minimum while maintaining the dose of the β_2-agonists. They next lower the sympathomimetic agents. This regimen is financially less expensive for the patient. There are few data that demonstrate the superiority of one approach over the other, nor are there data on the minimal effective quantities of steroids or cromolyn that will maintain remission.

If the patient is going to have problems, lung function will diminish before symptoms occur, and the PEFR will begin to show increased circadian variations. If these changes occur and the patient is asymptomatic, no further therapeutic adjustments should be made until function returns to normal. This may take several weeks. If the patient becomes symptomatic, he or she should again receive the lowest effective quantities of medication. When a patient's disease is unresponsive to intensive bronchodilator and antiinflammatory therapy, or when the dosage of such a therapeutic regimen cannot be reduced, alternative or concomitant reasons for the patient's pulmonary abnormalities, such as upper airway obstruction, embolic phenomena, vasculitis, congestive cardiac disease, or chronic subacute bacterial or fungal infections, should be explored.

References

1. McFadden ER Jr, Stevens JB: A history of asthma, in Middleton E, Reed C, Ellis E, (eds): *Allergy: Principles and Practice,* ed 2. St Louis, Mosby–Year Book, 1983, pp 805–809.
2. *National Asthma Education Program Expert Panel Report.* Guidelines for the diagnosis and management of asthma. U.S. Depart of Health and Human Services Publication No. 01:3042, 1991, pp 35–43.
3. Konig P, Godfrey S: Prevalence of exercise induced bronchial lability in families of children with asthma. *Arch Dis Child* 1973; 48:513–518.
4. Deal EC Jr, McFadden ER Jr, Ingram RH Jr, et al: Airway responsiveness to cold air and hyperpnea in normal subjects and in those with hay fever and asthma. *Am Rev Respir Dis* 1980; 121:621–628.
5. Silverman M, Hobbs FDR, Gordeon IRS, et al: Cystic fibrosis, atopy and airway lability. *Arch Dis Child* 1978; 53:873–877.
6. Ramsdell JW, Nachtwey FS, Moser KM: Bronchial hyperreactivity in chronic obstructive bronchitis. *Am Rev Respir Dis* 1982; 126:829–832.
7. Weiss KB, Gergen PJ, Hodgson TA: An economic evaluation of asthma in the United States. *N Engl J Med* 1992; 326:862–866.
8. Evans R, Mullally DI, Wilson RW, et al: National trends in the morbidity and mortality of asthma in the United States. Prevalence, hospitalization, and mortality of asthma over two decades, 1965–1984. *Chest* (Suppl) 1987; 91:65S–74S.
9. Weiss KB, Wagner DK: Changing patterns of asthma mortality identifying target populations at high risk. *JAMA* 1990; 264:1683–1687.
10. Johnson AJ, Nunn AJ, Somner AR, et al: Circumstances of death from asthma. *Brit Med J* 1984; 288:1870–1872.
11. Sears MR, Rea HH, Rosswell RPG, et al: Asthma mortality: Comparison between New Zealand and England. *Brit Med J* 1986; 293:1342–1345.
12. McFadden ER Jr, Gilbert IA: Asthma. *N Engl J Med* 1992; 327:1928–1937.
13. Boulet LP, Cartier A, Thomson NC, et al: Asthma and increases in nonallergic bronchial responsiveness from seasonal pollen exposure. *J Allergy Clin Immunol* 1983; 71:399–406.
14. Cartier A, Thomson NC, Frith PA, et al: Allergen-induced increases in bronchial responsiveness to histamine: Relationship to the late asthmatic response and change in airway caliber. *J Allergy Clin Immunol* 1982; 70:170–177.
15. Platts-Mills TAE, Mitchell EB, Nock P, et al: Reduction of bronchial hyperreactivity during prolonged allergen avoidance. *Lancet* 1982; 2:675–677.
16. Hargreave FE, Ryan G, Thomson NC, et al: Bronchial responsiveness to histamine of methacholine in asthma: Measurement and clinical significance. *J Allergy Clin Immunol* 1981; 68:347–355.
17. Empey DW, Laitinen LA, Jacobs J, et al: Mechanisms of bronchial hyperreactivity in normal subjects after upper respiratory tract infection. *Am Rev Respir Dis* 1976; 113:131–139.
18. Holtzman MI, Cunningham JH, Sheller JR, et al: Effect of ozone on bronchial

reactivity in atopic and non-atopic subjects. *Am Rev Respir Dis* 1979; 120:1059–1067.

19. Orehek J, Massari JP, Gayrard P, et al: Effect of short-term, low-level nitrogen dioxide exposure on bronchial sensitivity of asthmatic patients. *J Clin Invest* 1976; 57:301–307.
20. Sheppard D, Epstein J, Bethel RA, et al: Tolerance to sulfur dioxide-induced bronchoconstriction in subjects with asthma. *Environ Res* 1983; 30:412–419.
21. Mussaffi H, Springer C, Godfrey S: Increased bronchial responsiveness to exercise and histamine after allergen challenge in children with asthma. *J Allergy Clin Immunol* 1986; 77:48–52.
22. Thorpe JE, Steinberg D, Bernstein IL, et al: Bronchial reactivity increases soon after the immediate response in dual-responding asthmatic subjects. *Chest* 1987; 91:21–25.
23. Zawadski DK, Lenner KA, McFadden ER Jr: Effects of exercise on non-specific airway reactivity in asthmatics. *J Appl Physiol* 1988; 64:812–816.
24. Smolensky MH, Barnes PJ, Reinberg A, et al: Chronobiology and asthma. I. Day-night differences in bronchial patency and dyspnea and circadian rhythm dependencies. *J Asthma* 1986; 23:321–343.
25. Turner-Warwick M: On observing patterns of airflow obstruction in chronic asthma. *Br J Dis Chest* 1977; 71:73–86.
26. Hetzel MR, Clark TJH: Comparison of normal and asthmatic circadian rhythms in peak expiratory flow rate. *Thorax* 1980; 35:732–738.
27. Turner-Warwick M: Epidemiology of nocturnal asthma. *Am J Med* (Suppl 1B) 1988; 85:6–8.
28. Messer J, Peters GA, Bennet WA: Cause of death and pathological findings in 304 cases of bronchial asthma. *Dis Chest* 1960; 38:616–624.
29. Dunnill MS: The pathology of asthma with special reference to changes in the bronchial mucosa. *J Clin Pathol* 1960; 13:27–33.
30. *International consensus report on diagnosis and treatment of asthma.* US Department of Health and Human Services, Publication No. 92–2082.
31. Laitinen LA, Heino M, Laitinen A, et al: Damage of the airway epithelium and bronchial reactivity in patients with asthma. *Am Rev Respir Dis* 1985; 131:599–606.
32. Lozewicz S, Gomez E, Ferguson H, et al: Inflammatory cells in the airways in mild asthma. *Brit Med J* 1988; 297:1515–1516.
33. Beasley R, Roche WR, Roberts JA, et al: Cellular events in the bronchi in mild asthma and after bronchial provocation. *Am Rev Respir Dis* 1989; 139:806–817.
34. Jeffery PK, Wardlaw AJ, Nelson FC, et al: Bronchial biopsies in asthma, an ultrastructural, quantitative study and correlation with hyperreactivity. *Am Rev Respir Dis* 1989; 140:1745–1753.
35. Djukanovic R, Wilson JW, Britten KM, et al: Quantitation of mast cells and eosinophils in the bronchial mucosa of symptomatic atopic asthmatics and healthy control subjects using immunohistochemistry. *Am Rev Respir Dis* 1990; 142:863–871.
36. Lozewicz S, Wells C, Gomez E, et al: Morphological integrity of the bronchial epithelium in mild asthma. *Thorax* 1990; 45:12–15.
37. Brewster CEP, Howarth PH, Djukanovic R, et al: Myofibroblasts and subepithelial fibrosis in bronchial asthma. *Am J Respir Cell Mol Biol* 1990; 3:507–511.
38. Gilbert IA, Logan LS, Abdul-Karim F, et al: Inter-relationships between air-

way inflammation, morphology and asthma severity. *Clin Res* 1992; 40:(3) A696.

39. Woolcock AJ, Ollerenshaw SL: Characteristics of the inflammation in biopsies from large airways of subjects with asthma and subjects with chronic airflow limitation. *Am Rev Respir Dis* 1992; 145:922–927.
40. Djukanovic R, Roche WR, Wilson JW, et al: Mucosal inflammation in asthma. *Am Rev Respir Dis* 1990; 142:434–457.
41. Leff AR, Hamann KJ, Wegner CD: Inflammation and cell-cell interactions in airway hyperresponsiveness. *Am J Physiol* 1991; 260(Lung Cell Mol Physiol 4):L189–L206.
42. Kay AB: Asthma and inflammation. *J Allergy Clin Immunol* 1991; 87:893–910.
43. Wasserman SI: Mediators of immediate hypersensitivity. *J Allergy Clin Immunol* 1983; 72:101–115.
44. Barnes PJ: Neuropeptides and asthma. *Am Rev Respir Dis* 1991; 143:S28–S32.
45. Kaliner M: Asthma and mast cell activation. *J Allergy Clin Immunol* 1989; 83:510–520.
46. Drazen JM, Austen KF: Leukotrienes and airway responses. *Am Rev Respir Dis* 1987; 136:985–998.

46a. Corrigan CJ, Haczku A, Gemold-Engesaeth V, et al: CD_4 T-lymphocyte activation on asthma as accompanied by increased serum concentrations of interleukin-5. Effect of glucocorticoid therapy. *Am Rev Respir Dis* 1993; 147:504–507.

47. Kaplan AP, Haak-Frendscho M, Fauci A, et al: Histamine-releasing factor from activated human mononuclear cells. *J Immunol* 1985; 235:2027–2032.
48. Kelley J: Cytokines of the lung. *Am Rev Respir Dis* 1990; 141:765–788.
49. Soloperto M, Mattoso VL, Fasoli A, et al: A bronchial epithelial cell-derived factor in asthma that promotes eosinophil activation and survival as GM-CSF. *Am J Physiol* 1991; 260:L530–L538.
50. Howell CJ, Pujol JL, Crea AEG, et al: Identification of an alveolar macrophage-derived activity in bronchial asthma that enhances leukotriene C_4 generation by human eosinophils stimulated by ionophore A23187 as a granulocyte-macrophage colony-stimulating factor. *Am Rev Respir Dis* 1989; 140:1340–1347.
51. Hamid Q, Azzawi M, Ying S, et al: Expression of mRNA for interleukin-5 in mucosal bronchial biopsies from asthma. *J Clin Invest* 1991; 87:1541–1546.
52. Sedgwick JB, Calhoun WJ, Gleich GJ, et al: Immediate and late airway response of allergic rhinitis patients to segmental antigen challenge: Characterization of eosinophil and mast cell mediators. *Am Rev Respir Dis* 1991; 144:1274–1281.
53. Georas SN, Liu MC, Newman W, et al: Altered adhesion molecule expression and endothelial cell activation accompany the recruitment of human granulocytes to the lung after segmental antigen challenge. *Am J Respir Cell Mol Biol* 1992; 7:261–269.
54. Frigas E, Loegering DA, Solley GO, et al: Elevated levels of eosinophil granule major basic protein in the sputum of patients with bronchial asthma. *Mayo Clinic Proc* 1981; 56:345–353.
55. Bousquet J, Chanez P, Lacoste JY, et al: Eosinophilic inflammation in asthma. *N Engl J Med* 1990; 323:1033–1039.
56. Wardlaw AJ, Dunnette S, Gleich GJ, et al: Eosinophils and mast cells in

bronchoalveolar lavage in subjects with mild asthma. Relationship to bronchial hyperreactivity. *Am Rev Respir Dis* 1988; 137:62–69.

57. Adelroth E, Rosenhall L, Johansson SA, et al: Inflammatory cells and eosinophilic activity in asthmatics investigated by bronchoalveolar lavage. The effects of antiasthmatic treatment with budesonide or terbutaline. *Am Rev Respir Dis* 1990; 142:91–99.
58. Nadel JA, Borson DB: Modulation of neurogenic inflammation by neutral endopeptidase. *Am Rev Respir Dis* 1991; 142:S33–S36.
59. Brusasco V, Crimi E, Gianiorio P, et al: Allergen-induced increase in airway responsiveness and inflammation in mild asthma. *J Appl Physiol* 1990; 69:2209–2214.
60. Foresi A, Bertorelli G, Pesci A, et al: Inflammatory markers in bronchoalveolar lavage and in bronchial biopsy in asthma during remission. *Chest* 1990; 98:528–535.
61. Godard P, Bousquet J, Lebel B, et al: Bronchoalveolar lavage in the asthmatic. *Bull Eur Physiopathol Respir* 1987; 23:73–83.
62. Nagy L, Lee TH, Kay AB: Neutrophil chemotactic activity in antigen-induced late asthmatic reactions. *N Engl J Med* 1982; 306:497–501.
63. Westcott JY, Smith HR, Wenzel SE, et al: Urinary leukotriene E_4 in patients with asthma. Effect of airways reactivity and sodium cromoglycate. *Am Rev Respir Dis* 1991; 143:1322–1328.
64. Stenton SC, Court EN, Kingston WP, et al: Platelet-activating factor in bronchoalveolar lavage fluid from asthmatic subjects. *Eur Respir J* 1990; 3:408–413.
65. Liu MC, Bleecker ER, Lichtenstein LM, et al: Evidence for elevated levels of histamine, prostaglandin D_2 and other bronchoconstricting prostaglandins in the airways of subjects with mild asthma. *Am Rev Respir Dis* 1990; 142:126–132.
66. Jarjour NN, Calhoun WJ, Schwartz LB, et al: Elevated bronchoalveolar lavage fluid histamine levels in allergic asthmatics are associated with increased airway obstruction. *Am Rev Respir Dis* 1991; 144:83–87.
67. Wenzel SE, Westcott JY, Smith HR, et al: Spectrum of prostanoid release after bronchoalveolar allergen challenge in atopic asthmatics and in control groups. An alteration in the ratio of bronchoconstrictive to bronchoprotective mediators. *Am Rev Respir Dis* 1989; 139:450–457.
68. Lam S, Chan H, LeRiche JC, et al: Release of leukotrienes in patients with bronchial asthma. *J Allergy Clin Immunol* 1988; 81:711–717.
69. Casale TB, Wood D, Richerson HB, et al: Elevated bronchoalveolar lavage fluid histamine levels in allergic asthmatics are associated with methacholine bronchial hyperresponsiveness. *J Clin Invest* 1987; 79:1197–1203.
70. Murray JJ, Tonnel AB, Brash AR, et al: Release of prostaglandin D_2 into human airways during acute antigen challenge. *N Engl J Med* 1986; 315:800–804.
71. Smith LJ: The role of platelet-activating factor in asthma. *Am Rev Respir Dis* 1991; 143:S100–S102.
72. Cuss FM, Dixon CMS, Barnes PJ: Effect of inhaled platelet activating factor on pulmonary function and bronchoresponsiveness in humans. *Lancet* 1986; 2:189–192.
73. Rubin A-HE, Smith LJ, Patterson R: The bronchoconstrictor properties of platelet-activating factor in humans. *Am Rev Respir Dis* 1987; 136:1145–1151.
74. Lai CKW, Jenkins JR, Polosa R, et al: Inhaled PAF fails to induce airway hy-

perresponsiveness to methacholine in normal human subjects. *J Appl Physiol* 1990; 68:919–926.

75. Wasserman SI, Soter NA, Center DM, et al: Cold urticaria. Recognition and characterization of neutrophil chemotactic factor which appears in serum during experimental cold challenge. *J Clin Invest* 1977; 60:189–196.
76. Soter NA, Wasserman SI, Austen KF, et al: Release of mast-cell mediators and alterations in lung function in patients with cholinergic urticaria. *N Engl J Med* 1980; 302:604–608.
77. Chung KF, Barnes PJ: Effects of platelet activating factor on airway calibre, airway responsiveness and circulating cells in asthmatic subjects. *Thorax* 1989; 44:108–115.
78. O'Byrne PM, Dolovich J, Hargreave FE: Late asthmatic responses. *Am Rev Respir Dis* 1987; 136:740–751.
79. Lee TH, Nagakura T, Papageorgiou N, et al: Exercise-induced late asthmatic reactions with neutrophil chemotactic activity. *N Engl J Med* 1983; 308:1502–1505.
80. Cockcroft DW, Murdock KY: Comparative effects of inhaled salbutamol, sodium, cromoglycate, and beclomethasone dipropionate on allergen-induced early asthmatic responses, late asthmatic responses, and increased bronchial responsiveness to histamine. *J Allergy Clin Immunol* 1987; 79:734–740.
81. Mattoli S, Foresi A, Corbo GM, et al: Effects of two doses of cromolyn on allergen-induced late asthmatic response and increased responsiveness. *J Allergy Clin Immunol* 1987; 79:747–754.
82. Church MK, Hiroi J: Inhibition of IgE-dependent histamine release from human dispersed lung mast cells by antiallergic drugs and salbutamol. *Br J Pharmacol* 1987; 90:421–429.
83. Kraan J, Koeter GH, van der Mark TW, et al: Changes in bronchial hyperreactivity induced by 4 weeks of treatment with antiasthmatic drugs in patients with allergic asthma: a comparison between budesonide and terbutaline. *J Allergy Clin Immunol* 1985; 76:628–636.
84. Kerrebijn KF, van Essen-Zandvliet EEM, Neijens HJ: Effects of long term treatment with inhaled corticosteroids and beta-agonists on the bronchial responsiveness in children with asthma. *J Allergy Clin Immunol* 1987; 79:653–659.
85. Dutoit JI, Salome CM, Woolcock AJ: Inhaled corticosteroids reduce the severity of bronchial hyperresponsiveness in asthma, but oral theophylline does not. *Am Rev Respir Dis* 1987; 136:1174–1178.
86. Schleimer RP, Schulman ES, MacGlashan DW, et al: Effects of dexamethasone on mediator release from human lung fragments and purified human lung mast cells. *J Clin Invest* 1983; 71:1830–1835.
87. McFadden ER Jr: Beta receptor agonists: metabolism and pharmacology. *J Allergy Clin Immunol* 1981; 68:91–97.
88. Stiles GL, Caron MG, Lefkowitz RJ: β-adrenergic receptors: biochemical mechanisms of physiological regulation. *Physiol Rev* 1984; 64:661–743.
89. Nadel JA, Davis B: Autonomic regulation of mucus secretion and ion transport in airways, in Lictenstein LM, Austen KF (eds): *Asthma: Physiology, Immunopharmacology, and Treatment,* New York, Academic Press 1977, pp 197–210.
90. Santa Cruz R, Landa J, Hirsch J, et al: Tracheal mucus velocity in normal man and in patients with obstructive lung disease, effects of terbutaline. *Am Rev Respir Dis* 1974; 109:458–461.
91. Basran GS, Paul W, Morley J, et al: Adrenoceptor-agonist inhibition of hista-

mine-induced cutaneous response in man. *Br J Dermatol* (Suppl 23) 1982; 107:140–142.

92. Rhoden KJ, Meldrum LA, Barnes PJ: Inhibition of cholinergic neurotransmission in human airways by β_2-adrenoceptors. *J Appl Physiol* 1988; 65:700–705.
93. Nelson HS: Adrenergic therapy of bronchial asthma. *J Allergy Clin Immunol* 1986; 77:771–785.
94. Rossing TH, Fanta CH, Goldstein DH, et al: Emergency therapy of asthma: comparison of the acute effects of parenteral and inhaled sympathomimetics and infused aminophylline. *Am Rev Respir Dis* 1980; 122:365.
95. Haahtela T, Jarvinen M, Kava T, et al: Comparison of a β_2-agonist, terbutaline, with an inhaled corticosteroid, budesonide, in newly detected asthma. *N Engl J Med* 1991; 325:388–392.
96. Laitinen LA, Laitinen A, Haahtela T: A comparative study of the effects of an inhaled corticosteroid, budesonide, and a β_2-agonist, terbutaline in newly diagnosed asthma: A randomized, double-blind, parallel group controlled trial. *J Allergy Clin Immunol* 1992; 90:32–42.
97. Pearlman DS, Chervinsky P, LaFarce C, et al: A comparison of salmeterol with albuterol in the treatment of mild to moderate asthma. *N Engl J Med* 1992; 327:1420–1451.
98. Measen FP, Smeets JJ, Gubbelmans HLL, et al: Bronchodilator effect of inhaled formoterol vs salbutamol over 12 hours. *Chest* 1990; 97:590–594.
99. Wong BJ, Dolovich J, Ramsdale EH, et al: Formoterol compared with beclomethasone and placebo on allergen-induced asthma responses. *Am Rev Respir Dis* 1992; 146:1156–1160.
100. Derem EY, Pauwels RA, Van Der Straeten MEF: The effect of inhaled salmeterol on methacholine responsiveness in subjects with asthma up to 12 hours. *J Allergy Clin Immunol* 1992; 89:811–815.
101. Twentyman OP, Finnerty SP, Harris A, et al: Protection against allergen-induced asthma by salmeterol. *Lancet* 1990; 336:1338–1342.
102. O'Shaughnessy KM, Taylor CK, Fuller RW: β_2-agonists in asthma. *Lancet* 1991; 337:45–46.
103. Leitch AG, Clancy LJ, Costello JF, et al: Effect of intravenous infusion of salbutamol on ventilatory response to carbon dioxide and hypoxia and on heart rate and plasma potassium in normal man. *Br Med J* 1976; 1:365–367.
104. Kallenbach J, Joffe BI, Zwi S, et al: Metabolic and cardiovascular effects of salbutamol in atopic subjects with and without asthma. *Scand J Respir Dis* 1979; 60:44–48.
105. Nogrady SG, Hartley JPR, Seaton A: Metabolic effects of intravenous salbutamol in the course of acute severe asthma. *Thorax* 1977; 32:559–561.
106. Leslie D, Coates PM: Salbutamol-induced diabetic ketoacidosis. *Br Med J* 1977; 3:768–770.
107. Coady TJ, Stewart CJ, Davies HJ: Synchronization of bronchodilator release. *Practitioner* 1976; 217:273–275.
108. Shim C, Williams MH: The adequacy of inhalation of aerosol from canister nebulizers. *Am J Med* 1980; 69:891–894.
109. Crompton G: Problems patients have using pressurized aerosol inhalers. *Eur J Respir Dis* 1982; 63(suppl 119):101–104.
110. Kelling JS, Strohl KP, Smith RL, et al: Physician knowledge in the use of canister nebulizers. *Chest* 1983; 83:612–614.
111. Guidry GG, Brown WD, Stogner SW, et al: Incorrect use of metered dose inhalers by medical personnel. *Chest* 1992; 101:31–33.

112. Crompton GK: New inhalation devices. *Eur Respir J* 1988; 1:679–680.
113. Nicklas RA: Paradoxical bronchospasm associated with the use of inhaled β-agonists. *J Allergy Clin Immunol* 1990; 85:959–964.
114. Jackson R, Sears MR, Beaglehole R, et al: International trends in asthma mortality: 1970–1985. *Chest* 1988; 94:914–919.
115. Crane J, Flatt A, Jackson R, et al: Prescribed fenoterol and death from asthma in New Zealand, 1981–83: Case-control study. *Lancet* 1989; 917–922.
116. Pearce N, Granger J, Atkinson M, et al: Case control study of prescribed fenoterol and death in New Zealand, 1977–81. *Thorax* 1990; 45:170–175.
117. Granger J, Woodman K, Pearce N, et al: Prescribed fenoterol and death from asthma in New Zealand, 1981–1987: a further case-control study. *Thorax* 1991; 46:105–111.
118. Spitzer WO, Suissa S, Ernst P, et al: The use of β-agonists and the risk of death and near death from asthma. *N Engl J Med* 1992; 326:501–506.
119. CSM. Working party. β-agonist use in asthma. *Curr Problems* 1992; No. 33.
120. Sears MR, Rea HH, Fenwick J, et al: Deaths in asthmatics prescribed home nebulizers. *Br Med J* 1987; 294:477–480.
121. Weber RW, Smith JA, Nelson HS: Aerosolized terbutaline in asthmatics: development of subsensitivity with long-term administration. *J Allergy Clin Immunol* 1982; 70:417–422.
122. Repsher LH, Anderson JA, Bush RK, et al: Assessment of tachyphylaxis following prolonged therapy of asthma with inhaled albuterol aerosol. *Chest* 1984; 85:34–38.
123. Vathenen AS, Knox AJ, Higgins RG, et al: Rebound increase in bronchial responsiveness after treatment with inhaled terbutaline. *Lancet* 1988; i:554–557.
124. van Schayck CP, Graafsma SJ, Visch MB, et al: Increased bronchial hyperresponsiveness after inhaling salbutamol during 1 year is not caused by subsensitization to salbutamol. *J Allergy Clin Immunol* 1990; 86:793–800.
125. Tattersfield AE: Tolerance to β-agonists. *Bull Eur Physiopathol Respir* 1985; 21:1S–5S.
126. Page CP: One explanation of the asthma paradox: inhibition of natural autoinflammatory mechanism by β_2-agonist. *Lancet* 1991; 337:717–720.
127. Sears MR, Taylor DR, Print CG, et al: Regular inhaled β-agonist treatment in bronchial asthma. *Lancet* 1990; 336:1391–1396.
127a. Taylor DR, Sears MR, Herbison GP, et al: Regular inhaled β-agonist in asthma. Effects on exacerbations and lung function. *Thorax* 1993; 48:134–138.
128. Shepherd GL, Hetzel MR, Clark TJH: Regular versus symptomatic aerosol bronchodilator treatment of asthma. *Br J Dis Chest* 1981; 75:215–217.
129. Cheung D, Timmers MC, Zwinderman AH, et al: Long-term effects of a long-acting β_2-adrenoceptor agonist, salmeterol, on airway hyperresponsiveness in patients with mild asthma. *N Engl J Med* 1992; 327:1198–1203.
129a. Chapman KR, Kesten S: Asthma control and the regular versus as needed use of inhaled salbutamol. *Am Rev Respir Dis* 1993; 147:A59.
130. Hendles L, Weinberger M: Theophylline: A state of the art review. *Pharmacotherapy* 1983; 3:2–44.
131. Persson CG: Overview of effects of theophylline. *J Allergy Clin Immunol* 1986; 78:780–787.
132. Weinberger M, Hendeles L: Experience with theophylline for the management of chronic asthma. *Eur J Respir Dis* 1980; 61(suppl 109):120–133.

133. Hambelton G, Weinberger M, Taylor J, et al: Comparison of cromoglycate (cromolyn) and theophylline in controlling symptoms of chronic asthma. *Lancet* 1977; 1:381–385.
134. Nassif EG, Weinberger M, Thompson R, et al: The value of maintenance theophylline in steroid-dependent asthma. *N Engl J Med* 1981; 304:71–75.
135. Bundgaard A, Weeks B: Long-term treatment with oral sustained-release theophylline. *Allergy* 1982; 37:149–154.
136. Suedmyr K: β_2-Adrenoceptor stimulants and theophylline in asthma therapy. *Eur J Respir Dis* (suppl) 1981; 116:1–48.
137. Tsiu SJ, Self TH, Burnes R: Theophylline toxicity: Update. *Ann Allergy* 1990; 64:241–257.
138. Greening AP, Baillie E, Gribbin HR, et al: Sustained release oral aminophylline in patients with airflow obstruction. *Thorax* 1981; 36:303–307.
139. Rachelefsky GS, Wo J, Adelson J, et al: Behavior abnormalities and poor school performance due to oral theophylline use. *Pediatrics* 1986; 78:1133–1138.
140. Lindgren S, Lakshin B, Stromquist A, et al: Does asthma or treatment with theophylline limit children's academic performance? *N Engl J Med* 1992; 327:926–930.
141. Gross NJ: Ipratropium bromide. *N Engl J Med* 1988; 319:486–494.
142. Cockcroft DW, Ruffin RE, Hargreave FE: Effect of Sch1000 in allergen-induced asthma. *Clin Allergy* 1978; 8:361–372.
143. Howard PH, Durham SR, Lee TH, et al: Influence of albuterol, cromolyn sodium and ipratropium bromide on the airway and circulating mediator responses to allergen bronchial provocation in asthma. *Am Rev Respir Dis* 1985; 132:986–992.
144. Rebuck AS, Chapman KR, Abboud R, et al: Nebulized anticholinergic and sympathomimetic treatment of asthma and chronic obstructive airways disease in the emergency room. *Am J Med* 1987; 82:59–64.
145. Shenfield GM: Combination bronchodilator therapy. *Drugs* 1982; 24:414–439.
146. Baigelman W, Chodosh S, Pizzuto D, et al: Sputum and blood eosinophils during corticosteroid treatment of acute exacerbations of asthma. *Am J Med* 1983; 75:929–936.
147. Flowers RJ: Lipocortin and the mechanism of action of the glucocorticoids. *Br J Pharmacol* 1988; 94:987–1015.
148. Ellul-Micallef R, Fenech FF: Intravenous prednisolone in chronic bronchial asthma. *Thorax* 1975; 30:312–315.
149. McFadden ER Jr, Kiser R, DeGroot W, et al: A controlled study of the effect of single doses of hydrocortisone on the resolution of acute attacks of asthma. *Am J Med* 1976; 60:52–59.
150. Molema J, Lammers J-WJ, van Herwaarden CLA, et al: Effects of inhaled beclomethasone dipropionate on β_2-receptor function in the airways and adrenal responsiveness in bronchial asthma. *Eur J Clin Pharmacol* 1988; 34:577–583.
151. Ellul-Micallef R, Borthwick RC, McHardy GJR: The time-course of response to prednisolone in chronic bronchial asthma. *Clin Sci Mole Med* 1974; 47:105–117.
152. Klaustermeyer WB, Hale FC: The physiologic effect of an intravenous glucocorticoid in bronchial asthma. *Ann Allergy* 1976; 37:80–86.
153. Britton MG, Collins JV, Brown D, et al: High-dose corticosteroids in severe acute asthma. *Brit Med J* 1976; 2:73–74.

154. Sue MA, Kwong FK, Klaustermeyer WB: A comparison of intravenous hydrocortisone, methylprednisolone, and dexamethasone in acute bronchial asthma. *Ann Allergy* 1986; 56:406–409.
155. Pierson WE, Bierman CW, Kelley VC: A double-blind trial of corticosteroid therapy in Status Asthmaticus. *Pediatrics* 1974; 54:282–288.
156. Collins JV, Clark TJH, Brown D, et al: The use of corticosteroids in the treatment of acute asthma. *Quart J Med* 1975; 174:259–273.
157. Haskell RJ, Wong BM, Hansen JE: A double-blind, randomized clinical trial of methylprednisolone in Status Asthmaticus. *Arch Intern Med* 1983; 143:1324–1327.
158. Fanta CH, Rossing TH, McFadden ER Jr: Glucocorticoids in acute asthma, A critical controlled trial. *Am J Med* 1983; 74:845–851.
159. Ramsdell JW, Berry CC, Clausen JL: The immediate effects of cortisol on pulmonary function in normals and asthmatics. *J Allergy Clin Immunol* 1983; 71:69–74.
160. Kattan M, Gurwitz D, Levison H: Corticosteroids in Status Asthmaticus. *J Pediat* 1980; 96:596–599.
161. Storr J, Barrell E, Barry W, et al: Effect of a single oral dose of prednisolone in acute childhood asthma. *Lancet* 1987; ii:879–882.
162. Harfi H, Hanissian AS, Crawford LV: Treatment of Status Asthmaticus in children with high doses and conventional doses of methylprednisolone. *Pediatrics* 1978; 61:829–831.
163. McFadden ER Jr: Dosages of corticosteroids in asthma: A clinical commentary. *Am Rev Respir Dis* (in press).
164. Brogden RN, Heel RC, Speight TM, et al: Beclomethasone dipropionate. A reappraisal of its pharmacodynamic properties and therapeutic efficacy after a decade of use in asthma and rhinitis. *Drugs* 1984; 28:99–126.
165. Bernstein IL, Chervinsky P, Falliers CJ: Efficacy and safety of triamcinolone acetonide aerosol in chronic asthma. *Chest* 1982; 81:20–26.
166. Slavin RG, Izu AE, Bernstein IL, et al: Multi-center study of flunisolide aerosol in adult patients with steroid-dependent asthma. *J Allergy Clin Immunol* 1980; 66:379–385.
167. Rafferty P, Tucker LG, Frame MH, et al: Comparison of budesonide and beclomethasone dipropionate in patients with severe chronic asthma: assessment of relative prednisolone-sparing effects. *Br J Dis Chest* 1985; 79:244–250.
168. American Academy of Allergy and Immunology Study Group, Reed CE, Chairman: Treatment of mild to moderate asthma: Comparison of aerosol beclomethasone and oral theophylline. *Am Acad Respir Dis* 1991; 143:A625.
168a. Salmeron J, Guerin J-C, Godard P: High doses of inhaled corticosteroids in unstable chronic asthma. A multicenter, double-blind, placebo controlled study. *Am Rev Respir Dis* 1989; 140:167–171.
169. Brogden RN, Pinder RM, Sawyer PR, et al: Beclomethasone dipropionate inhaler: a review of its pharmacology, therapeutic value and adverse effects. I. Asthma. *Drugs* 1975; 10:166–210.
170. Juniper EF, Kline PA, Vanzieleghem MA, et al: Effect of long-term treatment with an inhaled corticosteroid (Budesonide) on airway hyperresponsiveness and clinical asthma in nonsteroid-dependent asthmatics. *Am Rev Respir Dis* 1990; 142:832–836.
171. Vathenen AS, Knox AJ, Wisniewski A, et al: Time course of change in bronchial reactivity with an inhaled corticosteroid in asthma. *Am Rev Respir Dis* 1991; 143:1317–1321.

172. Kraan J, Koeter GH, Van Der Mark TH W, et al: Dosage and time effects of inhaled budesonide on bronchial hyperreactivity. *Am Rev Respir Dis* 1988; 137:44–48.
173. Easton JG: Effect of inhaled corticosteroid on methacholine airway reactivity. *J Allergy Clin Immunol* 1981; 67:388–390.
174. Jeffery PK, Godfrey RW, Adelroth E, et al: Effects of treatment on airway inflammation and thickening of basement membrane reticular collagen in asthma: a quantitative light and electron microscopic study. *Am Rev Respir Dis* 1992; 145:890–899.
175. Jenkins CR, Woolcock AJ: Effect of prednisone and beclomethasone dipropionate on airway responsiveness in asthma: a comparative study. *Thorax* 1988; 42:378–384.
176. Djukanovic R, Wilson JW, Britten KM, et al: Effect of an inhaled corticosteroid on airway inflammation and symptoms of asthma. *Am Rev Respir Dis* 1992; 145:669–674.
176a. Bhagat R, Grunstein MM: Effect of corticosteroids on bronchial responsiveness to methacholine in asthmatic children. *Am Rev Respir Dis* 1985; 131: 902–906.
177. Wiebicke W, Jorres R, Magnussen H: Comparison of the effects of inhaled corticosteroids on the airway response to histamine, methacholine, hyperventilation, and sulfur dioxide in subjects with asthma. *J Allergy Clin Immunol* 1990; 86:915–923.
178. Svendsen UG, Frolund L, Madsen F, et al: A comparison of the effects of sodium cromoglycate and beclomethasone dipropionate on pulmonary function and bronchial hyperreactivity in subjects with asthma. *J Allergy Clin Immunol* 1987; 80:68–74.
179. Molema J, van Herwaarden CLA, Folgering HTM: Effects of long-term treatment with inhaled cromoglycate and budesonide on bronchial hyperresponsiveness in patients with allergic asthma. *Eur Respir J* 1989; 2:308–316.
180. De Baets FM, Goeteyn M, Kerrebijn KF: The effect of two months of treatment with inhaled budesonide on bronchial responsiveness to histamine and house-dust mite antigen in asthmatic children. *Am Rev Respir Dis* 1990; 142:581–586.
181. Juniper EF, Kline PA, Vanzieleghem MA, et al: Reduction of budesonide after a year of increased use: a randomized controlled trial to evaluate whether improvements in airway responsiveness and clinical asthma are maintained. *J Allergy Clin Immunol* 1991; 87:483–489.
182. Bel EH, Timmers MC, Zwinderman AH, et al: The effect of inhaled corticosteroids on the maximal degree of airway narrowing to methacholine in asthmatic subjects. *Am Rev Respir Dis* 1991; 143:109–113.
183. Toogood JH: High-dose inhaled steroid therapy for asthma. *J Allergy Clin Immunol* 1989; 83:528–536.
184. Salmeron S, Guerin JC, Godard P, et al: High doses of inhaled corticosteroids in unstable chronic asthma: a multicenter, double-blind, placebo controlled study. *Am Rev Respir Dis* 1989; 140:167–171.
185. Malo JL, Cartier A, Merland N, et al: Four-times-a-day dosing frequency is better than a twice-a-day regimen in subjects requiring a high-dose inhaled steroid, budesonide, to control moderate to severe asthma. *Am Rev Respir Dis* 1989; 140:624–628.
186. Toogood JH, Jennings B, Greenway RW, et al: Candidiasis and dysphonia complicating beclomethasone treatment of asthma. *J Allergy Clin Immunol* 1980; 65:145–153.

187. Williams AJ, Baghat MS, Stableforth DE, et al: Dysphonia caused by inhaled steroids: recognition of a characteristic laryngeal abnormality. *Thorax* 1983; 38:813–821.
188. Smith MJ, Hodson ME: Effects of long term inhaled high dose beclomethasone dipropionate on adrenal function. *Thorax* 1983; 38:676–681.
189. Law CM, Marchant JL, Honour JW, et al: Nocturnal adrenal suppression in asthmatic children taking inhaled beclomethasone dipropionate. *Lancet* 1986; 1:942–944.
190. Kewley GD: Possible association between beclomethasone diproprionate aerosol and cataracts. *Aust Pediatr J* 1980; 16:117–118.
191. Pouw EM, Prummel MF, Oosting H, et al: Beclomethasone inhalation decreases serum osteocalcin concentrations. *Br Med J* 1991; 302:627–628.
192. Wolthers OD, Pedersen S: Growth of asthmatic children during treatment with budesonide: a double blind trial. *Br Med J* 1991; 303:163–165.
193. Capewell S, Reynolds S, Shuttleworth D, et al: Purpura and dermal thinning associated with high dose inhaled corticosteroids. *Br Med J* 1990; 300:1548–1551.
194. Diaz P, Galleguillos FR, Gonzalez MC, et al: Bronchoalveolar lavage in asthma: The effect of disodium cromoglycate (cromolyn) on leukocyte counts, immunoglobulins, and complement. *J Allergy Clin Immunol* 1984; 74:41–48.
195. Auty RM: Pharmacologic modulation of bronchial hyperreactivity. *Immunol Allergy Practice* 1983; 3:47–54.
196. Long-term study of disodium cromoglycate in treatment of severe extrinsic or intrinsic bronchial asthma in adults: Brompton Hospital/Medical Research Council Collaboration Trial. *Br Med J* 1972; 4:383–388.
197. Murphy S, Kelly HW: Cromolyn sodium: a review of mechanisms and clinical use in asthma. *Drug Intell Clin Pharm* 1987; 21:22–35.
198. Hoag JE, McFadden ER Jr: Long-term effect of cromolyn sodium on nonspecific bronchial hyperresponsiveness: a review. *Ann Allergy* 1991; 66:53–63.
199. Godfrey S, Konig P: Inhibition of exercise-induced asthma by different pharmacological pathways. *Thorax* 1976; 31:137–143.
200. Breslin FJ, McFadden ER Jr, Ingram RH: The effects of cromolyn sodium on the airway response to hyperpnea and cold air in asthma. *Am Rev Respir Dis* 1980; 122:11–16.
201. Sheppard D, Nadel JA, Boushey HA: Inhibition of sulfur dioxide-induced bronchoconstriction by disodium cromoglycate in asthmatic subjects. *Am Rev Respir Dis* 1981; 124:257–259.
202. Butcher BT, Karr RM, O'Neil CE, et al: Inhalation challenge and pharmacologic studies of toluene diisocyanate (TDI)-sensitive workers. *J Allergy Clin Immunol* 1979; 64:146–152.
203. Latimer KM, O'Byrne PM, Morris MM, et al: Bronchoconstriction stimulated by airway cooling—better protection with combined inhalation of terbutaline sulphate and cromolyn sodium than with either alone. *Am Rev Respir Dis* 1983; 128:440–443.
204. Numeroso R, Torre FD, Radaelli C, et al: Effect of long-term treatment with sodium cromoglycate on non-specific bronchial hyperreactivity in non-atopic patients with chronic bronchitis. *Respiration* 1983; 44:109–117.
205. Auty RM, Holgate ST: Nedocromil sodium: A review of its anti-inflammatory properties and clinical activity in the treatment of asthma, in Kay AB (ed): *Allergy and Asthma: New Trends and Approaches to Therapy,* Boston, Blackwell Scientific Publications, 1989, pp 171–188.

206. Rebuck AS, Kesten S, Boulet LP, et al: A 3-month evaluation of the efficacy of nedocromil sodium in asthma: A randomized, double-blind, placebo-controlled trial of nedocromil sodium conducted by a Canadian multicenter study group. *J Allergy Clin Immunol* 1990; 85:612–617.
207. Bone MF, Kubik MM, Keaney NP, et al: Nedocromil sodium in adults with asthma dependent on inhaled corticosteroids: a double-blind, placebo controlled study. *Thorax* 1989; 44:654–659.
208. Goldin JG, Bateman ED: Does nedocromil sodium have a steroid sparing effect in adult asthmatic patients requiring maintenance oral corticosteroids. *Thorax* 1988; 43:982–986.
209. Mullarkey MF, Blumenstein BA, Andrade WP, et al: Methotrexate in the treatment of corticosteroid-dependent asthma. A double-blind crossover study. *N Engl J Med* 1988; 318:603–607.
210. Dyer PD, Vaughan TR, Weber RW: Methotrexate in the treatment of steroid-dependent asthma. *J Allergy Clin Immunol* 1991; 88:208–212.
211. Shiner RJ, Nunn AJ, Chung KF, et al: Randomized, double-blind, placebo-controlled trial of methotrexate in steroid-dependent asthma. *Lancet* 1990; 336:137–140.
212. Erzurum SC, Leff JA, Cochran JE, et al: Lack of benefit of methotrexate in severe, steroid-dependent asthma. A double-blind, placebo-controlled study. *Ann Int Med* 1991; 114:353–360.
212a. Trigg CJ, Davies RJ: Comparison of methotrexate 30 mg per week with placebo in chronic steroid-dependent asthma. A 12-week double-blind, cross over study. *Respir Med* 1993; 87:211–216.
213. Mullarkey MF, Webb R, Pardee NE: Methotrexate in the treatment of steroid-dependent asthma. *Ann Allergy* 1986; 56:347–350.
214. Mullarkey MF, Lammert JK, Blumenstein BA: Long-term methotrexate treatment in corticosteroid-dependent asthma. *Ann Int Med* 1990; 112:577–581.
215. Bernstein DI, Bernstein IL, Bodenheimer SS, et al: An open study of auranofin in the treatment of steroid-dependent asthma. *J Allergy Clin Immunol* 1988; 81:6–16.
216. Muranaka M, Miyamoto T, Shida T, et al: Gold salt in the treatment of bronchial asthma—a double-blind study. *Ann Allergy* 1978; 40:132–137.
217. Klaustermeyer WB, Noritake DT, Kwong FK: Chrysotherapy in the treatment of corticosteroid-dependent asthma. *J Allergy Clin Immunol* 1987; 79:720–725.
218. Holgate ST, Finnerty J: Antihistamines in asthma. *J Allergy Clin Immunol* 1989; 83:537–547.
219. Rafferty P, Holgate ST: Histamine and its antagonists in asthma. *J Allergy Clin Immunol* 1989; 84:144–151.
220. Tinkelman DC, Webb CS, Vanderpool CC, et al: The use of ketotifen in the prophylaxis of seasonal allergic asthma. *Ann Allergy* 1986; 56:213–217.
221. Loftus BG, Price JF: Long-term, placebo-controlled trial of ketotifen in the management of preschool children with asthma. *J Allergy Clin Immunol* 1987; 79:350–355.
222. Busse WW, Gaddy JN: The role of leukotriene antagonists and inhibitors in the treatment of airway disease. *Am Rev Respir Dis* 1991; 143:5103–5107.
223. Israel E, Rubin P, Pearlman H, et al: 5-Liposygenase inhibitor by zibenton causes acute bronchodilation in asthma. *Am Rev Respir Dis* 1992; 145:A16.
224. Benton G, Thomas RC, Nickerson BG, et al: Experience with a metered-dose inhaler with a spacer in pediatric emergency department. *AJDC* 1989; 143:678–681.

225. Bowton DL, Goldsmith WM, Haponik EF: Substitution of metered-dose inhalers for hand-held nebulizers. *Chest* 1992; 101:305–308.
226. Littenberg B, Gluck EH: A controlled trial of methylprednisolone in the emergency treatment of acute asthma. *N Engl J Med* 1986; 314:150–152.
227. Chapman KR, Verberk PR, White JG, et al: Effect of a short course of prednisone in the prevention of early relapse after the emergency room treatment of acute asthma. *N Engl J Med* 1991; 324:788–794.
228. Stein LM, Cole RP: Early administration of corticosteroids in emergency room treatment of acute asthma. *Ann Inf Med* 1990; 112:822–827.
229. Fiel SB, Swartz NA, Glanz K, et al: Efficacy of short-term corticosteroid therapy in outpatient treatment of acute bronchial asthma. *Am J Med* 1983; 75:259–262.
230. Shapiro GG, Furukawa CT, Pierson WE, et al: Double-blind evaluation of methylprednisolone versus placebo for acute asthma episodes. *Pediatrics* 1983; 71:510–514.
231. Harris JB, Weinberger MM, Nassif E, et al: Early intervention with short courses of prednisone to prevent progression of asthma in ambulatory patients incompletely responsive to bronchodilators. *J Peds* 1987; 110: 627–633.
232. Shapiro GG, Sharpe M, DeRouen TA, et al: Cromolyn versus triamcinolone acetonide for youngsters with moderate asthma. *J Allergy Clin Immunol* 1991; 88:742–748.

NO POSTAGE
NECESSARY
IF MAILED
IN THE
UNITED STATES

BUSINESS REPLY MAIL

FIRST CLASS MAIL PERMIT No. 762 CHICAGO, IL

POSTAGE WILL BE PAID BY ADDRESSEE

Chris Hughes
Mosby-Year Book, Inc.
200 N. LaSalle Street
Suite 2600
Chicago, IL 60601-9981

NO POSTAGE
NECESSARY
IF MAILED
IN THE
UNITED STATES

BUSINESS REPLY MAIL

FIRST CLASS MAIL PERMIT No. 762 CHICAGO, IL

POSTAGE WILL BE PAID BY ADDRESSEE

Chris Hughes
Mosby-Year Book, Inc.
200 N. LaSalle Street
Suite 2600
Chicago, IL 60601-9981

The Techniques of Molecular Biology and Their Application to the Cardiomyopathies

Adolph Mares, Jr., M.D.

Fellow, Section of Cardiology, Baylor College of Medicine, Houston, Texas

Robert Roberts, M.D.

Professor of Medicine and Cell Biology, Chief of Cardiology, Baylor College of Medicine; Director, Bugher Foundation Center for Molecular Cardiology, Houston, Texas

We are witnessing a tremendous increase in our understanding of many diseases spanning all areas of medicine due in part to the development and application of new technology. The application of the techniques of molecular biology and molecular genetics has perhaps provided the greatest impetus for this progression. The unraveling of the genetic code, the development of cloning techniques, the ability to sequence nucleic acids, and the recent development of polymerase chain reaction to amplify DNA fragments have been key discoveries in accelerating our acquisition of new knowledge.[1] With the use of these techniques, many chromosomal markers have been identified to provide the DNA landmarks necessary for chromosomal mapping and identification of disease-related genes. The cardiomyopathies, defined as disease in which the primary defect is in the myocardium, as opposed to ischemic heart disease where the primary defect is in the coronary artery, have until recently been largely ignored. It has been known for some time that several of the cardiomyopathies are familial, but until the techniques of molecular genetics were developed, there was very little hope of elucidating the primary defect. The first primary myocardial disease to succumb was hypertrophic cardiomyopathy (HCM) when, in 1989,[2, 3] the chromosomal locus on which the gene responsible for this disease resides was mapped and subsequently identified.[4] The techniques of molecular genetics are being applied to cardiac disorders at a greatly accelerated pace. In just 3 years, the locus or the gene or both have been identified for several cardiomyopathies. It is estimated that more than 80 diseases affecting the heart are familial, and with the advent of molecular genetics and the global effort to map the human genome,[5–7] chromosomal mapping and isolation of disease-related genes are likely to undergo a major boost. This comes at a propitious time, when the techniques to unravel the physiological and biochemical significance of genes and their mutations are also being revolutionized through their overexpression in transgenic animals and their elimination through homologous recombination.

This review is designed to provide the practicing clinician with an increased awareness of the techniques of molecular genetics and their application to isolate and identify genes responsible for diseases of the heart. Several genetic disorders, in which a cardiomyopathy is either the primary disease or a significant feature, will be reviewed emphasizing their pathophysiology and our present knowledge of the molecular genetic hereditary defect. HCM will be used as a model to illustrate the successful application of the techniques of molecular genetics.

Overview of Molecular Genetics and Linkage Analysis

Until recently, isolation of a gene responsible for hereditary disease was not feasible unless the defective protein responsible for the disease was known. The human genome contains 3 billion base pairs (bp), which is probably sufficient DNA to generate 10 million genes; however, it is estimated that man has at the most 100,000 and perhaps more likely in the range of 40,000 to 50,000 genes. Thus, most of the DNA, in fact more than 95%, does not code for proteins, which makes it more difficult to isolate a specific gene for a specific disorder. In simple terms, the difficulty in isolating a gene is the lack of landmarks on the 46 chromosomes. To isolate a gene requires that one must map the locus on the chromosome on which the gene resides. Chromosomal mapping of genes responsible for familial diseases was greatly accelerated in the 1980s with the development of a technique initially referred to as reverse genetics and now more appropriately termed positional cloning, since it involves cloning of a disease-related gene from knowing only its chromosomal position.[8, 9] The basic concept was to develop a large number of chromosomal DNA markers whose position on the chromosome could be determined and then to show from DNA analysis of two or three generations whether the marker is co-inherited with the disease more often than by chance. Once a marker is known to be co-inherited with a disease (genetically linked), additional markers are developed in the region with the hope of flanking the fragment of DNA that contains the gene. Once the gene is in close proximity to the markers, the DNA encompassed by the markers is cloned. Following isolation and identification of the gene, one can determine the specific mutations and ultimately develop an assay for genetic diagnosis.

Chromosomal Mapping Using DNA Markers and Linkage Analysis

The process of chromosomal mapping of disease-related genes by reverse genetics or positional cloning was accelerated by the development of chromosomal markers and improved computerized techniques to perform genetic linkage analysis. The first boost came with the increased availability of chromosomal markers based on restriction fragment-length polymorphism (RFLP).[9, 10] Enzymes referred to as restriction endonucleases cut the DNA in smaller fragments by recognizing specific sequences that contain anywhere from 3 to 8 bp. Analysis of DNA by this technique provides what is often referred to as a restriction map, since the number of recognition sites for a particular enzyme will determine the number and length of fragments which gives a particular pattern easily recognized on electrophoresis that is specific for each enzyme. It was recognized that for every 250 to 300 bp of DNA, there are regions of polymorphism defined as a change in the sequence of the bases between the two homologous chromosomes. This change may include a single base pair or several. If the polymorphism involves one of the recognition sites for a restriction endonuclease, it will eliminate that site, or if it alters the sequence elsewhere, it could induce a new recognition site. The former would lead to a decrease in the number of fragments and an increase in their length, while the latter would lead to more fragments of lesser length, and hence, the term restriction fragment length polymorphism. The particular pattern produced by a restriction enzyme can be easily recognized by electrophoresis. In simple terms, then, if someone were to analyze the DNA of a family of two or more generations and show that a particular restriction pattern shows up in individuals affected with the disease with more than 50% frequency, it would imply that the gene responsible for the disease and the marker are inherited together. This process is referred to as genetic linkage analysis and would mean the gene is on the same chromosome and in close physical proximity to the marker and thus gives the chromosomal locus of the gene relative to the locus of the known chromosomal marker. Many markers based on RFLP were developed and are easily detected by southern blotting.[11] The availability of markers was further increased with the recognition of a large number of sequences repeated in tandem of 15 to 20 bp or more in length referred to as satellites or short repeats and consisting of dinucleotides or trinucleotides (microsatellites). The length of the repetitions varies significantly between homologous chromosomes, which makes them highly polymorphic, hence, their use as chromosomal markers. With use of the polymerase chain reaction, it is possible to amplify the region of repeats and after electrophoresis after staining with ethidium bromide to identify the fragments and determine if there is variation in the length of repetitions (polymorphism) and whether it is co-inherited with the disease. The advantage of variable repeat sequences and detection by polymerase chain reaction (PCR) rather than RFLPs detected by southern blotting are several: (1) requires only nanograms of quantities of DNA as opposed to micrograms; (2) detected by electrophoresis, which requires only hours as opposed to days for southern blotting; (3) better resolution than southern blotting; and (4) more informative for genetic linkage, since there are usually multiple alleles as opposed to only two alleles for RFLPs. The number of markers have increased exponentially, and there are well over 12,000 markers of known chromosomal location. Given that there are 3 billion bp, it would mean that, on the average, there is a marker every 250,000 bp. Unfortunately, they are not evenly distributed and some chromosomes have stretches of 50 million bp without a marker. The basis for genetic linkage and how these markers are analyzed to determine genetic linkage will be discussed in the subsequent paragraph.

Since man inherits two sets of autosomal chromosomes (diploid), all of the genes have two forms referred to as alleles. The two alleles occupy the same chromosomal locus, but the loci are on different chromosomes (homologous), which gives rise to the terminology of homologous loci on homologous chromosomes. One allele comes from the mother and the other from the father. In a Mendelian-dominant disease, the individual with the disease will have one defective allele that is responsible for the disease and a normal allele. In some individuals, despite the presence of the disease-related gene (genotype), there is no clinical evidence of the disease (phenotype). Thus the genotype is that of the disease, but the phenotype is normal. The percentage of individuals with the disease-related gene who exhibit some feature of the disease is referred to as the penetrance of the disease. This is to be distinguished from expressivity which refers to the variable nature of the clinical features. Penetrance is an all or none phenomenon, meaning any manifestations of the disease due to the defective gene means the penetrance is complete, whereas expressivity refers to the variability of the clinical findings (phenotype) in those individuals in whom the disease is present.

Generally, the ratio of observed phenotypes expressed during transmission of two unrelated nonallelic genes is 1:1:1:1; thus, all phenotypic combinations are equally likely.[12, 13] However, when these two nonallelic loci are located in close proximity to one another on a chromosome, there is a deviation from this expected ratio, and the parenteral phenotypes are inherited more frequently than by chance alone. When alleles at two different loci are coinherited more frequently than expected, the loci are said to be genetically linked, meaning that the genes comprising these loci are coinherited more than 50% of the time. For practical purposes, genetic linkage means that the loci are on the same chromosome and in reasonably close proximity.

The concept of linkage analysis is illustrated in Figure 1. Shown on the left panel is an illustration of genetic linkage between a locus for a DNA

FIG 1.
Illustrated here is the difference between two genetically linked loci *(left panel)* and two loci that are not linked *(right panel)*. In the *left panel,* the loci designated **A** represents the location of two homologous genes and that designated **B** is a separate locus for two homologous genes. The other pair of homologous chromosomes with loci designated **a** and **b** represent the homologous genes from the other parent. Loci **A** and **B** as are **a** and **b** are very far apart and upon the formation of a chiasma, the chromosome exchanges identical portions with the result that the portion containing the **B** locus now recombines with **a** locus. In genetic parlance, recombination has occurred whereby the two loci, **A** and **B,** are now on separate chromosomes as are **a** and **b.** In contrast, in the *right panel* the loci **A** and **B,** and **a** and **b** are in close physical proximity. During the formation of chiasma and re-

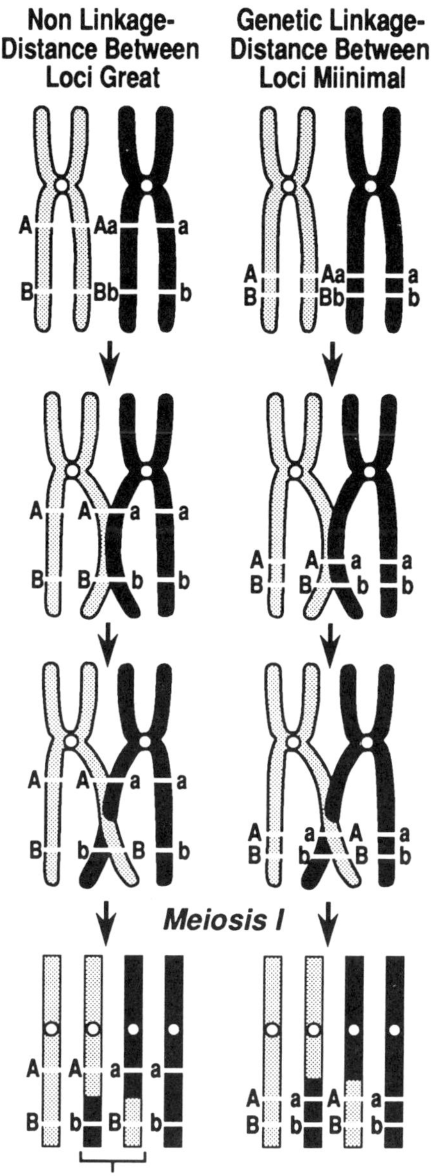

combination, because the two loci are so close together, they both move to the other chromosome. Thus, **A** and **B,** as are **a** and **b,** are genetically linked, namely, that **A** and **B** loci will stay together more frequently than by chance alone, meaning for more than 50% of the meioses. It should not be construed, however, that if two markers are genetically linked that recombination never occurs. As the two markers are very close together such as a few 100 kbp, they may never separate. Whereas if there are 20,000 kbp, they would be expected to separate with a frequency of 20% in subsequent meioses. (From Mares A Jr, Towbin J, Bies R, et al: Molecular biology for the cardiologist, in O'Rourke RA (ed): *Current Problems in Cardiology,* vol 17. St Louis, Mosby–Year Book, 1992. Used by permission.)

marker and that of a disease that is inherited in a Mendelian dominant fashion. The locus designated with an "A" carries the allele responsible for the disease. The corresponding locus "a" on the homologous chromosome has the allele that codes for the same protein but has not undergone a mutation and is thus the normal allele and is referred to as the wild type. The loci designated "B" and the other "b" represent alleles of a DNA marker of known location that has nothing to do with the disease. In the left panel the disease and the marker loci are so close that they tend to be coinherited within the family, whereas in the right panel, the DNA marker of known location is so far from the locus carrying the disease allele that it is far less likely they will be co-inherited. Prior to meioses, homologous chromosomes, and only homologous chromosomes, come together and form bridges (chiasmata) between them so that segments of equal proportion are exchanged between them giving rise to crossover of various genes. This separates various loci with their genes that otherwise would have been co-inherited. This is the basis for genetic diversity within the species. However, it is important to point out that even with crossover, the location occupied by the allele after crossing over will correspond to the same location (locus) as it had on the previous homologous chromosome. Thus, although two homologous alleles can exchange positions between the two homologous chromosomes, the actual position on either chromosome referred to as the locus remains the same for any particular allele. In genetic parlance, crossing over is referred to as recombination, namely, a segment of one chromosome has broken away and recombined with its homologous chromosome. The recombination frequency or fraction (θ) between two markers is the ratio of the number of crossover events to the total number of meioses. The lower the recombination frequency between the locus of a marker and that of a disease-related gene the closer those two must be in physical distance on the chromosome. Even though the locus of the marker and that of the disease-related gene are in close enough proximity to be genetically linked, recombination may occur, and the extent to which recombination does occur reflects roughly the physical distance between the two loci. Theoretically, if two loci are co-inherited more than 50% of the time they are said to be genetically linked. There is a 50% chance of co-inheritance of two loci even if they are not linked and even if they are on different chromosomes. However, genetic linkage means they are not only on the same chromosome, but that they are also in reasonably close physical proximity. The recombination fraction is used to develop a means of estimating the genetic distance between the linked loci, and the unit of measurement used is that of the centimorgan. A recombination frequency of one percent corresponds to a distance of one centimorgan (cM). It has also been determined that 1 cM is approximately 1 million bp in physical distance. This method of placing markers on chromosomes and estimating their distance in centimorgans derived from the recombination frequency is referred to as a genetic map as opposed to a physical map, which can only be determined by sequencing the bases. The correlation between the distance derived from a genetic map and actual distance (physical) is variable from chromosome to chromosome and from region to region even on the same chromosome. For example, recombination is more common in the telomeric than in the centromeric portion of the chromosome. If the marker locus and the disease-related locus are close, such as 5 to 10 cM, then a single crossover may be uncommon and a double crossover rare. However, two loci may be 20 to 40 cM apart and a double crossover occurs, which recombines the locus with the original chromosome leading to co-inheritance of the two loci (linkage of the two loci). When this occurs, the genetic distance is misleading and represents a gross underestimation of the true physical distance between the two loci.

A genetic map is constructed arithmetically by genetic-linkage analysis. A computer analysis is used to establish whether a marker locus is linked to a disease-related locus within a family. The most commonly used method is the Maximum Likelihood Estimation method, which estimates the probability of occurrence of a particular inheritance pattern for a set of markers based on a set recombination frequency within a particular family. This probability is compared with the probability that the same inheritance pattern occurs if the marker and the disease-related locus were not linked. The ratio of these two probabilities is called the odds ratio for linkage at the set recombination frequency. This ratio or "lod score" is determined by calculating the logarithm of the odds ratio. Two loci are said to be linked when the determined lod score is greater than or equal to +3.0 which indicates that the marker locus used is 1,000 times more likely to be located on close proximity to the locus of interest. On the other hand, a lod score of −2.0 represents nonlinkage between the marker and the disease-related locus. While a lod score of 3 represents a 1,000:1 odds in favor of linkage, it does not take into account the strong apriori odds against linkage. Since there are 22 autosomes, the chances of any two randomly selected loci being on different autosomes are about 20 times more likely than not. This makes the apriori odds against linkage about 50:1. This explains why a lod score of −2.0 is adequate to exclude genetic linkage, which actually represents an odds of 1:2,000 against linkage (not 1:100).

Axioms Fundamental to Linkage Analysis

The concept of linkage analysis and a appreciation of how to apply it in analyzing chromosomal DNA markers is often difficult in part because certain axioms are not emphasized. The axioms in applying linkage analysis to a dominantly inherited disease, as summarized from a previous publication,[14] are as follows: (1) In reference to genes on autosomal chromosomes, every individual has two forms of the gene referred to as alleles one being inherited from the mother the other from the father. In individuals with dominant disease one allele is defective and the other is normal. (2) The DNA marker of known chromosomal location to which a disease gene is linked also has two alleles, one from the father and one from the mother. (3) When a DNA marker and a disease-related gene are said to be genetically linked, it means that the two loci are linked. (4) Since the two loci are linked and not the alleles, which allele a particular offspring gets is totally by chance since the inheritance of either or both alleles at a particular locus is independent of each other. (5) Neither of the alleles at the marker locus has anything to do with causing the disease. Both alleles of the marker locus occur in the general population and do not themselves cause disease. They simply reside at a locus which is in close enough physical proximity to the locus that contains the disease-producing gene to be coinherited together more often than by chance. (6) To facilitate linkage analysis the alleles of the marker locus and the disease-related locus must be heterozygous. This means that the two alleles at the marker locus must not have an identical nucleotide sequence for the probe being utilized for their detection but be polymorphic and similar for the disease locus one allele must be normal and the other mutant. (7) Linkage of a marker locus and that of a disease-related locus implies that the two are co-inherited more often than by chance alone, which means more often than 50% of the time. It does not mean, however, that the two loci are always co-inherited and, in fact, only if they are extremely close would this be true. (8) It follows from previous axioms that in analyzing the DNA of the marker locus of individuals within families affected with the disease, the same pattern may be seen in an individual without the disease as in those individuals with the disease, and this is why computer analysis is necessary to ascertain whether the disease allele is more commonly inherited with one or more of the alleles at the marker loci than would be expected by chance. (9) Crossover or recombination occurs between, and only between, homologous chromosomes so the position of the allele that crosses over or recombines occupies the same locus on its new chromosome as it did on the previous.

The Role of the Clinician

The role of the clinician is pivotal in our attempt to isolate the genes responsible for the hereditary cardiomyopathies and unravel the pathophysiology of how the various phenotypes are induced. This is evident from the following outline[15] for chromosomal mapping by linkage analysis and subsequent identification of the gene: (1) collection of data from families affected by the specific disease; (2) accurate diagnosis of the disease using consistent and objective criteria to separate normal individuals from those affected and those that are indeterminate or unknown; (3) collection of blood samples from normals and those affected for immediate DNA analysis and to develop lymphoblastoid cell lines for a renewable source of DNA; (4) construction of a pedigree of the family; (5) DNA analysis for markers of known chromosomal loci that span the human genome in an attempt to find a locus linked to the disease; (6) development of flanking markers around the region containing the disease locus; (7) isolation and cloning of the region of DNA containing the gene; (8) identification of the

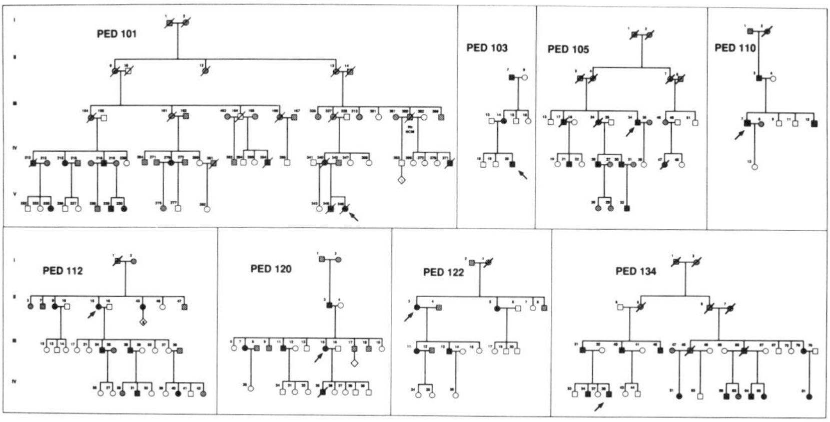

FIG 2.
Schematic diagram showing inheritance of familial hypertrophic cardiomyopathy in eight pedigrees. *Squares* denote male members, *circles* denote female members, *Open* symbols indicate family member unaffected; *solid* symbols denote family members affected with hypertrophic cardiomyopathy; and *hatched* symbols indicate members in whom the diagnosis is unknown. *Slashes* indicate deceased individuals, and *arrows* denote probands. *PED* = pedigree. (From Mares A Jr, Towbin J, Bies R, et al: Molecular biology for the cardiologist, in O'Rourke RA (ed): *Current Problems in Cardiology*, vol 17. St Louis, Mosby–Year Book, 1992. Used by permission.)

gene; (9) sequence analysis of the gene to identify the precise mutation(s) causing the disease; (10) demonstration of a causal relationship between the defective protein and the disease; (11) development of a convenient test to screen for the mutations. The clinician must be much more motivated and inquisitive about obtaining a family history and possible clues to the familial nature of the disease. It is imperative that a pedigree be made of the family history and the appropriate information be correctly noted. When it is uncertain whether an individual is affected, a category of undetermined should be clearly maintained for those individuals until the genotype is known (Fig 2). The first primary hereditary myocardial disease to succumb to molecular genetic techniques was HCM, which was not until 1989, yet in this short interval, subsequent efforts have been successful in identifying the chromosomal locus and/or gene in several cardiomyopathies (Table 1).

Techniques of Molecular Biology

Extensive reviews of the techniques of molecular biology and molecular genetics for the beginner have recently been published and will be covered here only briefly.[14–16]

TABLE 1.
Cardiomyopathies Caused by Inherited Defects

Disease	Chromosome
Hypertrophic cardiomyopathy (HCM)	14q1
Congenital long QT syndrome	11
X-linked cardiomyopathy	Xp21
Emery-Dreifuss dystrophy	Xq28
Duchenne muscular dystrophy	Xp21
Myotonic muscular dystrophy	19q13
Mitochondrial cardiomyopathy	MIT DNA

Isolation of DNA

Blood samples must be taken for DNA analysis. Since the genes are the same in all cells, it makes it convenient to isolate DNA from leucocytes. These cells are easy to isolate and enough DNA (approximately 200 μg) can be isolated from 10 to 20 mL of blood. The DNA may be isolated by a manual technique or through one of the more commonly used automated techniques.[17]

Transformed Lymphoblast Cell Lines

In addition to obtaining DNA immediately from the white cells, lymphocytes are convenient cells that can be transformed so that a permanent cell line can be kept which provides a renewable source of DNA. Peripheral blood of 10 to 15 mL drawn from the patient in tubes containing heparin or acid citrate dextrose (ACD) may be immortalized by transformation with Epstein Barr virus and cyclosporin A. A standard method is now available for transforming the cells, which then may be used directly for DNA extraction or may be frozen in storage as a renewable supply of high-quality genomic DNA.[3]

Digestion of DNA with Restriction Endonucleases

As indicated earlier, DNA molecules are large and the restriction endonuclease enzymes are used to cut the DNA molecules into smaller fragments of predetermined size. These enzymes recognize specific sequences of three to eight nucleotides and break the polynucleotide change within that sequence to create discrete fragments of defined length and sequence. These enzymes are used routinely to digest DNA and to insert DNA fragments into vectors for cloning (Fig 3). They are also essential to a variety of other manipulations. There are well over 300 commercially available enzymes, and each has a specific restriction site that leads to a particular restriction map of any given piece of DNA.

Separation and Identification of DNA Fragments by Gel Electrophoresis

Fortunately, DNA fragments are negatively charged because of a net negative charge carried by the phosphate group, which induces the fragment to migrate towards the anode at a rate that correlates approximately with the length of the fragment. Thus, the digested DNA can be loaded onto a gel such as agarose or polyacrylamide and the various fragments separated by electrophoresis. The fragments are then stained with ethidium bromide

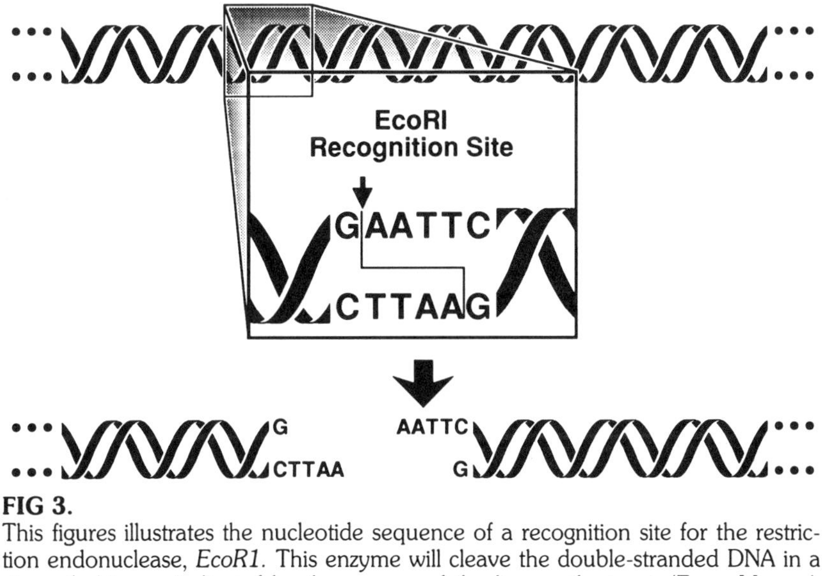

FIG 3.
This figures illustrates the nucleotide sequence of a recognition site for the restriction endonuclease, *EcoR1*. This enzyme will cleave the double-stranded DNA in a zigzag fashion as indicated by the *arrow* and the *line* on the inset. (From Mares A Jr, Towbin J, Bies R, et al: Molecular biology for the cardiologist, in O'Rourke RA (ed): *Current Problems in Cardiology*, vol 17. St Louis, Mosby–Year Book, 1992. Used by permission.)

which intercalates between the bases and fluoresces under UV illumination from which photographs of the DNA are taken. Electrophoresis through agarose will separate double-stranded DNA fragments varying from 70 to 100,000 bp. Polyacrylamide is used to separate DNA fragments from 6 to 1,000 bp. Utilizing these gels, one can depict bands of as little as 1 ng and a difference between fragments of 0.5% of their size. Most recently a new technique has been developed (referred to as pulse gel electrophoresis), in which molecules as large as 1 to 2 million base pairs can be separated by electrophoresis.

Southern, Northern and Western Blotting

Southern blotting, named after its inventor, E.M. Southern,[11] utilizes several techniques including restriction digestion of the DNA and separation of the DNA fragments by electrophoresis. Southern found that, following separation of the DNA by electrophoresis, it was possible to transfer the DNA by buffer via capillary action from the gel to a filter. The DNA binds to the filter and following heating or UV, it is fixed permanently to the filter. Since the DNA is single-stranded, it is possible with a complementary DNA fragment tagged with a radioactive or fluorescent label to isolate the DNA of interest. A piece of single-stranded DNA that is complementary to the piece of DNA of interest is then brought into contact with the filter. If indeed the piece of complementary DNA is present, it will bind to the probe. An autoradiogram is then obtained of the filter, and the only area where radioactivity will be detected is that area in which the probe has bound to complementary foreign DNA. Instead of an autoradiogram, with all of the fragments stained as was the case with ethidium bromide, one now has a band only where there is a DNA fragment of interest (Fig 4). This has high resolution and is referred to as Southern blotting, which is used frequently to isolate and identify DNA. If the same procedure is used to isolate and identify RNA[18] rather than DNA, it is referred to as northern blotting. A similar procedure can be used to identify proteins where the probe is frequently that of a specific polyclonal or monoclonal antibody, and the process is referred to as western blotting.

Generation of a cDNA from mRNA

Messenger RNA (mRNA), present in the cytoplasm of the cell, is dedicated to one specific function, namely, to encode for a specific polypeptide. The mRNA contains the protein coding sequences (exons) of a discrete gene designed to perform the specific function of providing the template for synthesis of a specific polypeptide. The discovery of the enzyme reverse transcriptase made it possible to go from mRNA to DNA referred to as complementary DNA (cDNA). When DNA is copied from mRNA, it is single stranded but one can, with the use of DNA polymerase, convert it to double-stranded DNA, which can be inserted into the DNA of a vector and subsequently into a host to be cloned. The discovery of reverse tran-

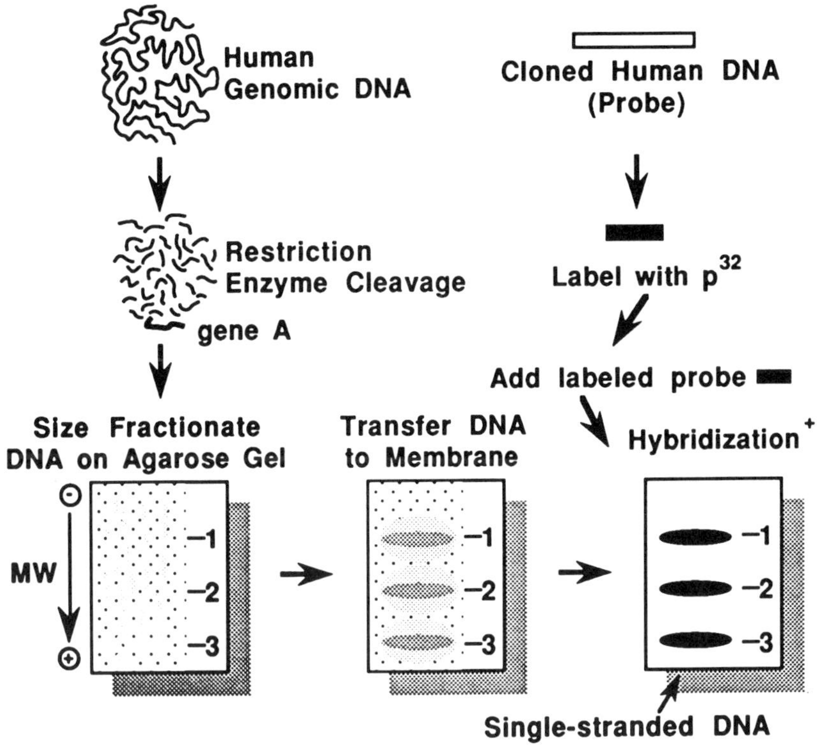

FIG 4.
Illustration of the Southern blotting technique. The DNA is cleaved with an appropriately selected restriction endonuclease. The digested fragments are separated by electrophoresis on agarose gel, and the fragments of *gene A* are located at positions *1, 2,* and *3,* but cannot be seen against the background of many other randomly occurring DNA fragments. The DNA is denatured and transferred to a membrane in an identical pattern to what it was on the agarose gel. It is difficult to manipulate anything on a soft gel or to remove it. Once transferred to the membrane (filter) a solid support system the DNA is much easier to handle. A DNA probe (cDNA) that has been labeled with ^{32}P is hybridized to its complementary DNA and visualized after exposure of the nylon membrane to an autoradiograph. The transfer of the DNA from the gel to the membrane developed by Southern was a major innovation and is illustrated in Fig 5. (From Mares A Jr, Towbin J, Bies R, et al: Molecular biology for the cardiologist, in O'Rourke RA (ed): *Current Problems in Cardiology,* vol 17. St Louis, Mosby–Year Book, 1992. Used by permission.)

scriptase and the ability to generate a cDNA from mRNA was essential to the subsequent development of cloning. An example of the application of the technique was that of recombinant tissue plasminogen activator (rt-PA), which initially was cloned in a bacterium and later into a mammalian cell line, which is now used to produce rt-PA in commercial quantities. It is important to recognize the difference between DNA generated from mRNA as opposed to DNA obtained from genomic material of the nucleus. When DNA is obtained from the nucleus, it contains introns (spliced out during the formation of mRNA and not leaving the nucleus) together with exons which are spliced together and exit the nucleus in the mature mRNA to code for protein synthesis. Thus, the cDNA made from mRNA contains only the exons and is devoid of any of the introns. The cDNA can be inserted into a vector and subsequently into a host and then be stimulated to produce large quantities of the particular polypeptide.

DNA Cloning

The method of DNA cloning is a direct result of the discovery and isolation of enzymes used to cleave (restriction endonucleases) and repair (ligases) DNA in bacteria. Cloning (Fig 5) essentially refers to the amplification of a foreign-specific segment of DNA (insert) through its association with genetic material capable of independent replication such as a plasmid (vector) within an unrelated host (bacteria). Under optimal conditions, one can expect to clone a million copies of the DNA fragments. There are several prerequisites basic to cloning: (1) an isolated fragment of DNA to serve as an insert; (2) a vector, such as a bacterial plasmid which can propagate independently of the host DNA; (3) a restriction endonuclease to modify both the insert and vector resulting in their compatibility; (4) a DNA ligase to ligate the compatible ends of the insert and vector; and (5) a means to differentiate the host cells that have incorporated the vector containing the insert from those that have not. Restriction endonucleases recognize specific series of nucleotides which restrict their cleaving activity to only that particular sequence. DNA ligase rejoins two DNA fragments together and the reaction is termed ligation.

Conventional vectors fall into three classes: (1) plasmids harvested from bacteria, which contain the genes inducing resistance to antibiotics such as ampicillin, chloramphenicol, and neomycin, and genes regulating the metabolism of particular sugars; (2) bacteriophages (virus) that invade and multiply in bacterial hosts; and (3) combinations of both of these, called cosmids. The limitations of cloning are generally related to the size of the insert. Plasmids can only accommodate inserts up to 15,000 bp, phage up to 25,000 bp, and cosmids up to 45,000 bp.

Once DNA fragments have been isolated after appropriate modification with restriction endonucleases, the fragments are ligated to the compatible vector in a ligation reaction. The ligation products are introduced into bacterial hosts, transforming these cells into a new phenotype dictated by the genes carried in the vector. Monoclonal cell colonies are then isolated on the basis of antibiotic resistance and sugar metabolism, both properties indicating the successful incorporation of a plasmid harboring the inserted foreign DNA, respectively. Recently a new cloning technique[19] has been developed in yeast whereby the DNA insert is packaged as a yeast artificial chromosome and is referred to as a YAC and can accommodate DNA fragments up to 2 million bp.

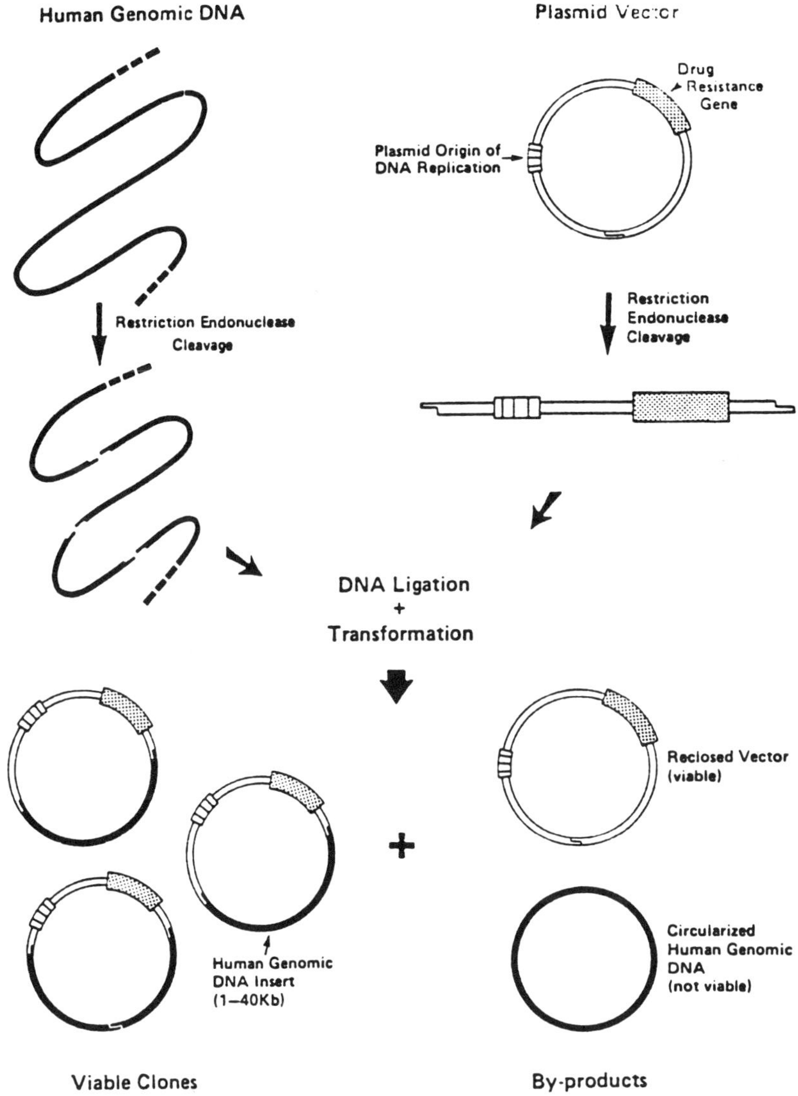

FIG 5.
The cloning of a DNA fragment utilizing a plasmid as the vector. (From Mares A Jr, Towbin J, Bies R, et al: Molecular biology for the cardiologist, in O'Rourke RA (ed): *Current Problems in Cardiology,* vol 17. St Louis, Mosby–Year Book, 1992. Used by permission.)

Development of Gene Libraries

Gene libraries are collections of individual fragments grown in a suitable host such as *E. coli*. These libraries can be either genomic (fragments of nuclear DNA), chromosomal (fragments derived from a specific chromosome), or a cDNA library (derived from mRNA). It is possible to develop a cDNA library specific for one organ or one tissue of an organ. Again, as emphasized previously, a genomic library has the same genes regardless of the source from which it is derived and contains both introns and exons, whereas cDNA represents only DNA that was made from mRNA and codes for protein. In addition, a cDNA library is specific for the source from which it is derived.

Nucleic Acid Sequencing

The ultimate goal of molecular biology is to define the exact nucleic acid composition of genes. In fact, there is a unified international effort to define the entire nucleic acid sequence of DNA of humans through the multimillion Human Genome Project. Definition of the gene sequence will allow the identification of mutations causing disease and subsequent manipulation of the DNA sequence in an attempt to correct the abnormality produced by the mutation. Nucleic acid sequencing was once a tedious, time-consuming task, but presently it is automated allowing segments of at least 300 to 5,000 bp to be defined. Sequencing is accomplished by either a chemical[20] or an enzymatic method.[21]

Polymerase Chain Reaction

The polymerase chain reaction is the newest advance[22] in the molecular techniques which have revolutionized the approach to molecular biology and molecular genetics. Polymerase chain reaction is an automated in vitro repetitive reaction which is able to amplify in a logarithmic manner a single copy of a target fragment of DNA up to a millionfold in a matter of hours (Fig 6). The discovery of a heat-stable DNA polymerase in the bacterium

FIG 6.

Polymerase chain reaction. The three steps to be followed once the primers have been added includes denaturation, which separates the double-stranded DNA into single strands and the primers from their respective complementary strands; reannealing, the phase during which the primers anneal to their respective complementary base pairs on each strand; and extension, the phase catalyzed by the enzyme polymerase during which the nucleotides are added to the primers, in one case in the sense direction and the other in the antisense direction. The cycle is repeated and DNA has now been denatured, so that the primers break away from the strands and the double strands separate into single strands. Then the primers again reanneal in their appropriate position and one sees now the stage is set to develop proportionately more of the short segments of DNA. In *Cycle 3* one sees now that the short DNA segments are being amplified preferentially over the long segments

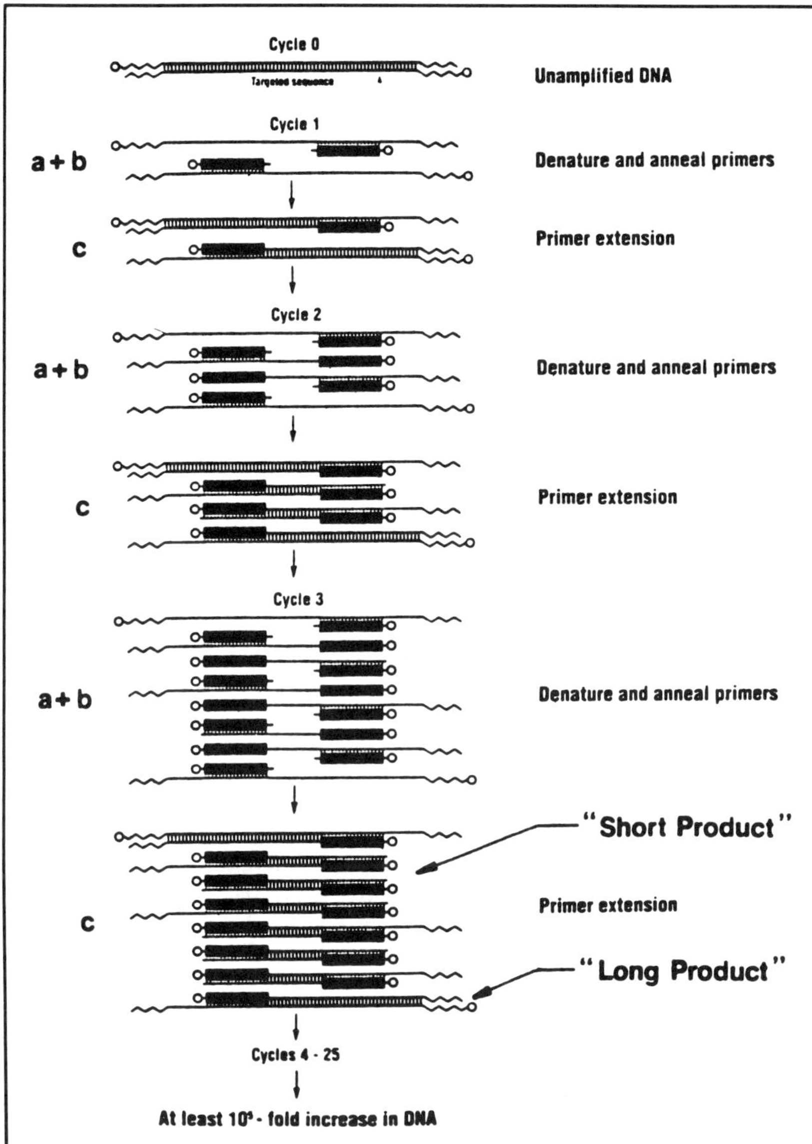

and this increases exponentially so that by *Cycle 4 and 5,* amplification of the short segments of interest predominates and the proportion contributed by the long segments become less and less important, thus, the main product at the end of 20 to 30 cycles will be the short DNA segment of interest. One increases the temperature to around 95° C for denaturation, but for reannealing, the temperature is decreased to about 50° C, and during the extension cycle the temperature is increased to 72° C so the reaction proceeds rapidly and then it is again recycled, namely, denaturation, reannealing, and extension. (From Mares A Jr, Towbin J, Bies R, et al: Molecular biology for the cardiologist, in O'Rourke RA (ed): *Current Problems in Cardiology,* vol 17. St Louis, Mosby–Year Book, 1992. Used by permission.)

Thermus aquaticus allows multiple reaction cycles consisting of: (1) heat denaturation at 94° C of a single double stranded DNA template; (2) annealing of primers to specified regions on each of the single-stranded templates; and (3) extension of the primer sites in the 5′ to 3′ direction by DNA polymerase to yield two double-stranded products. Further advances in PCR amplification have come from improving the fidelity of the polymerase action due to a proofreading ability correcting for any mistakes during the amplification.

One limitation to PCR is that one must know a short stretch of nucleotide sequences flanking both the 5′ and 3′ ends of the desired segment of DNA in order to design primers that limit the area of amplification. Another limitation is the fragment being amplified is limited to about 2,000 bp. A primer is an oligonucleotide whose sequence is complementary to small regions of both strands of target DNA (template) located both at the 5′ and 3′ ends. A sense primer is designed with a sequence identical to the 5′ end of the template and an antisense primer is designed having the sequence of the strand that is the complement to the 3′ end of the template. Primers of 18 and 24 bp have a significant affinity for only the target template which assures that the vast majority of the reaction product is specific. As indicated previously, amplification of polymorphic satellite repeat sequences has greatly boosted the number of chromosomal DNA markers as well as reduced the time necessary for analysis.

Polymerase chain reaction has many other applications. For example, PCR may in part substitute for some portions of classical cloning procedures simply by modifying the 5′ ends of both primers with sequences harboring restriction sites. The generated segment of DNA can then be easily incorporated into subcloning procedures avoiding lengthy and tedious preparatory steps. Full-length cDNA can be generated from single-copy mRNA of expressed genes by combining procedures of reverse transcription and PCR (RT-PCR). Reverse transcription PCR sequentially combines the activity of the enzyme reverse transcriptase (RT) to generate a cDNA from the mRNA, and the activity of DNA polymerase is used to amplify the cDNA product. Mutant genes can be created by designing primers containing modified mutant sequences in a procedure called site-directed mutagenesis. The effect of the mutant gene product can then be evaluated after it is inserted and expressed in the appropriate host. Mutations in cDNA and genomic DNA sequences can be detected by forming double-stranded hybrids between the PCR products of the test target and those of a normal target. Single-nucleotide mismatches in the hybrid can be identified by chemical cleavage at the site of the mismatch after electrophoresis on an acrylamide gel. Similarly, changes in the mobility pattern of amplified PCR products compared with normal migration patterns can be identified after electrophoresis, suggesting a change in the nucleotide sequence. These are just a few of the potential applications of PCR, and it is certain that PCR will continue to have its impact on medicine for years to come.

Chromosomal Walking and Jumping to Isolate Genes

As outlined previously, following collection of the family's DNA, one utilizes markers and computerized techniques to do linkage analysis to chromosomally map the locus on the chromosome on which the gene resides. Once the locus responsible for the disease has been mapped to a particular chromosome, one must then attempt to isolate the DNA fragment containing the specific gene. This is sometimes a very difficult task and may take several years to complete as in the case of Huntington's chorea where, despite the locus having been mapped for 10 years, the gene has yet to be isolated. A common approach (once the locus has been determined) is to attempt by various markers to get within a few hundred thousand base pairs of the specific gene and then to attempt to isolate the whole segment containing the gene by cloning overlapping regions of the DNA.[23–25] This requires extreme skill and ingenuity in terms of ultimately putting the fragments together to get the intact gene. Once the whole DNA fragment containing the gene has been cloned, the specific gene is identified using approaches such as identifying start and stop codons that would correspond to the beginning and end of the gene as well as comparing it to known sequences with the hope of identifying the protein for which the genes encodes. This and other procedures are utilized in an attempt to finally identify the gene and from that derive the sequences of the protein encoded by the gene. This ultimately leads to the identification of the protein that determines whether it is a structural or regulatory protein. The next step is to determine whether the mutation is a deletion, an addition, or a missense mutation whereby often only a single base has been altered and substituted by another base that changes the codon for that amino acid, thereby leading to an alteration in the encoded protein. The techniques available to screen for mutations are indicated in the next paragraph.

Techniques to Screen for Mutations

Once a gene has been identified, it often is a tedious procedure to identify the mutation, particularly when it is of the missense type. The mutation is ultimately confirmed by determining the nucleotide sequence. Major deletions are easy to detect and are visible upon electrophoresis such as southern blotting. Detecting simple base changes that induce many of the hereditary disorders is much more difficult. Each of the procedures utilized to detect mutations are cumbersome and tedious and fall into one of the following categories: (1) denaturing gradient gel electrophoresis; (2) single-strand confirmational analysis; and (3) formation of heteroduplexes[26] between the wild type and the mutant allele. The heteroduplexes may be formed using DNA or RNA and are based on the concept of identifying the mismatch of the sequences between the wild and mutant forms. A specific form of this method, referred to as chemical cleavage, utilizes the properties of either osmium tetroxide or hydroxylamine to further increase the vulnerability of the nucleotide mismatches to chemical cleavage by piperidine. Chemical cleavage is claimed to be the most sensitive and specific of the techniques.[27]

The Molecular Genetics of Various Cardiomyopathies

Familial Hypertrophic Cardiomyopathy

Hypertrophic cardiomyopathy is a hereditary primary myocardial disease with the hallmark of hypertrophy affecting primarily the septum of the left ventricular cavity, but it may involve the free wall or occasionally be localized to the free wall or apex.[28] Histologically, there is increased muscle mass with structurally intact sarcomeres but markedly disarrayed fibers. Hypertrophic cardiomyopathy has been referred to by different names including idiopathic hypertrophic subaortic stenosis (IHSS), asymmetric septal hypertrophy (ASH), and hypertrophic obstructive cardiomyopathy (HOCM).

Hypertrophic cardiomyopathy exhibits a spectrum of clinical manifestations ranging from asymptomatic to sudden cardiac death. In fact, HCM is the most common cause of sudden cardiac death in young people,[29, 30] particularly athletes. It is estimated that, in the United States, 24,000 people die of HCM every year.[29] The most common symptom affecting 90% of the patients is dyspnea, primarily due to increased ventricular wall stiffness leading to elevated left ventricular end diastolic pressure resulting in pulmonary congestion. Three fourths of symptomatic patients experience angina pectoris despite the absence of atherosclerotic occlusive disease. This may be caused by microvascular ischemia resulting from the hypercontractile left ventricle. Other nonspecific symptoms include fatigue, palpitations, paroxysmal nocturnal dyspnea, and, less frequently, cardiac failure and dizziness. The obstructive nature of the interventricular septum causes some symptoms to be exacerbated by exertion, thus presyncope is experienced by 50% of symptomatic patients and presumably is the forerunner of syncope and sudden death.

Physical examination shows a laterally displaced, forceful apical impulse. There may be a prominent presystolic apical impulse secondary to a forceful atrial contraction manifested as a systolic thrill at the apex or left lower sternal border. On auscultation the first heart sound is normal, usually with a fourth heart sound preceding it. The second heart sound is normally split; however, patients having severe outflow gradients may have a single second sound or may even exhibit paradoxical splitting. There is a harsh crescendo-decrescendo systolic murmur beginning well after S1 that is heard best between the apex and left sternal border. The murmur may be labile in intensity and duration, but, when present, often radiates to the left sternal border, axilla, and base but not the carotids.

The diagnosis of HCM is made primarily from findings on physical examination, together with those on the electrocardiogram and echocardiogram. Electrocardiographic findings include voltage criteria for left ventricular hypertrophy, with 40% to 50% of affected patients having Q waves in addition to nonspecific ST segment and T wave changes in leads II, III, aVF, and/or precordial leads V4-6. Frequently, the PR interval may be short followed by slurring of a tall R wave with a normal QRS interval.

The criteria having the greatest sensitivity and specificity for the diagnosis of HCM utilize 2-D echocardiography together with Doppler.[3] A septal wall thickness of 13 mm or a septal wall to ventricular free wall thickness ratio of 1.5 without other cause for hypertrophy is adequate for the diagnosis in the adult. Systolic anterior motion of the anterior mitral leaflet and a infraaortic valvular pressure gradient may also be present on echocardiographic analysis.

Classically, HCM has been genetically described as an autosomal dominant disease with variable degrees of penetrance (see Fig 2). However, until recently, it was not possible to determine the true penetrance since the responsible gene was not known. Hypertrophic cardiomyopathy was the first familial primary myocardial disease for which the gene was identified. In 1989, genetic linkage analysis mapped the locus responsible for HCM to the long arm of chromosome 14 in kindreds of a French-Canadian family residing in North America.[2] The gene was identified as β-myosin heavy chain (βMHC) located in the chromosomal region 14q1.[31] Shortly thereafter, seven families[3] from regions distributed throughout North America were also linked to the same locus showing it to be a major locus for this disease in North America.[2] Several other families in the United States have since been linked to the locus,[32, 33] including a family from Newfoundland, Canada.[34]

The β myosin heavy chain (βMHC) gene consists of about 23,000 bp (23 kbp) forming 40 exons and is separated from the gene for βMHC by only 4.5 kbp.[35, 36] The βMHC gene transcribes a mRNA of approximately 6.0 kb, that encodes for a protein of 1939 amino acids with a molecular weight of 223,000. The βMHC molecule, which is a major contractile protein of cardiac and skeletal muscle, forms the thick filament of the sarcomere unit. Its molecular structure consists of a globular head, a long rod, and an adjoining tail coiled in an α-helix which in turn is coiled with another βMHC molecule. Attached to the head of each myosin molecule are two myosin light chains. Most of the known functional domains are in the head of the molecule as shown in Figure 7. The major domains are the binding site for actin, adenosine triphosphate generation site, thiol groups, the hinge regions, binding sites for myosin light chains and the tail which is responsible for the formation of the filaments. It is estimated that 400 to 600 molecules of myosin are joined together by their tails through the terminal two to three amino acids of the tail to form the thick filament.

Despite the gene not being isolated until 1990, several mutations have been identified as shown in Table 2. Essentially all of the mutations have been of the missense type except for one which is a deletion[37] involving the 3′ end of the βMHC gene. The deletion which consists of 2.3 kb encodes for the tail of the myosin including all of the 3′ nonprotein coding sequences and the poly-A recognition site as shown in Figure 8. All of the missense mutations in contrast have been found in the myosin head. Evi-

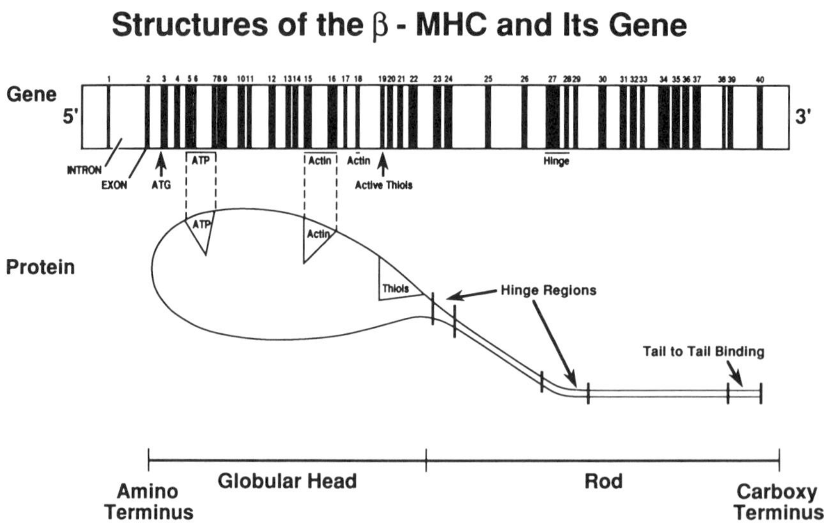

FIG 7.
Structures of the β-myosin heavy chain (βMHC) and its gene. Shown are the βMHC gene *(top)* and the globular protein of βMHC *(bottom)*. The *open areas* on the gene referred to as introns, consist of DNA which will be spliced out and are not used to code for the βMHC protein. Whereas the enclosed *blackened areas* referred to as exons represent the portion of the gene which will be included in the messenger RNA and codes for the βMHC protein. The exons are numbered from 1 to 40, and all of the mutations have been found in that portion of the gene coding for the globular head except for one mutation, a deletion, which involves exon 39 and 40. The prominent functional domains of the βMHC gene are indicated together with the corresponding portion of the βMHC protein for which they encode. (From Mares A Jr, Towbin J, Bies R, et al: Molecular biology for the cardiologist, in O'Rourke RA (ed): *Current Problems in Cardiology*, vol 17. St Louis, Mosby–Year Book, 1992. Used by permission.)

dence that these mutations are likely responsible for the disease are as follows: (1) the families show genetic linkage to the βMHC locus; (2) the mutation is observed in affected individuals, but not in normals; (3) each mutation involves a change in the amino acid of the protein; (4) in the one family in which the proband was sporadic, the disease was passed on to the offspring[38]; and (5) the missense mutation in exon 13 in which glutamine substitutes for arginine in position 403 was shown to be expressed in the βMHC mRNA obtained from an endomyocardial biopsy of an individual affected with the disease.[39] The same mutation has also been shown to be expressed in the βMHC mRNA of skeletal muscle[40] and more recently shown to be expressed in the βMHC protein of the skeletal muscle[41] of an individual affected with HCM.

The ability to detect specific mutations makes it possible to determine the genotype and correlate it with clinical features. Until the present, no

TABLE 2.
Missense Mutations in the β-Myosin Heavy Chain Gene

Exon Affected	Nucleotide Change	Amino Acid Change	No. of Families
5	cytosine → thymidine	threonine → isoleucine	1
9	guanine → adenine	arginine^{249} → glutamine	1
13	guanine → adenine	arginine^{403} → glutamine	5
14	cytosine → thymidine	arginine^{453} → cysteine	2
16	guanine → adenine	valine → methionine	1
16	guanine → cytosine	glycine^{584} → arginine	2
16	guanidine → adenine	valine^{606} → methionine	3
20	guanine → cytosine	glycine → arginine	1
23	cytosine → guanine	leucine^{908} → valine	1
23	guanine → adenine	glutamine^{924} → lysine	1
23	guanine → adenine	glutamine^{949} → lysine	1

one of the clinical features was predictive of outcome such as sudden death. In most individuals, the disease is not present until puberty even on echocardiography. The ability to determine if the mutated gene is present before or immediately after birth has significant diagnostic, etiologic, and therapeutic implications. The ability to determine the genotype early in life makes it possible to determine whether certain mutations will be predictive of clinical manifestations and this has already been shown for several mutations.[33, 34, 42] We[43] recently studied three families with HCM. In two of

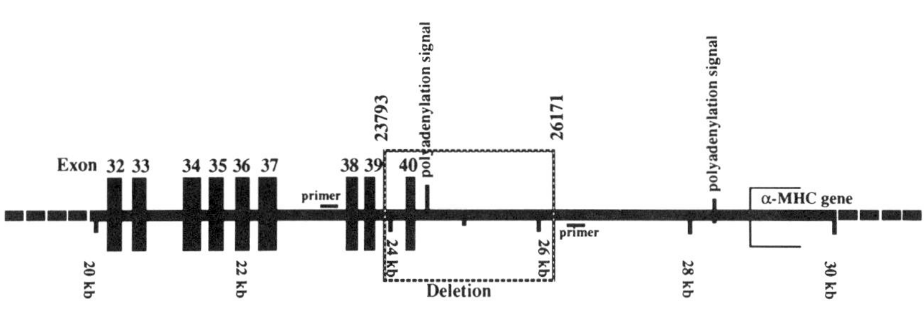

FIG 8.
Diagram showing the location of the deletion in the β-myosin heavy chain (βMHC) gene. Deletion involves part of intron 39, exon 40, including 3′-untranslated region and the polyadenylation signal. It also extends 1.8 kb into the β/α intergenic region. (From Mares A Jr, Towbin J, Bies R, et al: Molecular biology for the cardiologist, in O'Rourke RA (ed): *Current Problems in Cardiology*, vol 17. St Louis, Mosby–Year Book, 1992. Used by permission.)

the families there was the same missense mutation in exon 13 of the βMHC gene in which adenine substitutes for guanine at position 1208 of the coding sequence resulting in substitution of glutamine for arginine at position 403 of the βMHC protein (Arg 403 Gln). In the other family the missense sequence was in exon 23 consisting of the substitution of an adenine for guanine residue at position 2788 of the coding sequence. This mutation results in the substitution of lysine for glutamic acid at position 930 of the βMHC protein (Glu 930 Lys). The contrasting clinical features of these two mutations are summarized in Table 3. The outstanding feature to be noted is that the missense mutation in position 403 is clearly

TABLE 3.
Clinical Characteristics of Families With Known Missense Mutations

	Arg 403 Gln Mutation	Glu 930 Lys Mutation
Families	155 & 2	152
No. of individuals	58	35
No. with HCM	21	16
No. dead	11	2
No. of SCD	8	2
Mean age at time of SCD	33	—
βMHC Mutation	G1208A	G2788A
Mutant exon	13	23
Genotype present	9/9	12/12
Symptomatic	12/13	3/14
Mean age at onset of symptoms	23.7	—
Chest pain	6/12	1/14
Dyspnea	8/12	2/14
Syncope	3/12	—
Palpitation	6/12	1/14
ECG abnormality	10/12	—
Atrial fibrillation	6/12	0/14
Mitral regurgitation	5/12	0/14
Mean septal thickness	18.8 ± 5.8	18.5 ± 5.0
Mean posterior wall thickness	10.9 ± 4.0	10.0 ± 1.0
ASH	8/12	11/14
Concentric hypertrophy	4/12	3/14
LVOT gradient	6/12	—
Mean gradient	70 mmHg	—
Myomectomy	3/12	—
Mean LVEF	>65%	>60%

associated with a very high incidence of premature sudden death with about half of the family members being dead by the second or third decade. In contrast, the mutation in position 903 is associated with a very low incidence of premature death. There are other significant features such as the presence of left ventricular outflow tract obstruction in two thirds of the patients with missense 403, while this is extremely uncommon with mutation 903. The onset of patient symptoms was much earlier with mutation 403 than with mutation 903, and the severity of the symptoms were clearly much more severe with mutation 403. Two other families[33, 42] have been reported with the 403 mutation, and they consistently observed the high incidence of premature sudden death, the early onset of symptoms, and the increased severity of symptoms, as compared with several other mutations. Thus, mutations that predict severe symptoms such as premature onset of sudden death are being recognized, as are seemingly more benign mutations that can be determined within the first few days of life and can be utilized for appropriate treatment and counseling. It is recommended at this time that all families with HCM be screened for known mutations. If a mutation such as 403 is detected that is predictive of sudden death, the information should be utilized to counsel children away from combative sports, which are known to exaggerate and precipitate premature sudden death. Although many mutations have been identified, it is highly likely that many more are yet to be identified in the βMHC gene, and clinical correlations of significant diagnostic and therapeutic value will be determined in the very near future. It is important to emphasize that the genetic diagnoses can be made from a single blood test for those mutations that have been characterized. The dramatic difference in the lifespan of individuals with the two mutations, 403 and 903, is illustrated by the Kaplan Meier life tables in Fig 9.

The complexity of the genetics of HCM have significantly increased in recent months with the recognition of genetic heterogeneity.[44–46] While it is evident that many families in North America with HCM have disease shown to be due to mutations in the βMHC gene, it is also clear that several families do not link to the chromosome 14 locus. This would indicate there are other genes that are responsible for this disease as the phenotypes of the families linked to chromosome 14 appear to be virtually identical to those observed in families that are not linked to chromosome 14. There is currently an intense investigative effort under way to identify other loci with the hope of characterizing the responsible gene and its mutations. In one particular family, which is not linked to chromosome 14, we[47] have shown that there appears to be parental imprinting. In this family most of the affected children have inherited the mutant gene from their mother, while the offspring who inherit the defective gene from the father appear not to develop the disease (phenotype). Parental imprinting has been noted in only a couple of other diseases and, thus, this becomes a very interesting phenomenon. The mechanism responsible for this remains an enigma, although there is speculation that it is methylation of the cytosine residues, which prevents gene expression.

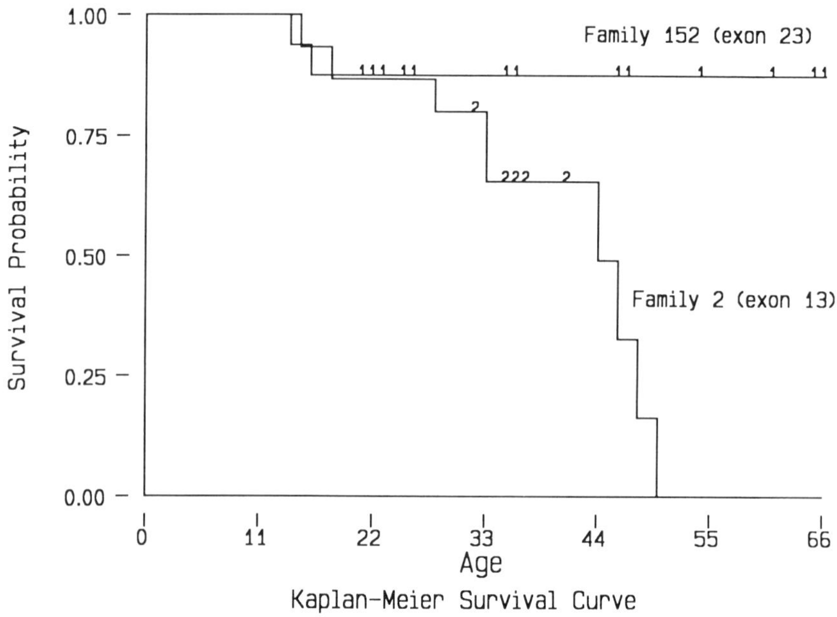

FIG 9.
Kaplan-Meier survival curves for Family 152 with the G2788A mutation and Family 2 with G1208A mutation. There is a high attrition rate in the third and fourth decade of life of the affected individuals with the exon 13 missense mutation. (From Mares A Jr, Towbin J, Bies R, et al: Molecular biology for the cardiologist, in O'Rourke RA (ed): *Current Problems in Cardiology,* vol 17. St Louis, Mosby–Year Book, 1992. Used by permission.)

Certain hypotheses have been postulated[39, 42] regarding the role of the mutations in producing disease. The occurrence of mutations affecting highly conserved regions of the MHC is thought to be a significant precursor to the development of disease. Additionally, mutations yielding a change in amino acid charge within the polypeptide are thought to produce significant conformational changes in secondary and tertiary structures of the polypeptide resulting in an abnormally functioning protein. Expression and incorporation of the mutant MHC into thick filaments or the subsequent interference of the formation of thick filaments or sarcomeres may cause the formation of mutant and defective myofibrils in patients with HCM. These abnormal myofibrils may lead to the myofibrillar disarray long recognized as the cardinal pathologic feature of the myocardium of patients with HCM.

The rational basis whereby mutations in the βMHC gene would lead to the phenotype observed in patients with HCM regardless of the type of mutation remains an enigma. The complexity of understanding the pathophysiology of this disease is further complicated by the localization of the phenotypic manifestations. Although βMHC is the major contractile protein of both right and left ventricles as well as skeletal muscle, the hypertrophy is primarily localized to the ventricular septum, seldom involves the right ventricle, and only occasionally involves the free wall. While the mutation is expressed in skeletal muscle and there may be some abnormal function in skeletal muscle, it does not appear to be a significant abnormality in most patients with HCM. Furthermore, the characteristic, consistent clinical observation of these patients is that the contractility of the heart if anything is increased, as manifested by increased ejection fraction, increased emptying time, and a significant increase in cardiac output. Several observations regarding the structure and composition of the contractile proteins have been made in patients with HCM prior to the discovery of the genetic defect. These studies[48] consistently showed that myosin and actin were normal and there appeared to be no abnormality either in composition or in the quality of the myosin adenosine triphosphatase activity. In an attempt to further assess the protein composition, we[49] performed biopsies on two patients with the known 403 mutation. Light microscopy was performed, and myosin and actin were analyzed by specific antibodies. These findings are notable in that the architecture of the sarcomere in terms of myofilament assembly appears to be normal. Thus, the disarray of the myocytes relate to myofibril disarray, but not to any disarray or abnormality in myofilament assembly. Second, the ratio of actin to myosin was normal as was the ratio of βMHC to αMHC. Similar findings were observed in the skeletal muscle biopsy both in terms of normal myofilament formation and normal myosin and actin composition. On gel electrophoresis, we did observe certain other minor protein bands which appear to have decreased intensity relative to that of the normal cardiac and skeletal muscle, but this may be due to in vitro proteolysis, and whether this really has significance remains to be determined. Based on these findings and clinical observations, we postulate that the defect is clearly functional rather than structural, and, also, it may well be that the hypertrophic response is a secondary phenomenon rather than a primary one. There is clinical evidence in favor of this hypothesis,[50] namely, it has been observed that children examined prior to puberty who did not have any cardiac hypertrophy subsequently developed it and became symptomatic. The primary defect, however, leading to cardiac hypertrophy may be defective function and the hypertrophy is compensatory growth, or it may, in fact, be that the contractility is altered in such a way that there is increased velocity or contraction, which in turn alters the stress or strain relationships in the ventricle leading to secondary hypertrophy.[39] The alterations in stress and strain are in keeping with some of the clinical observations. The hypertrophy is localized to the septum in most individuals, certainly in the initial years of this disease. Thus, if it were simply a secondary phenomenon without any change in the stress or strain of the ventricle, one would expect the hypertrophy to be concentric rather than localized to the septum. It has also been postulated that there is in some way a necrotic factor that is produced that leads to the destruction of the myocytes. One can only postulate potential mechanisms to explain the pathophysiology. However, we must keep in mind certain observations, namely, that the sarcomere appears to be assembled properly, and second, there is normal contractility in the initial stages of this disease and the hypertrophy is localized. Ultimate documentation of how these mutations induce the disease in man will probably require an intense investigation with the use of animal models (such as transgenic animals) as well as gene elimination experiments with homologous recombination. The understanding of the pathophysiology will perhaps be significantly delayed because the models that are available for transgenic manipulation or homologous recombination are of rodents, in which the adult myosin is αMHC rather than βMHC. The recent documentation[40] that the mutation is indeed expressed in the skeletal muscle does open up other avenues of investigation such as utilizing the slow twitch skeletal muscle fiber from patients affected with the disease.[51] One can assess contractility and function in these fibers which may provide a significant understanding of how these mutations induce the disease. In the final analysis unraveling the pathophysiology at the DNA level is most likely going to help in the diagnosis and treatment of the disease. In addition, it should also help us in our understanding of ventricular modeling and compensatory growth (hypertrophy) following acquired diseases such as myocardial infarction, hypertension, or valvular disease. It is perhaps worthy to note that although the heart does not replicate and simply enlarges in response to injury, it does however, turn itself over every 4 or 5 days just from constitutive maintenance growth. This constitutive baseline growth is important in the remodeling of the heart in response to injury in which there may be very minimal increase in muscle mass or hypertrophy, but the overall regulation and modulation of its architecture involves gene regulation at multiple levels. It is, thus, highly likely that whatever we learn from HCM in addition to the diagnostic and therapeutic application, we are likely to also add to our understanding of cardiac growth hypertrophy.

Myotonic Muscular Dystrophy

Myotonic muscular dystrophy (DM), like HCM, is inherited in an autosomal-dominant fashion with variable degrees of penetrance and expressivity, and it is the most prevalent form of muscular dystrophy in adults.[52] The incidence of DM is estimated at 13.5 per 100,000 live births,[53] with a prevalence of 2.4 to 5.5 per 100,000 in North America, Europe and Japan.[54] The primary clinical pattern consists of significant progressive distal muscle weakness, atrophy, and myotonia primarily of the distal muscle groups, but also involving the bulbar muscles. Characteristic hatchet facies are common due to weakness of the facial, temporalis, and sternocleidomastoid muscles, accompanied by bilateral ptosis. Interestingly, if the affected patient is male, frontal baldness is prominent, and 70% to 90% have some cardiac involvement. Other organ systems affected in this disease include the endocrine, testes, optic lens, central nervous system, peripheral nerves, the gastrointestinal system, and the skin.

Although myotonic muscular dystrophy has been considered a primary disease of skeletal muscle like Duchenne, it has a high incidence of serious cardiac involvement. Sudden cardiac death remains the single most important cause of death, and the incidence of cardiac involvement is described as anywhere from 20% to 90% consisting of a dilated cardiomyopathy. Clinical cardiac dysfunction usually appears after the disease is evident in the peripheral muscle, although in certain individuals, it may be the first manifestation. Pathological analysis of hearts from patients with DM have shown heterogeneous replacement of the myocardium and conduction system by fatty and fibrous tissue. The most frequently observed lesions consist of fibrosis, fatty infiltration, atrophy of the cardiac conduction system, and the ventricular myocardium. The distribution of the lesions in the conduction system tend to correlate with electrocardiographic abnormalities, which include prolonged PR interval, intraventricular conduction defects, and bundle branch block. It is of note that the Purkinje system, which appears to be specifically affected in this disease, is a highly differentiated form of muscle that conducts electrical impulses to provide uniform and rapid excitation of the heart. Identification and isolation of the protein responsible for DM should provide significant insight at the molecular level into defective conduction and its pathogenetic role in sudden death. Until the molecular defect has been elucidated, it is not possible to determine whether the sudden death is primarily related to the diffuse cardiomyopathy or secondary to the predominant involvement of the Purkinje system. However, it is highly likely that it is a combination of both, since the conduction system is simply a specialized form of muscle tissue and, therefore, one would expect the defect throughout the myocardium.

The typical inheritance pattern of DM manifests itself in two clinical scenarios. The most recognized scenario occurs in adults manifesting the clinical picture described earlier.[55] However, the other pattern of manifestation occurs in neonates born with congenital myotonic dystrophy syndrome. Interestingly, congenital myotonic dystrophy syndrome occurs only when the child inherits the disease from its mother.[56] Fifty percent of the mothers, on the other hand, are completely asymptomatic or have minimal symptoms that never require medical attention.

The genetics of DM were uncovered within the past year and have proved to be quite interesting. Conventional genetic linkage analysis and subsequent physical mapping placed the DM locus on chromosome 19q13.2-13.3.[57,58] Observations on large pedigrees with affected individuals have shown a phenomenon in which the severity of disease worsens or manifestations of the disease occur earlier with successive generations, referred to as genetic anticipation.

GCT, a particular type of polymorphic marker and a triplet repeat was the key to the identification of myotonin protein kinase (MT-PK) as the gene causing DM.[58–60] The mRNA of the MT-PK gene appears to be approximately 5 kb, with a sequence which predicts domains such as an adenosine triphosphate–binding site, a serine/threonine catalytic protein kinase domain, as well as structural and transmembrane protein domains. The CCT repetition exists in the 3′ untranslated portion of the MT-PK gene in sets of 50 to 100 in normals and in patients with few or no symptoms of DM. The GCT repeats in patients manifesting the disease are present in sets of up to several thousand and presumably are unstable. The appearance of greater number of repeats in general correlates with the phenomenon of anticipation, with a higher number of repetitions in successive generations.

The discovery of the unstable GCT repeat allows for more efficient diagnosis. Polymerase chain reaction amplification of the repeat locus is a rapid and efficient method to quantitate the extent of repeat instability. Endonuclease digestion of genomic DNA using Bam HI digestion results in a digestion fragment of 1.4 kb containing the GCT repeat in normals after conventional southern DNA hybridization analysis with a larger fragment being evident in affected individuals. Elucidation of how the GCT repeats induce the disease has yet to be determined.

Recent studies[61] indicate that patients with myotonic dystrophy exhibit decreased mRNA and protein levels for the gene product (myotonin protein kinase) encoded at the DM locus. Furthermore, there is a strong correlation with the extent of this decrease and the clinical phenotype, i.e., patients with more severe symptoms exhibit a greater decrease in the level of myotonin protein kinase than patients with mild symptoms. The biochemical consequences of the change in expression, as well as the identity of substrates of this novel protein kinase, are presently unknown.

Duchenne's and Becker's Muscular Dystrophies

Duchenne's and Becker's muscular dystrophies are X-linked recessive disorders manifesting as progressively deteriorating musculoskeletal systems affecting only males within a family. There is multisystem involvement. However, the associated cardiac pathology accounts for a significant proportion of the mortality. Recent epidemiological studies indicate that the incidence of Duchenne's muscular dystrophy (DMD) is about 30 per 100,000 live born males and is fairly uniform throughout the world. Both DMD and Becker's muscular dystrophies (BMD) are due to aberrations in the same musculoskeletal protein, dystrophin.[62, 63]

The onset of DMD is usually appreciated at the appearance of delay in developmental milestones, which manifests itself as late walking.[64–66] Once walking is accomplished, there is a tendency to fall in addition to clumsiness. One of the earliest signs of the disease is weakness of the neck flexor muscles, with inability to raise the head against gravity. During the first 6 years of life, the affected boy demonstrates a wide-based waddling gait with an exaggerated lumbar lordosis. Gower's sign is apparent when the child arises from the floor—the legs are spread, the buttocks are elevated, and the patient climbs up the thighs with his hands. Pseudohypertrophy of the calf, quadricep, gluteal, and deltoid muscle groups may be evident. Muscle groups affected by decreasing order of severity include the proximal musculature of the lower extremities, the proximal muscles of the upper extremity, usually sparing the plantar flexors, ankle invertors, and cranial nerve musculature. Contractures of the iliotibial bands, hip muscles, and heel cords are present by age 6 years while contractures of the knee, elbow and wrist appear by 8 years. Contractures of the shoulders are usually not evident until late in the course of the disease. Between the ages of 5 and 15 years, a progressive deterioration in muscle strength is evident as an inability to climb stairs, stand from the floor, and walk independently. The child is committed to wearing long-leg braces by age 10, with wheelchair dependence occurring by the age of 20 years. Progression of the kyphoscoliosis, contractures, and weakening of the respiratory muscles compromise the pulmonary function. By about age 20 years, the weakness and musculoskeletal abnormalities leave the patient with little use of the extremities, and death ensues shortly thereafter.

Cardiac involvement is that of a dilated cardiomyopathy usually occurring toward the later stages of the disease. Autopsy studies show that there is extensive fibrosis of the posterobasal free wall of the left ventricle with relative sparing of the interventricular septum, the right ventricle, and atria.[67–70] There is significant involvement of the Purkinje system, and as many as 90% of patients demonstrate electrocardiographic abnormalities. The most frequent and distinctive pattern includes increased R/S ratio in the right precordial leads and deep narrow Q waves in leads I, aVL, and the left precordial leads. Conduction system abnormalities affect the intra-atrial system to a much greater extent than the atrioventricular node and infranodal systems. There may be persistent sinus arrhythmias or labile sinus tachycardias. Congestive cardiac failure and significant arrhythmias may manifest in the later stages of the disease.

Elucidation of the molecular abnormality in DMD began in the 1970s after the identification of several X chromosome translocations[71–74] using cytogenetic techniques. Genetic linkage of DMD was subsequently established in 1982 to the distal region of the short arm of the X chromosome, Xp21.[72, 75, 76] In 1985, a clone containing a DNA fragment corresponding to Xp21 was isolated, and after chromosome walking, the gene for dystrophin was cloned[77–79] and its protein product determined.[80]

The gene for dystrophin is comprised of approximately 2.5 million bp, which are transcribed into a 14 kb mRNA molecule.[81] Deletion mutations[63, 82, 83] account for the abnormality in greater than 50% of affected persons. Mutations in the dystrophin gene result in either low level production of a nonfunctional protein or complete absence of the protein in heart[84] and skeletal muscle[85] of affected persons.[62] Dystrophin has been localized to the cytoplasmic surface of the sarcolemma and is believed to be a cytoskeletal protein that is associated with several integral membrane glycoproteins.[86] The glycoprotein/dystrophin complex is hypothesized to be involved in the regulation of intracellular calcium, because dystrophin-deficient muscle has abnormally elevated levels of intracellular calcium and an elevated calcium channel leak has been observed at the cell membrane.[87]

Skeletal muscle and brain tissue contain different isoforms of dystrophin implicating a tissue-specific function.[85] Alternative splicing of the dystrophin mRNA transcript during posttranscriptional modification is responsible for the functional diversity of the dystrophin molecule. Different isoforms of dystrophin have been detected in human cardiac Purkinje fibers,[84, 88] a finding that may explain the development of cardiac arrhythmias in this disorder.

Becker's muscular dystrophy[89, 90] appears to also result from mutations in the dystrophin gene. More than 30% of patients with BMD have no family history of the disease and are thought to represent spontaneous mutations. The incidence is approximately 10 times less than DMD, at approximately 3 per 100,000.[91] The clinical pattern of muscle weakness in BMD closely resembles that of DMD.[90] Pelvic girdle and thigh muscles are predominantly involved with upper extremity weakness developing after the onset of leg weakness. Hypertrophy of the calf muscles is a predominant component in BMD, whereas the development of contractures plays less of a role. Disease progression differentiates BMD from DMD.[90] BMD patients initially become symptomatic between ages 5 and 15, and few are wheelchair bound before 16 years. Greater than 90% of patients are alive at age 20, and the majority survive into their fourth and fifth decades. In addition, the cognitive abilities are not impaired as commonly as in DMD.

Diagnosis of these dystrophies depends on clinical observations, pedigree analysis, and dystrophin gene analysis.[92–95] Creatine kinase activity is elevated from 50 to greater than 100 times normal around age 3 years, and thereafter, it decreases about 20% per year.[64, 96, 97] The identification of deletions and the advent of probes specific for these mutations make the diagnosis in prenatal and new onset cases much more accurate than previous methods. Importantly, carrier females may be identified and offered appropriate genetic counseling. This is particularly true in BMD, since these patients are likely to reproduce. As in DM, elucidation of all mutations in the dystrophin gene will allow the possibility of gene therapy to become a reality in these diseases.

Romano-Ward Long QT Syndrome

Romano-Ward Long QT Syndrome (LQTS), like HCM, is an autosomal dominant disease responsible for stress-induced syncope, malignant ventricular arrhythmias such as torsade de pointes[98–101] and ventricular fibrillation, and sudden death independently described by Romano[102] and Ward.[103] Electrocardiographic findings associated with this syndrome are an elongated QT interval and inverted T waves.

Recently, genetic linkage analysis of the largest kindred documented to be affected with LQTS placed the locus on the short arm of chromosome 11 (11p15).[104] A candidate locus was determined using the Harvey *ras*-1 gene as a marker which detects highly polymorphic variable number tandem repeats.[105] Harvey *ras*-1 is a protooncogene which in association with guanosine triphosphatase–activating protein has been shown in a cell-free system to regulate atrial potassium channels and thus has a rational basis for altering the electrical conduction of the heart and prolonging its electrical repolarization.[106] However, this does not appear to be the gene, and all attempts so far have been unsuccessful in isolating the gene.

Similar to HCM, LQTS has been shown to be genetically heterogeneous by documenting nonlinkage to chromosome 11p in 4 of 11 families,[93] thus necessitating the continued search for other associated loci.

X-linked cardiomyopathy (XCLM) is a rapidly progressive, dilated cardiomyopathy affecting only males during their late teen years or early into their third decade.[107] Affected males usually present with evidence of mitral regurgitation and show echocardiographic evidence of a dilated cardiomyopathy. Dysrhythmias such as ventricular tachycardia have been noted in several patients. The progression is rapid, leading to death or cardiac transplantation within 1 year. In contrast, female carriers may manifest a mild cardiomyopathy without rapid deterioration. Pathologic findings include marked ventricular dilatation and widespread patchy fibrosis particularly in the posterior ventricular wall. Electron microscopy reveals normal mitochondrial structure.

Genetic linkage was established in two pedigrees to the dystrophin locus Xp21 at the most proximal 5′ terminal end.[108, 109] Cardiac tissue showed absent or greatly reduced levels of dystrophin when antibodies to the N-terminus of dystrophin were used for immunofluorescence, while antibodies to the C-terminus showed normal levels.[84] Towbin et al. have speculated that XLCM is caused by an abnormality within the central portion of the dystrophin gene, due either to a pretranscriptional or a posttranscriptional event. Two pretranscriptional abnormalities that may result in abnormal dystrophin include a missense mutation in the proximal region of the dystrophin coding sequence preferentially affecting the myocardium or a cardiac-specific promoter mutation that alters expression. Posttranscriptional splicing aberrancies result in an altered arrangement that interferes with normal cardiac expression of the dystrophin gene.

Friedreich's Ataxia

Friedreich's ataxia is the most common of the inherited ataxias. The disease is inherited in an autosomal recessive pattern and has a carrier frequency of nearly 1 in 100 and a prevalence of 2 per 100,000.

Ataxia becomes apparent in late childhood or adolescence with progression in most patients to a loss of ability to walk around 15 years after presentation. Clinical findings include loss of deep tendon reflexes, limb ataxia, Babinski's sign, cerebellar dysarthria, distal sensory deficits of the limbs, abnormal vibratory and proprioceptive sense in the lower extremities, distal muscle group wasting, nystagmus, optic atrophy, deafness, and pes cavus. Supraventricular arrhythmias such as labile sinus tachycardia, atrial fibrillation, and paroxysmal supraventricular tachycardia are associated with hypertrophic cardiomyopathy[105, 110, 111] deteriorating to congestive heart failure and death in most affected patients.

Electrocardiographic signs are present in about 90% of cases and can be detected in children at the time of onset of the neurological symptoms. The most frequent finding is T wave inversion in the left precordial and inferior limb leads. Pathologic findings show muscle fiber hypertrophy, interstitial fibrosis, and small intramural coronary artery obliteration.

Genetic linkage with lod scores greater than 50 has been obtained for the chromosomal locus of 9q13-21.1[112] using two anonymous DNA markers D9S5 and D9S15; however, a candidate gene for this disorder has not yet been established.

Idiopathic Dilated Cardiomyopathy

This syndrome represents a large proportion of patients with cardiomyopathies and cardiac failure.[113, 114] The essential clinical features are those of chronic cardiac congestive failure in which the heart is dilated, and on histological examination there are varying degrees of fibrosis and hypertrophy. Attempts to chromosomally map the locus have been stymied by the large proportion of patients who seemingly have similar syndromes due to acquired diseases such as ischemic heart disease or hypertension. In a recent study, it was estimated that more than 20% of the cases are familial.[115, 116] It is perhaps not meaningful to generalize about the incidence, until at least a gene has been isolated. Linkage analysis will be further hampered in this disease by genetic heterogeneity, because it is most likely that there are multiple loci. Nevertheless, this is likely to represent fertile areas for molecular genetics and should present us with exciting pathophysiology. Why cardiomyopathies, whether familial or acquired, tend to be either hypertrophic or dilated is an enigma, and the molecular defects leading to such consistent patterns of cardiac growth and remodeling will be very insightful both in terms of diagnosis and treatment.

References

1. Roberts R: Molecular biology and its impact for the future. *Am J Cardiol* 1991; 68:3C–5C.
2. Jarcho JA, McKenna W, Pare JAP, et al: Mapping a gene for familial hypertrophic cardiomyopathy to chromosome 14q1. *N Engl J Med* 1989; 321:1372–1378.
3. Hejtmancik JF, Brink PA, Towbin J, et al: Localization of gene for familial hypertrophic cardiomyopathy to chromosome 14q1 in a diverse U.S. population. *Circulation* 1991; 83:1592–1597.
4. Solomon SD, Geisterfer-Lawrance AA, Vosberg HP, et al: A locus for familial hypertrophic cardiomyopathy is closely linked to the cardiac myosin heavy chain genes, CRI-L436 and CRI-L329, on chromosome 14 at q11-q12. *Am J Hum Genet* 1990; 47:389–394.
5. *Report of the Committee on Mapping and Sequencing the Human Genome.* Washington, National Academy Press, 1988.
6. Adam MD, Kelley JM, Gocayne JD, et al: Complementary DNA sequencing: Expressed sequence tags and human genome project. *Science* 1991; 252:1651–1656.
7. Friedmann T: Opinion: The human genome project—Some implications of extensive "reverse genetic" medicine. *Am J Hum Genet* 1990; 46:407–414.
8. Orkin SH: Reverse genetics and human disease. *Cell* 1986; 47:845–850.
9. Botstein D, White RL, Skolnick M, et al: Construction of a genetic linkage map in man using restriction fragment length polymorphisms. *Am J Hum Genet* 1980; 32:314–331.

10. Nakamura Y, Leppert M, O'Connell P, et al: Variable number of tandem repeat (VNTR) markers for human gene mapping. *Science* 1987; 235:1616–1622.
11. Southern EM: Detection of specific sequences among DNA fragments separated by gel electrophoresis. *J Mol Biol* 1975; 98:503–517.
12. Risch N: Genetic linkage: Interpreting lod scores. *Science* 1992; 255:803–804.
13. Ott J: *Analysis of Human Genetic Linkage.* Baltimore, The Johns Hopskins University Press, 1991.
14. Roberts R, Towbin J, Parker TG, et al: *A Primer of Molecular Biology.* New York, Elsevier Science Publishing Co, Inc, 1992, p 202.
15. Roberts R (ed): *Molecular Basis of Cardiology.* Cambridge, Mass, Blackwell Scientific, 1993, pp 1–518.
16. Mares A Jr, Towbin J, Bies RD, et al: Molecular biology of the cardiologist, in O'Rourke R, McCall D (eds): *Current Problems in Cardiology.* St. Louis, Mosby–Year Book, 1992.
17. Blin N, Stafford DW: A general method for isolation of high molecular weight DNA from eukaryotes. *Nucleic Acids Res* 1976; 3:2303.
18. Alwine JC, Kekmp DJ, Stark GR: Method for detection of specific RNAs in agarose gels by transfer to diazobenzyloxymethyl-paper and hybridization with DNA probes. *Proc Natl Acad Sci USA* 1977; 75:5350.
19. Burke DT, Carl GF, Olson MV: Cloning of large segments of exogenous DNA into yeast by means of artificial chromosome vectors. *Science* 1987; 236:806–809.
20. Maxam AM, Gilbert W: A new method of sequencing DNA. *Proc Natl Acad Sci USA* 1977; 74:560–564.
21. Sanger F, Nicklen S, Coulson AR: DNA sequencing with chain-terminating inhibitors. *Proc Natl Acad Sci USA* 1977; 74:5463–5467.
22. Mullis KB, Faloona F: Specific synthesis of DNA in vitro via a polymerase catalyzed chain reaction. *Methods Enzymol* 1987; 144:335.
23. Bender W, Spierer P, Hogness D: Gene isolation by chromosomal walking. *J Supramolec Struct* 1979; 10:32.
24. Poutska A, Phol TM, Barlow DP, et al: Constructure and use of human chromosome jumping libraries from Notl-digested DNA. *Nature* 1987; 325:353.
25. Collins FS, Drumm ML, Cole JL, et al: Construction of a general human chromosome jumping library with application to cystic fibrosis. *Science* 1987; 235:1046.
26. Myers RN, Larin Z, Maniatis T: Detection of single base substitutions by ribonuclease cleavage at mismatches in RNA:DNA duplexes. *Science* 1985; 230:1242.
27. Cotton RGH, Rodrigues NR, Campbell RD: Reactivity of cytosine and thymine in single base pair mismatches with hydroxylamine and osmium tetroxide and its application to the study of mutations. *Proc Natl Acad Sci USA* 1988; 85:4397–4401.
28. Sasson Z, Rakowski H, Wigle ED: Hypertrophic cardiomyopathy. *Cardiol Clinics* 1988; 6:233–288.
29. Maron BJ, Epstein SE, Roberts WC: Causes of sudden death in competitive athletes. *J Am Coll Cardiol* 1986; 7:204–214.
30. Maron BJ, Roberts WC, Edwards JE, et al: Sudden death in patients with hypertrophic cardiomyopathy: Characterization of 26 patients without functional limitation. *Am J Cardiol* 1978; 41:803–810.

31. Geisterfer-Lawrance AA, Kass S, Tanigawa G, et al: A molecular basis for familial hypertrophic cardiomyopathy: A beta-cardiac myosin heavy chain gene missense mutation. *Cell* 1990; 62:999–1006.
32. Mares A, Jr, Marian AJ, Yu QT, et al: Genetic screening of 75 families with hypertrophic cardiomyopathy show missense mutations the most common genetic defect. *Circulation* 1992; 86:1–228.
33. Epstein ND, Cohn GM, Cyran F, et al: Differences in clinical expression of hypertrophic cardiomyopathy associated with two distinct mutations in the β-myosin heavy chain gene: A 908 Leu-Val mutation and a 403 Arg-Gln mutation. *Circulation* 1992; 86:345–352.
34. Marian AJ, Kelly D, Mares A, Jr, et al: The missense mutation in exon 13 of the β-myosin heavy chain gene, a genetic marker for sudden cardiac death in patients with familial hypertrophic cardiomyopathy (abstract). *Circulation* 1992; 86:1–16.
35. Liew CC, Sole MJ, Yamauchi-Takihara K, et al: Complete sequence and organization of the human cardiac β-myosin heavy chain gene. *Nucleic Acids Res* 1990; 18:3647–3651.
36. Jaenicke T, Diedrich KW, Haas W, et al: The complete sequence of the human heavy chain gene and a comparative analysis of its product. *Genomics* 1990; 8:194–206.
37. Marian AJ, Yu QT, Mares A, Jr, et al: Detection of a new mutation in the beta myosin heavy chain gene in an individual with hypertrophic cardiomyopathy. *J Clin Invest* 1992; 90:2156–2165.
38. Watkins H, Thierfelder L, Hwang DS, et al: Sporadic hypertrophic cardiomyopathy due to de novo myosin mutations. *J Clin Invest* 1992; 90:1666–1671.
39. Perryman MB, Yu QT, Marian AJ, et al: Expression of a missense mutation in the mRNA for β-myosin heavy chain in myocardial tissue in hypertrophic cardiomyopathy. *J Clin Invest* 1992; 90:271–277.
40. Yu QT, Ifegwu J, Marian AJ, et al: Hypertrophic cardiomyopathy mutation is expressed in mRNA of skeletal as well as cardiac muscle. *Circulation* 1993; 87:406–412.
41. Epstein ND, Zhu W-S, Cuda G, et al: Mutant message and myosin protein in skeletal muscle of hypertrophic cardiomyopathy patients with distinct mutations in the beta-myosin heavy chain gene. *Circulation* 1992; 86:1–229.
42. Watkins H, Rosenweig A, Hwang D, et al: Characteristics and prognostic implications of myosin missense mutations in familial hypertrophic cardiomyopathy. *N Engl J Med* 1992; 326:1108–1114.
43. Marian AJ, Mares A, Jr, Kelly D, et al: Sudden death in hypertrophic cardiomyopathy: Contrasting incidence in families with novel and known mutations. *N Engl J Med,* in press.
44. Epstein ND, Fananapazir L, Lin HJ, et al: Evidence of genetic heterogeneity in five kindreds with familial hypertrophic cardiomyopathy. *Circulation* 1992; 85:635–647.
45. Bachinski LL, Czernuszewicz G, Elstein E, et al: Identification of a Canadian family with hypertrophic cardiomyopathy that it is not genetically linked to chromosome 14 locus using polymorphic satellite markers (abstract). *Circulation* 1992; 86:1–230.
46. Solomon SD, Jarcho JA, McKenna W, et al: Familial hypertrophic cardiomyopathy is a genetically heterogeneous disease. *J Clin Invest* 1990; 86:993–999.

47. Elstein E, Clarke LA, Rakowski H, et al: Genomic imprinting in the inheritance of familial hypertrophic cardiomyopathy. *Circulation* 1992; 86:1–272.
48. Schier JJ, Adelstein RS: Structural and enzymatic comparison of human cardiac muscle myosins isolated from infants, adults, and patients with hypertrophic cardiomyopathy. *J Clin Invest* 1982; 69:816–825.
49. Vybiral T, Roberts R, Deitiker PR, et al: Accumulation and assembly of myosin in the Arg-Gln β-MHC hypertrophic cardiomyopathy mutant. *Circ Res* 1992; 71:1404–1409.
50. Clark CE, Henry WL, Epstein SE: Familial prevalence and genetic transmission of idiopathic hypertrophic subaortic stenosis. *N Engl J Med* 1973; 289:709–714.
51. Cuda G, Fananapazir L, Epstein ND, et al: Abnormal myosin in-vitro motility activity in two hypertrophic cardiomyopathy kindreds with distinct cardiac beta myosin heavy chain gene mutations. *Circulation* 1992; 86:1–229.
52. Harper P: *Myotonic Dystrophy*. Philadelphia, WB Saunders, 1989.
53. Todorov A, Jequier M, Klein D, et al: Segregation analysis of myotonia atrophica. *J Genet Hum* 1970; 18:387–406.
54. Pinessi L, Bergamini L, Cantello R, et al: Myotonia congenita and myotonic dystrophy: Descriptive epidemiological investigation in Turin, Italy (1955–1979). *Ital J Neurol Sci* 1982; 3:207–210.
55. Harper PS: Congenital myotonic dystrophy in Britain. II. Genetic basis. *Arch Dis Child* 1975; 50:514–521.
56. Howeler CJ, Busch HF, Geraedts JP, et al: Anticipation in myotonic dystrophy: fact or fiction? *Brain* 1989; 112:779–797.
57. Tsilfidis C, MacKenzie AE, Shutler G, et al: D19S51 is closely linked with and maps distal to the myotonic dystrophy locus on 19q. *Am J Hum Genet* 1991; 49:961–965.
58. Harley HG, Brook JD, Rundle SA, et al: Expansion of an unstable DNA region and phenotypic variation in myotonic dystrophy. *Nature* 1992; 355: 545–546.
59. Fu Y-H, Pizzuti A, Fenwick RG, Jr, et al: An unstable triplet repeat in a gene related to myotonic muscular dystrophy. *Science* 1992; 255:1256–1258.
60. Brook JD, McCurrack ME, Harley HG, et al: Molecular basis of myotonic dystrophy: Expansion of a trinucleotide (CTG) repeat at the 3′ end of a transcript encoding a protein kinase family member. *Cell* 1992; 68:799–808.
61. Fu Y-H, Friedman DL, Richards S, et al: Decreased expression of myotonin-protein kinase mRNA and protein in adult form of myotonic dystrophy. *Science* 1993; 260:235–238.
62. Kao L, Krstenansky J, Mendell J, et al: Immunological identification of a high molecular weight protein as a candidate for the product of the Duchenne muscular dystrophy gene. *Proc Natl Acad Sci USA* 1988; 85:4491–4495.
63. Kunkel LM: Analysis of deletions in DNA from patients with Becker and Duchenne muscular dystrophy. *Nature* 1986; 322:73–77.
64. Brooke MH, Fenichel GM, Griggs RC, et al: Clinical investigation in Duchenne dystrophy: 2. Determination of the "power" of therapeutic trials based on the natural history. *Muscle Nerve* 1983; 6:91–103.
65. Meryon E: On granular and fatty degeneration of the voluntary muscles. *Med Chir Trans* 1852; 35:73.
66. Gowers WR: *A Manual of Diseases of the Nervous System*. London, Churchill, 1886.

67. Frankel KA, Rosser RJ: The pathology of the heart in progressive muscular dystrophy: Epimyocardial fibrosis. *Hum Pathol* 1976; 7:375–386.
68. Perloff JK, Roberts WC, De Leon AC, Jr, et al: The distinctive electrocardiogram of Duchenne's progressive muscular dystrophy. An electrocardiographic-pathologic correlative study. *Am J Med* 1967; 42:179–188.
69. Sanyal SK, Johnson WW, Thapar MK, et al: An ultrastructural basis for electrocardiographic alterations associated with Duchenne's progressive muscular dystrophy. *Circulation* 1978; 57:1122–1129.
70. Perloff JK, De Leon AC, O'Doherty D: The cardiomyopathy of progressive muscular dystrophy. *Circulation* 1966; 33:625–648.
71. Jacobs PA, Hunt PA, Mayer M, et al: Duchenne muscular dystrophy (DMD) in a female with an X/autosome translocation: further evidence that the DMD locus is at Xp21. *Am J Hum Genet* 1981; 33:513–518.
72. Lindenbaum RH, Clarke G, Patel C, et al: Muscular dystrophy in an X; 1 translocation female suggests that Duchenne locus is on X chromosome short arm. *J Med Genet* 1979; 16:389–392.
73. Verellen C, Freund M, DeMeyer R, et al: Progressive muscular dystrophy of the Duchenne type in a young girl associated with an aberration of chromosome X. *Exerpta Medica ICS* 1977; 426:42.
74. Zatz M, Vianna Morgante AM, Campos P, et al: Translocation (X;6) in a female with Duchenne muscular dystrophy: Implications for the localisation of the DMD locus. *J Med Genet* 1981; 18:442–447.
75. Davies KE, Pearson PL, Harper PS, et al: Linkage analysis of two cloned DNA sequences flanking the Duchenne muscular dystrophy locus on the short arm of the human X chromosome. *Nucleic Acids Res* 1983; 11:2303–2312.
76. De Martinville B, Kunkel LM, Bruns G, et al: Localization of DNA sequences in region Xp21 of the human X chromosome: Search for molecular markers close to the Duchenne muscular dystrophy locus. *Am J Hum Genet* 1985; 37:235–249.
77. Koenig M, Hoffman EP, Bertelson CJ, et al: Complete cloning of the Duchenne muscular dystrophy (DMD) cDNA and preliminary genomic organization of the DMD gene in normal and affected individuals. *Cell* 1987; 50:509–517.
78. Burghes AH, Logan C, Hu X, et al: A cDNA clone from the Duchenne/Becker muscular dystrophy gene. *Nature* 1987; 328:434–437.
79. Monaco AP, Neve RL, Colletti Feener C, et al: Isolation of candidate cDNAs for portions of the Duchenne muscular dystrophy gene. *Nature* 1986; 323:646–650.
80. Hoffman EP, Brown RH, Jr, Kunkel LM: Dystrophin: The protein product of the Duchenne muscular dystrophy locus. *Cell* 1987; 51:919–928.
81. Koenig M, Hoffman EP, Bertelson CJ, et al: Complete cloning of the Duchenne muscular dystrophy (DMD) cDNA and preliminary genomic organization of the DMD gene in normal and affected individuals. *Cell* 1987; 50:509–517.
82. Monaco AP, Bertelson CJ, Middlesworth W, et al: Detection of deletions spanning the Duchenne muscular dystrophy locus using a tightly linked DNA segment. *Nature* 1985; 316:842–845.
83. Ray PN, Belfall B, Duff C, et al: Cloning of the breakpoint of an X;21 translocation associated with Duchenne muscular dystrophy. *Nature* 1985; 318:672–675.

84. Bies RD, Friedman DL, Roberts R, et al: Expression and localization of dystrophin in human cardiac purkinje fibers. *Circulation* 1992; 86:147–153.
85. Chamberlain JS, Pearlman JA, Muzny DM, et al: Expression of the murine Duchenne muscular dystrophy gene in muscle and brain. *Science* 1988; 239:1416–1418.
86. Campbell KP, Kahl SD: Association of dystrophin and an integral membrane glycoprotein. *Nature* 1989; 388:259–262.
87. Fong P, Turner PR, Danatclau WF, et al: Increased activity of calcium leak channels in myotubes of Duchenne human and mdx mouse origin. *Science* 1990; 250:673–676.
88. Bies RD, Phelps SF, Cortez MD, et al: Human and murine dystrophin mRNA transcripts are differentially expressed during skeletal muscle, heart and brain development. *Nucleic Acids Res* 1992; 20:1725–1731.
89. Bradley WG, Jones MZ, Mussini J-M, et al: Becker-type muscular dystrophy. *Muscle Nerve* 1978; 1:111.
90. Emery AE, Skinner R: Clinical studies in benign (Becker type) X-linked muscular dystrophy. *Clin Genet* 1976; 10:189–201.
91. Kloepfer HW, Emery AE: Genetic aspects of neuromuscular disease, in Walton JN (ed): *Disorders of Voluntary Muscle.* Edinburg, Churchill Livingston, 1974.
92. Chamberlain JS, Gibbs RA, Ranier JE, et al: Deletion screening of the DMD locus via multiplex DNA amplification. *Nucleic Acids Res* 1988; 16:11141–11156.
93. Beggs AH, Koenig M, Boyce FM, et al: Detection of 98% of DMD/BDM deletions by PCR. *Hum Genet* 1990; 86:45–48.
94. Bulman DE, Murphy EG, Zubrzycka Gaarn EE, et al: Differentiation of Duchenne and Becker muscular dystrophy phenotypes with amino- and carboxy-terminal antisera specific for dystrophin. *Am J Hum Genet* 1991; 48:295–304.
95. Hejtmancik JF, Harris SG, Tsao CC, et al: Carrier diagnosis of Duchenne muscular dystrophy using restriction fragment length polymorphisms. *Neurology* 1986; 36:1553–1562.
96. Perloff JK: Cardiac rhythm and conduction in Duchenne's muscular dystrophy: a prospective study of 20 patients. *J Am Coll Cardiol* 1984; 3:1263–1268.
97. Munsat TL, Baloh R, Pearson CM, et al: Serum enzyme alterations in neuromuscular disorders. *JAMA* 1973; 226:1536–1543.
98. Schwartz PJ, Periti M, Malliani A: The long Q-T syndrome. *Am Heart J* 1975; 89:378–390.
99. Moss AJ, Schwartz PJ: Sudden death and the idiopathic long Q-T syndrome. *Am J Med* 1979; 66:6–7.
100. Moss AJ: Prolonged QT-interval syndromes. *JAMA* 1986; 256:2985–2987.
101. Schwartz PJ, Bonazzi O, Locati E, et al: Pathogenesis and therapy of the idiopathic long QT syndrome, in Hashiba K, Moss AJ, Schwartz PJ (eds): *QT Prolongation and Ventricular Arrhythmias.* New York, Ann NY Acad Sci, 1992.
102. Romano C: Congenial cardiac arrhythmia. *Lancet* 1965; 1:658–659.
103. Ward OC: A new familial cardiac syndrome in children. *J Indian Med Assoc* 1964; 54:103–106.
104. Keating M, Dunn C, Atkinson D, et al: Consistent linkage of the long-QT syndrome to the Harvey ras-1 locus on chromosome 11. *Am J Hum Genet* 1991; 49:1335–1339.

105. Hardin AE, Hewer RL: The heart disease of Friedreich's ataxia: A clinical and electrocardiographic study of 115 patients with an analysis of serial electrocardiographic changes in 30 cases. *Q J Med* 1983; 52:489–502.
106. Yatani A, Okabe K, Polakis P, et al: Ras p21 and GAP inhibit coupling of muscarinic receptors to atrial potassium channels. *Cell* 1990; 61:769–776.
107. Berko BA, Swift M: X-linked dilated cardiomyopathy. *N Engl J Med* 1987; 316:1186–1191.
108. Towbin JA, Brink PA, Gelb B, et al: X-linked cardiomyopathy: Molecular genetic evidence of linkage to the Duchenne muscular dystrophy locus. *Pediatr Res* 1990; 27:25A.
109. Towbin JA, Zhu XM, Gelb BD, et al: X-linked dilated cardiomyopathy (XLCM): Molecular pathogenesis. *Pediatr Res* 1991; 29:25A.
110. Geoffrey G, Barbeau A, Breton G, et al: Clinical description of roentgenologic evaluation of patients with Friedrich's ataxia. *Can J Neurol Sci* 1976; 3:279–287.
111. Malone S, Giunta A, Mansi D, et al: Cardiac abnormalities in Friedreich's ataxia patients and first-degree relatives: Evidence of hypertrophic cardiomyopathy in obligate heterozygotes. *Acta Neurol* 1980; 35:354–356.
112. Chamberlain S, Shaw J, Rowland A, et al: Mapping of mutation causing Friedreich's ataxia to human chromosome 9. *Nature* 1988; 334:248–250.
113. Codd MB, Sugrue DD, Gersh BJ, et al: Epidemiology of idiopathic dilated and hypertrophic cardiomyopathy: A population-based study in Olmsted County, Minnesota, 1975–1984. *Circulation* 1989; 80:564–572.
114. Schmidt MA, Michels W, Edwards WD, et al: Familial dilated cardiomyopathy. *Am J Med Genet* 1988; 31:135–143.
115. Michels W, Driscoll DJ, Miller FA, Jr: Familial aggregation of idiopathic dilated cardiomyopathy. *Am J Cardiol* 1985; 55:1232–1233.
116. Michels W, Moll PP, Miller FA, et al: The frequency of familial dilated cardiomyopathy in a series of patients with idiopathic dilated cardiomyopathy. *N Engl J Med* 1992; 326:77–82.

Medical Management of Coronary Artery Disease After Angioplasty and Thrombolytic Therapy

David P. Faxon, M.D.

Professor of Medicine, University of Southern California School of Medicine, Chief, Division of Cardiology, University of Southern California Medical Center, Los Angeles, California

Thomas J. Ryan, M.D.

Professor of Medicine, Evans Department of Clinical Research and Department of Medicine, Chief of Cardiology, Section of Cardiology, University Hospital, Boston University Medical Center, Boston, Massachusetts

Medical Management After Percutaneous Transluminal Coronary Angioplasty

In-Hospital Management After Angioplasty

The management of any patient after percutaneous transluminal coronary angioplasty (PTCA) should be individualized and determined by the patient's clinical status, the angiographic features of the lesions dilated, and the clinical outcome of the procedure. These issues will be discussed in more detail later in this chapter. However, there are standard practices that are utilized in nearly all patients to avoid the major cardiac complications that arise following the procedure (Table 1). These complications include abrupt closure and subacute closure, vasospasm, and recurrent ischemia.

Abrupt closure is the most important complication of angioplasty, occurring in 5% to 10% of patients undergoing the procedure.[1–11] It is defined as a complete or nearly complete closure of the vessel following an initially successful dilation.[12] In about one half of patients, abrupt closure occurs in the cardiac catheterization laboratory; in the remainder of patients abrupt closure occurs within the next 24 hours. When abrupt closure occurs beyond this time point, it is frequently referred to as *subacute closure.*[13] It is extremely unusual for subacute closure to occur after a balloon angioplasty, but it is not unusual after placement of a coronary stent; the incidence ranges from 5% to 15%.[13] The importance of abrupt closure is that

TABLE 1.
Routine Medical Therapy After Angioplasty

Drug	Dose	Duration
1. Aspirin	80–325 mg/d	24 hr prior; continue indefinitely
or		
Dipyridamole	100 mg qid	24 hr prior; continue 1–2 wk
or		
Sulfinpyrazone	200 mg bid	24 hr prior; continue 1–2 wk
2. Heparin	5,000 U bolus 1,000 U/h adjust to partial thromboplastin time (1.5 times normal)	Just prior; continue for 2 to 24 hr after
3. Calcium antagonist		
Nifedipine	10 mg tid or higher	24 hr prior or 10 mg SL just prior
Verapamil	80 mg tid or higher	24 hr prior; continue 1–2 wk
Diltiazem	30 mg tid or higher	24 hr prior; continue 1–2 wk
4. Nitroglycerin	100–200 mg intracoronary 20–150 mg/min IV	Just prior and just after 1–24 hr after

it accounts for nearly half of all the major complications of angioplasty. In a recent report by Detre et al.[6] from the National Heart, Lung, and Blood Institute's (NHLBI) PTCA Registry, the mortality of a patient who developed abrupt closure was 5%, while the entire patient population had a 1% incidence of death. This observation has been confirmed by other studies, where the mortality of abrupt closure ranges from 5% to 10%.[1–5] In addition, the incidence of acute myocardial infarction (MI) in patients with abrupt closure is 20% to 50%, and at least 30% require an emergency bypass operation.

The pathophysiologic mechanism of abrupt closure is related to the underlying mechanism of angioplasty itself. It is now recognized that angioplasty enlarges the lumen of the vessel by stretching the wall.[14, 15] Because the components of the atherosclerotic plaque are largely noncompressible, the entire vessel enlarges, creating a fusiform localized aneurysm. As a consequence of the stretching, the neointimal layers tear and create flaps that fold into the lumen, a finding verified by pathologic, angioscopic, and ultrasound studies.[15] Experimental studies show that immediately after deflation of the balloon, platelets adhere and then aggregate, forming small thrombi within the crevices of the tears. The greater the local damage, the greater the degree of platelet thrombi that are formed.[16, 17] It is likely that this process occurs in nearly all patients, yet only a small percentage of thrombi go on to occlude the vessel.[18] Unless there is a continuing stimulus to thrombus formation, as occurs with metallic stents, the vessel becomes less thrombogenic over a 24-hour period, although the endothelial lining and neointimal tears are still present. This process has been referred to as *passivation*. This event closely parallels the risk period of abrupt closure in humans.

Clinical factors that are associated with an increased incidence of abrupt closure include unstable angina and female gender[1, 6, 7] (Table 2). Studies have shown that females have a threefold increased mortality with angioplasty. Women, however, are older, have more risk factors, and have more severe coronary disease than men who undergo the procedure.[19] Gender is still a risk, however, even after these differences are taken into account. This increased risk is in part attributable to women's smaller body size, but not all of the differences can be explained by size alone.[20] It appears that women may be more susceptible to abrupt closure, which results in their higher mortality. The preprocedural angiographic factors predisposing a patient to abrupt closure are the amount of myocardium at jeopardy and the angiographic features of the lesion.[1–12] Lesion factors include bifurcation lesions, lesions on bends or in tortuous vessels, and lesions showing irregular or complex contours or thrombosis. These latter lesion characteristics and unstable angina are recognized to be associated with intracoronary thrombosis, which is a major risk factor for abrupt closure.[12] The most important angiographic factor associated with abrupt closure after angioplasty is angiographic evidence of coronary dissection.[21] The presence of a large dissection is associated with a fourfold increased risk of abrupt closure. If blood flow is also reduced, the risk increases to nearly 50%.[22]

The medical management at the time of angioplasty and within the first 24 hours of the procedure is aimed at reducing recurrent ischemia caused by coronary spasm as well as preventing the occurrence of abrupt closure. All patients receive calcium antagonists prior to angioplasty and immediately following the procedure for at least 48 hours for this reason.[23] Most patients are given these agents for 1 to 2 weeks. It is not necessary to continue use of the calcium antagonists beyond this time unless there are other medical indications for continuation. While coronary spasm is rare even in the absence of treatment with calcium antagonists, it is associated with a significant risk of severe ischemic complications.[24] In addition, recent animal and clinical studies have shown that angioplasty causes diffuse nonocclusive spasm of the vessel distal to the stenosis.[25] Experimental studies suggest that this may be due in part to platelet deposition and thrombosis.[17] Reduced blood flow can lead to further thrombosis, setting in motion a vicious circle leading to abrupt closure. For these reasons, intravenous and/or intracoronary nitroglycerin is routinely given to all patients during the procedure.[25] Administration of nitroglycerin is often con-

TABLE 2.
Risk Factors for Abrupt Closure After Angioplasty*

Clinical
Female gender
High risk for bypass surgery
Unstable
Angiographic
Multivessel disease
ACC/AHA lesion class
Long stenosis
Bifurcation lesions
Other stenosis in same artery
Collaterals
Complex lesion
Pre-PTCA % stenosis
Thrombus
Procedural
Post-PTCA % stenosis
Gradient >20 mm/hg
Dissection

*Modified from Ellis SG, Roubin GS, King SB III, et al: Angiographic and clinical predictors of acute closure after native vessel angioplasty. *Circulation* 1988; 77:372–379; Detre KM, Holmes DR, Holubkov R, et al: Incidence and consequences of periprocedural occlusion. The 1985–1986 National Heart, Lung, and Blood Institute Percutaneous Transluminal Coronary Angioplasty Registry. *Circulation* 1990; 82:739–750; de Feyter PJ, van den Brand M, Laarman GJ, et al: Acute coronary artery occlusion during and after percutaneous transluminary coronary angioplasty: Frequency, prediction, clinical course, management and follow-up. *Circulation* 1991; 83:927–936.

tinued afterward if spasm or poor distal flow is present. Long-term use of oral or topical nitrates is not usually necessary unless the patient has documented coronary spasm or variant angina. These patients are at particularly high risk for subsequent abrupt closure or restenosis if not adequately treated. However if the spasm is effectively treated with calcium antagonists, the incidence of complications is similar to that in patients without spasm.[24]

The prevention of thrombosis by the use of aspirin or other newer antiplatelet agents is an essential component of the management of the PTCA patient. In the absence of an antiplatelet agent, the risk of abrupt closure is 15% to 20%.[17] The risk is reduced to 5% when antiplatelet agents are used. Most PTCA operators will not do a PTCA when an antiplatelet agent cannot be used. Alternative agents that have been used in aspirin-allergic patients include the phosphodiesterase inhibitors, dipyridamole and sulfinpyrazone, and the experimental antiplatelet agent, ticlopidine.

Equally essential is adequate anticoagulation with heparin. Commonly the patient is given a bolus of heparin prior to dilation. A continuous drip is then started to maintain the activated coagulation time at higher than 300 seconds. Following the procedure, heparin is usually maintained at the same level for 2 to 24 hours and adjusted to the activated coagulation time or partial thromboplastin time. The duration of heparin is determined at the time of the procedure. Heparin is used for a prolonged period if a significant dissection is present or if the risk of abrupt closure is felt to be high. In the absence of these factors, heparin is continued for 2 hours with sheath removal in 4 hours or when the activated coagulation time is normal (<140 seconds). When an intracoronary stent has been placed, heparin is continued for 3 to 5 days as coumadin therapy is begun.[26] In the patient who has received a stent, the risk of subacute closure can be greatly reduced by meticulously maintaining the partial thromboplastin time to 1.5 to 2.0 times control.[13] Recently, several reports have suggested that elevation of certain markers of thrombus formation (e.g., fibrinogen F1 and F2) can identify patients at higher risk of subacute thrombosis after stent placement and that these patients should be even more aggressively anticoagulated.[27]

Following the procedure, the sheaths in the femoral artery and vein are removed and the patient remains in bed with a sandbag or pressure dressing on the entry site for at least 6 hours. Then the patient can be ambulatory and discharged from the hospital, often within 24 hours of the procedure. The groin should be carefully inspected for bleeding or evidence of retroperitoneal bleeding in every patient. In addition, the occurrence of an arteriovenous fistula is rare but more common following angioplasty or other interventional procedures, because the sheaths and catheters are very large (8 to 12 French).

The medical therapy at the time of discharge usually consists of aspirin and a calcium antagonist. While there is no evidence that long-term aspirin therapy reduces late restenosis, it is common practice to continue use of aspirin for its general benefit in the secondary prevention of MI in patients with known coronary disease.[28]

The use of noninvasive testing in the management of the patient immediately following PTCA is quite variable. Early in the development of angioplasty, it was recommended that all patients undergo an exercise test within several days to assess the adequacy of the procedure. However it has been suggested that there may be a high risk of abrupt closure if an exercise test is done early, presumably because of extension of a coronary dissection that may have occurred at the time of angioplasty.[29] However, a recent randomized trial has shown that it is safe to perform an exercise test early after the procedure and that the information derived from the test is helpful in guiding the activity level of the patient over the next few weeks.[29]

If the test is not done early, it is advisable to have one done within the first month. A positive test at 1 month is predictive of restenosis.[30] It can also help in assessing the adequacy of revascularization when complete revascularization was not achieved at the time of the PTCA. The vast majority of patients with multivessel disease have incomplete revascularization. This most often results because only one lesion, believed to be responsible for the patient's symptoms, is dilated (so-called culprit lesion angioplasty).[31, 32] In this setting, an exercise test or other noninvasive tests, such as a dipyridamole thallium test, can help in assessing the need for further revascularization.[32] Even when incomplete revascularization is present, a negative thallium exercise test predicts a favorable long-term outcome.[33]

Out-of-Hospital Management

Physical Activity and Return to Work

There is no general agreement as to when a patient should resume normal physical activity and return to work following a successful angioplasty. In a recent survey of physicians at our institution, there was a wide variation in the recommendations concerning return to work and resumption of normal physical activity.[29] In general, patients can resume normal activities after 1 week if the patient has not suffered a myocardial infarction. In patients who do not perform heavy physical work, a few days of rehabilitation are necessary. One recent study reported an unexpectedly long time between the procedure and the return to work.[34] The best predictor of return to work was self-efficacy score, a psychosocial concept that reflects the patient's degree of self-confidence to perform the job he or she previously had. Dr. Andreas Gruentzig, the first to describe coronary angioplasty, spent a great deal of time counseling his patients on an early return to work and was very successful in doing so. The minimal morbidity of the procedure lends itself to rapid rehabilitation, and this may be one of the major advantages of the procedure over bypass surgery.

For patients with a myocardial infarction, the management should be similar to that for any patient with an MI. However, the course of recovery can be much more rapid given the improved revascularization status of these patients.

Management of Recurrent Chest Pain Following Angioplasty

The most common reason for recurrent chest pain within the first 6 months after angioplasty is incomplete revascularization or the presence of restenosis at the site of the angioplasty.[35] Incomplete revascularization occurs in the majority of patients with multivessel disease.[36] In a recent report, Bourassa and colleagues[37] reported that nearly 70% of patients with triple vessel disease are incompletely revascularized by angioplasty. In this study, incomplete revascularization, whether intended or not, was associated with a less favorable 1-year outcome. Other recent studies confirm these findings but indicate that the functional degree of revascularization is more important than achieving anatomic revascularization.[38]

Regardless of the cause of the recurrent angina, it is appropriate to investigate the cause of the symptom. If the patient has had a symptom-free interval and the chest pain is typical for angina, then repeating catheterization and PTCA, if restenosis is present, is the best course of action. If the symptoms are equivocal or the patient has remained asymptomatic, then noninvasive testing may be helpful in determining the need for repeat catheterization. In patients with incomplete revascularization and symptoms since the angioplasty, maximal medical therapy should be first instituted; if symptoms persist, PTCA should be repeated for lesions not previously dilated to achieve complete revascularization, or surgical revascularization should be attempted if angioplasty is not possible.

Repeat PTCA is the treatment of choice for restenosis.[39] Despite reports of angiographic evidence of restenosis in 35% to 50% of patients who have undergone angioplasty, repeat PTCA occurs in only 20% of patients during the first 6 months postoperatively.[39, 40] Of these patients, 70% undergo the procedure for restenosis and the remainder undergo it for another lesion not previously dilated. After 5 years, nearly 30% of all patients will have had a repeat PTCA. Beyond 1 year, the most common reason to have another PTCA is dilation of a new stenosis. Percutaneous transluminal coronary angioplasty can be repeated multiple times, because the success is more favorable and complications are fewer the more times the procedure is done.[39] However, the incidence of restenosis rises after each procedure. In a study by Glazier et al.,[39] the incidence of restenosis rose from 22% to 28% to 33% to 50% as successive angioplasties were done on the same lesion.[39] Despite the increased morbidity and cost, a strategy of repeat PTCA for restenosis is not associated with any greater morbidity or cost than is bypass surgery. It is reasonable, however, to consider bypass for patients who have had three angioplasties for the same stenosis or in whom the interval between the procedures is less than 2 months, particularly if this time interval is shortening. These factors have been shown to predict a restenosis rate of more than 50%.[40–42]

The process that leads to restenosis is complex but is a natural response to the injury that occurs as a result of the angioplasty. It is a process that is analogous to generalized wound healing.[43] Angioplasty works by stretching the vessel wall and in the process tears the neointima, creating fissures in the vessel. These are generally not visible angiographically but occur in 70% of patients, as shown by intravascular ultrasound imaging.[44] The balloon also removes the endothelial lining, and circulating platelets immediately adhere to this denuded surface.[14, 16] Small thrombi form with the tears within minutes to hours as previously described.[16] The majority of the smooth muscle cells within the vessel wall are in a quiescent but contractile state. Following injury, a large number of cytokines and mitogens are released; they stimulate the smooth muscle cells to migrate, to proliferate, and to produce extracellular matrix. The most important mitogens appear to be platelet-derived growth factor, fibroblast growth factor and transforming growth factor beta.[43] The proliferative phase repairs the damaged vessel but in the process frequently renarrows the lumen, leading to recurrence of symptoms.

Despite our much greater understanding of the mechanisms responsible for restenosis, an extensive list of drugs has been used in an attempt to prevent this problem.[45] Antiplatelet drugs, aspirin, both high-dose (1,000 mg/d) and low-dose (100 mg/d), ticlopidine, ciprostene, dipyridamole, and prostacyclin have been ineffective in all reported trials.[35, 45] Perhaps the one agent that has shown some effect has been the omega 3 fatty acid or fish oil.[45] Of the seven trials done to date, three have found omega 3 to have a positive effect on restenosis, while in four results have been negative. A large multicenter trial is currently ongoing. In addition the calcium antagonists, nifedipine, verapamil, and diltiazem, have shown either negative results or equivocal results. Finally, results of trials with antiproliferative agents, including steroids, colchicine, angiotensin-converting enzyme (ACE) inhibitors, and heparin, have also been disappointingly negative. Many of these trials have been criticized for study design problems or for inadequate drug administration.[45] The early studies enrolled an extremely small number of patients and therefore were unlikely to show a beneficial effect. Assuming that a single drug could reduce the restenosis rate from 40% to 25%, it is now estimated that at least 2,000 patients need to be studied to show a positive effect.[33] In addition, animal studies have indicated that a beneficial effect is usually not seen unless very high doses of each drug are used.[45] This has led many to investigate techniques that would allow local drug administration.[46, 47] Balloon catheters that release drugs or are coated with drugs as well as biodegradable stents that can deliver drugs over a prolonged period of time are being actively studied.[45] Currently, there is no effective means of reducing restenosis pharmacologically. However, because aspirin significantly reduces abrupt closure and may reduce the incidence of subsequent MI, it is standard practice to have the patient continue the use of aspirin indefinitely.

Our studies and those of others have shown that the majority of patients with restenosis present with exertional angina[48] (Table 3). Less than 2% present with a myocardial infarction. In most patients, a gradual increase in symptoms occurs that allows time to institute medical therapy and evaluate the patient. However almost 12% of patients develop severe unstable angina requiring immediate hospitalization and repeat PTCA if feasible. Patients who initially present with an acute myocardial infarction or unstable angina are more likely to present in a similar way if they develop restenosis. It is well recognized that 20% to 30% of patients with angiographic demonstration of restenosis are asymptomatic and would not have been recognized if they had not undergone cardiac catheterization for other reasons.[49] Approximately half of these patients have a positive exercise test although, in our series, repeat PTCA was done in less than 2% for angiographic restenosis in the absence of symptoms. Patients with asymptomatic

TABLE 3.
Clinical Presentation at the Time of Restenosis (n = 123)

Exertional angina	85.5%
Canadian Heart Class	2.6 ± 1 class
Unstable angina	11.4%
Acute myocardial infarction	2.6%
Asymptomatic plus exercise test	1.6%

restenosis do very well and are not at risk of serious cardiac complications that are unheralded by some clinical sign. This is probably due to the mechanism of asymptomatic restenosis. Angiographic studies indicate that asymptomatic restenosis is usually caused by the development of a borderline stenosis that does not restrict blood flow (e.g., a 50% to 60% stenosis) or the presence of abundant collateral vessels that supply an adequate amount of blood to the myocardium. Accordingly, we do not recommend cardiac catheterization in all patients following angioplasty. We would, however, recommend cardiac catheterization for any symptomatic patient, no matter how minimal the symptoms were. In addition we would suggest catheterization for patients who are asymptomatic but for whom a routine exercise test is markedly positive. It is not unreasonable to follow all other patients carefully to ensure that they do not develop symptoms.

Chest pain outside of the window of restenosis, particularly after 1 year, is more likely caused by progression of coronary disease than by restenosis.[41] In this case, the patient can be managed in a similar manner to any patient with symptomatic coronary disease.

Noninvasive Testing

As discussed earlier, the proper timing and use of noninvasive testing after PTCA is controversial. Exercise testing lacks the sensitivity to predict restenosis.[32] Califf et al.[33] reported that a positive test results in only a moderate predictive accuracy in identifying patients with angiographically documented restenosis while a negative test provides a high level of assurance that restenosis is absent. Thallium and more recently sestimibi can improve the predictive value of the exercise tests. Other tests, such as dipyridamole, thallium, or dobutamine echo testing, have not been evaluated adequately to determine their value in predicting restenosis. In addition, the proper timing of these tests is unclear. Nearly 80% of patients will develop restenosis by 3 months; however, earlier evaluation may identify patients at higher risk of developing restenosis.[50] Current practice is to do an exercise test within 1 month of the procedure to ensure that the patient had an initially successful procedure and then to repeat the test if the patient develops symptoms or at 6 months to reassure the patient that he or she does not have restenosis.

Long-Term Outcome

The long-term outcome of angioplasty has been shown to be excellent.[51–56] Gruentzig et al.[51] reported on the first 169 patients undergoing PTCA to be followed for 5 to 8 years. The overall survival was 96%. A second angioplasty was required in 27 patients and coronary bypass surgery in 19. Event-free survival occurred in 79% at 6 years. However, only a minority of the patients had multivessel disease. Data from the NHLBI PTCA registry indicate that 6 years after PTCA, 9% of patients with single vessel disease and 15% of patients with multivessel disease have died.[52, 56] Myocardial infarction occurred in 12% and 20% and revascularization (PTCA or coronary artery bypass graft) in 38% and 53%, respectively. The experiences of other large centers parallel these observations.[53]

The factors that are associated with a less favorable outcome include age, female gender, diabetes, congestive heart failure, severe concomitant disease, incomplete revascularization, multivessel coronary disease, and left ventricular function.[56, 57] Of all these factors, congestive heart failure and age impart the greatest influence, increasing the risk of death fivefold or sixfold. In a study by Vandormael and colleagues,[57] when only initially successful patients were analyzed, the only independent predictor of cardiac mortality was poor left ventricular function as measured by a wall motion score.

Angioplasty is usually done to relieve angina and improve the quality of life rather than to reduce mortality. Numerous studies have shown it to be highly effective in this regard. More than 80% of patients enrolled in the NHLBI PTCA registry were asymptomatic and were taking no long-acting angina medication at a mean of 6 years of follow-up (personal communication, K. Detre M.D., Ph.D.). Only 9% had angina that was the same as or worse than before the procedure. Consistent with this are the observations of Mulcahy et al.[58] that both PTCA and coronary artery bypass graft are effective in improving exercise-induced ischemia and reducing the number of ambulatory ST-segment changes seen during a 24-hour monitoring period.

Although PTCA is widely accepted as the treatment of choice for patients with single-vessel disease, it is not at all clear which revascularization strategy is best for treatment of multivessel disease. A number of nonrandomized trials have been reported. Nearly all have shown a similar mortality and recurrent infarction rate.[58–64] Most have shown a significantly higher incidence of repeat revascularization with PTCA because of restenosis. In an evaluation of the national Medicare experience, Hartz et al.[62] showed that bypass was associated with a risk-adjusted relative risk of death of 1.72 compared with PTCA. In low-risk patients this relative risk was 2.15 and in high-risk patients this was 0.9. These data suggest that low-risk patients have a better chance of survival with PTCA than with bypass but high-risk patients have similar risk with either procedure. A recent report also supports this, showing that for less severe disease the outcome is better with PTCA, and for more severe vessel disease the outcome is better with bypass.[65]

The importance of this question has lead to the initiation of six large randomized trials comparing PTCA with coronary artery bypass graft in patients with multivessel disease.[66] The Emory Angioplasty vs. Surgery Trial (EAST) is the only single-center trial. The primary endpoint of the trial is a combined endpoint that includes freedom from death, Q-wave myocardial infarction, and a large thallium defect on exercise testing. The Bypass Angioplasty Revascularization Investigation (BARI) is an NIH-sponsored trial involving 16 centers. It is also the largest, having randomized 1,800 patients. The primary endpoint of this study is mortality; angina, quality of life, MI, repeat revascularization, and economic impact are secondary endpoints. The Randomized Intervention Treatment of Angina (RITA), the Coronary Artery Bypass Revascularization Investigation (CABRI), and the German Angioplasty Bypass Intervention Trial (GABI) are being conducted in Europe. The results of these trials will not be known for several years and, until then, clinical judgment will need to be the best guide in choosing a revascularization strategy for patients with multivessel disease.

There has been only one randomized trial comparing PTCA with medical therapy. The ACME trial was conducted in eight Veterans Administration hospitals. Two hundred twelve patients with mild angina and single-vessel disease were randomized to PTCA or to medical therapy.[67] At 6 months 64% of the PTCA patients were free of angina, while 46% of the medical patients were free of angina. The PTCA patients also had a longer duration of exercise; however the initial hospital costs were more and the complications were greater. The study emphasized that, while PTCA can effectively reduce angina, it is associated with a small but important risk. Thus it seems most appropriate to reserve the procedure for patients with disabling angina or for those who are intolerant of medical therapy.

Medical Management After Thrombolytic Therapy

In-Hospital Management

Rationale for Adjunctive Medical Therapy

Two of the most important advances in cardiology over the last decade have been the development of angioplasty and thrombolysis. The latter therapy has dramatically changed the treatment of acute myocardial infarction.[68] It is widely accepted that all eligible patients should receive a thrombolytic agent to improve long-term survival, presumably by reducing the extent of the myocardial infarction and improving its subsequent healing. Thrombolysis does have a number of significant limitations. It is applicable to less than 50% of all patients hospitalized in the United States with a diagnosis of acute myocardial infarction, because of conventional contraindications to thrombolytic therapy and the difficulty of diagnosing acute myocardial infarction on admission in a substantial number of people. Thrombolysis fails to restore blood flow in 20% to 30% of patients. A low but important incidence of reocclusion and recurrent ischemia results in a need for revascularization in 15% to 20% of patients during the initial hospitalization.[68] Recent randomized trials have suggested that angioplasty is an effective alternative to thrombolysis, and angioplasty is particularly attractive for the patient who is not a candidate for fibrinolytic therapy.[70] The management of the patient who undergoes PTCA without thrombolysis should be similar to other patients undergoing angioplasty as previously described. The management of the patients after thrombolysis is aimed at improving reperfusion, improving ventricular remodeling, and reducing reocclusion and recurrent ischemia (Table 4).

Therapy to Improve Reperfusion

Improved thrombolytic regimens have improved the acute reperfusion rates but still have not been able to achieve better than an 80% patency rate 90 minutes after drug administration, possibly because other mechanisms, such as plaque rupture, are responsible for the occlusion or because thrombolysis is inadequate.[71, 72] To improve reperfusion, a number of studies have evaluated the role of adjunctive PTCA in patients with a persistent total occlusion of the infarct artery. Ellis and colleagues[73] recently reviewed the data available on "rescue angioplasty" and in a meta-analysis demonstrated an 80% success rate for PTCA in thrombolytic failures. However, the procedure was completed by a high reocclusion rate (18%) and a mortality of 10.6%. Compared to that of patients receiving only thrombolysis and not rescue angioplasty, the mortality was no different, nor was there any obvious difference in myocardial function. However, these studies were not randomized and reperfusion theoretically should be of benefit to these patients as well. A large multicenter trial is currently ongoing. Although the role of rescue angioplasty remains uncertain, our policy is not to perform rescue PTCA, given the available information on the risks vs. the benefits.

The ISIS II study compared administration of intravenous streptokinase (SK), oral aspirin, both, or neither, in 17,187 patients with suspected acute MI.[74] The results showed that SK, aspirin, or both reduced 5-week mortality compared with the rate when there was no therapy (Fig 1). The combination of SK and aspirin was significantly better than SK alone, and it is now standard practice to administer aspirin to all patients immediately on presentation. Administration of the drug is continued during the hospital stay and in most instances indefinitely. The mechanism for this synergistic effect is likely a lower incidence of reocclusion and an improved reperfusion rate, because platelet hyperreactivity is recognized to be associated with a less favorable outcome.[75]

The use of other antiplatelet agents in patients with an acute MI have not been well studied. These alternative agents however may be equally

TABLE 4.
Routine Medical Management After Thrombolysis

Drug	Dose	Duration
Heparin	5,000 U bolus	SK—follow partial thromboplastin time; start when less than 2 times
	1,000 U/hr; adjust to partial thromboplastin time (1.5 times)	control rtPA—start simultaneously APSAC—start 4–6 hr after With all, continue for 5–7 days
Aspirin	160–325 mg/d	Start with or prior to thrombolytic; continue indefinitely
Nitroglycerin	20–200 mg/mm IV adjust to blood pressure: >90 <130 systolic	24–48 hr
β-Blocker		
Metoprolol	5–15 mg IV; 25–50 mg po qid	Start immediately if no contraindication
Propranolol	1–5 mg IV; 10–40 mg po qid	
Angiotensin enzyme inhibitors (e.g.)		
Captopril	1.25–25 mg tid	Begin 5–7 days after MI
Enalapril	5–20 mg qd	With large MI or congestive heart failure can be started on day 1

effective. Potential adjunctive drugs, as shown in Table 5, include dipyridamole, a phosphodiesterase inhibitor, and the anti-inflammatory agent, sulfinpyrazone, has been used in aspirin-allergic patients.[76] More recent attention was focused on the more powerful platelet, glycoprotein receptor antagonists. The GPIIb/IIIa receptor is important in the adhesion of platelets to other platelets and to von Willebrand's factor. Experimental studies have shown that the combination of an antibody to the GPIIb/IIIa receptor and recombinant tissue-type plasminogen activator (rtPA) results in a much more rapid and complete thrombolysis.[77] The investigational agent

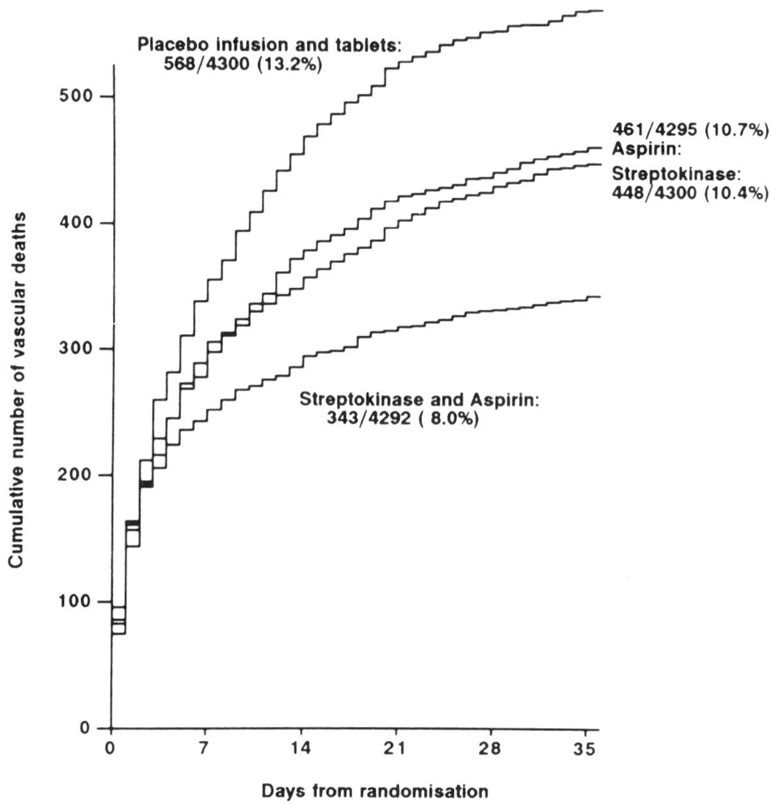

FIG 1.
The cumulative vascular mortality in days 0 to 35 in patients randomized to placebo, streptokinese, aspirin, or both in the ISIS II trial. (From Yusuf S, Sleight P, Held P, et al: Routine medical management of acute myocardial infarction. *Circulation* 1990; 82(suppl II):II117–II134. Used by permission.)

ticlopidine is also a powerful antiplatelet agent but has not been fully investigated in the setting of an acute myocardial infarction.

The role of heparin following thrombolysis is more controversial (Fig 2). It is generally agreed that heparin should be started either simultaneously with the thrombolytic agent in the case of rtPA or at the conclusion of the intravenous administration of SK or APSAC when the partial thromboplastin time falls to one and a half times control. Despite the routine use of heparin, the Third International Study of Infarct Survival (ISIS-III) and the International Study Group failed to find a benefit from the addition of heparin to either SK or tissue plasminogen activator (tPA) plus aspirin in 41,299 and 20,891 randomized patients, respectively.[78, 79] Administration of 12,500 U of heparin subcutaneously twice daily was begun 12 hours after administration of the fibrinolytic agent; critics have argued that the late administration and route might have obscured a benefit. Five trials

TABLE 5.
Potential Adjunctive Therapy in Acute Myocardial Infarction*

- I. Agents to improve reperfusion
  - A. Platelet antagonists
    1. Thromboxane A_2 inhibitors or receptor antagonists
    2. Aspirin
    3. Serotonin antagonists (Katanserin)
    4. Prostaglandins
    5. Prostaglandins I_2 and E
    6. Glycoprotein IIb/IIIa receptor blockers (7E3)
    7. Disintegrins
    8. von Willebrand's factor antibodies
    9. Dipyridamole
    10. Ticlopidine
    11. Sulfinpyrazone
    12. Fish oil (eicosapentenoic acid)
  - B. Thrombin inhibitors
    1. Heparin
    2. Low-molecular-weight heparin
    3. Hiruden, hirilog, hirugen
    4. Argotoban
    5. PPAC
    6. Tick anticoagulation peptide
- II. Agents to improve healing and remodeling
  - A. β-Blockers
  - B. Angiotensin-converting enzyme inhibitor
  - C. Calcium channel blockers
  - D. Oxygen-free radical scavengers
  - E. Neutrophil inhibitors
    1. Adenosine
    2. Ibuprofen
    3. Prostacyclin
    4. Perflurochemicals
  - F. Nitrates (IV, oral, or topical)
- III. Agents to reduce ischemia and recocclusion
  - A. Thrombolysis (for reocclusion)
  - B. Nitrates
  - C. β-adrenergic blockers
  - D. Calcium antagonists

*Modified from Popma JJ, Topol EJ: Adjuncts to thrombolysis for myocardial reperfusion. *Ann Intern Med* 1991; 115:34–44.

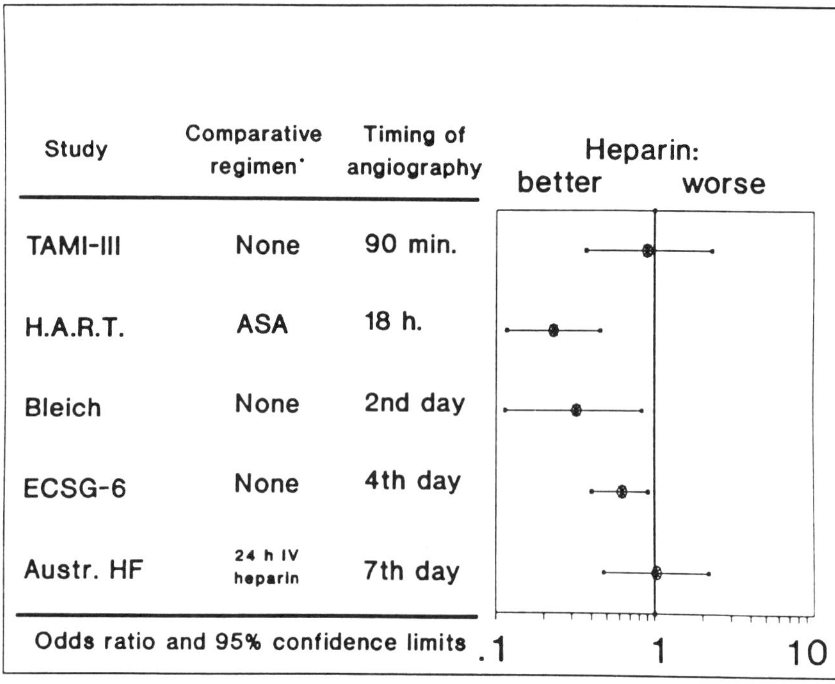

FIG 2.
The influence of heparin in patency of the infarct artery following rtPA in five randomized trials. Two trials, the TAMI-III and the National Heart Foundation of Australia trials, showed no benefit, while the HART trial and the trial by Bleich et al.[81] and the ECSG-6 trial did. (From ISIS-2 Collaborative Group: Randomized trial of intravenous streptokinase, oral aspirin, both or neither among 17,987 cases of suspected acute myocardial infarction: ISIS 2. *Lancet* 1988; 2:349. Used by permission.)

have evaluated the influence of heparin on patency of the infarct-related artery in patients who received rtPA.[74, 80–83] The Heparin–Aspirin Reperfusion Trial (HART) demonstrated that patency was better 18 hours postlysis when heparin was used. Likewise the Sixth European Cooperative Study Group (ECS6-VI) trial and a study reported by Bleich et al.[82] also showed heparin to have a benefit. Two other trials, the Thrombolysis and Angioplasty in Myocardial Infarction (TAMI-III)[81] and the Australian Heart Foundation study showed only a trend toward benefit. The large European trials, such as the ISIS III trial, evaluated the combination of SK and subcutaneous heparin.[78] The lack of a difference seen between SK and tPA in these trials may be due to the route of heparin administration, because tPA may require early intravenous heparin to prevent the recognized higher incidence of reocclusion. For this reason, the Global Utilization of Streptokinase and rtPA for Occluded Arteries (GUSTO) is being conducted to help evaluate this question. The study is comparing various thrombolytic combinations as well as intravenous vs. subcutaneous heparin. Another benefit of intravenous heparin is significant reduction in left ventricular thrombi, as revealed by echocardiography. In some studies, heparin can reduce the incidence by one half to two thirds.[83] Prins and Hirsch[84] have shown that intravenous heparin in a dose of 1,200 U/h following a bolus of 5,000 U adequately anticoagulates 80% of patients, while 12,500 U of subcutaneous heparin fails to do so in the majority of patients.

The major complication of intravenous heparin is a recognized increased risk of bleeding, which can be kept at a minimum if the partial thromboplastin time is kept at one and a half times normal. Currently the most common practice in the United States is to use continuous intravenous heparin for 5 to 7 days in addition to aspirin and then to continue with aspirin only thereafter. Alternatively, coumadin can be given, but it is usually reserved for patients with complicated MIs or atrial fibrillation and for those with evidence of mural thrombi. However, recent studies have shown routine coumadin use to favorably effect long-term outcome.[85] Patients with large anterior MIs are particularly at high risk for increased bleeding, and routine echocardiograms looking for left ventricular clots should be done in these patients.

Thrombin inhibitors are currently undergoing extensive investigation as adjunctive therapy for acute MI[86, 87] (see Table 5). Hirudin is a naturally occurring component of leech saliva. It binds with thrombin to prevent thrombin-induced platelet activation, and activation of factors V, VII, and XIII. Another thrombin inhibitor is hirugen. Argatroban is another synthetic competitive inhibitor of thrombin. These agents have a great potential for improved thrombolysis as well as treatment of other clinical situations associated with thrombosis, such as unstable angina. A large number of clinical trials to evaluate the effectiveness of these antithrombin agents are ongoing.

Therapy to Improve Ventricular Healing and Remodeling

Following a myocardial infarction, ventricular healing begins almost immediately. This healing process is complex but again shares similarities to generalized wound healing.[88] The final shape of the ventricle is related to ventricular remodeling. If the ventricular scar stretches as it heals (so-called infarct expansion) then the final size will be larger, the ventricular volume greater, and the long-term outcome less favorable.[89–93] A number of agents that influence this process have been studied: β-blockers, calcium blockers, and ACE inhibitors. β-Adrenergic blockers benefit the MI patient by reducing myocardial ischemia through a reduction in heart rate and myocardial oxygen consumption as well as recurrent atrial and ventricular arrhythmias (Fig 3). These effects result in a reduction in infarct size and improved healing. Numerous clinical trials of β-blockers in the secondary prevention of an MI have shown a reduced mortality from long-term β-blockade use.[94–100] It has also been demonstrated that earlier intravenous administration within the first 8 hours is also beneficial, particularly in patients who are given thrombolytic agents. In a review of 27 randomized trials including more than 27,000 patients, there was a 13% reduction in

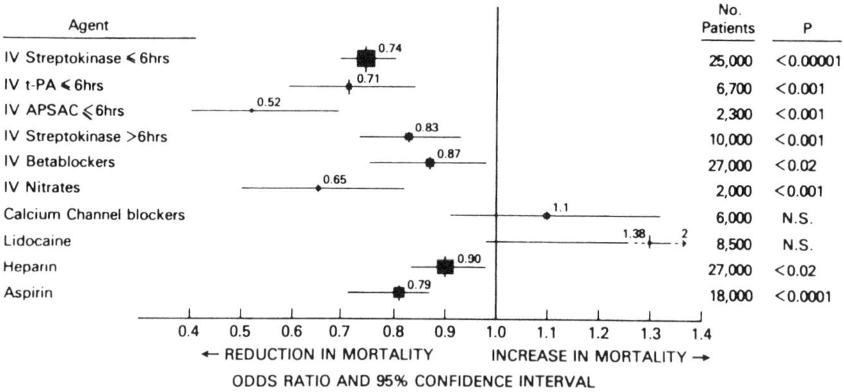

FIG 3.
The effect of various treatments on mortality after acute myocardial infarction.

mortality.[94] Importantly, the greatest benefit was most apparent during the first 2 days postinfarction. There was not only a reduction in mortality but also a decrease in infarction rate (19% and 10%, respectively). These benefits appear to be present whether or not the infarct artery is patent. The great benefit also appears to be in the higher-risk patients, and the development of new β-adrenergic blocking drugs with vasodilator properties may be advantageous in these patients.[99, 100]

The NHLBI TIMI-II study included a subrandomization to early β-blockers or not.[101] Fifty-two percent of patients were excluded for significant bradyarrhythmia, congestive heart failure, or other contraindications to acute β-blocker therapy. Of 3,262 in the trial, 1,390 were eligible for this substudy. One half received 15 mg of intravenous metoprolol followed by oral drugs and remainder received only oral therapy at the time of hospital discharge. The groups had a similar incidence of in-hospital and 42-day mortality and left ventricular function. However, in the group that received intravenous metoprolol, 16 patients had a nonfatal MI and 107 had recurrent ischemia as compared to 31 and 147 in the nontreated patients ($P = .02$ and $P = .05$), respectively. The greatest benefit was seen in patients who received tPA within 2 hours of the onset of symptoms. The long-term benefit of β-blockers was not evaluated in this study, because all patients received metoprolol at the time of hospital discharge.

The use of calcium antagonists is more controversial.[102–108] Studies done prior to thrombolysis use showed no benefit from nifedipine and verapamil in reduction of infarct size. However, the utility of these drugs in combination with thrombolytic agents has not been well studied. One small study of nifedipine failed to show a benefit.[107] The Multicenter Diltiazem Reinfarction Trial studied patients who had a subendocardial infarction.[108] The incidence of subsequent recurrent ischemia and infarction was less in the treated group than in the placebo group (Fig 4).

However, the benefit was restricted to those with good left ventricular function. In those with ejection fractions less than 50%, the mortality was greater in the treatment group. Based on these studies and others it seems best to recommend calcium antagonists only in patients who develop recurrent ischemia and those with a subendocardial MI and good left ventricular function.

Angiotensin-converting enzyme inhibitors are effective antihypertensive agents and might be expected to reduce ventricular afterload and improve healing and remodeling.[109] Angiotensin-converting enzyme inhibitors have also been shown to improve coronary blood flow and reduce myocardial demand in patients with coronary disease.[110] Recent interest has also focused on their vascular and antiatherogenic effects.[111] Since the left ventricle progressively enlarges in 40% to 50% of patients, reduction in afterload can reduce left ventricular size and improve healing and lead to improved

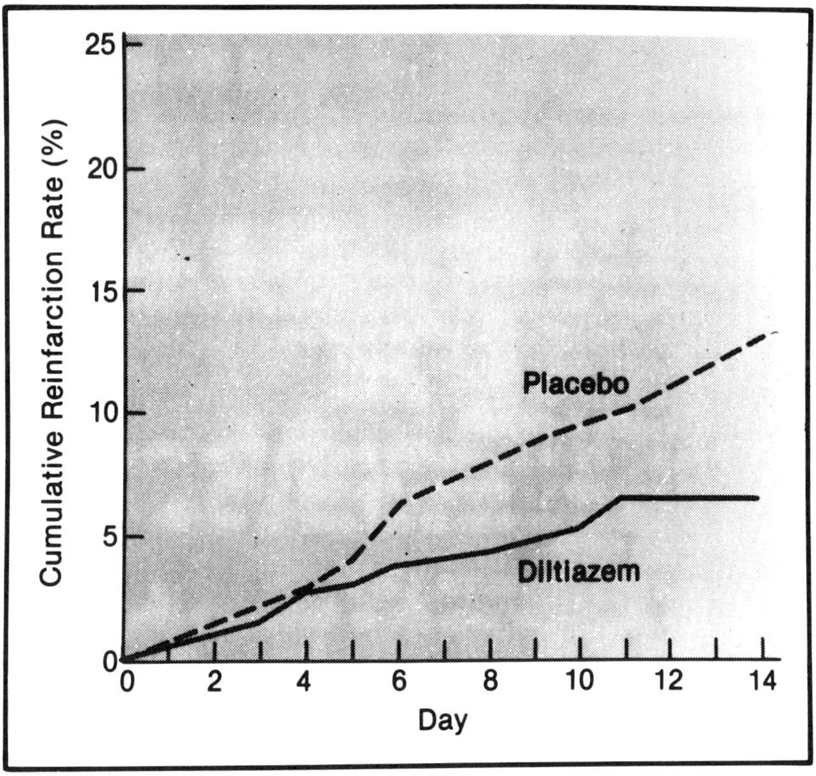

FIG 4.
The cumulative reinfarction rate in patients with non–Q-wave MI randomized into groups receiving diltiazem or placebo. (From the Multicenter Diltiazem Postinfarction Trial Research Group: The effect of diltiazem on mortality and reinfarction after myocardial infarction. *N Engl J Med* 1988; 319:385–392. Used by permission.)

survival. A large multicenter trial recently reported by Pfeffer and colleagues,[112] indicated that captopril, given 7 to 14 days after an MI in 1,500 patients, reduced overall and cardiac mortality by 25% over a 2-year period. In addition, ventricular size was smaller, consistent with an effect of the drug on remodeling and infarct expansion. The benefit was not observed until 6 months after the MI and increased with time. A study of the effects of ACE inhibitors in patients with congestive heart failure showed a lower incidence of recurrent MI in the treatment group.[113] Contrary to these studies, the consensus II study showed that enalapril started within 24 hours of the onset of an acute MI did not improve survival during the first 6 months.[114] The difference in type of ACE inhibitor used or the longer follow-up period may explain the difference in the results. Taken together, these studies raise the possibility that ACE inhibitors not only may affect ventricular remodeling by a reduction in left ventricular size but also may affect the underlying atherosclerotic process itself. Based on these results, current practice is to treat all eligible patients with ACE inhibitors. Those that are likely to benefit the most are patients with large MIs and reduced left ventricular function.

Therapy to Reduce Ischemia and Reocclusion

The most frequent adverse event to occur after thrombolysis is recurrent ischemia, which occurs in 20% to 50% of patients in the hospital and in up to 70% during the first 6 months.[115] Reocclusion within the first few days occurs in 5% to 20% of patients and is associated with a high mortality rate. As previously mentioned, the use of aspirin and heparin are important in reducing this complication. Unfortunately no acute clinical or angiographic features are predictive of reocclusion.

The management of recurrent ischemia or reocclusion in the hospital should be aggressive, because the mortality is significantly increased (Fig 5). In a study of 303 patients who had successful reperfusion, the in-hospital mortality for patients without recurrent ischemia was 2% while it was 14.9% for patients with recurrent ischemia.[115] This rate was not as high as that for patients who did not achieve acute reperfusion at all (32.1%). In addition, left ventricular function did not improve in those who had recurrent ischemia. However, if early successful reperfusion was achieved with either repeat thrombolysis or PTCA, the mortality was reduced to 0% in that study.[115] Those reperfused later than 90 minutes after the onset of recurrent symptom had a mortality of 20.8%, comparable to those who failed reperfusion (24%). It is clear that in patients developing symptoms of reocclusion early and effective therapy is imperative. We currently recommended readministration of a thrombolytic agent; if the patient does not show clinical signs of reperfusion (such as resolution of chest pain and a decrease in ST-segment elevation) then the patient should be brought to the catheterization laboratory and an angioplasty should be performed if the vessel remains occluded. In patients who are not eligible for thrombolysis, we recommend proceeding directly to PTCA.

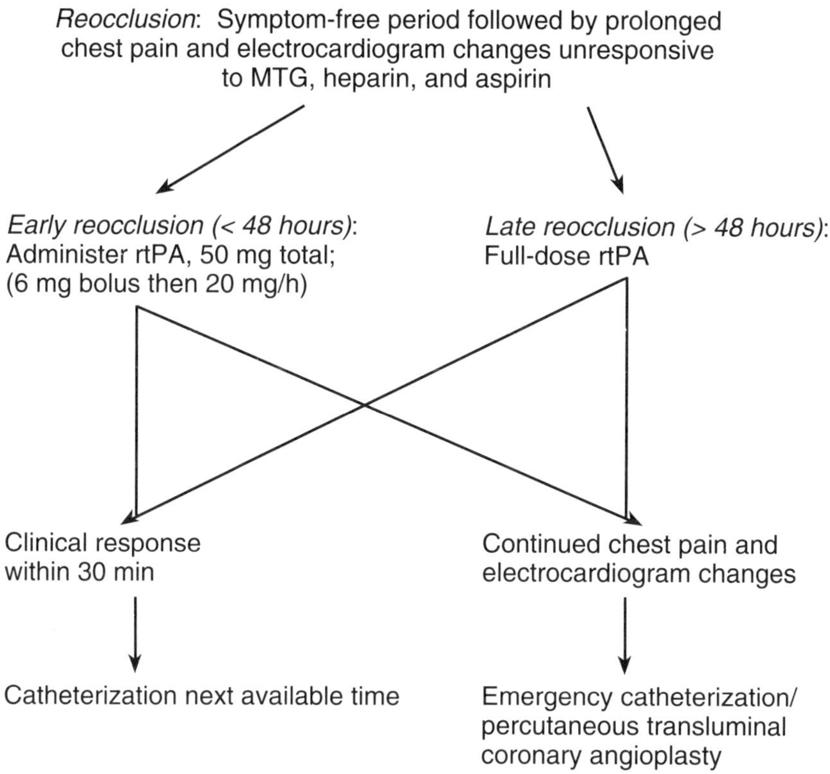

FIG 5.
Management of reocclusion.

Postinfarction angina in the hospital is also not an infrequent occurrence. Among the 1,626 patients in the conservatively treated group of the TIMI II study, 20.7% needed revascularization with either angioplasty or bypass surgery within the first 21 days.[101] By 1 year, 35.5% had received a revascularization procedure.[116] However routine angioplasty did not result in an improved long-term outcome (Fig 6). The recommendations of the trial were that waiting for the patient to develop recurrent ischemia is the optimum strategy, because there is no increased risk with this approach and it is less complex and less costly than providing routine angioplasty for all patients.

It has been suggested that an open infarct-related artery, regardless of the infarct size, is associated with a better long-term outcome than a closed artery. The current hypothesis is that the incidence of sudden death is lower in the open-artery patients because of improved healing and fewer late potentials, known to predispose patients to cardiac arrhythmias. Randomized trials are being proposed to evaluate this question. Currently, however, only patients with recurrent ischemia need be considered for re-

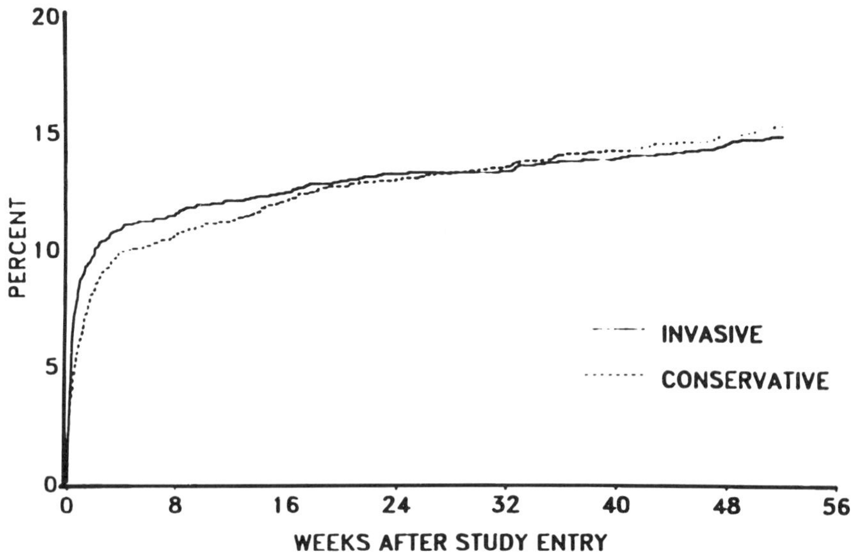

FIG 6.
The cumulative Kaplan-Meier event rate for death and myocardial infarction through 1 year in patients assigned to an invasive strategy or conservative therapy in the TIMI-II trial. (From Williams DO, Braunwald E, Knatterud G, et al: One-year results of the Thrombolysis in Myocardial Infarction Investigation (TIMI) phase II trial. *Circulation* 1992; 85:533–542. Used by permission.)

vascularization. Our practice is to be aggressive, referring any patient who has even mild angina or a positive exercise test during the initial hospitalization for PTCA or a bypass procedure prior to discharge.

Other Therapy

Antiarrhythmics are well recognized to control atrial and ventricular arrhythmias following an acute MI. However, a number of studies have shown that routine use of antiarrhythmics has no benefit and that they should be used only when clinically indicated for life-threatening arrhythmias.[117–121] In particular, a recent trial indicated that flecainide and encainide may increase mortality.[121]

Recent studies have suggested that magnesium may reduce the 1-year mortality after MI, perhaps through a reduction in arrhythmias.[122] For this reason, the ongoing ISIS IV trial will be evaluating use of intravenous magnesium in addition to ACE inhibitors following thrombolysis.

The role of digitalis in acute MI has also been previously studied. Hemodynamic studies have shown that indexes of left ventricular function improve following intravenous digitalis preparation, but no evidence exists that chronic oral therapy reduces infarct size or improves clinical outcome.[123–126] Its uses in patients with congestive heart failure and arrhythmias are well established but a long-term benefit cannot be demonstrated.[123]

The Role of Noninvasive Testing

The goal of noninvasive testing following an MI is to identify those patients who need further invasive treatment or intensified medical management as well as to provide some prognostic information to assist the physician and patient in future management. Multiple studies have evaluated the prognostic value of the exercise test, thallium-201, scintigraphy, two-dimensional echocardiography, radionuclide ventriculography, Holter monitoring, and cardiac catheterization.[127–131] Recently, Candell-Riera and colleagues[131] evaluated the prognostic role of combined cardiac studies in patients with a first MI. Of the 69 patients studied, 60% developed complications. Comparing four different possible decision models, the researchers concluded that the use of a test to evaluate residual ischemia and a test assessing ventricular function resulted in the greatest prognostic information. The addition of a cardiac catheterization did not improve the predictive power of the noninvasive tests. They did not evaluate stress echocardiography or Sestimibi-gated ventricular function and perfusion imaging. Both tests would provide information about ischemia and function in the same test, further simplifying the workup of the patient. In their study, a patient with an uncomplicated MI and a negative noninvasive evaluation had a 30% chance of a complication, and severe complications occurred in 12%.[131] Some would argue that this is not low enough and that a cardiac catheterization could provide more information than the noninvasive tests.[132] Although there is some logic to this argument, the cost and unproven benefit of catheterization has persuaded most physicians to recommend noninvasive testing instead of routine cardiac catheterization.

Patients without complications can be safely discharged from the hospital early. In a study by Topol et al.,[133] 80 patients with an uncomplicated acute MI and a negative exercise test were randomized to be discharged from the hospital either early (day 3) or conventionally (days 5 to 7). The early discharge group returned to work earlier and had a $5,000 saving in the hospital charges without a higher 30-day mortality or rehospitalization rate.

Long-Term Management

Long-term medical management is an extension of the in-hospital management, with continuation of therapy initiated in the hospital. Anticoagulation with coumadin is continued for at least 6 months, at which time the patient can be switched to aspirin. For the majority of patients, aspirin therapy should be continued indefinitely based on the results of the secondary prevention trials.[94] Other therapy is initiated or discontinued at the discretion of the physician and based on the patient's symptoms.

Noninvasive testing should include a full exercise test at 6 weeks to fully evaluate functional capacity and the presence of inducible ischemia. If ischemia is present, the patient should be considered for cardiac catheterization. A thallium exercise test may provide more prognostic information in this setting. In a study by Gibson, the degree of positivity on a thallium exercise test highly predicted long-term outcome and was better than an exercise test alone.[134]

Revascularization should be considered in any patient with recurrent angina that is poorly controlled by medical therapy. In patients with minimally positive exercise tests or in patients with mild angina, the need for revascularization is less certain. While patients with a recent MI are at higher risk for events early after their MI, the risks diminishes with time and is similar to that for patients without an MI after 6 months. The onset of angina early (within 6 weeks) after hospital discharge is a harbinger of future adverse cardiac events, and such patients should undergo catheterization. Beyond this time period, the management should be similar to that of other patients with coronary disease.

References

1. Ellis SG, Roubin GS, King SB III, et al: Angiographic and clinical predictors of acute closure after native vessel angioplasty. *Circulation* 1988; 77:372–379.
2. Meyerovitz MF, Friedman PL, Ganz P, et al: Acute occlusion developing during or immediately after percutaneous transluminal coronary angioplasty: Nonsurgical treatment. *Radiology* 1988; 169:491–494.
3. Sinclair JN, McGabe CH, Sipperly ME, et al: Predictors, therapeutic options and long-term outcome of abrupt reclosure. *Am J Cardiol* 1988; 61:61G–66G.
4. Steffenino G, Meier B, Finci L, et al: Acute complications of elective coronary angioplasty: A review of 500 consecutive procedures. *Br Heart J* 1988; 59:151–158.
5. Goldbaum T, DiSciascio G, Cowley MJ, et al: Early occlusion following successful coronary angioplasty: Clinical and angiographic observations. *Cathet Cardiovasc Diagn* 1989; 17:22–32.
6. Detre KM, Holmes DR, Holubkov R, et al: Incidence and consequences of periprocedural occlusion. The 1985–1986 National Heart, Lung, and Blood Institute Percutaneous Transluminal Coronary Angioplasty Registry. *Circulation* 1990; 82:739–750.
7. de Feyter PJ, van den Brand M, Laarman GJ, et al: Acute coronary artery occlusion during and after percutaneous transluminal coronary angioplasty: Frequency, prediction, clinical course, management and follow-up. *Circulation* 1991; 83:927–936.
8. Hollman J, Gruentzig AR, Douglas JS, et al: Acute occlusion after percutaneous transluminal coronary artery angioplasty: A new approach. *Circulation* 1983; 68:725–732.
9. Simpfendorfer C, Belardi J, Bellamy G, et al: Frequency, management and follow-up of patients with acute coronary occlusions after percutaneous transluminal coronary angioplasty. *Am J Cardiol* 1987; 59:267–269.
10. Gabliani G, Deligonul U, Kern MJ, et al: Acute coronary occlusion occurring after successful percutaneous transluminal coronary angioplasty. Temporal

relationship to discontinuation of anticoagulation. *Am Heart J* 1988; 116:696–700.

11. Gaul G, Hollman J, Simpfendorfer C, et al: Acute occlusion in multiple lesion coronary angioplasty: Frequency and management. *J Am Coll Cardiol* 1989; 13:283–288.
12. de Feyter PJ, de Jaegere PPT, Murphy ES, et al: Abrupt coronary artery occlusion during percutaneous transluminal coronary angioplasty. *Am Heart J* 1992; 123:1633–1642.
13. Bucz JJ, Scheerder I, Beatt K, et al: The importance of adequate anticoagulation to prevent early thrombosis after stenting of stenosed venous bypass grafts. *Am Heart J* 1991; 121:1389–1396.
14. Sanbron TA, Faxon DP, Haudenschild CC, et al: The mechanism of angioplasty: Evidence for aneurysm formulation in experimental atherosclerosis. *Circulation* 1983; 68:1136–1140.
15. Faxon DP, Sanbron TA, Haudenschild CC: Mechanism of angioplasty and its relation to restenosis. *Am J Cardiol* 1987; 60:5B–9B.
16. Wilentz JR, Sanbron TA, Haudenschild CC, et al: Platelet accumulation in experimental angiography: Time course and relation to vascular injury. *Circulation* 1987; 75:636–642.
17. Ip JH, Fuster V, Israel D, et al: The role of platelets, thrombin and hyperplasia in restenosis after coronary angioplasty. *J Am Coll Cardiol* 1991; 17:77B–88B.
18. Ellis SG, Roubin GS, King SB III, et al: In-hospital cardiac mortality after acute closure after coronary angioplasty: Analysis of risk factors from 8,207 procedures. *J Am Coll Cardiol* 1988; 11:211–216.
19. Kelsey SF, James M, Holubkov AL, et al: Results of percutaneous transluminal coronary angioplasty in women. *Circulation,* 1993; 87:1–8.
20. McEniery PT, Hollman J, Knezinek V, et al: Comparative safety and efficacy of percutaneous transluminal coronary angioplasty in men and in women. *Cathet Cardiovasc Diagn* 1987; 13:364–371.
21. Ischinger T, Gruentzig AR, Meier B, et al: Coronary dissection and total coronary occlusion associated with percutaneous transluminal coronary angioplasty: Significance of initial angiographic morphology of coronary stenoses. *Circulation* 1986; 74:1371–1378.
22. Leitschuh ML, Mills RM, Jacobs AK, et al: Outcome after major dissection during coronary angioplasty using the perfusion balloon catheter. *Am J Cardiol* 1991; 67:1056–1060.
23. Leitschun ML, Currier J: Management of the patient after angioplasty, in Faxon D (ed): *Practical Angioplasty.* New York, Raven Press, in press.
24. Bertrand ME, LaBlanche JM, Fourrier JL, et al: Percutaneous transluminal coronary angioplasty in patients with spasm superimposed on atherosclerotic narrowing. *Br Heart J* 1987; 58:469–472.
25. Fischell TA, Derby G, Tse TM, et al: Coronary artery vasoconstriction routinely occurs after percutaneous transluminal coronary angioplasty. *Circulation* 1988; 78:1323–1334.
26. Schatz R, Baim D, Leon M, et al: Clinical experience with the Palmaz-Schatz coronary stent. *Circulation* 1991; 83:147–162.
27. Erbel R, Swars H, Hafner L, et al: Reduction of subacute thrombotic stent occlusion by improved anticoagulation monitoring. *Circulation* 1991; 84:II-588.
28. Antiplatelet Trialists' Collaboration: Secondary prevention of vascular disease by prolonged antiplatelet treatment. *Br Med J* 1988; 296:320.

29. Leitschuh ML, Balady GJ, Jacobs AK, et al: Safety and utility of early exercise testing after PTCA: Results of a randomized trial. *J Am Coll Cardiol* 1991; 17:237A.
30. Breisblatt WM, Barnes JV, Weiland F, et al: Incomplete revascularization in multivessel percutaneous transluminal coronary angioplasty: The role for stress thallium-201 imaging. *J Am Coll Cardiol* 1988; 11:1183–1190.
31. Wohlgelernter D, Cleman M, Highman HA, et al: Percutaneous transluminal coronary angioplasty of the "culprit lesion" for management of unstable angina pectoris in patients with multivessel coronary artery disease. *Am J Cardiol* 1986; 58:460–464.
32. Deligonul U, Vandormael MG, Shah Y, et al: Prognostic value of early exercise stress testing after successful coronary angioplasty: Importance of the degree of revascularization. *Am Heart J* 1989; 117:509–514.
33. Califf RM, Ohman EM, Frid DJ, et al: Restenosis: The clinic issues, in Topol E (ed): *Textbook of Interventional Cardiology.* Philadelphia, WB Saunders, 1990, pp 199–223.
34. Fitzgerald ST, Becker DM, Celentano DD, et al: Return to work after percutaneous transluminal coronary angioplasty. *Am J Cardiol* 1989; 64:1108–1112.
35. Joelson JM, Becker DJ, Most A, et al: Initial presentation predicts clinical manifestation of restenosis after successful coronary angioplasty. *Circulation* 1988; 78:II–633.
36. De Feyter PJ. PTCA in patients with stable angina pectoris and multivessel disease: Is incomplete revascularization acceptable? *Clin Cardiol* 1992; 15:317–322.
37. Bourassa MG, Holubkov R, Yeh W, et al: A strategy of complete revascularization in patients with multivessel coronary artery disease. (A report from the 1985–1986 NHLBI PTCA Registry). *Am J Cardiol* 1992; 123: 173–178.
38. Faxon DP, Ghalilli K, Jacobs AK, et al: The degree of revascularization and outcome after multivessel coronary angioplasty. *Am J Cardiol* 1992; 123:853–859.
39. Glazier JJ, Varricchione TR, Ryan TJ, et al: Outcome in patients with recurrent restenosis after percutaneous transluminal balloon angioplasty. *Br Heart J* 199; 61:485–488.
40. Glazier JJ, Varricchione TR, Ryan TJ, et al: Factors predicting recurrent restenosis after percutaneous transluminal coronary balloon angioplasty. *Am J Cardiol* 1989; 63:902–905.
41. Faxon DP, Jacobs AK, Yeh W, et al: The relationship between repeat PTCA and time from initial procedure: A report from the NHLBI PTCA registry. *Circulation* 1992; 86:I-255.
42. Black AJR, Anderson HV, Roubin GS, et al: Repeat coronary angioplasty: Correlates of a second restenosis. *J Am Coll Cardiol* 1988; 11:714–718.
43. Forrester JS, Fishbein M, Helfant R, et al: A paradigm for restenosis based on cell biology: Clues for the development of new preventive therapies. *J Am Coll Cardiol* 1991; 17:758–769.
44. Honye J, Mahon DJ, Jain A, et al: Morphological effects of coronary balloon angioplasty in vivo assessed by intravascular ultrasound imaging. *Circulation* 1992; 85:1011–1025.
45. Franklin S, Faxon D. Pharmacologic prevention of restenosis after coronary angioplasty: Review of the randomized clinical trials coronary artery disease. *Coronary Artery Disease* 1993; 4:232–242.

46. Currier JW, Haudenschild CC, Faxon DP: Pathology of restenosis: Clinical implications, in Ischinger T, Gohlke H (eds): *Strategies in Primary and Secondary Prevention of Coronary Artery Disease.* Munich, W. Zuckschwerdt Verlag, 1992, pp 181–192.
47. Wolinsky H, Lin CS: Use of the perforated balloon catheter to infuse marker substances into diseased coronary artery walls after experimental postmortem angioplasty. *J Am Coll Cardiol* 1991; 17:174B–178B.
48. Currier JW, Litschuh ML: The management of patients following successful coronary angioplasty, in Faxon D (ed): *Practical Angioplasty.* New York, Raven Press, in press.
49. Berman JN, Hankin BR, Jacobs AK, et al: Silent restenosis (abstract). Presented at the XIV InterAmerican Congress of Cardiology, Orlando, Fla, May 1992.
50. Manyari DE, Knudtson M, Kloiber R, et al: Sequential thallium-201 myocardial perfusion studies after successful percutaneous transluminal coronary artery angioplasty: Delayed resolution of exercise-induced scintigraphic abnormalities. *Circulation* 1988; 77:86–95.
51. Gruentzig AR, King SB III, Schlumpf M, et al: Long-term follow-up after percutaneous transluminal coronary angioplasty. *N Engl J Med* 1987; 316:1127–1132.
52. Detre K, Holubkov R, Kelsey S, et al: One-year follow-up results of the 1985–1986 National Heart, Lung, and Blood Institute's Percutaneous Transluminal Coronary Angioplasty Registry. *Circulation* 1989; 80:421–428.
53. Talley JD, Hurst JW, King SP III, et al: Clinical outcome 5 years after attempted percutaneous transluminal coronary angioplasty in 427 patients. *Circulation* 1988; 77:820–829.
54. Finci L, Meier B, Favre J, et al: Long-term results of successful and failed angioplasty for chronic total coronary arterial occlusion. *Am J Cardiol* 1990; 66:653–662.
55. Webb JG, Myler RK, Shaw RE, et al: Bidirectional crossover and late outcome after coronary angioplasty and bypass surgery: 8 to 11 year follow-up. *J Am Coll Cardiol* 1990; 16:57–65.
56. Kent K, Cowley M, Detre K, et al: Report of one year outcome for 1977–81 and 1985–86. NHLBI PTCA registry. *Circulation* 1982; 86:I-55.
57. Vandormael M, Deligonul U, Taussig S, et al: Predictors of long-term cardiac survival in patients with multivessel coronary artery disease undergoing percutaneous transluminal coronary angioplasty. *Am J Cardiol* 1991; 67:1–6.
58. Mulcahy D, Keegan J, Phadke K, et al: Effects of coronary artery bypass surgery and angioplasty on the total ischemic burden: A study of exercise testing and ambulatory ST segment monitoring. *Am Heart J* 1992; 123:597–603.
59. Vacek JL, Rosamond TL, Stites HW, et al: Comparison of percutaneous transluminal coronary angioplasty versus coronary artery bypass grafting for multivessel coronary artery disease. *Am J Cardiol* 1992; 69:592.
60. Wong JB, Sonnenberg FA, Salem DN, et al: Myocardial revascularization for chronic stable angina. *Ann Intern Med* 1990; 113:852.
61. Kramer JR, Proudfit WL, Loop FD, et al: Late follow-up of 781 patients undergoing percutaneous transluminal coronary angioplasty or coronary artery bypass grafting for an isolated obstruction in the left anterior descending coronary artery. *Am Heart J* 1989; 118:1144.
62. Hartz AJ, Kuhn EM, Pryor DB, et al: Mortality after coronary angioplasty and coronary artery bypass surgery (The National Medicare Experience). *Am J Cardiol* 1992; 70:179–185.

63. Weintraub WS, Jones EL, King SB, et al: Changing use of coronary angioplasty and coronary bypass surgery in the treatment of chronic artery disease. *Am J Cardiol* 1990; 65:183–188.
64. Akins CW, Block PC, Palacios IF, et al: Comparison of coronary artery bypass grafting and percutaneous transluminal coronary angioplasty as initial treatment strategies. *Ann Thorac Surg* 1989; 4:507–516.
65. Mark DB, Nelson CL, Frank EH, et al: Improved survival benefits with coronary angioplasty and coronary bypass surgery: Assessment using a new coronary prognostic index. *Circulation* 1992; 86:I-536.
66. Lembo NJ, King SB III: Randomized trials of percutaneous transluminal coronary angioplasty, coronary artery bypass grafting surgery, or medical therapy in patients with coronary artery disease. *Coronary Artery Dis* 1990; 1:449–454.
67. Parisi AF, Folland ED, Hartigan P: A comparison of angioplasty with medical therapy in the treatment of single-vessel coronary artery disease. *N Engl J Med* 1992; 326:10–16.
68. Topol EJ: Thrombolytic intervention, in Topol E (ed): *Textbook of Interventional Cardiology.* Philadelphia, WB Saunders, 1990, pp 76–120.
69. Muller DWM, Topol EJ: Selection of Patients with Acute Myocardial Infarction for Thrombolytic Therapy. Ann Intern Med 1990; 113:949–960.
70. Grives C, Browne K, Vandermael M, et al: Primary angioplasty in myocardial infarction (PAMI) trial. *Circulation* 1992; 86:I-641.
71. Richardson SG, Allen DC, Morton P, et al: Pathological changes after intravenous streptokinase treatment in eight patients with acute myocardial infarction. *Br Heart J* 1989; 61:390–395.
72. Jang Ik, Gold HK, Ziskind AA, et al: Differential sensitivity of erythrocyte-rich and platelet-rich arterial thrombi to lysis with recombinant tissue-type plasminogen activator. A possible explanation for resistance to coronary thrombolysis. *Circulation* 1989; 79:920–928.
73. Ellis SG, Van de Wert F, Riberio-DaSalva E, et al: Present status of rescue coronary angioplasty: current polarization of opinion and randomized trials. *J Am Coll Cardiol* 1992; 19:681–686.
74. ISIS-2 Collaborative Group: Randomized trial of intravenous streptokinase, oral aspirin, both, or neither among 17,187 cases of suspected acute myocardial infarction: ISIS-2. *Lancet* 1988; 349–360.
75. Trip MD, Cats Manger V, van Capelle FJL, et al: Platelet hyperreactivity and prognosis in survivors of myocardial infarction. *New Engl J Med* 1990; 322:1549–1554.
76. Popma JJ, Topol EJ: Adjuncts to thrombolysis for myocardial reperfusion. *Ann Intern Med* 1991; 115:34–44.
77. Gold HK, Coller BS, Yasuda T, et al: Rapid and sustained coronary artery recanalization with combined bolus injection of recombinant tissue-type plasminogen activator and monoclonal antiplatelet GPIIb/IIIa antibody in a canine preparation. *Circulation* 1988; 77:670–677.
78. ISIS-3 Collaborative Group: ISIS-3: A randomized comparison of streptokinase vs tissue plasminogen activator vs anistreplase and of aspirin alone among 41,299 cases of suspected acute myocardial infarction. *Lancet* 1992; 339:1–18.
79. International Study Group: In-hospital mortality and clinical course of 20,891 patients with suspected acute myocardial infarction randomized between alteplase and streptokinase with or without heparin. *Lancet* 1990; 336:71–75.

80. Hsia J, Hamilton WP, Kleiman N, et al: A comparison between heparin and low-dose aspirin as adjunctive therapy with tissue plasminogen activator for acute myocardial infarction. *New Engl J Med* 1990; 323:1433–1437.
81. Topol EJ, George BS, Kereiakes DJ, et al: A randomized controlled trial of intravenous tissue plasminogen activator and early intravenous heparin in acute myocardial infarction. *Circulation* 1989; 79:281–286.
82. Bleich SD, Nichols T, Schumacher R, et al: The role of heparin following coronary thrombolysis with tissue plasminogen activator (t-PA) (abstr). *Circulation* 1989; 80:II-113.
83. SCATI (Studio sulla Calciparina nell' Angina e nella Thrombosi Ventriculare nell' Infarto) Group. Randomized controlled trial of subcutaneous calcium-heparin in acute myocardial infarction. *Lancet* 1989; 2:182–186.
84. Prins MH, Hirsch J: Heparin as an adjunctive treatment after thrombolytic therapy for acute myocardial infarction. *Am J Cardiol* 1991; 67: 3A–11A.
85. Dmiyh P, Arnesen H, Holme I: The effect of warfarin on mortality and reinfarction after myocardial infarction. *New Engl J Med* 1990; 323:147.
86. Heras M, Chesebro JH, Penny WJ, et al: Effects of thrombin inhibition on the development of acute platelet-thrombus deposition during angioplasty in pigs. Heparin versus recombinant hirudin, a specific thrombin inhibitor. *Circulation* 1989; 79:657–665.
87. Jang IK, Gold HK, Ziskind AA, et al: Prevention of platelet-rich arterial thrombosis by selective thrombin inhibitor. *Circulation* 1990; 81:219–225.
88. Forman MB, Virmani R: Pathogenesis and modification of myocardial reperfusion injury, in *Current Topics in Cardiology*. Amsterdam, Elsevier Science Publishing, 1991, pp 349–370.
89. Pfeffer JM, Pfeffer MA, Fletcher PJ, et al: Progressive ventricular remodeling in rat with myocardial infarction. *Am J Physiol* 1991; 260:H1406–H1414.
90. Eaton LW, Weiss JL, Bulkley BH, et al: Regional cardiac dilatation after acute myocardial infarction: recognition by two-dimensional echocardiography. *N Engl J Med* 1979; 300:57–62.
91. McKay RG, Pfeffer MA,Pasternak RC, et al: Left ventricular remodeling after myocardial infarction: a corollary to infarct expansion. *Circulation* 1986; 74:693–702.
92. Gaudron P, Eilles C, Ertl G, et al: Early remodeling of the left ventricle in patients with myocardial infarction. *Eur Heart J* 1990; 11(suppl B):139–146.
93. Pfeffer MA, Braunwald E: Ventricular remodeling after myocardial infarction: experimental observations and clinical implications. *Circulation* 1990; 81:1161–1172.
94. Yusuf S, Sleight P, Held P, et al: Routine medical management of acute myocardial infarction: Lessons from overviews of recent randomized controlled trials. *Circulation* 1990; 82(suppl II):II-117–II-134.
95. Becker RC, Gore JM: Adjunctive use of beta-adrenergic blockers, calcium antagonists and other therapies in coronary thrombolysis. *Am J Cardiol* 1991; 67:25A–31A.
96. Glamann DB, Lange RA, Hillis LD: Beneficial effect of long-term beta blockade after acute myocardial infarction in patients without anterograde flow in the infarct artery. *Am J Cardiol* 1991; 68:150–154.
97. Ellis SG, Muller DW, Topol EJ: Possible survival benefit from concomitant beta—but not calcium—antagonist therapy during reperfusion for acute myocardial infarction. *Am J Cardiol* 1990; 66:125–128.

98. Sleight P: Beta blockade early in acute myocardial infarction. *Am J Cardiol* 1987; 60:6A–10A.
99. Pitt B: The role of beta-adrenergic blocking agents in preventing sudden cardiac death. *Circulation* 1992; 85(suppl I):I107–I111.
100. Popma JJ, Topol EJ: Adjuncts to thrombolysis for myocardial reperfusion. *Ann Intern Med* 1991; 115:34–44.
101. TIMI Study Group: Comparison of invasive and conservative strategies after treatment with intravenous tissue plasminogen activator in acute myocardial infarction. *New Engl J Med* 1989; 320:618–627.
102. Sirnes PA, Overskeid K, Pedersen TR, et al: Evolution of infarct size during the early use of nifedipine in patients with acute myocardial infarction: The Norwegian Nifedipine Multicenter Trial. *Circulation* 1984; 70:638–644.
103. Muller JE, Morrison J, Stone PH, et al: Nifedipine therapy for patients with threatened and acute myocardial infarction: A randomized, double-blind, placebo-controlled comparison. *Circulation* 1984; 69:740–747.
104. Branagan JP, Walsh K, Kelly P, et al: Effect of early treatment with nifedipine in suspected acute myocardial infarction. *Eur Heart J* 1986; 7:859–865.
105. Danish Study Group on Verapamil in Myocardial Infarction: Verapamil in acute myocardial infarction. *Eur Heart J* 1984; 5:516–528.
106. Gibson RS, Boden WE, Theroux P, et al: Diltiazem and reinfarction in patients with non-Q-wave myocardial infarction. Results of a double-blind, randomized, multicenter trial. *N Engl J Med* 1986; 315:423–429.
107. Erbel R, Pop T, Meinertz T, et al: Combination of calcium channel blocker and thrombolytic therapy in acute myocardial infarction. *Am Heart J* 1988; 115:529–538.
108. Multicenter Diltiazem Postinfarction Trial Research Group: The effect of diltiazem on mortality and reinfarction after myocardial infarction. *N Engl J Med* 1988; 319:385–392.
109. Pfeffer MA, Pfeffer JM, Steinberg C, et al: Survival after an experimental myocardial infarction: Beneficial effects of long-term therapy with captopril. *Circulation* 1985; 72:406–412.
110. Halperin JL, Creager MA, Faxon DP, et al: Coronary hemodynamic effects of angiotensin-converting enzyme inhibitor in congestive heart failure. *Am J Cardiol* 1982; 50:967–972.
111. Powell JS, Clozel J-P, Muller RKM, et al: Inhibitors of angiotensin-converting enzyme prevent myointimal proliferation after vascular injury. *Science* 1989; 245:186–188.
112. Pfeffer MA, Braunwald E, Moye LA, et al: Effect of Captopril in mortality and morbidity in patients with left ventricular dysfunction after myocardial infarction—results of the survival and ventricular enlargement trial. *New Engl J Med* 1992; 327:669–676.
113. SOLVD Investigators: Effect of enalapril on survival in patients with reduced left ventricular ejection fractions and congestive heart failure. *New Engl J Med* 1991; 325:293–302.
114. Swedberg K, Held P, Kjekshus J, et al: The effects of the early administration of enalapril on mortality in patients with acute myocardial infarction. *New Engl J Med* 1992; 327:678–684.
115. Ellis SG, DeBowey D, Bates ER, et al: Treatment of recurrent ischemia after thrombolysis and successful reperfusion for acute myocardial infarction: Effect on in-hospital mortality and left ventricular function. *J Am Coll Cardiol* 1991; 17:752–757.

116. Williams DO, Braunwald E, Knatterud G, et al: One-year results of the thrombolysis in myocardial infarction investigation (TIMI) Phase II trial. *Circulation* 1992; 85:533–542.
117. Mehra R, Zeiler RH, Gough WB, et al: Reentrant ventricular arrhythmias in the later myocardial infarction period. Electrophysiologic-anatomic correlation of reentrant circuits. *Circulation* 1983; 67:11.
118. May GS, Furberg CD, Eberlein KA, et al: Secondary prevention after myocardial infarction: A review of short-term acute phase trials. *Prog Cardiovasc Dis* 1983; 25:335.
119. May GS, Eberlein KA, Furberg CD, et al: Secondary prevention after myocardial infarction: A review of long-term trials. *Proc Cardiovasc Dis* 1982; 25:331.
120. Gottleib SH, Achuff SC, Mellits ED, et al: Prophylactic antiarrhythmic therapy of high risk survivors of myocardial infarction: Lower mortality at 1 month but not a 1 year. *Circulation* 1987; 75:792.
121. Cardiac Arrhythmia Suppression Trial (CAST) Investigators: Preliminary report: Effect of encainide and flecainide on mortality in a randomized trial of arrhythmia suppression after myocardial infarction. *N Engl J Med* 1989; 321:386.
122. Rasmussen HS, Gronbaek M, Cintin C, et al: One-year death rate in 270 patients with suspected acute myocardial infarction, initially treated with intravenous magnesium or placebo. *Clin Cardiol* 1988; 11:377.
123. Ryan TJ, Bailey KR, McCabe CH, et al: The effects of digitalis on survival in high-risk patients with coronary artery disease. *Circulation* 1983; 67:735.
124. Madsen EB, Gilpin E, Henning H, et al: Prognostic importance of digitalis after acute myocardial infarction. *J Am Coll Cardiol* 1984; 3:681.
125. Byington R, Golstein S, BHAT Research Group: Association of digitalis therapy with mortality in survivors of acute myocardial infarction: Observations in the beta-blocker heart attack trial. *J Am Coll Cardiol* 1985; 6:976.
126. Muller JE, Turi ZG, Stone PH, et al: Digoxin therapy and mortality after myocardial infarction. Experience in the MILIS Study. *N Engl J Med* 1986; 314:265.
127. Sutton JM, Topol EJ. Significance of a negative exercise thallium test in the presence of a critical residual stenosis after thrombolysis for acute myocardial infarction. *Circulation* 1991; 83:1278–1286.
128. Abraham RD, Freedman SB, Dunn RF, et al: Prediction of multivessel coronary artery disease and prognosis early after acute myocardial infarction by exercise electrocardiography and thallium-201 myocardial perfusion scintigraphy. *Am J Cardiol* 1986; 58:423–427.
129. Lavie CJ, Gibbons RJ, Zinsmeister AR, et al: Interpreting results of exercise studies after acute myocardial infarction altered by thrombolytic therapy, coronary angioplasty or bypass. *Am J Cardiol* 1991; 67:116–120.
130. Kulick DL, Rahimtoola SH: Risk stratification in survivors of acute myocardial infarction. Routine cardiac catheterization and angiography is a reasonable approach in most patients. *Am Heart J* 1991; 121:641–656.
131. Candell-Riera J, Permanyer-Miralda G, Castell J, et al: Uncomplicated first myocardial infarction: Strategy for comprehensive prognostic studies. *J Am Coll Cardiol* 1991; 18:1207–1219.
132. Butman SM: What would I want to know if my dad had a heart attack? Good sense versus dollars and cents. *J Am Coll Cardiol* 1991; 18:1220–1222.

133. Topol EJ, Burek K, O'Neill WW, et al: A randomized controlled trial of hospital discharge three days after myocardial infarction in the era of reperfusion. *New Engl J Med* 1988; 318:1083–1088.
134. Gibson RS, Watson DD, Craddock GB, et al: Prediction of cardiac events after uncomplicated myocardial infarction: A prospective study comparing predischarge exercise thallium-201 scintigraphy and coronary angiography. *Circulation* 1983; 68:321–336.

Coronary Artery Disease in Women: Diagnosis and Prevention

Peter Oettgen, M.D.

Charles A. Dana Research Institute, Harvard-Thorndike Laboratory of the Department of Medicine (Cardiovascular Division), Instructor of Medicine, Harvard Medical School, Codirector, Cardiovascular Health and Lipid Center, Beth Israel Hospital, Boston, Massachusetts

Pamela S. Douglas, M.D.

Charles A. Dana Research Institute, Harvard-Thorndike Laboratory of the Department of Medicine (Cardiovascular Division), Associate Professor of Medicine, Harvard Medical School, Director, Noninvasive Cardiology, Beth Israel Hospital, Boston, Massachusetts

The focus of this chapter is the diagnosis and treatment of heart disease in women. Because a review of all heart disease in women is beyond the scope of this chapter, we will discuss the major cause of heart disease in women, namely, coronary artery disease. Other forms of heart disease in women, including valvular heart disease and heart disease during pregnancy, are reviewed elsewhere.[1] We will begin by reviewing the epidemiology of coronary artery disease among women, followed by a discussion of the difficulties encountered in diagnosing the disease, including apparent gender differences in evaluation and treatment of the disease. Finally, the approach to medical management will emphasize the risk reduction afforded by aggressive treatment of modifiable contributing factors such as hypertension, smoking, obesity, hyperlipidemia, and menopause.

Epidemiology

Coronary artery disease (CAD) remains the leading cause of mortality among women, accounting for approximately 28% of deaths.[2] Despite a decreased trend in the total mortality from coronary artery disease for both men and women, the overall incidence of coronary heart disease (CHD) has been increasing among women.[3] In the Framingham Heart Study, the overall incidence of CHD morbidity and mortality among women is about one half that of men. The rate of CAD in women only begins to approximate that of men in old age (Fig 1).[4] Furthermore, when the incidences of

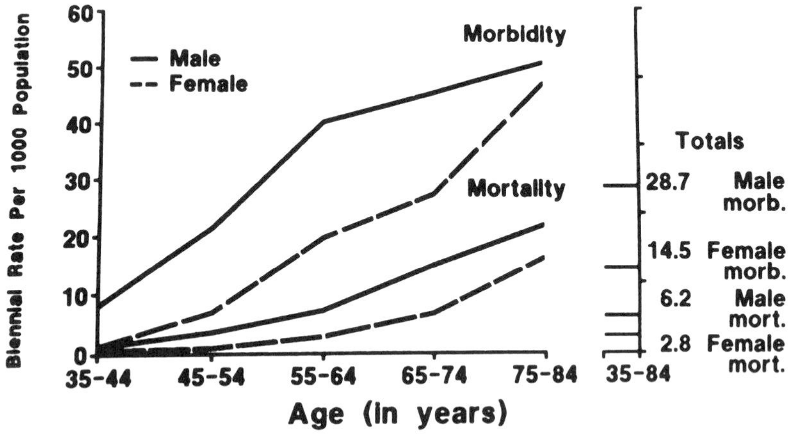

FIG 1.
Incidence of coronary heart disease morbidity and mortality by age and sex: 26-year follow-up, Framingham study. (From Lerner DJ, Kannel WB: *Amer Heart J* 1986; 111:383–390. Used by permission.)

CHD for men and women are grouped according to age, there is a striking fortyfold difference between the oldest age group and the youngest age group for women, whereas there is only a sixfold difference across these age groups for men. This is illustrated further by the marked disparity in the incidence of CHD occurring in men and women for the younger age groups. During the middle-age years this gap progressively diminishes. The difference in CHD mortality rate among women lags behind that for men by about 10 years. However, once women manifest the disease, there no longer appears to be a survival advantage over men. In fact, the case-fatality rate for women with CHD in the youngest age group (35–44 years) was 50%, compared to only 16% among men (Table 1).[4]

The clinical presentation of CHD differed significantly between men and women in the Framingham Heart Study. The incidences in this population for the most frequent presenting symptoms of CAD for men were myocardial infarction (14.1/1000), followed by angina (12.3/1000), and, least often, sudden death (3.1/1000). In contrast, women were twice as likely to present with angina than with a myocardial infarction and rarely with sudden death (8.3, 4.4, and 1.1/1000, respectively).[4] The higher prevalence of angina as the presenting symptom of CAD in women places a greater burden on diagnostic strategies than does the more easily recognized myocardial infarction in men.

The risk factors for the development of CHD among women are largely but not entirely the same as they are for men. The relative increased risk from the presence of hypertension, hyperlipidemia, obesity, and cigarette smoking all appear to be similar for men and women (Table 2). Glucose intolerance is a highly significant risk factor for women, but not for men. Finally, levels of high-density lipoprotein were inversely correlated with the

TABLE 1.
Sex- and Age-specific CHD Case Fatality Rates in Subjects Ages 35 to 84 Years: 26-year Follow-up, Framingham Study*†

	% Fatal	
Age (yr)	**Men**	**Women**
35–44	0.16	0.50
45–54	0.21	0.26
55–64	0.26	0.27
65–74	0.35	0.34
75–84	0.38	0.46
35–84	0.27	0.32

*From Lerner DJ, Kannel WB: Patterns of coronary heart disease morbidity and mortality in the sexes: A 26-year follow-up of the Framingham population. *Am Heart J* 1986; 111:383–390. Used by permission.

†Based on biennial rates/1000 population; case fatality rates reflect SD + non-SD ÷ MI + CI + SD + non-SD. (SD = sudden death; MI = myocardial infarction; CI = coronary insufficiency.)

incidence of CHD in women and are more strongly related than total serum cholesterol value. However, after controlling for these risk factors, men still appear to have a 2.5-fold greater risk of developing CHD than do women.[2]

Much of the increased incidence of CHD in women occurs after age 54. In women 55 years of age and older, there is a tenfold increase in CHD. The comparable increased risk for men over the same age span is only 4.6. This change in risk is thought to be largely related to the onset of menopause which occurs at an average age of 51.4 years. Interestingly, the incidence of CHD, excluding angina, was approximately fourfold greater for women who had undergone natural or surgical menopause compared to premenopausal women (Table 3).[2] Concomitant with this increased incidence of CHD is a marked increase in the total serum cholesterol values in women between the ages of 45 and 55 years (Fig 2).

Diagnosis

Unfortunately, the routinely available noninvasive tests used to screen for the presence of coronary artery disease have been relatively insensitive

TABLE 2.
Framingham Study: Ten-year Incidence of CHD Excluding Angina Pectoris Among Men and Women Aged 50 to 59 Years. Multiple Logistic Regression Analysis*

	Women†			Men‡		
Variable	**Coefficient**	**RR§**	***P*-Value**	**Coefficient**	**RR§**	***P*-Value**
Systolic blood pressure	0.01	1.24	<0.01	0.02	1.46	<0.001
Relative weight	0.01		n.s. ¶	0.00		n.s.
Serum cholesterol	0.01	1.28	<0.05	0.01	1.34	<0.001
Cigarette smoking	0.62	1.85	<0.01	0.59	1.80	<0.001
Glucose intolerance	1.15	3.17	<0.001	0.25		n.s.

*From Eaker ED, Packard B, Thom TJ: Epidemiology and risk factors for coronary heart disease in women, in Douglas PS (ed): *Heart Disease in Women*. Philadelphia, FA Davis Co., 1989. Used by permission.
†2017 women, 79 cases.
‡1545 men, 188 cases.
§Relative risks for the differences: systolic blood pressure: 20 mmHg; metropolitan relative weight: 20%; serum cholesterol: 50 mg/100 ml; cigarette smoking: smokers vs. nonsmokers; glucose intolerance: yes vs. no.
¶n.s. = not significant.

TABLE 3.
Ten-year Incidence of CHD (Excluding Angina Pectoris) Among Women Ages 50 to 59 years: Framingham Heart Study*

	All Women Menopausal Status		Postmenopausal Cause of Cessation		Surgical Menopause No. of Ovaries Removed		
	Before	**After**	**Natural**	**Surgical**	**0**	**1**	**2**
Incidence of CHD, %	1.0	4.3	4.1	4.5	4.7	6.0	4.5
(N)	(208)	(2335)	(1609)	(700)	(127)	(100)	(357)

*From Lerner DJ, Kannel WB: *Amer Heart J* 1986; 111:383–390. Used by permission.

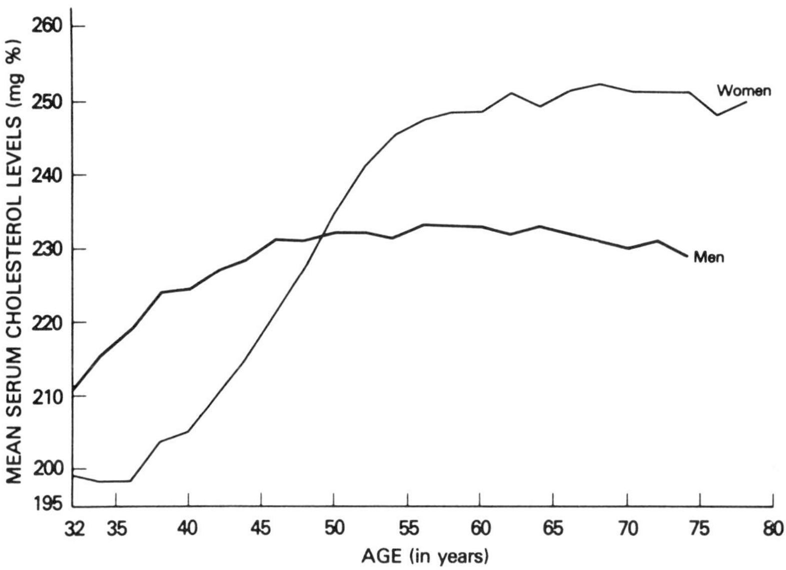

FIG 2.
Trends in serum cholesterol according to age for cohort data: Framingham Heart Study. (From Eaker ED, Packard B, Thom TJ, in Douglas PS (ed): *Heart Disease in Women*. Philadelphia, FA Davis Company, 1989. Used by permission.)

and nonspecific for women. The history alone may be particularly helpful in determining the likelihood of actual disease. In patients with chest pain syndromes without known CAD, women with "definite" or typical angina had a 70% incidence of angiographically documented CAD as compared to only 2% to 7% of those with atypical chest pain (Table 4). Those with probable angina had a 30% to 40% likelihood of angiographic CAD.[5]

The exercise ECG is particularly poor at detecting or excluding CAD in asymptomatic women, as ECG abnormalities are not associated with an increased incidence of CAD. Instead, there is a greater incidence of CAD among women with poor exercise tolerance.[6] Furthermore, in women with atypical chest pain who had positive stress ECGs, only 4.6% developed clinical CAD as compared to 18.3% for men after 3 to 7 years of follow-up.[7] These studies have been criticized because of a very low overall disease prevalence in women compared with men. However, even if one compares men and women with similar disease prevalences, the positive predictive value of a positive stress test for clinical events remains significantly greater for men than for women (77% vs. 47%).[8]

In patients with angina pectoris or a history of a prior myocardial infarction, the sensitivity of stress ECG is 98% for men compared with 75% for women.[9] Interestingly, when ECG criteria other than ST-segment depression are used to define a positive test for women, the diagnostic accuracy may improve. In one study the R-wave response to exercise was exam-

TABLE 4.
Prevalence of Coronary Artery Disease Among Women With Chest Pain and No Previous Myocardial Infarction*

		Prevalence, %			
Study	**Number of Women**	**Total**	**Definite Angina**	**Probable Angina**	**Nonspecific Chest Pain**
Chaitman et al.	2810	26	72	36	6
Weiner et al.	580	29	62	40	5
Guiteras Val et al.	112	37	75	36	2
Hung et al.	92	30	60	30	7

*From Chaitman BR, Bourassa MG, Lam J, et al: in Eaker ED, Packard B, Wenger N, et al (eds): *Coronary Heart Disease in Women*, New York, Haymarket Doymas Inc, 1987. Used by permission.

ined. The negative and positive predictive accuracies for a change in R-wave height were 94% and 100% respectively in women.[10] However, most studies investigating the diagnostic utility of exercise stress testing demonstrate a significantly lower accuracy for women than for men, and alternative diagnostic criteria are not widely applied.

One explanation for the differences is an overall lower disease prevalence among women. However, as mentioned earlier, when disease prevalence is corrected for, significant differences remain. Women may also have a greater prevalence of noncoronary causes of chest pain such as mitral valve prolapse and angina due to coronary vasospasm leading to false-positive diagnoses of CAD by stress testing.[11, 12] Possible physiological reasons include a blunted catecholamine response to exercise among women with disease as compared to an exaggerated or increased catecholamine response to exercise in the absence of disease. This may result in vasoconstriction and false-positive tests in the absence of disease and an overall decrease in positive tests among patients with disease.[13]

Other causes of false-positive tests include an abnormal resting electrocardiogram, low disease prevalence, and ECG changes related to standing or increased respiration. The hormonal status of women also influences the predictive value of exercise testing. Postmenopausal women not on estrogen replacement therapy (ERT) and males had similar positive predictive values, as compared to premenopausal or postmenopausal women supplemented with estrogens (76% vs. 17%; $P < 0.0001$).[14] Finally, endogenous estrogens have chemical similarity to digitalis which could in part explain false-positive, ST-segment depressions.[15] Reasons for more false negatives include the fact that women who are tested are generally elderly and more sedentary, thereby less likely to achieve an adequate exercise workload.

When exercise ECG is combined with thallium scintigraphy, the sensitivity in women increases to 75% to 85%, and the specificity increases to 85% to 95%.[16] One study suggests that single photon emission computed tomography (SPECT), a newer thallium-imaging modality, may be diagnostically worse than planar imaging for women.[17] The major limitation of thallium scans in women has been attenuation of the signal over the anterior wall of the heart secondary to breast shadowing, resulting in decreased accuracy.

One particularly promising new noninvasive test for women is exercise echocardiography. One recent study reported a sensitivity and specificity of 86%.[18] The advantages of this relatively inexpensive procedure include the avoidance of contrast agents, the simultaneous display of multiple images allowing easy detection of regional wall motion abnormalities, and its sensitivity to single vessel disease. Furthermore, breast attenuation does not appear to be a limiting factor. One of the major limitations of this procedure has been the difficulty to obtain sonographic images during or shortly after patients exercise. Considerable success has been achieved by using pharmacological means of simulating exercise such as dobutamine, in combination with echocardiography, making sonographic images much easier to obtain at peak stress. Furthermore, this procedure can also be used for men and women who cannot exercise, as is also the case with the persantine or adenosine thallium stress tests.[19]

Gender Bias

Over the past few years several studies have suggested that women with suspected coronary artery disease are referred less frequently for coronary angiography and coronary bypass surgery than are men. One of the earliest studies examining this issue was performed by Tobin et al. who compared the rates of referral of men and women with abnormal nuclear exercise tests for cardiac catheterization. The rates of referral among men and women were 40.2% and 4.2%, respectively. After controlling for age, prior myocardial infarction, abnormal test results, and degree of angina, male patients were 6.5 times more likely to be referred for catheterization than were female patients. Symptoms of ischemic heart disease were attributed to somatic or psychiatric causes in 27.5% of women as compared to only 12% of men.[20] This seems paradoxical in light of the fact that the noninvasive tests are less accurate in women and that the need for a "gold standard" such as angiography would be more desirable in women to define the presence or absence of disease. Perhaps the more likely explanation is that the clinician, when faced with abnormal results from tests which are generally less accurate for women and who generally have a lower disease prevalence, has a higher threshold for subjecting the patient to an invasive procedure with potential risks. However, one would also expect this process to limit referral to stress testing.

A more recent study performed by Ayanian et al. further supports the hypothesis that invasive diagnostic and therapeutic procedures are underutilized in women as compared to men. Over 80,000 men and women who were hospitalized for coronary heart disease in Massachusetts and Maryland were evaluated for referral for coronary angiography or revascularization. After correction for age, myocardial infarction, presence of diabetes, type of angina, and race, men were almost twice as likely to be referred for coronary angiography or a revascularization procedure.[21] In contrast, a smaller study performed by Krumholz et al. suggested that the referral for coronary angiography was similar for both men and women who were hospitalized with the principal diagnosis of a myocardial infarction, after correction for age.[22] This, however, might suggest that once the diagnostic dilemma is eliminated by clinical evidence of CAD such as a myocardial infarction for women, the use of invasive tests to further define the coronary anatomy equals that in men.

Further support for the underutilization of coronary arteriography in women comes from a retrospective analysis of patients enrolled in the Survival and Ventricular Enlargement Study (SAVE), in which patients with acute myocardial infarction and left ventricular dysfunction were randomly treated with an angiotensin-converting enzyme inhibitor. Men and women were compared as to their degree of functional disability as a result of angina, prior to their index infarction. Despite greater functional disability and equal rates of angina, women were much less likely to have been referred for cardiac catheterization than men; 15.4% vs. 27.3%, respectively ($P < 0.001$). This strongly suggests that clinicians may minimize anginal symptoms in women and are reluctant to proceed with more definitive diagnostic studies, despite an overall greater functional severity of symptoms.[23]

Similar trends with regard to revascularization are suggested by the study of Ayanian et al. in which men were more frequently referred for revascularization than were women by approximately 35%.[21] However, in the study by Krumholz et al., after correction for age and disease severity, men were no more likely to be referred for angioplasty than were women, and the difference in referral rates for coronary bypass surgery was of borderline significance.[22] The referral rates for revascularization were also similar in a Duke study, once coronary angiography had been performed.[24]

Perhaps the most striking example of gender bias is demonstrated in a study by Maynard et al. in which men and women with acute myocardial infarction were evaluated for eligibility for thrombolytic therapy. Although fewer women than men met the criteria for eligibility (16% vs. 25%), only 55% of eligible women vs. 72% of eligible men received thrombolytic treatment. The rates of patient refusal to receive thrombolytic therapy were similar for men and women.[25]

In conclusion, it appears that there is significant evidence for gender bias in the diagnosis and treatment of coronary artery disease in women. Until better noninvasive tests are routinely available for the diagnosis of coronary artery disease, clinicians may need to have a lower threshold for considering invasive diagnostic testing in women with possible coronary artery disease, particularly those with a history of typical angina.

Risk Factor Modification

Because women generally develop coronary artery disease at a later age than men, and because the "window of opportunity" during which the clinician can intervene to minimize the chance of a woman developing clinically evident CAD is wider, primary prevention by risk factor modification should be a major goal in the medical approach to heart disease in women. Many of the risk factors for the development of coronary artery disease apply to both men and women. Hypertension is such a risk factor. In 1988, approximately 16.6 million women were defined as having hypertension.[26] Because women come into contact with the health care system more frequently than do men, the chance for detection and treatment is greater for women than it is for men.[27] Furthermore, hypertension appears to be more easily controlled in women than in men, although most studies demonstrate treatment benefits among black, but not white women.[28] Among women who presented with symptoms of acute myocardial infarction or were candidates for bypass surgery, 50% to 60% were hypertensive.[23, 29, 30] The attributable risk for development of CHD is approximately 40%.[31]

Cigarette smoking is another risk factor common to both men and women. The increased risk of cigarette smoking and nonfatal myocardial infarction is well established. Furthermore, among women, the relative risk appears to be greatest for young women without other risk factors, especially those who take oral contraceptives.[27] Approximately 60% to 70% of myocardial infarctions in women below the age of 50 can be attributed to cigarette smoking. This may in part be related to a marked increase in susceptibility to coronary vasospasm.[32] Upon cessation of smoking, the relative risk of women developing CHD dissipates to that of nonsmokers within 2 to 3 years.[33] Unfortunately, despite national efforts directed toward promoting smoking cessation, the percentage of women smoking has only decreased by 6% over the last 20 years, compared to 19% for men over the same time period with no change in the percent of women smokers between 1965 and 1977 (Fig 3). Because such a large percentage of myocardial infarctions among women can be attributed to cigarette smoking, more progress needs to be made in educating women about the risk of smoking, and promoting the need for cessation.[26]

The presence of diabetes mellitus increases the relative risk of developing CHD for women by about threefold, thereby eliminating any advantage over men of the same age. However, the concurrent presence of other risk factors such as hypertension, hypercholesterolemia, and cigarette smoking may even more markedly affect the overall cardiovascular risk

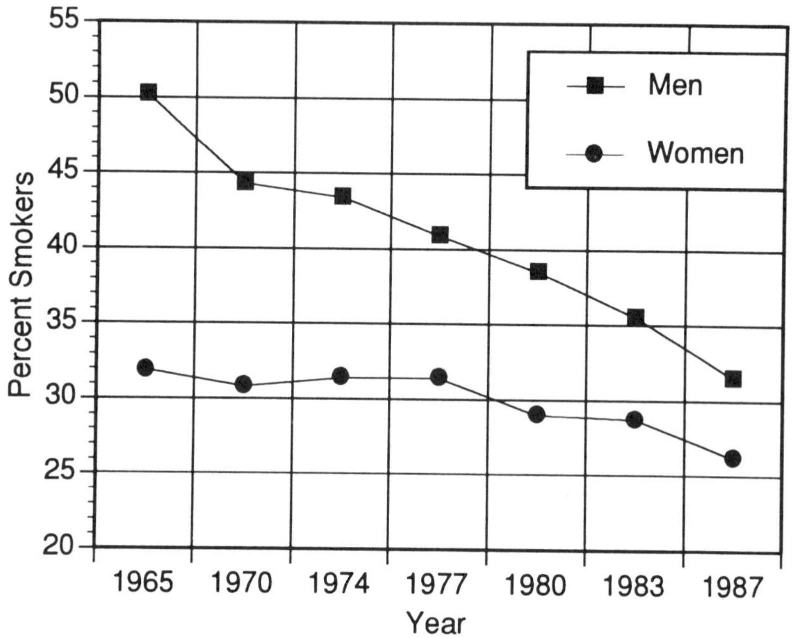

FIG 3.
Percentage of men and women smokers in the United States from 1965–1987. (Adapted from U.S. Bureau of the Census: Statistical Abstract of the United States, 1991.)

(Fig 4). Control of these risk factors may substantially improve the overall prognosis of diabetic patients.[34] A recent prospective study of middle-aged women in the United States with adult onset diabetes suggested that the increased relative risks of CHD and total cardiovascular mortality were 6.7 and 6.3, respectively. Although an independent effect of diabetes persisted, after correction for other risk factors, the relative risks of developing CHD with diabetes alone dropped to less than half of that with diabetes mellitus in the presence of other risk factors.[35] This study suggests that risk factor modification may considerably improve, but not eliminate, the increased risk of CHD in women with diabetes mellitus.

Data from the Framingham Heart Study have firmly established the relationship between lipid abnormalities and the risk for coronary heart disease for both men and women. Total serum cholesterol is a significant risk factor for women of all ages. There is a marked increase in mean total serum cholesterol values after menopause (Fig 2). In addition, high-density lipoprotein (HDL) levels tend to be approximately 10 mg/dl higher in women less than 50 years old than in similarly aged men, but gradually decrease after menopause. Because of the generally higher HDL levels in women than in men, it has been suggested that a better overall means of comparing CHD risk in women to men is to use the ratio of total serum

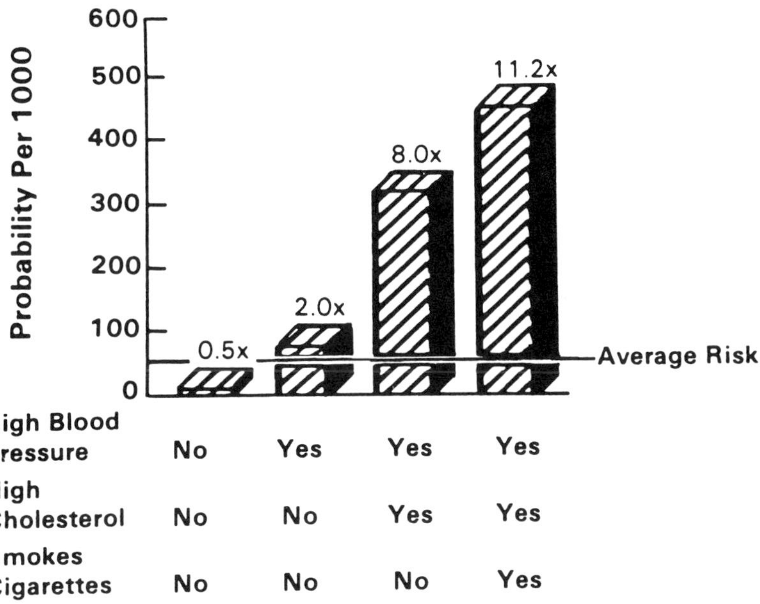

FIG 4.
Relative risk of cardiovascular disease among persons with glucose intolerance and other risk factors. (From Kannel WB: *Amer Heart J* 1987; 114:413–419. Used by permission.)

cholesterol to HDL cholesterol. At normal to moderately elevated ratios (up to 7.4), the relative risk of CHD for women is approximately half that of men. However, at ratios greater than or equal to 7.5, the age adjusted incidence of CHD was the same for men and women.[34] In comparison to men, women with CHD generally have higher serum cholesterol levels.[31] At least one angiographic study in women has suggested that the total cholesterol to HDL ratio is a better predictor of the presence, severity, and extent of CHD than the total cholesterol, HDL, or triglycerides alone.[36]

Multivariate analysis has demonstrated that the risk reduction conferred by an increase in HDL level is twice that of a corresponding reduction in total cholesterol in men and women.[37] Because postmenopausal women continue to have HDL levels which are 10 mg/dl higher than men (Fig 5), despite mean low-density lipoprotein (LDL) cholesterol levels which exceed those in men, may help to explain why the incidence of CHD remains twice as high in men as compared to women up to age 75 (Fig 3).[34]

Clearly lipoprotein levels in women are not solely determined by genetic factors, but also by other factors such as exercise, diet, cigarette smoking, and the onset of menopause. Women smokers had significantly lower HDL cholesterol levels and higher triglyceride levels than did nonsmokers.[38] Postmenopausal women receiving estrogen supplementation had significantly higher HDL levels than did those who were not supplemented

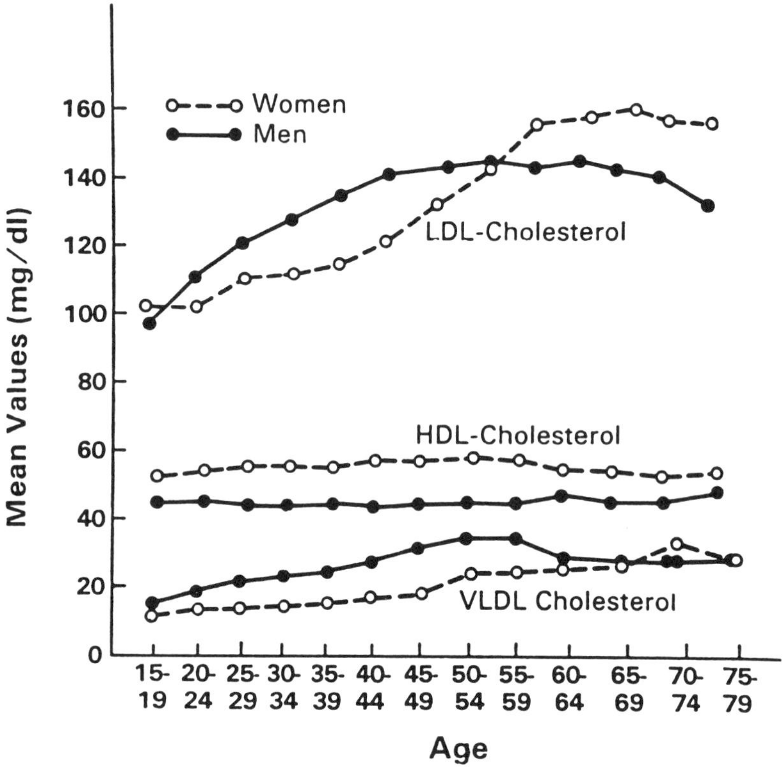

FIG 5.
Age trends in lipoprotein cholesterol fractions: Framingham Heart Study. (From Kannel WB: *Amer Heart J* 1987; 114:413–419. Used by permission.)

(63 ± 6 vs. 48 ± 2; $P < 0.01$).[39] Diet and exercise are the predominant causes of decreased total serum cholesterol and LDL levels.[40] Supplementation of estrogens in postmenopausal women and lifestyle modifications such as a low-fat, high-fiber diet, smoking cessation, and initiation of a regular exercise program may markedly improve the overall lipid profile and CHD risk.

Obesity is another significant risk factor for the development of CHD in women. Roughly 17 million women in the United States can be classified as being obese, that is, greater than 20% above their ideal body weight.[41] Obesity is associated with deterioration of the lipid profile, with elevation of triglycerides and LDL, and lowering of HDL. Furthermore, obesity, especially central adiposity, leads to insulin resistance, impaired glucose tolerance, and increases the likelihood of developing hypertension and adult-onset diabetes. All of these adverse effects improve with weight loss.[34] In a prospective study of 115,886 women age 30 to 55 who were initially free of CHD, the relative risk of developing CHD among the most obese women (top 20%) was 3.3 times that of their nonobese counterparts.[42] Besides dietary intervention, which is clearly warranted in the obese patient, it is also important to emphasize the role of physical activity on treatment and prevention of obesity. Aging is associated with weight gain in women. In a 3-year prospective study of 541 women, those who were physically active had the least weight gain and the least deterioration in their lipid profiles.[43] Finally, obese postmenopausal women receiving ERT generally tended to lose weight as compared to an overall weight gain among those who were not on ERT.[44]

The role of aspirin in the prevention of morbidity and mortality from coronary heart disease has become increasingly clear. However, most of the studies were performed in men. Women were included in the Aspirin Myocardial Infarction Study (AMIS). There was no clear benefit of aspirin in women in this trial, but the number of women in the study was small.[45] More conclusive evidence has been recently reported from the Nurses' Health Study, in which there was a significant reduction in the incidence of a first myocardial infarction in women taking aspirin. This was particularly true for women 50 years of age and older, who had a relative risk of developing a myocardial infarction of 0.61 compared to nonaspirin users. There did not appear to be a mortality difference over 6 years of followup.[46] A randomized trial of aspirin use in women is underway.

No area of investigation into women's health has received more attention in recent years than has ERT. From an epidemiological standpoint, myocardial infarction and CHD are rare prior to menopause, in the absence of diabetes mellitus or familial hypercholesterolemia.[47] Furthermore, it has been shown that the relative risk of developing CHD increases fourfold after either surgical or natural menopause. Thus it would appear that estrogen replacement therapy would be beneficial. However, the use of ERT in postmenopausal women has not been widespread because of early reports of the potential adverse effects of hormonal replacement. An initial epidemiological study suggested that there were significant deleterious effects of estrogens including increased risk of cardiovascular morbidity and incidence of cerebrovascular disease.[48] Furthermore, there was a suggestion of increased risk of breast cancer and uterine cancer with ERT. There has also been a suggestion of an increased thrombotic state and increased risk of hypertension with ERT, but these have not been borne out.

Discrepancies in the effects of estrogen reported in the literature can largely be explained by differences in preparations and dosages and populations treated. Estrogens used in contraceptives are synthetic and are generally ten times more potent than natural estrogens. Oral contraceptives (OCPs) have been associated with an increased risk for thrombotic events such as myocardial infarction, particularly among cigarette smokers.[49] However, there is no evidence to suggest that prior use of OCPs increases the risk of developing CHD.[50] Furthermore, the effects on coagulation appear to be dose dependent and are generally seen only with the more potent synthetic estrogens. When ERT with low-dose, natural estrogens was evaluated, there was no evidence of an increase in coagulation factors.[51, 52]

With regard to hypertension, the use of OCPs have been associated with an increased risk of developing hypertension. In contrast, the use of ERT in postmenopausal women was associated with significant decreases in both systolic and diastolic blood pressure.[51, 53] Furthermore, for progestins, there appears to be a vasodilatory effect of natural progestins compared to the synthetic progestins found in OCP's.[54]

The studies investigating the effects of estrogens on lipid metabolism have generally demonstrated a favorable effect on lipids, by lowering LDL and raising HDL. Even when estrogens were used in combination with progestins, a beneficial effect on lipids remained.[55] Percutaneous and vaginally administered estrogens appear to have little or no effect on lipid metabolism.[56, 57] The most favorable effects were seen with estrogen replacement alone. If combination therapy with a progestin is required, then the lowest dose and least androgenic progestin should be used. Nearly all studies investigating the role of ERT in preventing the development of CHD were performed without progestins.

Studies in the mid-1970s demonstrate that the use of unopposed estrogens resulted in an increased incidence of endometrial cancer. Subsequent studies have demonstrated that this effect was largely eliminated by the concurrent administration of a progestional agent. Thus, in postmenopausal women with intact uteri, ERT should be given in combination with a progestational agent.[47] Optimal monitoring for cancer risk (such as frequent surveillance endometrial biopsy) has not been established.

Similar concern was associated with the potential increased risk of women developing breast cancer while receiving ERT. In a recent meta-analysis, women who were taking low-dose ERT (0.625 mg/day) had a relative risk of 1.08 of developing breast cancer compared to nonusers. This relative risk increased to 2.0 when the dose was increased to 1.25 mg/day. Thus the relative risk of developing breast cancer secondary to ERT appears to be dose dependent and the increased risk is minimal at a dose of 0.625 mg/day.[58]

Finally, there has been a large body of evidence in support of a risk reduction of CHD morbidity and mortality with ERT. In a study of 8881 postmenopausal women followed for over 7 years, there was a 40% reduction in overall mortality among women receiving ERT.[59] Furthermore, the beneficial effect of ERT on decreased mortality appears to be particularly true for women with established coronary artery disease. In one study, women with at least a 70% stenosis of one coronary artery were treated with ERT and had a 10-year survival of 97% compared to 60% among those who never used ERT.[60] If borne out by other studies, these data suggest that ERT is among the most powerful interventions available for primary or secondary prevention of CHD.

In summary, menopause is associated with several metabolic changes which are associated with an increased incidence of CHD. Many of these adverse effects can be overcome with ERT. At the appropriate dosage level (0.625 mg/day), there are a small number of adverse side effects, whose incidence is overshadowed by the substantial reduction in CHD mortality. In the appropriate setting, concurrent use of a progestational agent is warranted.

Conclusion

Coronary artery disease remains the leading cause of death among women in the United States. Our ability to detect the presence of disease has been limited by the overall accuracy of the available noninvasive diagnostic tests. The advent of more sensitive and specific noninvasive diagnostic tests will allow for detection of significant CAD in patients with atypical clinical presentations. However, the majority of women with CHD present with a typical history of angina, and only a very small percentage of patients with atypical symptoms have significant coronary artery disease. A clinical history of angina should allow for detection of the large majority of women with significant disease. Finally, women who present with CAD tend to have more risk factors than men, such as cigarette smoking, obesity, diabetes, hypertension, and an estrogen-deficient state. This suggests that women may have a higher "threshold" for the development of CAD, and that no single risk factor is necessarily sufficient to result in the clinical development of the disease. Therefore, significant efforts aimed at primary and secondary prevention by modification of these risk factors, in women with and without established disease, may substantially reduce the morbidity and mortality from this disease.

References

1. Doublas PS (ed): *Cardiovascular Health and Disease in Women.* Philadelphia, WB Saunders, 1993.
2. Eaker ED, Packard B, Thom TJ: Epidemiology and risk factors for coronary heart disease in women, in Douglas PS (ed): *Heart Disease in Women.* Philadelphia, FA Davis Company, 1989.
3. Elveback LR, Connolly DC, Melton J: Coronary heart disease in residents of Rochester, Minnesota: *VII Incidence,* 1950 through 1982. *Mayo Clin Proc* 1986:896–900.
4. Lerner DJ, Kannel WB: Patterns of coronary heart disease morbidity and mortality in the sexes: A 26-year follow-up of the Framingham population. *Am Heart J* 1986; 111:383–390.
5. Chaitman BR, Bourassa MG, Lam J et al: Noninvasive diagnosis of coronary heart disease in women, in Eaker ED, Packard B, Wenger NK, et al. (eds): *Coronary Heart Disease in Women.* New York, Haymarket Doymas, 1987, pp 222–228.
6. Allen WH, Aronow WS, Goodman P, et al: Five-year follow-up of maximal treadmill stress test in asympatomatic men and women. *Circulation* 1980; 62:522.

7. Manga C, DeiCas L, Albertini D, et al: Different prognostic value of exercise electrocardiogram in men and women. *Cardiology* 1978; 63:312.
8. Barolsky SM, Gilbert CA, Fauqui A, et al: Differences in electrocardiographic response to exercise in women and men: A nonbaysian factor. *Circulation* 1979; 60:1021.
9. Detry JMR, Kapita BM, Cosyns J, et al: Diagnostic value of history and maximal exercise electrocardiography in men and women. *Circulation* 1977; 56:756.
10. Isley C, Canepa-Anson, Westgate C, et al: Influence of R wave analysis upon diagnostic accuracy of exercise testing in women. *Br Heart J* 1982; 48:161.
11. Wenger NK: Coronary heart disease in women: Clinical syndromes, prognosis, and diagnostic testing, in Douglas PS (ed): *Heart Disease in Women*. Philadelphia, FA Davis Company, 1989.
12. Selzer A, Langston M, Ruggeroli C, et al: Clinical syndrome of variant angina with normal coronary arteriogram. *N Engl J Med* 1976; 295:1343.
13. Lehman M, Berg A, Keul J: Sex-related differences in free plasma catecholamines in individuals of similar performance ability during graded ergometric exercise. *Eur J Applied Physiol* 1986; 55:54.
14. Dalal JN, Morise AP, Duval RD: The effect of estrogen status on positive predictive value in females undergoing diagnostic exercise electrocardiography. *Circulation* 1991; 84:II–574.
15. Osbakken MD: Exercise Stress Training in Women: Diagnostic Dilemma, in Douglas PS (ed): *Heart Disease in Women*. Philadelphia, FA Davis Company, 1989.
16. Friedman D, Green AC, Iskandrian AS, et al: Exercise thallium-201 myocardial scintigraphy in women: Correlation with coronary arteriography. *Am J Cardiol* 1982; 49:1632.
17. Fintel DJ, Links JM, Brinker JA, et al: Improved diagnostic performance of exercise thallium-201 single photon emission computed tomography over planar imaging in the diagnosis of coronary artery disease: A receiver operating characteristic analysis. *JACC* 1989; 13:600–612.
18. Sawada SG, Ryan T, Fineberg NS, et al: Exercise echocardiographic detection of coronary artery disease in women. 1989; 14:1440–7.
19. Bach DS, Armstrong WF: Dobutamine stress echocardiography. *Am J Cardiol* 1992; 69:90H–96H.
20. Tobin JN, Wassertheil-Smoller S, Wexler JP, et al: Sex bias in considering coronary bypass surgery. *Ann Intern Med* 1987; 107:19–25.
21. Ayanian JZ, Epstein AM: Differences in the use of procedures between women and men hospitalized for coronary artery disease. *New Engl J Med* 1991; 325:221–225.
22. Krumholz HM, Douglas PS, Lauer MS, et al: Selection of patients for coronary angiography and coronary revascularization early after myocardial infarction: Is there evidence for a gender bias? *Ann Intern Med* 1992; 116:785–790.
23. Steingart RM, Packer M, Hamm P, et al: Sex differences in the management of coronary artery disease. *New Engl J Med* 1991; 325:226–230.
24. Bickell NA, Pieper KS, Kerry LL, et al: Referral patterns for coronary artery disease treatment: gender bias or good clinical judgement? *Ann Intern Med* 1992; 116:791–797.
25. Maynard C, Althouse R, Cerqueira M, et al: Underutilization of thrombolytic therapy in eligible women with acute myocardial infarction. *Am J Cardiol* 1991; 68:529–530.

26. U.S. Bureau of the Census: Statistical abstracts of the United States, 1991, annual ed 111, Washington DC, US Government Printing Office, 1991.
27. Kindwall KE: Therapy for coronary heart disease in women, in Douglas PS (ed): *Heart Disease in Women.* Philadelphia, FA Davis Company, 1989.
28. Anastos K, Charney P, Charon RA, et al: Hypertension in women: What is really known? *Ann Intern Med* 1991; 115:287–293.
29. Greenland P, Reicher-Reiss, Goldbourt U, et al: In-hospital and 1-year mortality in 1524 women after myocardial infarction. *Circulation* 1991; 83:484–491.
30. Khan SS, Nessim S, Gray R, et al: Increased mortality of women in coronary artery bypass surgery: evidence for referral bias. *Ann Intern Med* 1990; 112:561–567.
31. Isles CG, Hole DJ, Hawthorne VM, et al: Relation between coronary risk and coronary mortality in women of the Renfrew and Paisley survey: Comparison with men. *Lancet* 1992; 339:702–706.
32. Caralis DG, Deligonul U, Kern MJ, et al: Smoking is a risk factor for coronary spasm in young women. *Circulation* 1992; 85:905–909.
33. Rosenberg L, Palmer JR, Shapiro S: Decline in the risk of myocardial infarction among women who stop smoking. *N Engl J Med* 1990; 322:213–217.
34. Kannel WB: Metabolic risk factors for coronary heart disease in women: Perspective from the Framingham Heart Study. *Am Heart J* 1987; 114:413–419.
35. Manson JE, Colditz GA, Stampfer MJ, et al: A prospective study of maturity-onset diabetes mellitus and risk of coronary heart disease and stroke in women. *Arch Intern Med* 1991; 151:1141–1147.
36. Hong MK, Romm PA, Reagan K, et al: Usefulness of the total cholesterol to high-density lipoprotein cholesterol ratio in predicting angiographic coronary artery disease in women. *Am J Cardiol* 1991; 68:1646–1650.
37. Kannel WB: High density lipoproteins: Epidemiologic profile and risks of coronary artery disease. *Am J Cardiol* 1983; 52:9b–72b.
38. Willet W, Hennekens CH, Castelli W, et al: Effects of cigarette smoking on fasting triglyceride, total cholesterol, and HDL-cholesterol in women. *Am Heart J* 1983; 105:417–421.
39. Hong MK, Romm PA, Reagan K, et al: Effects of estrogen replacement therapy on serum lipid values and angiographically defined coronary artery disease in postmenopausal women. *Am J Cardiol* 1992; 69:176–178.
40. Wood PD, Stefanick ML, Williams PT, et al: The effects on plasma lipoproteins of a prudent weight-reducing diet with or without exercise in overweight men and women. *N Engl J Med* 1991; 325:461–466.
41. National Institutes of Health Consensus Development Panel on Health Implications of Obesity. *Ann Intern Med* 1985; 103:1073–1077.
42. Manson JE, Colditz GA, Stampfer MJ, et al: A prospective study of obesity and risk of coronary heart disease in women. *N Engl J Med* 1990; 322:882–889.
43. Owens JF, Matthews KA, Wing RR, et al: Can physical activity mitigate the effects of aging in middle-aged women? *Circulation* 1992; 85:1265–1270.
44. Hart DM, Lindsay R, Purdie D: Vascular complications of long-term estrogen therapy. *Front Hormone Res* 1978; 5:174.
45. The Aspirin Myocardial Infarction Study Research Group: The aspirin myocardial infarction study: Final results. *Circulation* 1980; 62:V79–84.
46. Manson JE, Stanpfer MJ, Colditz GA, et al: A prospective study of aspirin use and primary prevention of cardiovascular disease in women. *JAMA* 1991; 266:521–527.

47. Barrett-Connor E, Bush TL: Estrogen replacement and coronary heart disease, in Douglas PS (ed): *Heart Disease in Women*. Philadelphia, FA Davis Company, 1989.
48. Wilson PWF, Garrision RJ, Castelli WP: Postmenopausal estrogen use, cigarette smoking, and cardiovascular morbidity in women over 50. The Framingham Heart Study. *N Engl J Med* 1985; 313:1038–1043.
49. Mann JI, Vessey MP, Thorogood M, et al: Myocardial infarction in young women with special reference to oral contraceptive practice. *Br Med J* 1975; 2:241–245.
50. Stampfer MJ, Willett WC, Colditz GA, et al: A prospective study of past use of oral contraceptive agents and risk of cardiovascular diseases. *N Engl J Med* 1988; 319:1313–1317.
51. Lind T, Cameron EC, Hunter WM, et al: A prospective controlled trial of six forms of hormone replacement therapy given to postmenopausal women. *Br J Obstet Gynaecol* 1979; 86:(suppl 3).
52. Chetkowswi RJ, Meldrum DR, Steingold KA, et al: Biological effects of transdermal estradiol. *N Engl J Med* 1986; 314:1615–1620.
53. Luotola H: Blood pressure and hemodynamics in postmenopausal women during estradiol 17beta substitution. *Ann Clin Res* 1983; 5:135.
54. Rylance PB, Brincat M, Lafferty K, et al: Natural progesterone and antihypertensive action. *Br Med J* 1985; 290:13.
55. Sherwin BB, Gelfand MM: A prospective one-year study of estrogen and progestin in postmenopausal women: Effects on clinical symptoms and lipoprotein lipids. *Obstet Gynecol* 1989; 73:759–766.
56. Fletcher CD, Farish E, Hart DM, et al: Long-term hormone implant therapy—effects on lipoprotein and steroid levels in post-menopausal women. *Acta Endocrinol (Copenh)* 1986; 111:419.
57. Mandel FP, Geola FL, Meldrum DR, et al: Biological effects of various doses of vaginally administered conjugated equine estrogens in postmenopausal women. *J Clin Endocrinol Metab* 1983; 57:133.
58. Dupont WD, Page DL: Menopausal estrogen replacement therapy and breast cancer. *Arch Intern Med* 1991; 151:67–72.
59. Henderson BE, Pananini-Hill A, Ross RK: Decreased mortality in users of estrogen replacement therapy. *Arch Intern Med* 1991; 151:75–78.
60. Sullivan JM, Vander Zwang R, Hughes JP, et al: Estrogen replacement and coronary artery disease. *Arch Intern Med* 1990; 150:2557–2562.

Approach to Treatment of the Patient With Heart Failure in 1994

Spencer H. Kubo, M.D.

Associate Professor of Medicine, Director, Heart Failure–Heart Transplantation Program, Cardiovascular Division, Department of Medicine, University of Minnesota Medical School, Minneapolis, Minnesota

Jay N. Cohn, M.D.

Professor of Medicine, Head, Cardiovascular Division, Department of Medicine, University of Minnesota Medical School, Minneapolis, Minnesota

Heart failure is a clinical syndrome characterized by left ventricular dysfunction (systolic and/or diastolic), fluid retention, exercise intolerance, and a reduced life expectancy. It has been estimated that there are 3,000,000 patients with heart failure in the United States[1] and that the incidence will likely increase given the advancing median age of the population and improvements in revascularization procedures and thrombolytic therapy. Heart failure is also associated with considerable morbidity and remains the most common indication for hospitalization in patients over the age of 65 years. Finally, heart failure is associated with high mortality rates and accounts for up to 400,000 deaths each year. Thus, there continues to be considerable interest in the management of this syndrome. Over the last decade, there have been important developments in our understanding of the pathophysiology of this syndrome. In addition, several multicenter trials have provided critical data that have greatly influenced treatment strategies. Thus, the treatment practices which are considered "state of the art" in 1994 are substantially different from the standard practice of 1984. It is therefore appropriate to review some of the more important data influencing treatment strategies and the current approach to therapy.

Treatment Endpoints and Patient Subgroups

Before discussing specific therapeutic indications, it is necessary to review two evolving concepts which have provided an important framework for the current approach to therapy. First, it is now widely held that one must critically examine the efficacy of all therapeutic interventions with respect to two different but equally important endpoints, including an improvement in the quality of life and prolonged survival. It is clear that therapeutic interventions do not necessarily have an equivalent beneficial effect on these two endpoints. For example, both digoxin and diuretics are very effective in reducing clinical signs and symptoms short-term, but their effects on survival are not presently known. In contrast, there are convincing data that vasodilators not only improve symptoms, reduce hospitalizations, and improve exercise tolerance but also prolong survival in patients with heart failure. Furthermore, the endpoint of survival benefit is complicated by the fact that treatment effects on death due to pump failure may not be in concert with the effects on death related to arrhythmias.

The second major concept involves a more precise targeting of patient groups to identify the specific population that is most likely to benefit from a particular intervention. This development is based on the recognition that pathophysiologic mechanisms and therapeutic endpoints may not be the same for all patients and that a standard "cookbook" of drug therapy is inappropriate. This targeting of patient groups includes the important distinction between systolic and diastolic dysfunction. Although relatively uncommon, patients with pure diastolic dysfunction can present with many of the signs and symptoms of heart failure associated with systolic dysfunction. However, certain pharmacologic agents may be contraindicated (e.g., digoxin) in this patient group. Thus, almost all patients will have a noninvasive measurement of ventricular function to assess the relative contributions of systolic and diastolic dysfunction and to direct the use of drugs that could be expected to have the greatest benefit.

The majority of patients with heart failure have systolic dysfunction as manifest by a reduced ejection fraction, and this chapter will largely focus on this population. Although there is considerable overlap, it is now appreciated that there may be three general subgroups of patients with systolic dysfunction (Table 1).

Group B is the largest subgroup and includes those patients with left ventricular systolic dysfunction, who also have mild to moderate signs and

TABLE 1.
Targeting of Specific Patient Subgroups

	LV Dysfunction	
A, NYHA I/II	**B, NYHA II/III**	**C, NYHA III/IV**
Prophylactic use of converting enzyme inhibitors	Combination therapy: Digitalis Diuretics Vasodilators Converting enzyme Inhibitors	Combination therapy plus: Inotropic agents Transplantation

symptoms of clinical heart failure, such as dyspnea, fatigue, edema, pulmonary congestion, and an S3 gallop. These patients most commonly gain symptom relief from combination therapy with digitalis, diuretics, and angiotensin-converting enzyme (ACE) inhibitors or vasodilators. For this group, the most important development is the clear documentation from several multicenter trials including studies of left ventricular dysfunction (SOLVD), vasodilators in heart failure trial (V-HeFT I and V-HeFT II) that some of these drugs also prolong survival.

Patients in Group C have persistent signs of disabling heart failure (New York Heart Association [NYHA] III/IV) despite this combination therapy and are often labeled as "refractory." For these patients, it is appropriate to consider more intensive measures such as heart transplantation. Heart transplantation, although limited to a small number of patients relative to the total population with heart failure, provides one of the most dramatic therapies and will be discussed from the perspective of an internist. In addition, many of these patients are hospitalized for decompensated heart failure and may require the use of intravenous vasodilators and inotropic agents for acute stabilization.

Perhaps the most exciting development, however, is the identification of important therapies for patients in group A. These patients have clear evidence of left ventricular dysfunction but either do not have signs or symptoms of heart failure (i.e., NYHA I) or have minimal symptoms of early heart failure that may not be recognized (NYHA II). It has been hypothesized that early "prophylactic" treatment in this group could have the greatest impact on health care expenditures and would be "cost effective" when compared to high intensity interventions for patients with advanced heart failure. The benefit of ACE inhibitors for this group of patients has been recently identified in multicenter trials.

This chapter will review the current approach to treatment for each of the three groups. In each section, we provide some of the most pertinent findings regarding pathophysiology, data from important clinical trials, and practical recommendations that will be useful in everyday clinical encounters.

Patients With Established Signs and Symptoms of Heart Failure—Group B

Diuretics

Pathophysiologic Mechanisms.—Diuretics are the cornerstones in the pharmacologic management of patients with heart failure. The principle indication for diuretics is to control excess extracellular fluid that is typically manifest as pulmonary congestion, peripheral edema, or ascites. These signs are in part related to avid sodium retention by the kidney, which is influenced by many neurohormonal and hemodynamic changes that are commonly observed in heart failure. Thus, decreased cardiac output, decreased renal blood flow, increased filtration fraction, redistribution of intrarenal blood flow to the salt-conserving medulla, enhanced renal sympathetic nerve activity, elevated antidiuretic hormone levels, and activation of the renin-angiotensin-aldosterone system all contribute to enhanced sodium and water retention by the kidney.[2–4]

Despite the wide acceptance of diuretics, they have a number of long-term adverse effects. In particular, diuretic administration is associated with activation of the renin-angiotensin system as manifest by increased levels of plasma renin activity and angiotensin II.[5–7] Increased angiotensin II will increase secretion of aldosterone which promotes sodium retention and therefore tends to counterbalance the diuretic action. Furthermore, increased vasoconstriction may have a positive feedback effect in which increased impedance to ventricular emptying results in greater systolic dysfunction. This effect may contribute to the association between increased levels of plasma renin activity and mortality in patients with heart failure.[8–9] The effect of diuretics on the renin-angiotensin system can be blocked by the concomitant administration of a converting enzyme inhibitor. With this combination therapy, one may obtain the beneficial effect of the diuretics but block the increase in angiotensin II and aldosterone levels.

Several clinical trials have now confirmed important benefits with this combination therapy compared to diuretic therapy alone and are reviewed in subsequent sections. For example, the Captopril-Digoxin Multicenter Trial[10] demonstrated that captopril and furosemide increased exercise time and decreased hospitalizations and NYHA functional class compared to patients on furosemide alone. Therefore, diuretics are still commonly used but only rarely as monotherapy.

Practical Considerations.—Table 2 summarizes the available diuretics and their usual dosages according to their site of action in the kidney. These include the loop diuretics (furosemide, ethacrynic acid, and bumetamide) which inhibit chloride and sodium reabsorption in the thick ascending limb of the loop of Henle. The nonloop diuretics (hydrochlorothiazide, chlorthalidone, and metolazone) inhibit sodium and chloride reabsorption in the distal tubule. There are two different types of potassium-sparing diuretics, including spironolactone, which is a direct antagonist to aldosterone, and triamterene and amiloride, which are direct inhibitors of collecting duct sodium reabsorption.

Patients with mild heart failure, who have slight or minimal symptoms of edema and pulmonary congestion, can often be managed with the combination of a sodium-restricted diet and a nonloop diuretic. Patients with more marked hemodynamic abnormalities, frequent hospitalizations, and more severe symptomatic impairment usually require a loop diuretic. In some patients with severe potassium wastage, the addition of a potassium sparing diuretic will allow these patients to reduce the dosage of potassium supplements to more tolerable levels.

Although diuretics can effectively control the manifestations of excess extracellular fluid, it is important to emphasize that they should be combined with dietary sodium restriction. It is abundantly clear that the magni-

TABLE 2.
Choice of Diuretic

Diuretic	Trade Name	Daily Dose
Loop diuretic		
Furosemide	Lasix	20–240 mg/day
Ethacrynic acid	Edecrin	50–200 mg/day
Bumetamide	Bumex	1–10 mg/day
Non-loop diuretic		
Hydrochlorothiazide	Hydrodiuril	25–100 mg/day
Chlorthalidone	Hygroton	25–100 mg/day
Metolazone	Zaroxolyn	2.5–10 mg/day
Potassium-sparing diuretic		
Spironolactone	Aldactone	25–200 mg/day
Triamterene	Dyrenium	37.5–200 mg/day
Amiloride	Midamor	2.5–10 mg/day

tude of edema formation is in part related to the magnitude of dietary sodium intake. Since almost all foods contain sodium, and since it is not possible to eliminate sodium entirely, *limitation* is the more useful goal. Many patients maintain that "I don't add any salt," but are unaware of the considerable sodium content of many foods, such as 122 mg in 8 ounces of milk and 1200 mg in 8 ounces of chicken noodle soup. It is advisable to carefully review dietary histories to identify hidden sources of sodium. We generally limit the daily total intake to approximately 2500 mg, although this amount can be modified to individual preferences and the severity of edema formation. This program provides patients with some flexibility as well as encouraging them to participate in their medical management. Some patients require additional instruction through a referral to a registered dietician.

There are several endpoints to monitor in patients treated with diuretics. Since the main medication is symptom relief, one may reduce the dose of diuretics to maintenance levels once there is a satisfactory reduction in dyspnea, orthopnea, and edema. An alternate strategy is to guide dosing based on normalization of the jugular venous pulse, which is thought by some to be an important factor in preventing progression of left ventricular dysfunction.

Some patients have refractory signs and symptoms and are frequently labeled "diuretic resistant."[11] Some patients may be noncompliant with their medication regimens or ineffective in limiting dietary sodium intake. In patients with obvious peripheral edema, significant bowel-wall edema may limit oral absorption, so that intravenous formulations (e.g. furosemide and/or chlorothiazide) may be effective in initiating a diuresis. In other patients, the problem is inadequate delivery to the tubular lumen due to reduced renal perfusion and impaired tubular secretion of diuretics. One approach to this problem is to combine therapy with a nonloop diuretic,[12] which exerts some effects on the proximal tubule resulting in increased delivery of sodium and chloride to the loop of Henle thereby facilitating the action of the loop diuretic.[13] The addition of a nonloop diuretic may also be used for transient episodes of fluid accumulation. This "booster pill" strategy allows one to keep the dose of the loop diuretic constant and minimize errors associated with frequent dose changes. Furthermore, by using the additional diuretic only on a temporary basis, one tends to reduce the amount of the diuretic that the patient will be exposed to long-term.

During long-term treatment, it is important to monitor levels of potassium, given the marked kaliuretic effects of diuretic drugs. One should also follow renal function since this parameter may be sensitive to changes in blood volume and/or vasoconstrictor hormones. Since diuretics are associated with a long list of adverse effects (Table 3), it is also advisable to use the lowest dose of diuretic necessary to maintain clinical stability.

Digitalis

Mechanisms of Action.—Digitalis inhibits the sodium potassium adenosine triphosphatase which results in the gradual accumulation of intracellular sodium and loss of intracellular potassium. The increase in intracellular sodium activates the sodium-calcium exchanger in sarcolemmal membranes leading to an increase in calcium influx. The increased availability of calcium for excitation-contraction coupling results in increased myocardial contractility. The inotropic effects of digitalis are well described in terms of the characteristic Frank Starling relationship. In heart failure,

TABLE 3.
Complications of Diuretic Therapy

Hypokalemia
Hyponatremia
Hypomagnesiumenia
Volume contraction
Renal insufficiency
Hyperuricemia
Hyperlipidemia
Metabolic alkalosis
Carbohydrate intolerance
Activation of the renin-angiotensin system

this relationship is depressed and flatter than normal, so that despite an increase in preload, cardiac output is still subnormal. The improvements in stroke volume and cardiac output have been established in numerous studies with precise hemodynamic measurements.[14, 15]

In addition to its direct inotropic action, digitalis may influence the circulation through its effects on sympathetic reflexes. Studies have demonstrated that digitalis may sensitize the depressed cardiopulmonary and aortic arch baroreceptors in heart failure.[16] This results in a net reduction in sympathetic activity and a potentiation of baroreceptor-mediated sympathetic mechanisms. However, the extent to which these effects contribute to the clinical efficacy of digitalis is not known.

Clinical Efficacy.—Although a great many physicians had personal experience with the favorable effects of digoxin in heart failure, there was considerable controversy in the early 1980s regarding the precise documentation of its clinical efficacy.[17, 18] It is therefore appropriate to review the more recent data from randomized placebo-controlled trials that have provided the firm scientific data to recommend the routine use of digoxin in patients with symptomatic heart failure.

Dobbs et al.[19] utilized a crossover design and demonstrated that 16 of 46 patients deteriorated when digoxin was changed to placebo. With a clinical score in 25 patients, Lee et al.[20] demonstrated that digoxin improved overall clinical signs and symptoms compared with placebo. Guyatt et al.[21] reported that digoxin prevented clinical deteriorations and led to improvements in echocardiographic assessments of left ventricular function and 6-minute-walk time in 20 patients. The prospective randomized study of ventricular failure and the efficacy of digoxin (PROVED) study utilized a randomized withdrawal design in 88 patients who were not taking converting enzyme inhibitors.[22] At the end of 12 weeks, patients withdrawn from digoxin were twice as likely to require an increase in diuretics or emergency room visits compared to digoxin-maintained patients. Furthermore, digoxin-withdrawal patients also had a significant deterioration in exercise treadmill time and ejection fraction.

DiBianco[23] reported a trial in which 230 patients treated with diuretics were randomized to placebo, digoxin, milrinone (a phosphodiesterase inhibitor inotropic agent), or the combination of digoxin and milrinone. When compared with placebo, digoxin reduced the incidence of worsening heart failure (15% vs. 47%) and significantly increased exercise time and ejection fraction. Interestingly, the effect of digoxin on exercise time was similar to milronine, a drug with more potent inotropic properties.

The Captopril Digoxin Multicenter Research Group compared digoxin with captopril in 300 patients treated with a diuretic.[10] Compared to placebo, digoxin significantly increased left ventricular ejection fraction and reduced the percentage of patients requiring hospitalizations and emergency room visits for the treatment of heart failure (15% vs. 20%). In contrast, captopril was associated with a significant improvement in functional class and exercise time compared with placebo, whereas these changes were not significant for digoxin. Other smaller studies[24, 25] have demonstrated improvements in a number of clinical variables with both digoxin and converting enzyme inhibitors.

The randomized assessment of (the effect of) digoxin on inhibitors of the angiotensin-converting enzyme (RADIANCE) study evaluated the effects of digoxin withdrawal in 178 patients who were treated with a converting enzyme inhibitor.[26] During the 12-week withdrawal phase, heart failure symptoms worsened in 28% of "digoxin-withdrawal" patients but only 6% of "digoxin-continuation" patients ($P < 0.05$). In addition, "digoxin-withdrawal" patients had more hospitalizations and emergency room visits for heart failure and decreased exercise tolerance. These data suggest that digoxin therapy produces clinical benefit even in patients treated with an ACE inhibitor.

Although there is no clear consensus regarding the relative superiority of digitalis or an ACE inhibitor, this issue has not been important in clinical practice. Since digoxin and ACE inhibitors have different mechanisms of action, most attention has focused on "triple-drug therapy" (i.e., digoxin, diuretics, and an ACE inhibitor), which has rapidly become the standard for patients with symptomatic heart failure.

In contrast to the effects of digitalis on short-term clinical parameters, the effects on mortality have been considerably more difficult to address. Virtually all of the clinical studies have been unable to assess an effect on survival because of inadequate sample size. Some but not all studies in patients recovering from acute myocardial infarction have shown that patients treated with digoxin had increased mortality rates when compared to patients who are not taking digoxin, even when corrected for the prevalence of symptomatic heart failure in digoxin-treated patients.[27–29] These specific effects of digitalis on mortality are currently being assessed in the Digitalis Investigation Group (DIG) trial, a randomized prospective study with an estimated enrollment of 8000 patients. It is hoped that this trial will provide firm evidence of whether or not the effects of digitalis on clinical parameters and survival are concordant.

In conclusion, the cumulative data from controlled trials would suggest that digitalis is associated with important clinical improvements and, therefore, is an integral part of the drug regimen for patients with left ventricular systolic dysfunction and significant heart failure. It is important to note, however, that digoxin should not be used in patients with heart failure primarily due to diastolic dysfunction, ongoing myocardial ischemia, or reduced ventricular compliance. Furthermore, there is no data to support the use of digitalis in patients who have asymptomatic left ventricular dysfunction.

Practical Considerations.—Previous practice typically involved the use of full digitalizing doses to more rapidly achieve therapeutic levels. However, this is usually not necessary for most patients who can be started on maintenance doses, ranging from 0.125 to 0.375 mg per day. The gelatin capsule increases oral bioavailability by up to 90%, so that there should be a 10% reduction in the total daily dose. Because drug elimination is primarily via the kidneys, digoxin doses must be adjusted in renal insufficiency. There are a number of drug interactions that can significantly influence the efficacy and toxicity of digoxin. Drugs known to increase digoxin levels include quinidine, verapamil, diltiazem, and amiodarone. It is common practice to empirically reduce digoxin doses when initiating therapy with these drugs with close follow-up of digoxin levels.[30]

Measurement of serum digoxin levels can be helpful especially in determining patients who are receiving subtherapeutic doses. Digitalis toxicity is usually a clinical diagnosis based on cardiac and extracardiac manifestations, rather than solely based on a digoxin level. Patients with advanced heart failure were once considered candidates for intensified digoxin therapy with doses occasionally pushed to the development of toxicity. With the availability of other treatments this is not a common practice currently.

Vasodilators

Mechanisms of Action.—One of the most important advances in the treatment of heart failure is the recognition that pump function in heart failure is critically dependent on the outflow resistance against which the ventricle must empty.[31] It is now well established that vasodilator drugs that relax peripheral arterioles shift the ventricular function curve upward and to the left. The end result in terms of hemodynamics is an increase in cardiac output without a large change in blood pressure. Moreover, drugs that increase the capacitance of the venous circulation redistribute blood volume from the central to peripheral reservoirs and therefore decrease the signs and symptoms of elevated cardiac filling pressures. Since these seminal discoveries, there have been an extraordinary number of clinical studies reviewed elsewhere[32–34] that have investigated the mechanisms of action as well as the systemic and regional hemodynamic effects of different vasodilators in patients with heart failure. These studies have characterized certain vasodilators that act predominantly on the arterioles leading to a reduction in impedance (e.g., hydralazine), vasodilators that act predominantly on venous tone (e.g., nitrates), and vasodilators that have a balanced effect on arterioles and veins (e.g., converting enzyme inhibitors).

Clinical Efficacy.—The V-HeFT trial tested the hypothesis that vasodilators could prolong survival when compared to placebo.[35] The vasodilators tested were prazosin, an alpha-adrenergic blocker, and the combination of hydralazine and isosorbide dinitrate. Both drug regimens were associated with acute hemodynamic benefit manifest by decreases in cardiac filling pressures and systemic vascular resistance and increases in cardiac output. The study included 642 males with reduced exercise capacity (peak oxygen consumption <25 mL/kg/min) and either a cardiothoracic ratio >0.55, a left ventricular internal dimension >2.7 mm, or a left ventricular ejection fraction $<45\%$. Over a mean follow-up of 2.3 years, the cumulative mortality rate was 25.6% in the hydralazine-isosorbide dinitrate group and 34.3% in the placebo group (risk reduction 34%; $P < 0.028$). In contrast, the mortality rate for the prazosin group was virtually identical to placebo.

V-HeFT was the first demonstration that vasodilator therapy could prolong survival in patients with heart failure. The beneficial effect of this combination was confirmed in the V-HeFT II, which will be discussed later. Despite these beneficial effects, this drug combination has not been used widely in practice. The action of both drugs are dose related, and many patients cannot tolerate the relatively large dosages (160 mg of isosorbide dinitrate and 300 mg of hydralazine) used in V-HeFT. Furthermore, the survival benefit with enalapril, a converting enzyme inhibitor, was greater than this drug combination in V-HeFT II. Nonetheless, this combination is often useful in patients with heart failure, especially those who are unable to tolerate a converting enzyme inhibition.

Flosequinan.—There has been recent interest in the potential clinical applications of flosequinan, an orally active quinolone derivative. Similar to all vasodilators, hemodynamic studies have demonstrated significant increases in cardiac output and stroke volume related primarily to a decrease in systemic resistance.[36] Flosequinan also has a balanced effect on venous capacitance as reflected by a decrease in right and left heart filling pressures and an increase in forearm venous capacitance.[36] Flosequinan may also have a positive inotropic effect as demonstrated in dogs[37] and in humans[38] using the left ventricular end systolic pressure-volume relationship as a relatively load independent measure of contractility. This inotropic action may be related to phosphodiesterase inhibition and observed only at very high drug concentrations.[39]

The clinical efficacy of flosequinan has been evaluated in several clinical trials. These trials have included 31 patients maintained on digoxin and diuretics,[40] 332 patients on digoxin, diuretics, and converting enzyme inhibitors,[41] and 88 patients in whom digoxin and diuretics were continued after a 2-week withdrawal of converting enzyme inhibitors.[42] These data indicate that flosequinan is associated with a statistically significant improvement in exercise duration and symptoms of heart failure. Flosequinan was released for general use in March 1993 for the management of patients with heart failure not responding adequately to diuretics (with or without digitalis), in patients who are already taking an ACE inhibitor, or patients who could not tolerate an ACE inhibitor. However, shortly after the release of flosequinan, the interim results of a large, multicenter placebo-controlled mortality trial indicated that patients receiving 100 mg/day of flosequinan had an increased risk of death compared to those patients treated with placebo. No excess deaths were noted in patients treated with 75 mg/day. At the present time, the appropriate role of flosequinan for patients with heart failure is unclear.

Calcium Channel Blockers.—Calcium channel blockers have been considered for patients with heart failure,[43] since these drugs have potent vasodilator actions and may also reduce ischemia in patients with left ventricular dysfunction due to coronary artery disease. Many hemodynamic studies have demonstrated that the acute administration of a calcium channel blocker can be associated with marked reductions in systemic vascular resistance and an increase in cardiac output.[44, 45] However, these acute hemodynamic effects have not been uniform, appear to be different among different calcium channel blockers, and have not been associated with short- or long-term clinical benefit.[46, 47]

The deleterious responses in patients with heart failure have been attributed to several mechanisms including a direct negative inotropic action and neurohormonal stimulation.[47] It has been speculated that the acute hemodynamic effect may reflect a larger role of afterload reduction, but that the direct negative inotropic action may predominate when given long-term. Newer calcium channel blockers such as nitrendipine, nicardipine, felodipine, and amlodipine have greater selectivity for vascular actions. The potential efficacy of felodipine and amlodipine for the treatment of heart failure is now being evaluated in multicenter studies. Calcium channel blockers can stimulate the release of neurohormones both directly and indirectly via a fall in blood pressure. Interestingly, aldosterone levels are not increased[44] possibly due to a direct effect on the adrenal gland. The long-term effects of these hormonal changes are not known.

Many clinicians have found that diltiazem is useful and well tolerated in some patients with heart failure, where it is often used for control of angina and myocardial ischemia in patients with left ventricular dysfunction and/or ischemic cardiomyopathy rather than for the treatment of heart failure per se. The long-term effects of diltiazem in the treatment of patients with heart failure are not known. Recently, a post hoc analysis of the Multicenter Diltiazem Postinfarction Trial demonstrated that diltiazem therapy was associated with an increased frequency of new or worsened heart failure in patients with an ejection fraction less than 40%.[48] Based on these cumulative data, and while awaiting the results of ongoing trials, calcium channel blockers should be used only with great caution in patients with heart failure.

Converting Enzyme Inhibitors

Mechanisms of Action.—The converting enzyme inhibitors have become the most widely used vasodilator in clinical practice. However, the exact mechanisms by which the converting enzyme inhibitors impart their clinical benefit in patients with heart failure are not known. These agents reduce angiotensin II-mediated vasoconstriction and aldosterone secretion.[49] However, they also increase bradykinin levels and reduce the presynaptic effects of angiotensin II in releasing norepinephrine.[50] Converting enzyme inhibitors also block the local generation of angiotensin I from tissue renin angiotensin systems which appears to mediate the blood pressure effects in some animal models of hypertension.[50] Finally, the effects of these agents may be mediated by an effect on production of nitric oxide and other endothelial derived relaxing factors.[51]

Clinical Efficacy.—Numerous prospective, placebo-controlled studies have demonstrated the beneficial effects of converting enzyme inhibitors on exercise tolerance, salt and water balance, clinical signs and symptoms, neurohormonal stimulation, and quality of life in patients with chronic heart failure.[52, 53] More recent studies have addressed the hypothesis that vasodilators also prolong survival in heart failure. The concordance of findings in these multicenter trials has provided a strong scientific basis for the expanding use of ACE inhibitors in the management of heart failure.

The CONSENSUS trial randomized 253 hospitalized patients with class IV symptoms to either enalapril or placebo in addition to treatment with digoxin, diuretics, and non-ACE vasodilators.[54] Based on an interim analysis, enalapril was associated with a highly significant survival benefit compared to placebo (36% vs. 52%). Therefore, this trial was prematurely terminated, since it was deemed unethical to continue a trial in which half of the participants could have been randomized to placebo.

V-HeFT II was designed to compare treatment with hydralazine-isosorbide dinitrate to enalapril in patients similar to those enrolled in V-HeFT I.[55] The enalapril group had a lower 2-year mortality rate compared with those patients randomized to hydralazine-isosorbide dinitrate (18% vs. 25%, mortality reduction 28%, $P = 0.016$). Interestingly, exercise time and left ventricular function improved to a greater degree in the patients randomized to hydralazine-isosorbide dinitrate.

SOLVD was a randomized, double-blind placebo-controlled trial in patients with an ejection fraction $\leq$ 35%.[56] The Treatment Trial of SOLVD enrolled 2567 patients who had signs and symptoms of heart failure and required treatment with digitalis and diuretics. After a mean follow-up of 41 months, there were significantly more deaths in the placebo group compared to the enalapril group (510 vs. 452; 16% mortality reduction). Furthermore, enalapril was associated with a significant 30% reduction in hospitalizations for heart failure. It is important to note that this mortality reduction likely underestimated the true effect of enalapril, since nearly 30% of the patients in the placebo group were taking open label converting enzyme inhibitors at the end of the trial.

Practical Considerations.—The most important problem to monitor during initiation of ACE inhibitors is hypotension. Marked hypotensive responses are more common in patients with activated renin-angiotensin systems and heightened levels of angiotensin II-mediated vasoconstriction.[57] Since assays for plasma renin activity and angiotensin II are difficult, most clinicians take advantage of the relatively tight inverse correlation between plasma renin activity and serum sodium concentration.[58, 59] Those patients with low serum sodium (<130 mEq/L) as well as patients who are volume depleted are more likely to develop hypotension during the initiation of therapy. These patients will often benefit by a reduction in diuretic dosage or by the use of very small doses initially followed by gradual dose titration.

The clinical use of the converting enzyme inhibitors has become more complicated with the recent addition of quinipril, ramipril, monopril, and benazapril. All these drugs are capable of inhibiting converting enzyme, but the clinical experience in patients with heart failure with the newer agents is more limited. The primary issue of whether the beneficial effects are class or drug specific has not been adequately addressed by appropriate clinical trials. In the absence of firm scientific data, clinical use is influenced by individual preference and occasionally by cost.

Tachyphylaxis or the attenuation of the beneficial effect is not a major problem during maintenance therapy. However, heart failure and the renin-angiotensin system are dynamic processes and are influenced by many factors, such as dietary sodium intake.[60] Patients with increased sodium intake frequently develop increased edema. Furthermore, because of suppressed renin activity, the hemodynamic changes following an ACE inhibitor are reduced. This patient might be considered a treatment "failure," when the primary problem is dietary salt intake.

Most patients who are treated with ACE inhibitors still require diuretic therapy. However, because ACE inhibitors will decrease levels of aldosterone, diuretic doses can frequently be decreased. In addition, since potassium levels may increase slightly, the dosage of potassium supplements should be closely monitored. Potassium-sparing diuretics should be used with caution because of the risk of hyperkalemia.

Many side effects of ACE inhibitors such as dysgeusia, skin rash, cough, and proteinuria are self limited or reversible with discontinuation of the drug. In many cases, the ACE inhibitor can be reinstituted without recurrence of the side effect. Although all ACE inhibitors share the same side-effect profile, it is not known if they have substantive differences in the incidence of side effects.

Renal insufficiency is the adverse effect that causes the greatest concern. However, the reported incidence of renal insufficiency in standardized trials is quite low.[61] Moreover, increases in blood urea nitrogen and creatinine levels after initiation of an ACE inhibitor are often related more to the coadministration of a nonsteroidal antiinflammatory drug (which reduces vasodilating prostaglandins) or diuretics (which may produce volume depletion) than to a side effect of the ACE inhibitor per se. Finally, a minor change in BUN and creatinine levels, if they do occur, may be acceptable if there are substantive improvements in symptoms, quality of life, and life expectancy.

Adjunctive Therapy

Anticoagulants.—It has been widely accepted that patients with dilated cardiomyopathy and symptomatic heart failure should be anticoagulated in the absence of a specific contraindication.[62] This recommendation was based on retrospective analyses which indicated that the incidence of peripheral emboli in such patients was high and that 18% of patients not taking anticoagulants experienced a peripheral embolism (3.5 emboli/100 patient-years) compared to no emboli in 32 patients given chronic anticoagulant treatment.[63] However, these recommendations are being reconsidered in view of recent data from multicenter trials. In V-HeFT II, there were only 46 embolic events in 804 patients followed an average of 2.56

years.[64] In SOLVD, only 5.3% of patients experienced an embolism during 39.2 months of follow-up.[65] Furthermore, the use of anticoagulants, as directed by individual physicians, was not associated with a reduced incidence of thromboembolic complications. Therefore, since the risk of thromboembolism and the benefits of anticoagulant therapy may not be as large as once considered, recommendations for anticoagulation for patients with heart failure should be made on an individual basis.

Antiarrhythmic Agents.—Although many patients with heart failure die of progressive left ventricular dysfunction, as many as 35% to 50% of deaths are sudden, presumably due to a malignant tachyarrhythmia.[66, 67] Therefore, there has been intense interest in the use of antiarrhythmic agents to potentially reduce the risk of sudden death.

Frequent ventricular premature contractions and nonsustained ventricular tachycardia on Holter recordings are almost universal in patients with heart failure.[66, 68] These arrhythmias are likely related to a number of factors including fibrosis, wall stress, left ventricular dilatation, electrolyte imbalances, and high levels of circulating catecholamines, as well as drug therapy such as digitalis. However, the association between ventricular arrhythmias and an increased risk of sudden death has not been uniform. This lack of consistent association may be due to the fact that ventricular arrhythmias may be a nonspecific manifestation of poor left ventricular dysfunction, rather than a specific arrhythmogenic substrate.[69] Furthermore, the mechanisms of sudden death in heart failure may also be related to ischemia or bradyarrhythmias.[70]

In addition, there are a number of adverse factors associated with the use of antiarrhythmic agents in patients with heart failure. There is a definite proarrhythmic effect in a significant number of patients.[71] The pharmacokinetics of drug distribution and elimination are frequently altered due to changes in splanchnic and renal blood flow. Almost all antiarrhythmic agents can depress ventricular function and aggravate heart failure.[72] Finally, the cardiac arrhythmia suppression trial (CAST) demonstrated that type I antiarrhythmic agents, although decreasing the frequency of ventricular ectopy, were actually associated with an increase in mortality in patients who had sustained a recent myocardial infarction.[73] Based on these findings, it is prudent to avoid the routine use of conventional antiarrhythmic drug therapy in the treatment of patients with heart failure.

There are two other interventions which may have a more favorable impact in patients with heart failure. Several studies have now suggested that amiodarone may substantially reduce the frequency and complexity of asymptomatic ventricular arrhythmias as well as total mortality in patients with chronic heart failure.[74–76] Although these studies had limited enrollment, many physicians favor the use of amiodarone, often directed by electrophysiologic testing, in patients considered at high risk for sudden death due to ventricular fibrillation and ventricular tachycardia.

There is increasing experience with the implantable cardioverter defibrillators for patients with symptomatic ventricular tachycardia and ventricular fibrillation. These devices can reliably detect and terminate these lethal rhythms and have dramatically changed the expected survival curves.[77, 78] Recent improvements include the ability to pace terminate arrhythmias and nonthoracotomy lead systems. At present, these devices are only indicated for patients with heart failure who have symptomatic ventricular arrhythmias.

Beta Blockers.—Beta blockers have been traditionally contraindicated in patients with heart failure because of concerns that the negative inotropic action could result in clinically important deteriorations. This dogma has recently been challenged by laboratory and clinical studies which suggest that beta-blockers may have important short- and long-term benefits for this patient population.

It is well established that the sympathetic nervous system is activated in heart failure, as manifest by plasma norepinephrine levels, norepinephrine kinetics, and direct nerve recordings,[58, 79, 80] and that activation is highly correlated with mortality.[81] Sympathetic activation is also associated with beta receptor "down-regulation," a complex sequence of biochemical and molecular events which results in a decreased number of surface beta receptors and uncoupling of the β receptor complex.[82, 83] With this background, several clinical trials have shown that carefully administered beta blockers can result in improved ventricular function, hemodynamics, functional class, and beta receptor density.[84] Most of these studies were small and open label,[85, 86] while others were placebo-controlled trials.[87, 88] Furthermore, two small trials[89, 90] suggested that beta blocker therapy may also be associated with a significant improvement in survival. The recent Metoprolol in Dilated Cardiomyopathy Trial,[91] however, did not show an improvement in survival with metoprolol. In that study, hemodynamic deterioration was markedly reduced in patients treated with metoprolol.

Although these cumulative data are provocative, there is still insufficient evidence to recommend the routine use of beta blockers in patients with heart failure. Additional studies are currently investigating alternate beta blocking agents (e.g., carvedilol) with additional pharmacologic properties.

Physical Training.—Recent interest has focused on the potential role of physical training as a treatment option for patients with heart failure. It is now well established that skeletal muscle structure and function are abnormal in heart failure and that these abnormalities contribute to deconditioning and exercise intolerance.[92–95] Small clinical trials have now suggested that regular physical exercise is associated with improvement in symptoms, clinical status, and exercise duration.[96, 97] Based on these findings and the atrophy and deconditioning that are often associated with advanced heart failure, most physicians recommended a program of regular exercise for their patients.

Orally Administered Inotropic Agents.—The last decade witnessed an extraordinary effort to develop orally administered inotropic agents for patients with advanced heart failure. Clinical studies investigating the efficacy of phosphodiesterase inhibitors, beta-adrenergic agonists, and other agents have been reviewed elsewhere in detail.[98–100] Although the phosphodiesterase inhibitors are associated with marked hemodynamic benefit acutely, the long-term administration of milrinone is associated with increased mortality.[101, 102] This adverse effect may be specifically due to an action of the phosphodiesterase inhibitors possibly mediated by increased cyclic adenosine monophosphate (cAMP). It has been postulated that inotropic agents with mechanisms of action that are not dependent on phosphodiesterase inhibition may not have such an adverse effect. Substantial clinical benefits in terms of exercise tolerance and quality of life were recently reported with pimobendan in a 12-week trial.[103] Vesnarinone is a quinolone derivative with very weak inotropic activity, but promising clinical efficacy has been demonstrated in short-term trials.[104, 105] Recently, a large multicenter randomized placebo-controlled trial demonstrated that vesnarinone, when added to conventional therapy, reduced morbidity, improved symptoms, and reduced mortality by 62%.[106] This agent is currently under FDA review.

Patients With Refractory or Persistent Signs and Symptoms of Heart Failure—Group C

Use of Intravenous Vasodilators and Inotropic Agents in the Intensive Care Unit

The most common indication for the use of intravenous vasodilators and inotropic drugs in the intensive care unit is the treatment of decompensated heart failure and low cardiac output syndrome, characterized by fatigue, shortness of breath, hypotension, pulmonary congestion, and multiorgan failure. It is important to note that there are no standard endpoints to guide therapy. One should carefully examine the entire spectrum of clinical (mental status, peripheral perfusion, urine output), laboratory (renal function, oxygenation, liver function), and hemodynamic (cardiac output, cardiac filling pressures, arterial pressure) endpoints to measure the efficacy of intravenous vasodilators and inotropic agents.[107] It is our strong preference to use right heart catheters and arterial cannulae at least for initial hemodynamic management. Although hemodynamic estimates can frequently be inferred from the examination and laboratory tests, precise data are critical for the accurate titration to desired endpoints and in order to avoid excessive doses.

Nitroprusside and Nitroglycerin.—Vasodilator drugs are used frequently in patients with decompensated heart failure primarily for their effects on reducing the loading conditions on the left ventricle. Drugs that increase venous capacitance lead to a redistribution of intravascular volume and decrease cardiac filling pressures while drugs that increase arterial compliance will lead to an increase in cardiac output. Some of these drugs exert additional effects on regional circulations so that their overall hemodynamic effects may be more complicated than their effects on left ventricular loading alone.

Nitroprusside is the most popular intravenous vasodilator because of its balanced effects on the venous and arterial systems. Infusions may be initiated at 15 to 20 μg/min, with increases by 20 μg/min at 5- to 10-minute intervals until the desired effect is achieved. The limiting factor in infusion increments is hypotension, which may compromise myocardial perfusion. Once the desired hemodynamic response has been achieved, the effect is generally stable, and continuous infusions for 2 to 5 days are usually well tolerated. Apart from hypotension, side effects are rare and include thiocyanate toxicity and methemoglobinemia.

Nitroglycerin is used less often because its effects are predominantly limited to venous capacitance. However, nitroglycerin relaxes conduit coronary arteries and may be useful when myocardial ischemia is an important concern. Infusions are also begun at 20 μg/min with similar dosage increments until the desired effect is achieved. Side effects include headache and nausea. Additional concerns have been raised about the development of vascular tolerance during continuous intravenous infusions.

Dobutamine and Dopamine.—The beta-adrenergic agonists increase cAMP formation which results in an increased delivery of calcium to the contractile proteins. Dobutamine is the most commonly used beta agonist. Compared with dopamine and isoproterenol, the selective $beta_1$ effects of dobutamine produce a larger increase in stroke volume with a smaller chronotropic effect. Unlike dopamine, dobutamine reduces left ventricular filling pressure, probably secondary to a combination of improved left ventricular systolic performance and venodilation.[108]

Intravenous infusions of dobutamine are usually started at a dose of 2.5 μg/kg/min, with dose increments of 2.5 μg until the desired hemodynamic effect is obtained. The onset of action occurs within 2 to 3 minutes with peak effects at approximately 10 minutes. Dobutamine has a half-life of approximately 2.5 minutes and is metabolized by catechol-o-methyltransferases and excreted by the kidney. Tolerance to infusions continued for more than 72 hours has been reported. The most common adverse effects include tachycardia, hypertension and hypotension, and atrial and ventricular arrhythmias.

Dopamine has several different dose-dependent hemodynamic effects. At doses smaller than 3 to 4 μg/kg/min, renal $dopamine_1$ postsynaptic receptors are activated resulting in increased renal blood flow, diuresis, and natriuresis. At 4 to 8 μg/kg/min, $beta_1$-adrenoceptors are activated, resulting in increased contractility and cardiac output. At doses greater than 8 μg/kg/min, there is vasoconstriction due to activation of vascular $alpha_1$-receptors.

Phosphodiesterase Inhibitors.—The phosphodiesterase (PDE) inhibitors amrinone and milrinone increase inotropy by inhibiting the breakdown of intracellular cAMP. Since they have both inotropic and vasodilating actions, the hemodynamic profile is characterized by increased cardiac output and decreased filling pressures. Mean arterial pressure is not uniformly decreased because of the associated increase in cardiac output. The vasodilating activity improves hemodynamics without increasing myocardial oxygen demand, which may be of benefit in patients with ischemic cardiomyopathy.[109]

Amrinone is administered in a loading dose of 0.75 mg/kg over 2 to 3 minutes, followed by a maintenance infusion of 5 to 10 μg/kg/min. Patients may be given additional bolus injections of 0.75 mg/kg up to a total daily dose of 10 mg/kg. The normal half-life of amrinone (2.5 hours) can be markedly prolonged in patients with heart failure, thus making rapid dose titration difficult. Side effects include arrhythmias (3%), thrombocytopenia (2%), abdominal pain (2%), fever (1%), and liver function abnormalities (<1%). The recently released milrinone[110] is more potent than amrinone, so that the loading dose (50 μg/kg) and maintenance infusions (0.50 μg/kg/min) are lower. The incidence of side effects may be lower, especially with regard to thrombocytopenia.

The PDE inhibitors may be particularly useful in patients who are refractory to beta-adrenergic agonists because of beta-receptor desensitization. Since the myocardial response to cAMP is intact, it may be anticipated that the maximal response to a beta agonist can be increased by the concomitant administration of a PDE inhibitor.[111] The combination of dobutamine and amrinone or milrinone may also permit the use of lower doses of each drug, thereby limiting the severity and incidence of adverse effects that can occur when a single drug is used in high concentrations.

Devices.—Additional measures for patients with refractory heart failure include intraaortic balloon pump and left ventricular assist device. Intraaortic balloon pumping decreases afterload and increases cardiac output. The augmentation of diastolic blood pressure improves coronary perfusion, which may be helpful in patients with significant hypotension and increased left ventricular end-diastolic pressure. However, these pumps are invasive, require the use of heparin, and are associated with infections, thrombosis, and thrombocytopenia. Since they cannot be used for prolonged periods, they are generally indicated for reversible processes or for temporary support before surgery. Left ventricular assist devices are generally reserved for cardiac transplantation candidates who have low-output heart failure that is refractory to intravenous inotropic therapy and intraaortic balloon counterpulsation. These devices require thoracotomy and are associated with thrombosis, hemolysis, and serious infections. Some of the limitations may be avoided with the permanent totally implantable devices which are currently under development.

Heart Transplantation

Heart transplantation is now a well-established treatment for patients with end-stage heart failure. Since the introduction of cyclosporine in 1984, the 5-year survival rates for heart transplant recipients now average between 70% and 80% at most centers, in marked contrast to the 20% to 30% survival rates for a comparable group of patients on medical therapy.[112, 113] Moreover, heart transplant recipients report an improvement in quality of life. Although final decisions regarding individual patients are generally made by a transplant center, it is important to review patient selection criteria so that appropriate patients can be referred in a timely fashion.

At the University of Minnesota, we require that all patients being considered for heart transplantation for end-stage heart failure fulfill five criteria (Table 4).[114] All patients should have evidence of severe left ventricular systolic dysfunction with an ejection fraction less than 35%. Most patients typically have an ejection fraction less than 20%, but this criterion can include patients with mitral insufficiency. Second, patients should be receiving maximal medical treatment including digitalis, diuretics, and vasodilators. If they are not able to tolerate these drugs, there should be at least two attempts to initiate therapy. Third, patients should report refractory or intolerable symptoms that limit the activities of daily life either at work or home. This criterion is often difficult to evaluate, since many patients will change their activity patterns to avoid symptoms, but it is important that the patient independently confirm the disability. Fourth, there should be no reversible factors, such as ischemia, surgically correctable valvular lesions, or noncompliance with medication regimens and dietary sodium restriction. Finally, all patients should have an estimated 1-year survival rate of less than 50%.[115] This criterion should focus efforts on the sickest patients, i.e., those with the highest mortality risk.

Since these criteria identify a very broad population of potential candidates, we search for other clinical characteristics which either indicate a poor short-term prognosis or corroborate a poor functional capacity (Table 5). Patients who have a peak exercise oxygen consumption of <14 mL/kg/min have severe aerobic impairment and markedly decreased survival rates.[116] Elevations in plasma norepinephrine >600 pg/mL have been shown to be an important independent predictor of mortality.[81] Anecdotal experience has suggested that cachexia, day-night reversal, use of inotropic agents, and decompensations with trivial events are often associated with progressive deteriorations and represent a more urgent need for transplantation. Patients who are intolerant of vasodilators have an increased mortality risk because of the lack of survival benefit provided by vasodila-

TABLE 4.
Selection Criteria for Heart Transplantation

1. Left ventricular ejection fraction <35%
2. Maximal medical treatment—digitalis, diuretics, vasodilators
3. Refractory/intolerable symptoms
4. Lack of reversible factors
5. Expected 1-year survival <50%

TABLE 5.
Other Important Clinical Findings Which Are Associated With a Poor Short-Term Prognosis or a Poor Functional Capacity.

1. Peak oxygen consumption < 14 mL/kg/min
2. Plasma norepinephrine > 600 pg/mL
3. Cachexia, ongoing weight loss
4. Intolerance of vasodilators
5. Day-night reversal, nocturnal wakefulness
6. Need for inotropic drug support
7. Decompensations with trivial events
8. Onset of atrial fibrillation
9. Familial dilated cardiomyopathy
10. Deterioration in objective measures

tor therapy. In addition, the inability to tolerate vasodilators because of hypotension may indicate the terminal lack of cardiac reserve.

Atrial fibrillation has been reported in some but not all studies[117, 118] to indicate an increased short-term mortality risk possibly due to severe reductions in left ventricular function and left atrial distention. Patients with familial dilated cardiomyopathy may also have a higher mortality risk when compared to patients with similar reductions in left ventricular function due to other causes.[119] Finally, in cases where transplantation has been deferred because of mild symptoms, it is our practice to repeat objective measures of ventricular function, hemodynamics, and aerobic capacity at 6- to 12-month intervals. A deterioration in these measures represents another indication for transplantation.

Although refractory heart failure is the most common indication for transplantation, there are a number of other conditions which have been successfully treated with transplantation. These indications account for only a small percentage of transplants and include: (1) refractory angina pectoris in the absence of anatomy suitable for angioplasty or bypass surgery, (2) life-threatening ventricular arrhythmias that are not controlled by implantable defibrillators and/or drug therapy, (3) uncorrectable congenital heart disease, (4) hypertrophic cardiomyopathy, and (5) restrictive cardiomyopathy. Heart transplantation has also been performed for infectious endocarditis, cardiac tumors and amyloid heart disease, but the results have not been uniform.

Table 6 lists the contraindications to transplantation that are used by most transplant centers. These contraindications have been extensively re-

TABLE 6.
Contraindications to Heart Transplantation

1. Age >60–65
2. Pulmonary hypertension
3. Infection
4. Irreversible renal/hepatic dysfunction
5. Co-morbid diseases, malignancy
6. Complicated diabetes mellitus
7. Severe lung disease
8. Symptomatic cerebral or peripheral vascular disease
9. Poor compliance; psychosocial issues

vised over the past decade. In most cases, a patient will be excluded because of a combination of factors.

The rationale for any upper age limit is related to the continued shortage of donor organs since several studies have demonstrated success rates in carefully selected elderly patients that are comparable to younger individuals.[120] Previous studies have shown that pulmonary hypertension and pulmonary vasoconstriction with a resting pulmonary vascular resistance of >6 Wood units and/or a transpulmonary gradient of >15 mm Hg are associated with increased early mortality due to perioperative right ventricular failure.[121] These patients are accepted only if pharmacologic interventions reduce the pulmonary vascular resistance to less than 4 Wood units.

Patients with irreversible renal and hepatic insufficiency are also high-risk candidates because of the known renal and hepatic toxicities of cyclosporine and azathioprine.[122] In general, patients are excluded for a serum creatinine >2.5 mg/dl, creatinine clearance <50 mL/min, bilirubin >2.0 mg%, transaminases >2 to 3 times normal, or with an elevated prothrombin time in the absence of anticoagulant therapy.

Co-morbid diseases are relatively strong contraindications, because they might independently limit survival or, as with severe lung disease, independently limit functional capacity. Despite case reports of satisfactory short-term results in patients with malignancies,[123] it is still prudent to consider transplantation only if there is demonstration of medical or surgical "cure," or at least a 3- to 5-year disease-free interval. Currently, insulin-dependent diabetics are considered only in the absence of retinopathy, neuropathy, nephropathy, and peripheral or cerebral vascular disease. Patients with symptomatic cerebrovascular and peripheral vascular disease are considered high risk because of the risk of stroke, seizure, and lower extremity ischemia associated with the use of cyclosporine and prednisone.

Finally, psychosocial issues and the ability to comply with a complex medical regimen are very important factors influencing the long-term success of transplantation. However, it is difficult to predict compliance and adherence to medical programs prior to transplantation. In the absence of well-defined criteria, the optimal candidates will have sufficient motivation and cognitive function to be able to independently administer medications and follow specific instructions.

Patients With Asymptomatic Left Ventricular Dysfunction—Group A

One of the most exciting developments in the treatment of patients with heart failure is the consideration of secondary prophylaxis. In the current framework, drug therapy is prompted by signs and/or symptoms, so that patients with asymptomatic left ventricular dysfunction do not necessarily require treatment. This treatment strategy is no longer used in hypertensive patients, since many studies have shown that drug therapy can reduce, delay, and/or prevent some of the known sequelae of hypertension. It has been hypothesized that a similar strategy employing early secondary prophylaxis in patients with asymptomatic left ventricular dysfunction could also have a great impact on the inexorable progression of heart failure.

The scientific rationale for this hypothesis is based on recent data regarding ventricular remodeling. The highly complex process of myocardial dilation and hypertrophy after discrete myocardial damage has been studied extensively in animal models as well as in humans following myocardial infarction and involves myocardial cell hyperplasia, new myofibrils formed predominantly in series as well as changes in the collagen matrix.[124–127] The exact signal initiating these cellular events is not known but likely involve circulating and local neurohormonal factors, wall stress, and loading conditions. Over time, an initial myocardial insult can progress to a poorly contracting, dilated, hypertrophied ventricle and the well-known sequelae of advanced heart failure. This progressive myocardial damage can occur in the absence of additional ischemic events, although such events would likely accelerate the progression.

Extensive animal studies have demonstrated that certain drugs can prevent ventricular remodeling and improve survival. Seminal findings were reported by Pfeffer[128, 129] in a rat model of myocardial infarction induced by ligature of the left anterior descending artery. In rats with mild or moderate infarct sizes, the prophylactic use of captopril not only reduced left ventricular size but also mortality. Studies in canine models of heart failure have also shown that nitrates and converting enzyme inhibitors will reduce the expected amount of hypertrophy.[130] Our laboratory has evaluated the canine model of discrete myocardial damage produced by external electrical shock.[131] This myocardial insult produces significant increases in left ventricular volume and mass which can be blocked by a converting enzyme inhibitor or by long-acting nitrates.[132]

Two studies demonstrated that the early use of ACE inhibitors had a beneficial effect on left ventricular dilatation and function in man. Pfeffer[133] and Sharpe[134] randomized survivors of myocardial infarction who had reduced ejection fraction to either captopril or placebo. After 1 year, the captopril-treated groups had lower ventricular volumes measured by contrast ventriculography or echocardiography. The final question was whether these changes in ventricular volumes and function would also be associated with an improvement in survival. Since the death rate in these asymptomatic patients was expected to be low, this question required large multicenter trials.

The SOLVD Prevention Trial[135] was run concurrently with the Treatment Trial and utilized the same experimental design except for the restriction to patients who had a left ventricular ejection fraction ≤35% but no treatment for clinically apparent heart failure. After an average follow-up of 37.4 months, there were 334 deaths in the placebo group compared to 313 in the enalapril group. This mortality reduction approached but did not achieve statistical significance. More impressive were the highly significant reductions in the first hospitalizations for heart failure (36%) and in the onset of heart failure requiring pharmacologic therapy (37%).

The Survival and Ventricular Enlargement (SAVE) Trial was similar to SOLVD except for differences in patient election and drug intervention.[136] All participating patients had survived an acute myocardial infarction, had a left ventricular ejection fraction ≤40%, and were enrolled 3 to 16 days after the event. In addition, the intervention used in SAVE was captopril. After a mean follow-up of 3.6 years, there were 274 deaths in the placebo group (24.6%) and 228 deaths in the captopril group (20.6%) for a significant 17% reduction in all-cause mortality. Moreover, hospitalizations and the onset of symptomatic heart failure were significantly reduced in the patients randomized to captopril.

The CONSENSUS II trial study randomly assigned patients with acute myocardial infarction within 24 hours of the event to either placebo or enalaprilat followed by oral enalapril.[137] At the 6-month endpoint, survival in two groups was comparable and the study was prematurely terminated since it was unlikely that it was going to be able to demonstrate a significant improvement with enalapril. Although this study was negative, it is very likely that the follow-up was too short, since the SAVE trial demonstrated that the beneficial effects of captopril were not evident until after the first year after the myocardial infarction. Moreover, the early use of a vasodilator may be deleterious as was demonstrated with the early experience with nitroprusside.[138]

These data have provided important information regarding the modification of the progressive nature of left ventricular dysfunction and the overall mortality that is characteristic of advanced heart failure. Additional studies designed to identify the molecular bases of these changes will also likely be important for other preventive therapies. An understanding of all of these developments certainly represents an enormous challenge for physicians caring for patients with heart failure. However, this difficulty is paralleled by the opportunity to make a significant impact on the morbidity and mortality associated with heart failure.

References

1. Smith MW: Epidemiology of congestive heart failure. *Am J Cardiol* 1985; 55:3A–8A.
2. Cody RJ, Covit AB, Schaer GL, et al: Sodium and water balance in chronic congestive heart failure. *J Clin Invest* 1986; 77:1441–1452.
3. Cody RJ, Ljungman S, Covit AB et al: Regulation of glomerular filtration rate in chronic congestive heart failure. *Kid Int* 1988; 34:3613.
4. Hollenberg NK: The role of the kidney in heart failure, in Cohn JN (ed): *Drug Treatment of Heart Failure.* Secaucus, NJ, Advanced Therapeutics Communications International, 1988, pp 105–126.
5. Francis GS, Siegel RM, Goldsmith SR, et al: Acute vasoconstrictor response to intravenous furosemide in patients with chronic congestive heart failure. *Ann Int Med* 1985; 103:1–6.
6. Ikram H, Chan W, Espiner EA, et al: Haemodynamic and hormone responses to acute and chronic furosemide therapy in congestive heart failure. *Clin Sci* 1980; 59:443–449.
7. Kubo SH, Clark M, Laragh JH, et al: Identification of normal neurohormonal activity in mild congestive heart failure and stimulating effect of upright posture and diuretics. *Am J Cardiol* 1987; 60:1322–1328.
8. Lee WH, Packer M: Prognostic importance of serum sodium concentration and its modification by converting enzyme inhibition in patients with severe chronic heart failure. *Circulation* 1986; 73:257.
9. Swedberg K, Emeroth P, Kjekshus J, et al: CONSENSUS Trial Study Group: Hormones regulating cardiovascular function in patients with severe heart failure and their relation to mortality. *Circulation* 1990; 82:1730–1736.
10. The Captopril-Digoxin Multicenter Research Group: Comparative effects of therapy with captopril and digoxin in patients with mild to moderate heart failure. *JAMA* 1988; 259:539–544.
11. Brater DC: Resistance to loop diuretics: Why it happens and what to do about it. *Drugs* 1985; 30:427–443.
12. Ellison DH: The physiologic basis of diuretic synergism: Its role in treating diuretic resistance. *Ann Int Med* 1991; 114:886–894.
13. Wollam GL, Tarazi RC, Bravo EL, et al: Diuretic potency of combined hydrochlorothiazide and furosemide therapy in patients with azotemia. *Am J Med* 1982; 72:929–938.
14. Arnold SB, Byrd RC, Meister W, et al: Long-term digitalis therapy improves left ventricular function in heart failure. *N Engl J Med* 1980; 303:1443–1448.
15. Ware JA, Snow E, Luchi JM, et al: Effect of digoxin on ejection fraction in elderly patients with congestive heart failure. *J Am Geriatr Soc* 1984; 32:631–635.
16. Ferguson DW, Berg WJ, Sanders JS, et al: Sympathoinhibitory responses to digitalis glycosides in heart failure patients. Direct evidence from sympathetic neural recordings. *Circulation* 1989; 80:65–77.
17. Gheorghiade M, Zarowitz BJ: Review of randomized trials of digoxin therapy in patients with chronic heart failure. *Am J Cardiol* 1992; 69:48G–63G.

18. Smith TW: Should digoxin be the drug of first choice after diuretics in chronic congestive heart failure? II. Protagonists viewpoint. *J Am Coll Cardiol* 1988; 12:267-271.
19. Dobbs SM, Kenyon WL, Dobbs RJ: Maintenance digoxin after an episode of heart failure: Placebo-controlled trial in outpatients. *Br Med J* 1977; 1:749–752.
20. Lee DC, Johnson RA, Bingham JB, et al: Heart failure in outpatients: A randomized trial of digoxin versus placebo. *N Engl J Med* 1982; 306:699–705.
21. Guyatt GH, Sullivan MJJ, Fallen EL, et al: A controlled trial of digoxin in congestive heart failure. *Am J Cardiol* 1988; 61:371–375.
22. Young JB, Uretsky BF, Shahidi FE, et al: on behalf of the PROVED Study Investigators: Multicenter, double-blind, placebo controlled randomized withdrawal trial of the efficacy and safety of digoxin in patients with mild to moderate chronic heart failure not treated with converting enzyme inhibitors (abstract). *J Am Coll Cardiol* 1992; 19:259.
23. DiBianco R, Shebetai R, Kostuk W, et al: Milrinone Multicenter Trial Group. A comparison of oral milrinone, digoxin, and their combination in the treatment of patients with chronic heart failure. *N Engl J Med* 1989; 320:677–683.
24. Alicandri C, Fariello R, Boni E, et al: Captopril versus digoxin in mild-moderate chronic heart failure: A crossover study. *J Cardiovasc Pharmacol* 1987; 9:S61–S67.
25. Beaune J, for the Enalapril Versus Digoxin French Multicenter Study Group: Comparison of enalapril versus digoxin for congestive heart failure. *Am J Cardiol* 1989; 63:22D–25D.
26. Packer M, Gheorghiade M, Young JB, et al: on behalf of the RADIANCE Study: Randomized, double blind, placebo controlled withdrawal study of digoxin in patients with chronic heart failure treated with converting enzyme inhibitors. *J Am Coll Cardiol* 1992; 19:260A (abstract).
27. Moss AJ, Davis HT, Conrad DL, et al: Digitalis associated cardiac mortality after myocardial infarction. *Circulation* 1981; 64:1150–1156.
28. Bigger JT, Fleiss JL, Rolnitsky LA, et al: Effect of digitalis treatment on survival after acute myocardial infarction. *Am J Cardiol* 1985; 55:623–630.
29. Muller JE, Turi ZG, Stone PH, et al and the MILIS Study Group: Digoxin therapy and mortality following myocardial infarction: Experience in the MILIS study. *N Engl J Med* 1986; 314:265–271.
30. Doherty JE. Use of digitalis and diuretics in the treatment of heart failure, in Cohn JN (ed): *Drug Treatment of Heart Failure.* Secaucus, NJ, Advanced Therapeutics Communications International, 1988, pp 127–146.
31. Cohn JN, Franciosa JA: Vasodilator therapy of cardiac failure. *N Engl J Med* 1977; 297:27–31, 254–258.
32. Packer M: Vasodilator and inotropic drugs in the treatment of chronic heart failure: Distinguishing hype from hope. *J Am Coll Cardiol* 1988; 12:1299–1317.
33. Chatterjee K: Vasodilator therapy for heart failure, in Cohn JN (ed): *Drug Treatment of Heart Failure.* Secaucus, NJ, Advanced Therapeutics Communications International, 1988, pp 199–226.
34. Parmley WE: Angiotensin converting enzyme inhibitors in the treatment of heart failure. in Cohn JN (ed): *Drug Treatment of Heart Failure.* Secaucus, NJ, Advanced Therapeutics Communications International, 1988, pp 227–250.

35. Cohn JN, Archibald DG, Ziesche S, et al: Effect of vasodilator therapy on mortality in chronic congestive heart failure. Results of a Veterans Administration Cooperative Study. *N Engl J Med* 1986; 314:1547–1552.
36. Haas GJ, Binkley PF, Carpenter JA, et al: Central and regional hemodynamic effects of flosequinan for congestive heart failure. *Am J Cardiol* 1989; 63:1354–1359.
37. Falotico R, Haertlein BJ, Lakas-Weiss CS, et al: Positive-inotropic and hemodynamic properties of flosequinan, a new vasodilator, and a sulphone metabolite. *J Cardiovasc Pharmacol* 1989; 14:412–418.
38. Burstein S, Semigran MJ, Dec GW, et al: Positive inotropic and lusitropic effects of intravenous flosequinan in patients with heart failure. *J Am Coll Cardiol* 1992; 20:822–829.
39. Roden RL, Bristow MR, Krall J, et al: Inotropic action of flosequinan in isolated human heart: Evidence for phosphodiesterase inhibition at high concentrations (abstract). *Circulation* 1992; 86:I–645.
40. Pinsky DJ, Wilson PB, Ahern D, et al: Flosequinan improves symptoms and excessive tolerance in heart failure. Results of placebo controlled trial (abstract). *Circulation* 9190; 82:III–322.
41. Massie BM, Berk MR, Brozena S, et al for the FACET investigators: Can further benefit be achieved by adding a vasodilator to triple therapy in CHF: Results of the flosequinan-ACE inhibitor trial (FACET) (abstract)? *Circulation* 1992; 86:I–645.
42. Packer M, Pitt B, on behalf of the REFLECT I and REFLECT II Study Groups: Efficacy of flosequinan in patients with heart failure who are withdrawn from therapy with converting-enzyme inhibitors: A double-blind controlled study (abstract). *Circulation* 1992; 86:I–644.
43. Colucci WS: Usefulness of calcium antagonists for congestive heart failure. *Am J Cardiol* 1987; 59:52B–58B.
44. Prida XE, Kubo SH, Laragh JH, et al: Evaluation of calcium-mediated vasoconstriction in chronic congestive heart failure. *Am J Med* 1983; 75:795–800.
45. Leier CV, Patrick TJ, Hermiller J, et al: Nifedipine in congestive heart failure: Effects on resting and exercise hemodynamics and regional blood flow. *Am Heart J* 1984; 108:1461–1468.
46. Agostoni PG, DeCesare N, Doria E, et al: Afterload reduction: A comparison of captopril and nifedipine in dilated cardiomyopathy. *Br Heart J* 1986; 55:391–399.
47. Packer M: Pathophysiological mechanisms underlying the adverse effects of calcium channel-blocking drugs in patients with chronic heart failure. *Circulation* 1989; 80(suppl IV):IV–59–IV–67.
48. Goldstein RE, Boccuzzi SJ, Cruess D, et al: the Adverse Experience Committee, and the Multicenter Diltiazem Postinfarction Research Group. Diltiazem increases late-onset congestive heart failure in postinfarction patients with early reduction in ejection fraction. *Circulation* 1991; 83:52–60.
49. Cody RJ, Laragh JH: The renin angiotensin aldosterone system in chronic heart failure: Pathophysiology and implications for treatment, in Cohn JN (ed): *Drug Treatment of Heart Failure*. Secaucus, NJ, Advanced Therapeutics Communications International, 1988, pp 79–104.
50. Dzau VJ: Circulating versus local renin angiotensin system in cardiovascular homeostasis. *Circulation* 1988; 77(suppl I):I–4–I–13.

51. Vanhoutte PM: Endothelium and control of vascular function: State of the art lecture. *Hypertension* 1986; 12:797–806.
52. Cohn JN: Current therapy of the failing heart. *Circulation* 1988; 78:1099–1107.
53. Parmley WW: Pathophysiology and current therapy of congestive heart failure. *J Am Coll Cardiol* 1989; 13:771–785.
54. The CONSENSUS Trial Study Group: Effects of enalapril on mortality in severe congestive heart failure. Results of the Cooperative North Scandinavian Enalapril Survival Study (CONSENSUS). *N Engl J Med* 1987; 316:1429–1435.
55. Cohn JN, Johnson G, Ziesche S, et al: A comparison of enalapril with hydralazine-isosorbide dinitrate in the treatment of chronic congestive heart failure. *N Engl J Med* 1991; 325:303–310.
56. The SOLVD Investigators: Effect of enalapril on survival in patients with reduced left ventricular ejection fractions and congestive heart failure. *N Engl J Med* 1991; 325:293–302.
57. Kubo SH, Cody RJ: Clinical and hemodynamic aspects of angiotensin converting enzyme inhibition for the management of congestive heart failure, in Fergusion RK, Vlasses PH (eds): *The Clinical Applications of the Angiotensin Converting Enzyme Inhibitors.* Mt. Kisco, NY, Futura Publishing Co, 1987, pp 87–136.
58. Kubo SH: Neurohormonal and activation and the response to converting enzyme inhibitors in congestive heart failure. *Circulation* 1990; 81(suppl III):III–107–114.
59. Levine TB, Franciosa JA, Vrobel T, et al: Hyponatremia as a marker for high renin heart failure. *Br Heart J* 1982; 47:161–166.
60. Cody RJ, Covit AB, Schaer GL, et al: Sodium and water balance in chronic congestive heart failure. *J Clin Invest* 1986; 77:1441–1452.
61. Ljungman S, Kjekshus J, Swedberg K, for the CONSENSUS Trial Group: Renal function in severe congestive heart failure during treatment with enalapril. *Am J Cardiol* 1992; 70:479–487.
62. Meltzer RS, Visser CA, Fuster V: Intracardiac thrombi and systemic embolization. *Ann Int Med* 1986; 104:689–698.
63. Fuster V, Gersch BJ, Giroliani ER, et al: The natural history of idiopathic dilated cardiomyopathy. *Am J Cardiol* 1981; 47:525–531.
64. Dunkman WB, Johnson GR, Carson PE, et al and the VA Cooperative Study Group: Incidence of thromboembolic events in congestive heart failure: Results from V-HeFT II (abstract). *Circulation* 1992; 86:I–252.
65. Cohn JN, Benedict CR, LeJemtel TH, et al, SOLVD Investigators: Risk of thromboembolism in left ventricular dysfunction: SOLVD (abstract). *Circulation* 1992; 86:I–252.
66. Francis GS: Should asymptomatic ventricular arrhythmias in patients with congestive heart failure be treated with antiarrhythmic drugs? *J Am Coll Cardiol* 1988; 12:274–283.
67. Podrid PJ, Fogel RI, Fuchs TT: Ventricular arrhythmia in congestive heart failure. *Am J Cardiol* 1992; 69:82G–98G.
68. Holmes J, Kubo SH, Cody RJ, et al: Arrhythmias in ischemic and nonischemic dilated cardiomyopathy: Prediction of mortality by ambulatory electrocardiography. *Am J Cardiol* 1985; 55:146–151.
69. Packer M: Lack of relation between ventricular arrhythmias and sudden

death in patients with chronic heart failure. *Circulation* 1992; 85(suppl I):I–50–I–56.
70. Luu M, Stevenson WG, Stevenson LW, et al: Diverse mechanisms of unexpected cardiac arrest in advanced heart failure. *Circulation* 1989; 80:1675–1680.
71. Velebit V, Podrid P, Lown B, et al: Aggravation and provocation of ventricular arrhythmias by antiarrhythmic drugs. *Circulation* 1982; 65:886–894.
72. Ravid S, Podrid PJ, Lampert S, et al: Congestive heart failure induced by six of the newer antiarrhythmic drugs. *J Am Coll Cardiol* 1989; 14:1326–1330.
73. Echt DS, Liebson PR, Mitchell LB, et al and the CAST Investigators: Mortality and morbidity in patients receiving encainide, flecainide, or placebo. The Cardiac Arrhythmia Suppression Trial. *N Engl J Med* 1991; 324:781–788.
74. Cleland JGF, Dargie HJ, Findlay IN, et al: Clinical, haemodynamic and antiarrhythmic effects of long term treatment with amiodarone of patients in heart failure. *Br Heart J* 1987; 57:436–445.
75. Neri R, Mestroni L, Salvi A, et al: Ventricular arrhythmias in dilated cardiomyopathy: Efficacy of amiodarone. *Am Heart J* 1987; 113:707–715.
76. Dargie HJ, Cleland JGF, Leckie BJ, et al: Relation of arrhythmias and electrolyte abnormalities to survival in patients with severe chronic heart failure. *Circulation* 1987; 75(suppl IV):98–107.
77. Winkle RA, Mead RH, Ruder MA, et al: Long-term outcome with the automatic implantable cardioverter-defibrillator. *J Am Coll Cardiol* 1989; 13:1353–1361.
78. Tchou PJ, Kadri N, Anderzin J, et al: Automatic implantable cardioverter defibrillators and survival of patients with left ventricular dysfunction and malignant ventricular arrhythmias. *Am Int Med* 1988; 109:529–534.
79. Ferguson DW, Berg WJ, Sanders JS: Clinical and hemodynamic correlates of sympathetic nerve activity in normal humans and patients with heart failure: Evidence from direct microneurographic recordings. *J Am Coll Cardiol* 1990; 16:1125–1134.
80. Hasking GJ, Esler MD, Jennings GL, et al: Norepinephrine spillover to plasma in patients with congestive heart failure: Evidence of increased overall and cardiorenal sympathetic nervous activity. *Circulation* 1986; 73:615–621.
81. Conn JN, Levine TB, Olivari MT, et al: Plasma norepinephrine as a guide to prognosis in patients with chronic congestive heart failure. *N Engl J Med* 1984; 311:819–823.
82. Fowler MB, Laser JA, Hopkins GL, et al: Assessment of the β-adrenergic receptor pathway in the intact failing human heart: Progressive receptor down-regulation and subsensitivity to agonist response. *Circulation* 1986; 74:1290–1302.
83. Colucci WS, Alexander RW, Williams GH, et al: Decreased lymphocyte beta-adrenergic receptor density in patients with heart failure and tolerance to the beta-adrenergic agonist pirbuterol. *N Engl J Med* 1981; 305:185–190.
84. Eichhorn EJ: The paradox of β-adrenergic blockade for the management of congestive heart failure. *Am J Med* 1992; 92:527–533.
85. Waagstein F, Hjalmarson A, Varnauskas E, et al: Effect of chronic beta-adrenergic receptor blockade in congestive cardiomyopathy. *Br Heart J* 1975; 37:1022–1036.
86. Heilbrunn SM, Shah P, Bristow MR, et al: Increased β-receptor density and improved hemodynamic response to catecholamine stimulation during long-term metoprolol therapy in heart failure from dilated cardiomyopathy. *Circulation* 1989; 79:483–490.

87. Engelmeier RS, O'Connell JB, Walsh R, et al: Improvement in symptoms and exercise tolerance by metoprolol in patients with dilated cardiomyopathy: A double-blind, randomized, placebo-controlled trial. *Circulation* 1985; 72:536–546.
88. Gilbert EM, Anderson JL, Deitchman D: Chronic β-blocker-vasodilator therapy improves cardiac function in idiopathic dilated cardiomyopathy: A double-blind, randomized study of bucindolol versus placebo. *Am J Med* 1990; 88:223–229.
89. Swedberg K, Waagstein F, Hjalmarson A, et al: Prolongation of survival in congestive cardiomyopathy by beta receptor blockade. *Lancet* 1979; 1:1374–1376.
90. Anderson JL, Lutz JR, Gilbert EM, et al: A randomized trial of low-dose beta-blockade therapy for idiopathic dilated cardiomyopathy. *Am J Cardiol* 1985; 55:471–475.
91. The MDC Trial Study Group: Metoprolol in dilated cardiomyopathy. Multicenter randomized placebo-controlled trial (abstract). *Circulation* 1992; 86:I–118.
92. Sullivan MJ, Green HJ, Cobb FR: Skeletal muscle biochemistry and histology in ambulatory patients with long-term heart failure. *Circulation* 1990; 81:518–527.
93. Massie BM, Conway M, Yonge R, et al: ^{31}P Nuclear magnetic resonance evidence of abnormal skeletal muscle metabolism in patients with congestive heart failure. *Am J Cardiol* 1987; 60:309–315.
94. Drexler H, Riede U, Münzel T, et al: Alterations of skeletal muscle in chronic heart failure. *Circulation* 1992; 85:1751–1759.
95. Buller NP, Jones D, Poole-Wilson PA: Direct measurement of skeletal muscle fatigue in patients with chronic heart failure. *Br Heart J* 1991; 65:20–24.
96. Sullivan MJ, Higginbotham MB, Cobb FR: Exercise training in patients with chronic heart failure delays ventilatory anaerobic threshold and improves submaximal exercise performance. *Circulation* 1989; 79:324–329.
97. Adamopoulos S, Coats AJS, Brunotte F, et al: Physical training improves skeletal muscle metabolism in patients with chronic heart failure. *J Am Coll Cardiol* 1993; 21:1101–1106.
98. Colucci WS, Wright RF, Braunwald E: New positive inotropic agents in the treatment of congestive heart failure. Mechanisms of action and recent clinical developments. *N Engl J Med* 1986; Jan:290–299, 349–358.
99. Hood WB: Controlled and uncontrolled studies of phosphodiesterase III inhibitors in contemporary cardiovascular medicine. *Am J Cardiol* 1989; 63:46A–53A.
100. DiBianco R, Shabetai R, Kostuk W, et al for the Milrinone Multicenter Trial Group: A comparison of oral milrinone, digoxin, and their combination in the treatment of patients with chronic heart failure. *N Engl J Med* 1989; 320:677–683.
101. Packer M, Carver JR, Rodeheffer RJ, et al for the PROMISE Study Research Group. Effect of oral milrinone on mortality in severe chronic heart failure. *N Engl J Med* 1991; 325:1468–1475.
102. Packer M: Effect of phosphodiesterase inhibitors on survival of patients with chronic congestive heart failure. *Am J Cardiol* 1989; 63:41A–45A.
103. Kubo SH, Gollub S, Bourge R, et al for the Pimobendan Multicenter Research Group: Beneficial effects of pimobendan on exercise tolerance and quality of life in patients with heart failure. Results of a multicenter trial. *Circulation* 1992; 85:942–949.

104. Kubo SH, Rector TS, Strobeck JE, et al: OPC-8212 in the treatment of congestive heart failure: Results of a pilot study. *Cardiovasc Drugs and Ther* 1988; 2:653–660.
105. Feldman AM, Baughman KL, Lee WK, et al: Usefulness of OPC-8212, a quinolinone derivative, for chronic congestive heart failure in patients with ischemic heart disease or idiopathic dilated cardiomyopathy. *Am J Cardiol* 1991; 68:1203–1210.
106. Feldman AM, Bristow MR, Parmley WW, et al for the OPC-8212 investigators and coordinators: Result of a multi-center study of OPC-8212 in chronic congestive heart failure. *Circulation* 1992; 86(suppl I):I–374.
107. Bank AJ, Kubo SH: Congestive heart failure: Inotropic agents, in Parillo JE (ed): *Current Therapy in Critical Care Medicine*. Philadelphia, BC Decker, Inc, 1991, pp 92–96.
108. Leier CV, Unverferth DV: Dobutamine. *Ann Intern Med* 1983; 99:490–496.
109. Colucci WS, Wright RF, Braunwald E: New positive inotropic agents in the treatment of congestive heart failure. *N Engl J Med* 1986; 314:290–299.
110. Anderson JL, Baim DS, Fein SA, et al. for the Milrinone Investigators and associates: Efficacy and safety of sustained (48 hour) intravenous infusions of milrinone in patients with severe congestive heart failure: A multicenter study. *J Am Coll Cardiol* 1987; 9:711–722.
111. Gage J, Rutman H, Lucido D, et al: Additive effects of dobutamine and amrinone on myocardial contractility and ventricular performance in patients with severe heart failure. *Circulation* 1986; 74:367–373.
112. Kaye MP: The registry of the International Society for Heart and Lung Transplantation: Ninth official report—1992. *J Heart Lung Transp* 1992; 11:599–606.
113. O'Connell JB, Bourge RC, Costanzo-Nordin MR, et al: Cardiac transplantation: Recipient selection, donor procurement, and medical follow-up. A statement for health professionals from the Committee on Cardiac Transplantation of the Council on Clinical Cardiology, American Heart Association. *Circulation* 1992; 86:1061–1079.
114. Kubo SH, Ormaza S, Francis GS, et al: Trends in patient selection for heart transplantation. *J Am Col Cardiol* 1993; 21:975–981.
115. Francis GS, Kubo SH. Prognostic factors affecting diagnosis and treatment of congestive heart failure. *Curr Probl Card* 1989; 14:631–671.
116. Mancini DM, Eisen H, Kussmaul W, et al: Value of peak exercise oxygen consumption for optimal timing of cardiac transplantation in ambulatory patients with heart failure. *Circulation* 1991; 83:778–786.
117. Middlekauff HR, Stevenson WG, Stevenson LW, et al: Adverse prognosis of atrial fibrillation in advanced heart failure: A study of 390 patients (abstract). *J Am Col Cardiol* 1991; 17:87.
118. Carson P, Fletcher R, Johnson G, et al and the V-HeFT I Study Group: Atrial fibrillation does not decrease survival in congestive heart failure (abstract). *J Am Coll Cardiol* 1991; 87:90.
119. Valantine HA, Hunt SA, Fowler MB, et al: Frequency of familial nature of dilated cardiomyopathy and usefulness of cardiac transplantation in this subset. *Am J Cardiol* 1989; 959–963.
120. Olivari MT, Antolick A, Kaye MP, et al: Heart transplantation in elderly patients. *J Heart Transp* 1988; 7:258–264.
121. Erickson KW, Costanzo-Nordin MR, O'Sullivan J, et al: Influence of preoperative transpulmonary gradient on late mortality after orthotopic heart transplantation. *J Heart Trans* 1990; 9:526–537.

122. Miller LW: Long-term complications of cardiac transplantation. *Prog Cardiovasc Dis* 1991; 33:229–282.
123. Edwards BS, Hunt SA, Fowler MB, et al: Cardiac transplantation in patients with pre-existing neoplastic diseases. *Am J Cardiol* 1990; 65:501–504.
124. Francis GS, McDonald KM: Left ventricular hypertrophy: An initial response to myocardial injury. *Am J Cardiol* 1992; 69:3G–9G.
125. Olivetti G, Capasso JM, Meggs LG, et al: Cellular basis of chronic ventricular remodeling after myocardial infarction in rats. *Circ Res* 1991; 68:856–869.
126. McKay RG, Pfeffer MA, Pasternak RC, et al: Left ventricular remodeling following myocardial infarction: A corollary to infarct expansion. *Circulation* 1986; 74:693–702.
127. Weber KT, Pick R, Silver MA, et al: Fibrillar collagen and remodeling of dilated canine left ventricle. *Circulation* 1990; 82:1387–1401.
128. Pfeffer MA, Braunwald E: Ventricular remodeling after myocardial infarction. Experimental observations and clinical implications. *Circulation* 1990; 81:1161–1172.
129. Pfeffer MA, Pfeffer JM, Steinberg C, et al: Survival after an experimental myocardial infarction: Beneficial effects of long-term therapy with captopril. *Circulation* 1985; 72:406–412.
130. Judgutt BI, Warnica JW: Intravenous nitroglycerin therapy to limit myocardial infarct size, expansion and complications: Effect of timing, dosage, and infarct location. *Circulation* 1988; 78:906–919.
131. McDonald KM, Francis GS, Carlyle PF, et al: Hemodynamic, left ventricular structural and hormonal changes after discrete myocardial damage in the dog. *J Am Coll Cardiol* 1992; 19:460–467.
132. McDonald K, Francis GS, Matthews J, et al: Long-term oral nitrate therapy prevents chronic ventricular remodeling in the dog. *J Am Coll Cardiol* 1993; 21:514–522.
133. Pfeffer MA, Lamas GA, Vaughan DE, et al: Effect of captopril on progressive ventricular dilatation after anterior myocardial infarction. *N Engl J Med* 1988; 319:80–86.
134. Sharpe N, Smith H, Murphy J, et al: Treatment of patients with symptomless left ventricular dysfunction after myocardial infarction. *Lancet* 1988; 1:255–259.
135. The SOLVD Investigators: Effect of enalapril on mortality and the development of heart failure in asymptomtaic patients with reduced left ventricular ejection fractions. *N Engl J Med* 1992; 327:685–691.
136. Pfeffer MA, Braunwald E, Moye LA, et al. on behalf of the SAVE Investigators: Effect of captopril on mortality and morbidity in patients with left ventricular dysfunction after myocardial infarction. Results of the survival and ventricular enlargement trial. *N Engl J Med* 1992: 327:669–677.
137. Swedberg K, Held P, Kjekshus J, et al. on behalf of the CONSENSUS II Study Group: Effects of the early administration of enalapril on mortality in patients with acute myocardial infarction. Results of the Cooperative New Scandinavian Enalapril Survival Study II (CONSENSUS II). *N Engl J Med* 1992; 327:678–684.
138. Cohn JN, Franciosa JA, Francis GS, et al: Effect of short-term infusion of sodium nitroprusside on mortality rate in acute myocardial infarction complicated by left ventricular failure: Results of a Veterans Administration Cooperative Study. *N Engl J Med* 1982; 306:1129–1135.

Obstructive Sleep Apnea

Allan I. Pack, M.B., Ch.B., Ph.D.

Professor of Medicine, Pulmonary and Critical Care Division, Director, Center for Sleep and Respiratory Neurobiology, University of Pennsylvania Medical Center, Philadelphia, Pennsylvania

Obstructive sleep apnea (OSA) is increasingly recognized as an extremely common condition.[1] It is a disease that is associated with significant morbidity. This morbidity occurs largely in two domains: (1) impact on daytime function with excessive daytime sleepiness and consequent increased risk of accidents, and (2) cardiovascular complications. Thus, sleep apnea is a major health problem.[2] It is important that physicians consider the disease in many different diagnostic situations. A relatively brief history is helpful in determining whether further investigation is warranted. As part of this history, the physician should ask about snoring. Habitual snoring, i.e., snoring every night or on several nights/weeks, is extremely common in patients with apnea. Not all snorers, however, have sleep apnea. Other complaints that should be inquired about are witnessed apneas from the bed partner and nocturnal awakenings. Patients may report waking up at night but usually they do not know why; they may, on occasion, report waking up snorting or gasping. Patients with obstructive sleep apnea will also report failing to feel refreshed in the morning when they awaken and feeling excessively sleepy during the day. The degree of sleepiness varies with the severity of the disease. Patients with mild disease report falling asleep in passive situations, e.g., watching TV in the evenings, although in other situations they will not fall asleep inappropriately. Patients with severe disease on the other hand will fall asleep in various active situations, e.g., in conversations, on the telephone, driving, etc. A brief standardized questionnaire for sleepiness, the Epworth Sleepiness Scale, has been validated; it allows a score to be assigned to the degree of sleepiness.[3] The questionnaire is simple to administer. More detailed questionnaires specifically for obstructive sleep apnea have also been developed.[4–6] The responses to these questionnaires are not sufficiently specific or sensitive for a diagnosis to be made based on the results.[5] But the results of questionnaires can be used to calculate a likelihood ratio that obstructive sleep apnea is present.[6]

Given the relative simplicity of the clinical history, and the high prevalence of disease that is discussed more fully in a later section (Prevalence of Obstructive Sleep Apnea), this history should be taken in a variety of clinical situations. These include the following: a routine physical examination; preoperative assessment of patients; evaluation of patients with obesity, since obesity is an important risk factor for the disease[1]; evaluation of patients with hypertension, since, as discussed later, hypertension and obstructive sleep apnea may be associated; and evaluation of patients with nocturnal angina, or those who have had acute cardiovascular events such as stroke, particularly if they occur during the night or early morning hours.

In this contribution, I provide a review of recent information about the diagnosis, pathogenesis, and treatment of this common disorder.

Varieties of Disease and Definitions

Obstructive sleep apnea syndrome is a disorder which results from recurrent decrements in breathing during sleep as a result of obstruction of the upper airway. An apnea is said to be present when there is a cessation of breathing for longer than 10 seconds. It is considered obstructive when there is absence of airflow but continuing respiratory effort; central, when both airflow and respiratory effort cease; and mixed, when there is an initial period of central apnea that becomes obstructive within the same episode. In general, obstructive and mixed apneas are considered together and their occurrence results in the disease obstructive sleep apnea. It is this disease which is discussed here. There are previous reviews about central sleep apnea to which the interested reader is referred.[7,8]

In the 1970s it was suggested that obstructive sleep apnea syndrome occurred when more than five apneas, as defined previously, occurred per hour of sleep.[9] This threshold was based on a study of a relatively small sample of healthy adults, all of whom had less than this frequency of apneas during sleep. But when this criterion is applied to other age groups, in particular the elderly, staggering prevalence rates are found (30% to 50%).[10,11] Thus, this criterion has been criticized.[12,13]

More recently it has been recognized that apneas do not need to occur for the clinical features of the disease to be present. Hypopneas can produce the same consequences.[14] A hypopnea is a decrement in breathing that leads to desaturation and arousal from sleep. (An arousal is a sudden change in sleep state to a lighter level. Recurrent arousals result in sleep fragmentation and contribute to the excessive daytime sleepiness of the disease.) The precise definition of hypopnea varies in different laboratories and reports. This variation relates largely to the magnitude of the decrement in airflow used in the definition. Gould et al.[14] showed that defining hypopneas on the basis of reductions in thoracoabdominal motion of at least 50% for greater than 10 seconds gives the best agreement with the number of episodes of desaturation with at least a 4% fall in oxygen saturation (Sa_{O_2}) and with the frequency of arousals. However, to evaluate desaturation episodes and arousals to then determine the decrement in airflow to be used in the definition is an indirect approach. Thus, an alternative definition is to consider a hypopnea as an episode where there is a clear decrement in respiratory airflow for 10 seconds or more that is associated with a 4% fall in oxygen saturation and/or is terminated by an arousal. The recognition that the same clinical consequences can result from recurrent hypopneas, without the presence of apneas, has led to use of the term "sleep hypopnea syndrome."[14]

The number of apneas plus hypopneas that need to occur before a definite abnormality is present is not precisely known. Studies of a small sample (n = 33) of normal subjects (ages 21 to 67 years) without sleep complaints show that all of them had fewer than 15 apneas plus hypopneas per hour of sleep.[14] This metric (number of apneas plus hypopneas per hour of sleep) is called the apnea/hypopnea index (AHI) or respiratory disturbance index (RDI). It has been proposed[14] that the definition of the sleep hypopnea syndrome should be the occurrence of at least 15 apneas plus hypopneas per hour of sleep when combined with two or more clinical features. The features included are excessive daytime sleepiness, loud snoring, disturbed sleep, and secondary polycythemia or ankle swelling without other known causes. This definition is now commonly used.

Defining abnormality has recently been further complicated by the proposal that neither apneas nor hypopneas are necessary for the clinical consequences to occur.[15, 16] Patients have been observed with a pattern of recurrent crescendo snoring, i.e., increases in intensity of snoring from breath to breath, that lead to recurrent arousals even in the absence of apnea or a major decrement in respiratory airflow (hypopnea) (Fig 1).[15, 16] With arousal, snoring declines but the pattern of snoring then reappears as the subject falls back to sleep. This phenomenon has been called the "Upper Airway Resistance Syndrome."[16] The diagnostic criteria for this syndrome are not fully established. There are patients with these features who have excessive daytime sleepiness that responds to treatment with, for example, nasal continuous positive airway pressure.[15, 16] There are, however, patients with this pattern of snoring who do not show objective improvements in sleepiness when they are treated for the disorder.[15] Thus, an important component of making this diagnosis is the demonstration that treatment of the disease with, for example, nasal continuous positive airway pressure, abolishes symptoms including excessive daytime sleepiness and improves objectively measured daytime sleepiness.

Three different syndromes have been described—sleep apnea syndrome, sleep hypopnea syndrome, and upper airway resistance syndrome. The major difference between them is the magnitude of the sleep-related change in respiration. All of these phenomena lead to recurrent arousals with sleep fragmentation. The magnitude of the resulting falls in oxygen, i.e., desaturation, will vary, however, with these different types of abnormality. Patients could demonstrate these different types of abnormality either within a single night or on different nights. There is night-to-night variability in the magnitude of the abnormality present,[17–19] particularly in those with milder forms of the disease.[17] This night-to-night variability can be clinically important. In particular, a single negative sleep study in a patient with a strong pretest suspicion of disease should not rule out the diagnosis.[20]

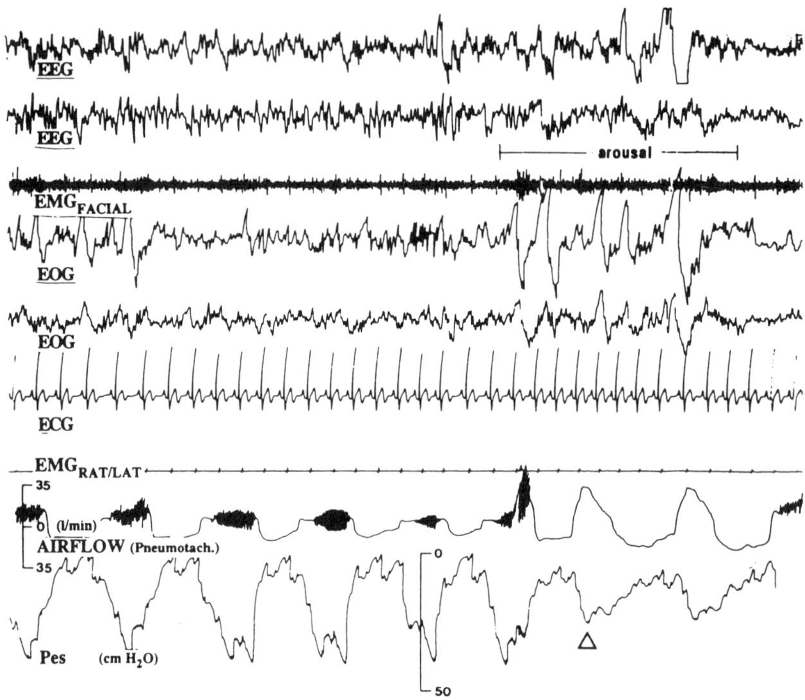

FIG 1.
Example of an episode associated with upper airway resistance syndrome. The figure shows from the top to bottom: 2 EEG traces, 1 EMG, 2 traces of EOG, 1 EKG, another EMG trace, airflow and esophageal pressure. The airflow trace shows the high frequency vibration associated with snoring. With arousal (marked), there is a reduction in upper airway resistance. There is an associated increase in airflow, abolition of snoring, and reduction and esophageal pressure (at *arrow* below bottom trace). In the last part of the record, snoring reappears. (Adapted from Guilleminault C, Stoohs R, Duncan S: Snoring. I. Daytime sleepiness in regular heavy snorers. *Chest* 1991; 99:40–48. Used by permission.)

Pathogenesis of Obstructive Sleep Apnea

No matter which type of abnormality is present, the underlying mechanism is likely to be similar, albeit varying in degree. A convenient way of thinking about the pathogenesis of obstructive sleep apnea is to consider that it has both an anatomical component, whereby the upper airway is reduced in size, and a neural component that allows airway collapse to occur during sleep.

Anatomical Component

In certain patients with this disease, the anatomical component is obvious; this includes patients with micrognathia,[21] acromegaly,[22, 23] or Down's syndrome.[24] In many patients obesity,[1] or more specifically increased collar size,[25, 26] is a predisposing factor. When all patients with the disease are studied in wakefulness using imaging techniques, certain abnormalities are found. The majority of studies,[27–31] although not all,[32] show that the airway of the sleep apneic is smaller than those in control subjects. This upper airway narrowing is predominantly in the lateral dimension. Thus, the airway of the apneic patient is more circular. In the normal individual it is elliptical with the long axis in the lateral dimension (Fig 2).[33, 34] The basis for this lateral narrowing is unknown. One theory is that in obese individuals with obstructive apnea, there is external compression of the lateral walls of the pharynx.[35–37] Parapharyngeal fat pads are adjacent to the lateral pharyngeal walls, and their size is increased in patients with sleep apnea.[36] (See location of parapharyngeal fats pads in Fig 3). It is somewhat difficult to conceive that these small structures could compress the muscular walls of the pharynx. Sleep apneics may be more susceptible to this effect, however, since the area enclosed by their mandibles is smaller than in normals.[37] Recent data suggest that the thickness of the lateral pharyngeal walls is increased in apneics leading to a compromise in airway size.[38] The basis for this increase in the thickness of these walls is unknown.

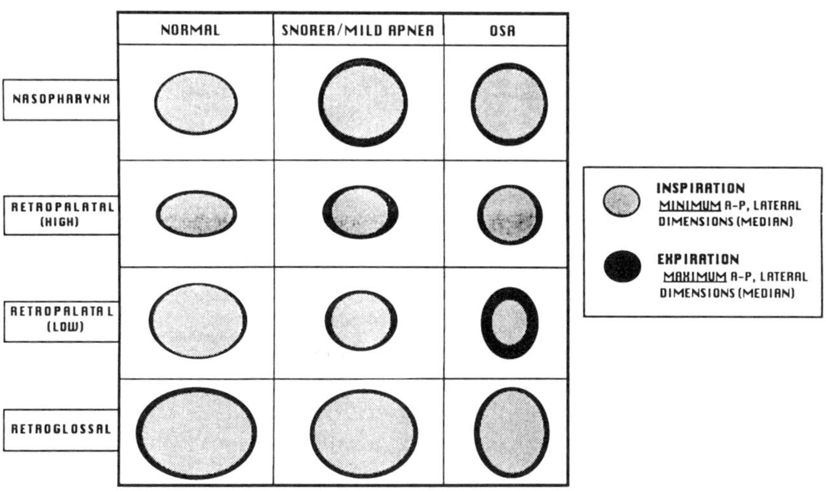

FIG 2.

Schematic showing the cross-sectional size of the airway at four anatomic levels—nasopharynx, retropalatal (high), retropalatal (low), and retroglossal—in three groups of subjects. The subject groups are normal subjects, those who snore or have mild apnea (RDI <15 events/hr), and those with obstructive sleep apnea. The darker shaded portion of each cross-section represents the difference in cross-sectional area between the minimum in inspiration and the maximum in expiration. The airway in apneics is more circular and the dimensional changes with respiration are larger. (From Schwab RJ, Gefter WB, Hoffman EA, et al: Dynamic upper airway imaging during respiration in normal subjects and patients with sleep disordered breathing. *Am Rev Respir Dis,* in press. Used by permission.)

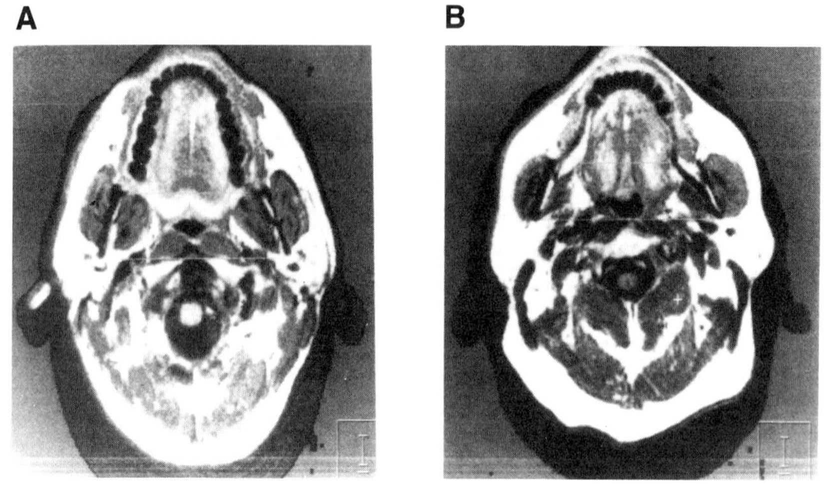

FIG 3.
Comparison of soft tissues and airway size in a normal subject **(A)** and subject with sleep apnea **(B)** as revealed by magnetic resonance imaging. The airway is the black area in the middle of each figure. Lateral to the airway are the pharyngeal walls and the parapharyngeal fat pads; the latter are white. These fat pads are larger in the apneic patient and their orientation is different. (From Shelton KE, Gay SB, Hollowell BE, et al: Mandible enclosure of upper airway and weight in obstructive sleep apnea. *Am Rev Respir Dis* 1993; 148:195–200. Used by permission.)

It is not only wall thickness that is increased in apneics, but also tongue size[39] and soft palate length.[39–42] Certain of these changes may be secondary to the disease rather than a primary abnormality. The soft tissues of the upper airway in an apneic patient are subjected to recurrent high levels of intraluminal pressures during the obstructive episodes. Thus, there is soft tissue edema that can resolve with therapy.[43]

The size as well as the function of the airway and surrounding structures is different in apneics in wakefulness. The airway of a sleep apneic is said to be more "compliant." It shows larger variation in size with changes in lung volume[44] and it is easier to collapse than is the airway of a normal subject.[45–47] Schwartz et al.[48] have argued that the upper airway can be regarded as a Starling resistor, whose collapsibility can be measured by one major parameter, Pcrit, i.e., the pressure necessary to collapse the airway. In normal individuals Pcrit is a high negative pressure, whereas in apneics, it is much less negative and may even be positive.[49] In the latter group, the airway tends to collapse passively unless collapse is prevented by positive intraluminal pressure.

These differences in the airway in wakefulness are reflected in different dynamic behavior of the airway during the respiratory cycle. This has been studied extensively by Schwab et al.[34, 50] Four stages of the normal respiratory cycle have been identified (Fig 4). In stage 1, at the onset of inspi-

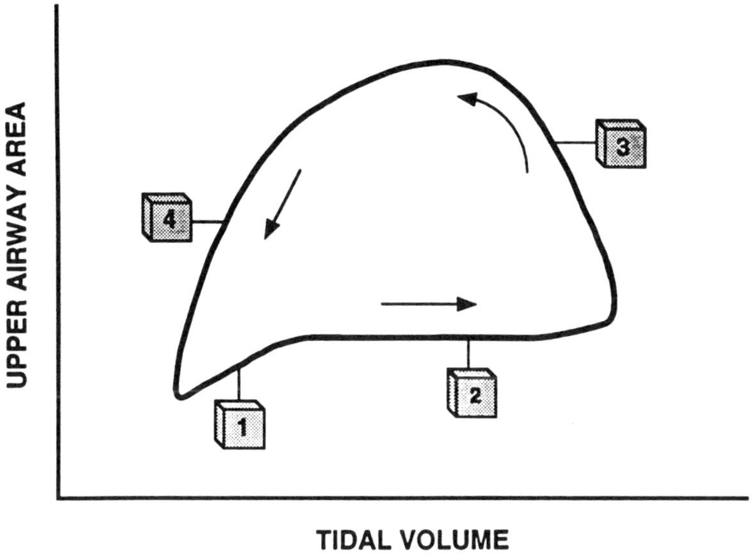

FIG 4.
Schematic of the changes in airway area during a respiratory cycle. The airway area is plotted as a function of tidal volume. The phase labeled *1* is at the onset of inspiration, while *2* is the remainder of inspiration. Phase *3* is the beginning of expiration, while phase *4* is the last part of expiration. (From Schwab RJ, Gefter WB, Hoffman EA, et al: Dynamic upper airway imaging during respiration in normal subjects and patients with sleep disordered breathing. *Am Rev Respir Dis,* in press. Used by permission.)

ration, there is an increase in the airway size of apneics, but not in normal subjects. This presumably reflects the effect of activation of upper airway dilator muscles. In patients with obstructive sleep apnea, there is increased activity of upper airway dilator muscles during wakefulness.[51] This increased activity must help compensate for the anatomical narrowing of the apneic airway. Later in inspiration, labeled stage 2, the airway size remains relatively constant. This must reflect a balance being established between the action of the negative intraluminal pressure tending to collapse the airway and the action of the airway dilator muscles opposing this collapse. During early expiration (phase 3 of the cycle), the airway increases in size presumably due to the effect of positive intraluminal pressure. This early expiratory increase in size is greater in apneics than in normal subjects, presumably reflecting the greater "compliance" of the airway discussed previously. Later in expiration (phase 4 of the cycle, see Fig 4), the airway narrows. The degree of narrowing is greater in apneics than in normal subjects. This narrowing must occur at the end of expiration, because there is neither the action of positive intraluminal pressure nor of airway dilator muscles to defend airway size. Thus, the late phase of expiration may be a particularly vulnerable period of the respiratory cycle for collapse. Obstruction of the airway during sleep in the expiratory phase has been reported.[52, 53]

While all of these differences have been demonstrated in wakefulness, we know less about the changes in the position of the soft tissue structures that occur during sleep. It is only recently that ultrafast magnetic resonance imaging (MRI) techniques have become available that would permit analysis of such changes. To date, such techniques have had only a limited application.[54] We do know that even in normal subjects, upper airway resistance increases with sleep.[55] The increase in resistance is much greater in subjects who snore.[56] In apneics the airway closes during sleep, but this closure takes place in different patients at different sites.[57] Some patients develop obstruction in the retropalatal region, while in others the obstruction occurs in the retroglossal area.[57] Within a subject, the site of obstruction tends to be constant from one episode of obstruction to the next.[57] Further studies are needed to clarify the precise biomechanical events that underlie airway obstruction.

Neural Component

No matter what the precise biomechanical events are, there is general agreement that the initiation of apnea is associated with reduction in the activity of upper airway dilator muscles.[58] The resumption of airflow at the end of apnea is associated with a massive increase in activity of the same airway dilator muscles that occurs with arousal. These changes have been documented both in studies in patients with the disease[58, 59] and in studies of sleep apnea in the English bulldog.[60, 61]

Sleep apneic individuals are more susceptible to the effects of sleep than are normal individuals. They have increased activity of their airway dilator muscles in wakefulness,[51] and hence they have a higher level of activity from which to fall. At least part of this increased activity in wakefulness is likely to be related to activation of upper airway reflex mechanisms. Negative intraluminal pressure augments the activity of upper airway dilator muscles; this effect has been demonstrated both in animal studies[62–66] and in human studies.[67, 68] In humans this reflex is markedly attenuated in sleep.[69, 70] Loss of this reflex would therefore contribute to reduction of activity of airway dilator muscles during sleep.

The central neural mechanisms underlying reduction of activity of airway dilator muscles with sleep are not fully elucidated. More is currently known about the mechanisms likely to be operative in rapid eye movement (REM) sleep. Much has been learned about such mechanisms from study of the carbachol model of REM sleep.[71] In REM sleep there is activation of cholinergic neurons in the brain stem.[72] These effects can, therefore, be simulated by microinjection of acetylcholine or appropriate agonists, i.e., carbachol, into the relevant brain stem region. Such microinjections produce depression of respiration and upper airway muscle activity both in chronically instrumented cats[73–75] and in decerebrate cats[76] or rats.[77]

This approach, therefore, provides a model to investigate mechanisms underlying the reduction in upper airway dilator muscle activity and other motor activity with sleep. It is known that pontine microinjections of carbachol lead to hyperpolarization of lumbar motoneurons. Such motoneurons have large inhibitory postsynaptic potentials[78] that are identical to those occurring in natural REM sleep.[79–81] This postsynaptic inhibition is mediated by glycine.[82] Somewhat surprisingly, however, fast synaptic inhibition does not play a role in the decrement in upper airway motor activity following microinjection of carbachol.[83] Since inhibition is not important, attention has recently focused on the potential role of withdrawal of an excitatory neural drive with sleep. One such drive is the serotonin input from the caudal raphe, a group of neurons in the midline of the brain stem. These neurons contain serotonin, thyrotropin releasing hormone (TRH), and substance P. There is a strong projection of caudal raphe neurons to upper airway motoneurons.[84] The firing of caudal raphe neurons declines with sleep particularly during REM sleep.[85] Moreover, both serotonin[86, 87] and TRH[88] excite hypoglossal motoneurons. Taken together, these observations lead to the working hypothesis that a major reason for the decline in upper airway motor activity with sleep is loss of an excitatory drive, mediated by serotonin and TRH, from caudal raphe neurons.

This hypothesis suggests that pharmacological manipulation of the serotonin system might be an approach to treat the disease. There is some support for this. Administration of L-tryptophan, a serotonin precursor, reduces the number of apneas[89] as does administration of a serotonin reuptake blocker,[90] at least in some patients. Further studies on the role of serotonin in state-related control of upper airway motoneurons are needed.

Diagnosis of Obstructive Sleep Apnea

Currently the diagnosis of sleep apnea is based on the results of tests on patients who stay overnight in a sleep laboratory—in-laboratory polysomnography. The indications and standards for this test have been described.[91] During this test, sleep stage is monitored by recording the electroencephalogram, submental electromyogram, and electrooculogram (the latter being used to record the rapid eye movements in sleep). Respiratory airflow, respiratory effort, and oxygen saturation ($Sa{O_2}$) are measured to monitor respiration. In addition, an electrocardiogram (ECG) is obtained to detect alterations in heart rate and/or arrhythmias, and electromyograms of the anterior tibialis muscles are recorded to detect nocturnal myoclonus (leg jerks). From these data, apneas, hypopneas, arousals, and episodes of oxygen saturation, etc. are identified. Metrics such as the respiratory disturbance index (RDI), i.e., number of apneas plus hypopneas per hour of sleep, are calculated.

The high prevalence of sleep apnea and the high cost of this test (around $1,000 per study)[92] have led to consideration of cheaper approaches to diagnosis. One approach is what has become known as the "split-night study." Here, the diagnosis is determined in the first part of the study, while the latter part of the night is used for titration of nasal continuous positive airway pressure (CPAP), the current first line treatment for the disease (see further information later). This approach obviates the need for one night in the sleep laboratory. Current practice is that one night in the sleep lab is used for establishing the diagnosis (diagnostic night), while the therapeutic CPAP pressure is established on another night (therapeutic night). The "split-night" approach, if adopted, would be estimated to save $30 million per year in the United States.[92] Use of "split-night" studies has, however, proved to be controversial.[93] Data supporting use of this approach are the following: (1) the respiratory disturbance index in the first part of the night is highly predictive of the index for the whole night (e.g., positive predictive value of an abnormal test, e.g., RDI > 15 events per hour, is 92%)[94]; and (2) in 78% of patients studied in this way a CPAP level can be determined for therapeutic purposes even though the testing time is shorter.[92] There are, however, arguments against the use of the approach. First, there is a suggestion that subsequent compliance with CPAP might be less if the split-night approach is used.[93] Second, 22% of patients who have a repeat CPAP titration study after a split-night study will need a re-adjustment of CPAP pressure of at least 2.5 cm H_2O, while 6% will require a change of 5.0 cm H_2O.[95] However, whether such changes are clinically relevant is unknown. Moreover, there are no comparable data for repeat studies with CPAP titration in patients having an initial full night of study. In my view, the data currently do suggest that split-night studies can be used. Certain patients who have high pretest probabilities of disease should be scheduled for such studies. Other patients might have split-night studied performed, if high respiratory disturbance indices are detected by the technologist in the first part of the night. The practitioner using this approach needs to be aware, however, of the possibility, albeit unproven, that more patients will have suboptimal levels of CPAP pressure prescribed. That CPAP pressure prescribed is not therapeutic is suggested by the continued presence of symptoms, e.g., excessive daytime sleepiness and observed snoring. Should this occur, a repeat CPAP titration study is warranted.

Split-night studies do not represent the major change in diagnostic strategy that use of in-home studies would produce. More major changes would result from use of various new technologies that allow unattended studies in the home. Here too, there is controversy, and there are major differences between the currently recommended practice in Europe[96] and in the United States.[97] Part of this difference reflects different philosophical approaches. On the one hand, diagnostic strategies have become established which consider the diagnosis of sleep apnea syndrome as an approach for all circumstances.[91] On the other hand, new approaches are evolving, which take account of the spectrum of abnormality.[96] At one end of the spectrum is the patient with obvious risk factors for the disease, e.g., increased collar size,[25, 26] who has all the symptoms of the disease—snoring, nocturnal awakenings, witnessed apneas, severe excessive daytime sleepiness. Such patients may be observed, moreover, having apneic episodes during naps in public places. In this type of patient with high pretest probability of disease, the diagnosis is not particularly challenging and a simple type of confirmatory study may be all that is required.[96] At the other end of the spectrum is the patient without obvious risk factors, with few, if any, clinical features, whom the patient's spouse persuades to seek medical advice, because of concern related to observed snoring. The majority of patients are between these extremes.

Given these different clinical scenarios, it seems reasonable to argue that the testing strategy should be appropriate to the question being posed—confirmation of the diagnosis in patients with rather obvious disease, establishing whether the disease exists, excluding the diagnosis in a patient with low pretest probability. The various measurements made during sleep might then be used in a different way dependent upon the question being posed. One of the measurements that has received the most attention is overnight oximetry.[98–103] Here oxygen saturation (Sa_{O_2}) is recorded continuously throughout sleep. Different approaches to analysis of such data have been employed. One approach is to have software count the frequency of occurrence of episodes of desaturation of fixed magnitude, e.g., 4% drops through the night.[98–102] When applied to all patients with sleep apnea, this approach leads to few (if any) false-positive diagnoses, but results in a larger number of false-negatives.[98–102] Thus, oximetry alone, analyzed in this way, can be used to confirm the diagnosis of sleep apnea in patients with high pretest probability of disease, but it cannot be used to exclude the diagnosis. In patients with a pretest probability of at least 50%, the finding of more than 15 episodes of 4% desaturation/hour has a positive predictive value for obstructive sleep apnea of greater than 90%.[102] Thus, this finding on its own, in the appropriate clinical setting, is sufficient to initiate therapy for the disease.

Another method of analyzing oximetry is to calculate the percentage of time spent below fixed values of saturation, e.g., 90%, 80%.[104] This approach is most likely to be useful in trying to exclude the diagnosis. When the percentage of time that the Sa_{O_2} is less than 90% is less than 1%, obstructive sleep apnea is practically excluded.[102]

A final approach to analyzing oximetry data is pattern recognition. In one study, recordings were simply scored as possible for sleep apnea or normal.[103] This approach leads to few false-negative diagnoses but many false-positives.[103] Thus, this approach could be useful for screening purposes. In another study, records were scored as being of three types: definite sleep apnea, possible sleep apnea, and no sleep apnea/hypopnea syndrome.[101] All patients with "definite" sleep apnea/hypopnea syndrome had a respiratory disturbance index greater than 15 events per hour. Thus, this particular pattern-recognition approach can be used to confirm the diagnosis.

If information like this can be gained from oximetry alone, the question is raised as to whether all of the variables recorded on a nocturnal sleep study are needed, in particular the electroencephalographic (EEG) data.

The latter are the most difficult to obtain in the home. Some would argue that EEG data are not needed. The respiratory disturbance index can be as accurately defined by calculating it per hour in bed as per hour of sleep.[101] However, this does not address whether information about arousals obtained from examination of the EEG data adds additional useful diagnostic information.

This discussion reveals that the diagnostic approach to patients with suspected obstructive sleep apnea is evolving. Simpler diagnostic strategies can be used to both confirm the diagnosis in patients with obvious disease and to exclude the diagnosis in patients with low pretest probabilities. We do not know, however, the actual role of these approaches in clinical practice. Adopting a two-stage approach to the diagnosis, i.e., simplified in-home test and in-laboratory polysomnography, might lead to significant cost savings by obviating a large number of in-laboratory tests. Alternatively, it might lead to increased costs by adding a large number of duplicate tests. Data are needed to address this issue. Moreover, the continued development of technology in this area will affect future diagnostic approaches. Technology is now available to allow all of the variables recorded in the laboratory, including the EEG, to be recorded during unattended monitoring in the home. Thus, the future is likely to bring a much larger role for in-home studies and a lesser role for in-laboratory studies. Further research incorporating clinical-decision-making approaches together with evaluation of costs is needed to determine the most cost-effective diagnostic strategies.

Prevalence of Obstructive Sleep Apnea

Prevalence studies show that obstructive sleep apnea is a common disease. Initial prevalence studies involving full nocturnal polysomnography were done in small samples of subjects who were selected because they complained of sleepiness,[105] snoring and sleepiness,[106] or had abnormal overnight oximetry.[107] These studies show prevalence rates for obstructive sleep apnea of the order of 0.89% (Israel), 1.3% (Sweden), and 0.3% (England), although the definition of obstructive apnea syndrome that was employed varies between these studies. Recently a much more complete prevalence study has been completed.[1] This study used a two-stage sampling approach described previously.[108] This investigation was done in Wisconsin as part of the Wisconsin Sleep Cohort study. In the study, a questionnaire survey was conducted of state employees. On the basis of the responses, subjects were divided into habitual snorers and nonhabitual snorers. Habitual snorers had loud snoring every night, witnessed apneas, or reported waking up snorting or gasping. All habitual snorers (n = 335) had full sleep studies as did 25% (n = 247) of nonhabitual snorers. Thus a sample "enriched" for the presence of apnea was studied. The results for the apnea/hypopnea indices in these two groups are shown in Figure 5. The number of subjects with high apnea/hypopnea scores is greater in the

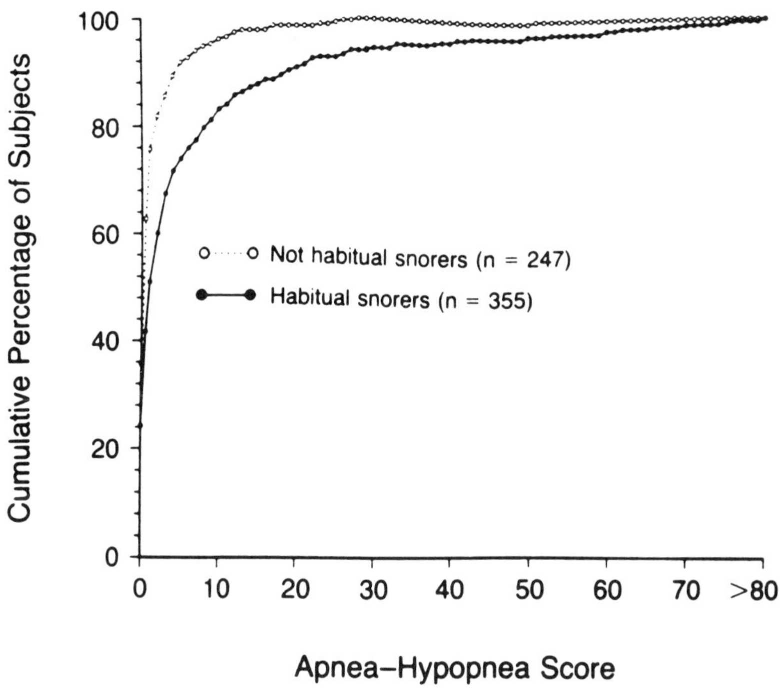

FIG 5.
Cumulative histogram of number of subjects with different values of apnea/hypopnea index (events per hour). The curves are shown for two groups of subjects—those who are not habitual snorers and those who are. The data are from the Wisconsin Sleep Cohort study. (From Young T, Palta M, Dempsey J, et al: The occurrence of sleep disordered breathing among middle-aged adults. *N Engl J Med* 1993; 328:1230–1235. Used by permission.)

habitual scoring group where the distribution is shifted to the right. In this group there is a "long tail" to the cumulative histogram, so that there is a fairly high percentage of subjects with high apnea/hypopnea indices. However, there are almost no nonhabitual snorers with apnea/hypopnea indices greater than 15 events per hour. Over the whole population studied, 9.1% of men and 4.0% of women had respiratory disturbance indices greater than 15 events per hour. Moreover, if only subjects with complaints of snoring, excessive daytime sleepiness, and a respiratory disturbance index of greater than 15 events per hour are counted (i.e., those subjects who fulfill the definition of the sleep hypopnea syndrome[14]), then 4% of middle-aged men and 2% of middle-aged women meet this definition. Another recent study of prevalence of obstructive sleep apnea in women in Iceland revealed a remarkably similar prevalence, i.e., 2.5%.[109] These numbers are large and thus sleep apnea is, as pointed out by Phillipson,[2] a major public health problem.

An extremely interesting observation in the Wisconsin Sleep Cohort study is that men were only 2.0 to 3.7 times more likely than women to have sleep-disordered breathing. This ratio is much lower than the ratio of men to women in clinic populations of patients with sleep apnea, which are typically 8:1 or 10:0.[110, 111] This suggests that there are a larger number of women with the disease who are undiagnosed. This is probably the result of two factors. First, since obstructive sleep apnea has been considered a predominantly male disease, the diagnosis may not be thought about in women. Second, complaints in women with obstructive sleep apnea are somewhat different than in men. Women more frequently complain of fatigue rather than more obvious excessive daytime sleepiness.[112]

The prevalence rates for this disease are likely to vary in different populations, since obesity is an important risk factor for the disease. In the Wisconsin Sleep Cohort study, an increase of 1 SD in any measure of body habitus increased the risk of sleep hypopnea syndrome by threefold. The increased risk of sleep-disordered breathing in obesity is more specifically related to fat in the neck. An increased collar size, rather than obesity, is a better predictor of the presence of apnea.[25]

Prevalence rates of individuals with sleepiness, as a result of sleep-disordered breathing, may be higher than even the Wisconsin results. As discussed earlier, there may be patients with snoring and upper airway resistance syndrome who are sleepy as a consequence.[15, 16] A population study in an English general practice revealed a strong association between self-reported "often" snoring and daytime sleepiness.[113] The sleepiness was not trivial since "often" snorers were 5.8 times more likely to admit to having had two or more car accidents while driving due to sleepiness.[113]

Mortality and Morbidity From Obstructive Sleep Apnea

Mortality

An important, and often-asked question by patients with OSA is whether it can lead to death during sleep. This is a difficult question to answer definitively. Indeed, we still know little of the natural history of this disease in either the treated or untreated form. Death could result from apnea because of profound hypoxemia and/or cardiac arrhythmias. But patients arouse to terminate apneic episodes, thereby preventing more profound hypoxemia and cardiovascular changes.

Current data on this question are somewhat controversial. Almost all of the current information is from incomplete retrospective studies. One study, albeit with a small sample size, rejected the hypothesis that patients with OSA are at increased risk of dying in their sleep.[114] Other studies with larger numbers of subjects did, however, find an increased mortality in essentially untreated patients with obstructive sleep apnea.[115–117] Patients treated with tracheostomy, the then more commonly used treatment for the disease, had lower mortality than did those untreated[117] or those treated with conservative measures (i.e., a recommendation for weight loss).[116, 117] Similarly, patients treated with weight loss only had a higher risk of new vascular accidents (stroke, myocardial infarction) and persistent, excessive, daytime sleepiness.[116]

In these retrospective studies, the increased mortality is related, at least to some degree, to the severity of disease.[117] Among 246 adult male patients, who were untreated and followed retrospectively, death rates were greater in the group with an apnea index greater than 20 events per hour as compared to those with an apnea index of less than 20 events per hour (Fig 6).[117] (When these patients had sleep studies, hypopneas were not routinely assessed.) There was, however, no difference in survival in the group whose apnea indices were between 21 and 40, as compared to those between 41 and 60, and above 60 events per hour. The causes of death in this study were not determined.

An alternative approach to the question, utilized in Finland,[118] is to examine the details of those who die suddenly and obtain retrospective information about symptoms suggestive of the presence of obstructive sleep apnea. These data too are suggestive that obstructive sleep apnea can be as-

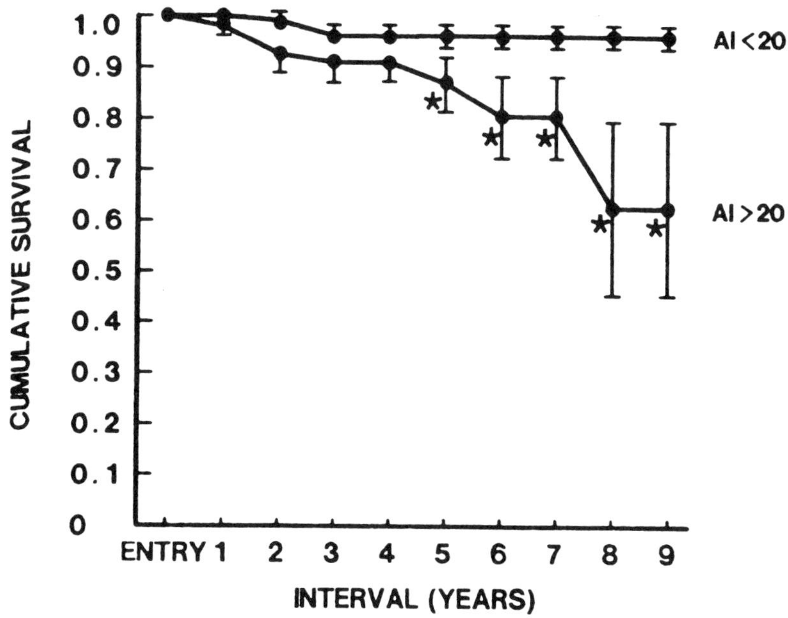

FIG 6.
Cumulative survival as function of number of years from initial diagnosis in two groups of patients with essentially untreated sleep apnea—those with an apnea index less than 20 events per hour *(AI < 20)* and those with apnea index greater than 20 events/hr *(AI > 20)*. The cumulative survival is significantly lower (*) in the group with more than 20 apneic episodes per hour of sleep. (From He J, Kryger MH, Zorick FJ, et al: Mortality and apnea index in obstructive sleep apnea. Experience in 385 male patients. *Chest* 1988; 94:9–14. Used by permission.)

sociated with sudden death. The number of subjects who had frequent evidence of witnessed apneas was surprisingly high—17.8% of the total. There was, however, no control group. Moreover, when relatives reported habitual snoring, such subjects died more often while sleeping than others in this series.

Taken together, the results of these somewhat imperfect studies lead one to the view that obstructive sleep apnea can cause sudden death. The exact magnitude of the risk is not defined. Better-designed prospective studies are needed.

Driving Accidents

One method by which patients with sleep apnea might die is from automobile accidents.[119] Patients with this disease can suffer from severe excessive daytime sleepiness.[120] That patients with sleep apnea have an increased risk of driving accidents has been shown in a number of ways. Patients with sleep apnea will report falling asleep while driving,[9] with the risk increasing with the severity of the disease. In our own practice, 32% of patients with respiratory disturbance indices greater than 60 events per hour report falling asleep while driving at least once per week (Maislin et al., unpublished observations). Several retrospective studies[114, 121–123] have shown an increased frequency of automobile accidents in patients with sleep apnea. The reported risk varies from a doubling of accidents[121] to a sevenfold increase.[122] The different results are probably related to two factors. First, some studies rely on self report of accidents[114, 121] while others use driving records from the state.[122, 123] The latter are more accurate. Second, the risk varies with severity of the disease.[123] There is no increased risk in patients with mild disease but there is in patients with severe apnea.[123] Patients with sleep apnea are also more likely to have more than one crash in which they are at fault, compared to controls.[122]

Difficulties with driving with OSA have been confirmed by studies using driving simulators.[124, 125] The performance of patients with OSA is much poorer in such tests than is the performance of control patients.[124, 125] In one driving simulation study[124] of 15 male drivers with nighttime snoring and excessive daytime sleepiness, the participants ran off the road a total of 101 times in a 60- to 90-minute simulated drive. A simpler form of a driving-like task has been developed to run on a personal computer.[125] This test can be used in one's office; it also confirms the poorer driving performance in patients with apnea.[125]

Accidents in sleep apnea patients can result in injury.[126] There are case reports of patients with unsuspected sleep apnea who fell asleep driving and sustained serious injuries.[126] Even though the risk of accidents is greater in sleep apnea, it is still not particularly high. Fewer than one third of the patients with the disease have reported automobile crashes during a 5-year period.[122] Thus, actual events are relatively uncommon, and even in those with severe apnea the accident rate is only 0.46 accidents per driver per 5-year period. The problem is, however, that while such accidents are somewhat uncommon, the consequences can be major. Fatalities are much more common in accidents in which the driver fell asleep.[127] This presumably relates to failure to take corrective actions.

The risk of driving accidents with the disease imposes an important challenge to the patient and to the physician. There are legal responsibilities that vary from state to state. This is an area of the law that is evolving, as lawyers and others become more aware of the risk of falling asleep while driving. It is an area of the law that is difficult for the physician. The physician has a responsibility to respect patient/physician confidentiality and also to protect society from highly impaired drivers.

An excellent discussion of this issue by Findley et al.[119] also presents guidelines. These authors point out that physicians have the responsibility to inform their patients of the known risks. The information should preferably be in writing. Patients who still drive, knowing that they are sleepy can be considered negligent. An example is given of a patient with sleep apnea, who had fallen asleep frequently while driving. The patient was convicted of reckless homicide and sentenced to a 3-year prison term after falling asleep, hitting a car, and killing a passenger.[128] Physicians should be aware of the relevant laws in their own state. Routine reporting of all patients with sleep apnea is not recommended. However, patients who continue to be severely sleepy should be reported to the appropriate state agency. Legal counsel should be sought before taking this step. In our own practice, we instruct patients not to drive at the time of their first visit, if they report falling asleep while driving and are a clear risk. This is particularly important in individuals who drive for a living, e.g., bus drivers, truck drivers. We study such patients early and institute therapy as soon as possible. It is likely, although unproven, that effective treatment of sleep apnea reduces the risk of accidents to an acceptable level. Thus, we tend to only report to the state those patients with severe continued sleepiness as a result, for example, of failure of therapy.

Hypertension and Other Cardiovascular Problems

Another important area of morbidity for patients with obstructive sleep apnea is cardiovascular complications. A number of different cardiovascular problems may occur. These have been the subject of recent reviews.[129–131] The role of sleep apnea in causation of certain of these problems, in particular daytime hypertension, remain the subject of debate. There are recent excellent, thoughtful syntheses of data in this area.[132–134]

During sleep in normal individuals, there are important changes in cardiovascular variables.[135] During non–rapid eye movement (NREM) sleep, the heart rate decreases by the order of 5% to 10%.[136–138] During REM sleep, the heart rate increases somewhat compared to NREM sleep and is more variable.[137, 138] On occasions in REM sleep, there can be sinus pauses with asystole of up to 9 seconds duration in otherwise healthy individuals.[139] These changes are part of the phasic changes in activities that are so characteristic of REM sleep.

Similar alterations occur in blood pressure. Blood pressure also declines in NREM sleep by the order of 10% to 20%.[137, 138, 140, 141] In REM sleep, blood pressure is somewhat higher and there is increased variability with periods of increased blood pressure.[137, 138] These increases in blood pressure in REM sleep are due to increases in peripheral vascular resistance due to vasoconstriction in skeletal muscle.[135]

The changes in cardiovascular variables during sleep are different in patients with obstructive sleep apnea. Characteristic changes occur in hemodynamic parameters in association with the apneic episodes.[142–151] First, cyclical changes in heart rate occur. Both increases[151] and decreases[146] in heart rate during apneic episodes in NREM sleep have been reported; during apneas in REM sleep, heart rate slows.[146, 151] In certain patients with obstructive sleep apnea, the changes in heart rate in association with the apneic episodes are more severe and arrhythmias can occur. Sinus pauses and second-degree atrioventricular block have been described.[145, 152–154] So too have ventricular tachyarrhythmias, which occur more commonly when Sa_{O_2} falls below 60% during the apneic episodes.[152, 153] Overall, however, serious arrhythmias during apneic episodes in sleep are relatively uncommon.[154]

Not only does heart rate show cyclical variations during apneic episodes, but so too does systemic blood pressure,[142–145, 149] pulmonary artery pressure,[142, 143, 145] cardiac index,[148] and pulmonary capillary wedge pressure.[147] If apneic episodes occur repetitively, these pressures may not return to normal between apneas, so that persistent elevations in pressure during sleep may occur.[142–145, 149] Cardiac output may also change during apneic episodes. Some studies report a fall in cardiac index by the order of 35% during apneic episodes with an abrupt increase with arousal at the onset of respiration.[148] Other studies report little change in cardiac output during apneas in NREM sleep, but report falls during apneas in REM sleep.[151] One mechanism that leads to a fall in cardiac output is the leftward shift of the interventricular septum with reduction in left ventricular volume occurring during apnea.[155] This is presumed to be secondary to the large increases in negative intrathoracic pressure.

The mechanisms for these hemodynamic changes are likely to be complex.[129–131, 133] During apneas there are progressive hypoxemia, progressive increases in negative intrathoracic pressure, and changes in autonomic function. Hypoxemia alone cannot be responsible for the cyclical changes in cardiovascular variables, because when hypoxia is prevented by breathing hyperoxic gas mixtures, cyclical changes in blood pressure persist.[156] Changes in sympathetic outflow must play an important role. Cyclical alterations in peripheral sympathetic nerve activity have been recorded in patients with sleep apnea in association with apneic episodes.[157] Moreover, patients with autonomic dysfunction, e.g., Shy-Drager syndrome, do not show cyclical changes in heart rate and blood pressure in association with apneas.[143, 145]

While there is no doubt that major hemodynamic changes occur during sleep in patients with obstructive sleep apnea, what is less certain is whether there are residual sustained effects during the daytime. One area that has received particular attention is systemic hypertension.[121–134] The relationship between obstructive sleep apnea and daytime hypertension has been approached in a number of ways. First, several studies have examined the prevalence of sleep apnea in hypertensive subjects.[158–164] The majority of these studies,[158–161, 163, 164] although not all,[162] contained a control group of normotensive subjects. The majority of the studies, albeit in relatively small numbers of subjects, in the range of 25–100, have found an increased prevalence of sleep apnea in patients with hypertension.[158–160, 162, 164] Two studies with an even smaller number of subjects did not find this.[161, 163] The results of these studies are difficult to compare since the patients were studied in various states of antihypertensive therapy; the definitions of hypertension and sleep apnea employed were, moreover, different. The latter was recognized by Hoffstein et al.,[134] who therefore reanalyzed the results of many of these studies. They showed that if sleep apnea was defined as an apnea index greater than 10 events per hour (in the majority of these studies hypopneas were not measured), then hypertension increased the relative risk of having sleep apnea. The odds ratios in different studies were between 1.5 to 40. Not all odds ratios were significant, but all were more than 1.0. Thus, Hoffstein et al.[134] concluded that "studies on the association between sleep apnea syndrome and systemic hypertension are consistent."

An alternative approach to this question is to examine the occurrence of hypertension in patients diagnosed with obstructive sleep apnea. A number of studies take this approach.[116, 153, 165] Shepard combined the results of these studies and estimated that 53% of the 401 predominantly male, middle-aged subjects with obstructive sleep apnea had hypertension.[131] More direct proof of the association would be the demonstration that treatment of sleep apnea alone eliminates hypertension. Unfortunately, however, here too, the data are not clear cut. Acute treatment of obstructive sleep apnea with nasal CPAP reduces markedly the variability of blood pressure during sleep that results from the cyclical oscillations in pressure in relation to apnea.[166, 167] Acutely, however, it has a minor effect[166] or no effect at all[167] on mean blood pressure during sleep. The longer-term effects of treatment of apnea on blood pressure are somewhat variable. Patients with obstructive sleep apnea and hypertension have been described who normalize their pressure following tracheostomy treatment.[168] Other studies report no change in blood pressure following this surgery.[169] The largest series of sleep apneics with hypertension who were treated with tracheostomy show a subset of patients whose hypertension was essentially cured by treatment of their obstructive apnea.[170] Similarly, when nasal CPAP therapy is used, the chronic effects on daytime pressure are on average small[171] or not significant.[150] However, there are some subjects in whom the reductions in blood pressure are larger and of clinical consequence.[150]

These studies do suggest that there are patients in whom sleep apnea plays an important role in the pathogenesis of their hypertension. This is not true, however, in all subjects. Since both hypertension and sleep apnea are common diseases, they may relatively frequently coexist. Moreover, risk factors for obstructive sleep apnea, such as obesity, may also be risk factors for hypertension. This will confound any attempt to establish a casual relationship.

Statistical approaches have been used, however, to try to dissect the role of obesity and apnea in causation of hypertension. These studies have examined, using multiple linear regression techniques, the relationship between hypertension and multiple variables such as age, degree of obesity, apnea/hypopnea index, degrees of oxygen desaturation during sleep, history of snoring etc.[165, 172, 173] Two of these studies were performed in clinic populations of patients with sleep apnea,[165, 172] while the other study was community-based and conducted in England.[173] Correlations were found between blood pressure and apnea/hypopnea index in one study[172] and between blood pressure and oxygen desaturation in two studies.[172, 173] However, all studies[165, 172, 173] show that the largest correlation for blood pressure is with the degree of obesity. Moreover, when relationships between blood pressure and respiratory variables are examined after allowing for the effect of obesity, they are either nonexistent[165, 173] or extremely small.[172] Thus, obesity, rather than sleep apnea, is, on the basis of these studies, the major predictor of daytime hypertension in this population.

This important association between obesity and hypertension on the one hand and obesity and sleep apnea on the other makes it extremely difficult to determine whether sleep apnea itself plays a causal role in the pathogenesis of hypertension. In many patients with sleep apnea and hypertension, the hypertension will be related to factors other than apnea per se. Nevertheless, the treatment studies discussed earlier do show that a subset of patients exist where the presence of obstructive sleep apnea plays an important role in genesis of their hypertension. The practicing physician needs to be aware of this association and take a detailed history of symptoms related to sleep apnea in all patients with hypertension. Moreover, the physician should be aware that treatment of sleep apnea can, in certain patients, cure their hypertension.

The cyclical changes in blood pressure associated with the falls in O_2 saturation that occur in relationship with apneic events might conceivably increase the risk for other acute cardiovascular events, e.g., stroke and myocardial infarction. Two major approaches to establishing this relationship have been adopted.

In the first approach the circadian variation of the time of acute cardiovascular events—sudden death,[174, 175] myocardial infarction,[176] stroke,[177–179] and deaths due to a number of causes[180] have been studied. Stroke secondary to brain infarction has been reported to be most common in the hours between 12:00 A.M. and 6:00 A.M.,[177] in the first 30 minutes after awakening,[178] and in the hours between 10:00 A.M. and 12:00 P.M.[179] Myocardial infarction also shows a marked circadian rhythm with a peak between 6:00 A.M. and 12:00 P.M.[176] Sudden cardiac death is also most common at these times with peaks between 7:00 to 11:00 A.M.[174] or 7:00 to 9:00 A.M.[175] Thus, circadian variation in acute cardiovascular events has been documented with the greatest vulnerability appearing to be in the first hours after awakening. The basis for this vulnerability is not known.

A more direct approach to establishing a relationship between sleep apnea and acute cardiovascular events is to examine the increased risk of such events in patients with apnea. Here there are limited data. Several studies have, however, examined the relative increased risk associated with habitual snoring using either a prospective study[181] or case-control methodology.[182, 183] The studies do show that habitual snoring is associated with increased risk of cerebral infarction,[182] ischemic heart disease and stroke,[181] and myocardial infarction.[183] This approach has been criticized, however.[132] It has been argued that the apparent association between snoring and cardiovascular disease could be related to bias, since subjects who are ill are more likely to be aware if they snore. The association could also be confounded by variables such as age and obesity.[132] Nonetheless, in recent studies, the increased risk is still found after adjusting for age, body mass index, and other factors.[181–183]

Moreover, in a study which examined overnight polysomnography in unselected male survivors of acute myocardial infarction and in controls, the increased relative risk of myocardial infarction (i.e., odds ratios, for those with apnea indices in the highest quartile) was extremely high, 23.3.[184] Thus, although the data are limited, they do suggest that sleep apnea is an important risk factor for acute vascular events. Further studies in this area are clearly needed.

Treatment of Obstructive Sleep Apnea

Underlying Causes and General Measures

In treating patients with obstructive sleep apnea, it is important to first consider that there may be an underlying cause. Important risk factors that should be thought about are obesity,[1] nasal problems, and hypothyroidism.[185, 186] Obese patients should be enrolled in weight management programs. Reduction in weight either by diet[187–189] or gastric surgery[188–190] reduces the apnea-hypopnea index and improves oxygenation during sleep. Weight reduction alters collapsibility of the pharynx.[188, 191] Alcohol also can be an important precipitant of apnea during sleep. Alcohol preferentially suppresses the activity of upper airway dilator muscles in comparison to the diaphragm.[192] Alcohol has, therefore, been shown to increase upper airway resistance.[193, 194] It increases the number of apneas in patients with the disease[195] or produces apneas in asymptomatic male snorers.[194] All patients with obstructive sleep apnea should be informed of this risk and advised to avoid alcohol in the evening.

Apneas during sleep may also be made worse by changes in body position. There are subjects who have apneas in the supine position, whose symptoms are markedly ameliorated or abolished by sleeping in the lateral position[196] or semi-upright.[197] Such patients are referred to as positional apneics. This diagnosis can be suspected by taking a careful history from the bed partner. They will report loud snoring and/or witnessed apneas in only the supine position. During polysomnography, body position should be monitored so that the respiratory disturbance index can be calculated separately for the supine and lateral positions. Patients with positional apnea will have high indices in the supine position (e.g., apnea/hypopneas in the range of 50 to 100 events per hour), but lower indices (e.g., <10 events per hour) in the lateral position.[198] Some laboratories have the patient select their sleeping position and then monitor it, while others, including our own, make an effort to obtain sufficient data during the study in the supine and lateral positions. There are no standards in this regard.

Patients with positional apnea can be treated with position therapy. In essence, patients are advised to sleep with a tennis ball attached to their pajamas at the level of their shoulder blades so that sleep in the supine position is uncomfortable. The long-term efficacy of this therapy is unknown. Alternatively, subjects can use a position-activated sound device that trains the patients with an auditory alarm to avoid supine sleep.[198] After training, some patients no longer sleep supine.[198]

Pharmacotherapy

With respect to more specific therapies, there is currently no satisfactory pharmacotherapy for obstructive sleep apnea. There are some reports of improvement in sleep apnea with acetazolamide,[199] nicotine,[200] and even strychnine.[201] Most attention has focused on use of two pharmacological approaches, medroxyprogesterone and protriptyline.

Medroxyprogesterone is a ventilatory stimulant[202] that stimulates ventilation by a hypothalamic mechanism that involves gene transcription.[203, 204] Medroxyprogesterone may still have some role in reducing P_{CO_2} in patients with obesity hyperventilation syndrome.[205, 206] Since its effects on ventilation are enhanced by simultaneous administration of estrogen,[203, 204] which upregulates progesterone receptors,[207] concurrent administration of estrogen would seem of value. But medroxyprogesterone is now very much a second-line therapy for obesity hypoventilation syndrome. The first-line approach is the use of noninvasive nocturnal ventilation through a nasal CPAP mask.[208] Medroxyprogesterone does not, however, exert specific effects on upper airway motor output. Its effects on obstructive sleep apnea are disappointing,[209, 210] and no benefit was found in a small double-blind randomized crossover study.[211] Thus, it has been concluded that medroxyprogesterone has no role in the treatment of obstructive sleep apnea in normocapnic patients.[212]

Protriptyline is another drug that has been employed. Its role of action is unknown, but animal studies do show that it increases the respiratory activity of nerves carrying motor output to upper airway muscles.[213] Protriptyline does decrease the respiratory disturbance index at least in some subjects.[90, 214–218] Some studies have suggested, however, that the major effect of protriptyline is through reduction in the amount of REM sleep[215, 217] in which apneas can be more frequent and associated with larger falls in oxygen saturation.[219] Whatever the mechanism of action, protriptyline is now seldom used. Its use is associated with side effects such as constipation, confusion, urinary retention, and in men, the inability to maintain an erection.[216, 217] Patients may develop tachyplaxis to the drug with time.[216] In our own practice, protriptyline is now used very much as a secondary line of therapy, and only in patients who have mostly apneas related to REM sleep.

Since pharmacotherapy is disappointing, current approaches to therapy are largely mechanical. These approaches are considered below, where we discuss use of nasal continuous positive airway pressure (CPAP), intraoral devices, and surgical treatments.

Nasal CPAP

The current treatment of choice for obstructive sleep apnea is the use of nasal continuous positive airway pressure (nasal CPAP). With this therapy, pressurized air is applied through the nares and acts as a "pneumatic splint" to maintain patency of the upper airway. The treatment was originally introduced by Sullivan et al. in 1981.[220] The treatment is remarkably effective in abolishing apneas, hypopneas, and arousals related to sleep-disordered breathing events.

While remarkably effective in normalizing respiration during sleep in a sleep laboratory, this therapy requires long-term, nightly use of the device.[221] This chronic use of CPAP is associated with a number of common complaints. These include waking up at night, mask discomfort, nasal discomfort, nasal congestion, rhinorrhea, nasal dryness, swallowing air, claustrophobia, and chest pain.[222–225] Certain of these side effects, such as nasal dryness, can be dealt with by simple remedies such as adding an in-line humidifier. Others, such as nasal congestion, may be transient. Infrequently, but more serious, side effects have been described and include pneumocephalus[226] and bacterial meningitis.[227]

These side effects impact on the usage of the therapy. A number of studies have retrospectively evaluated the patterns of use of CPAP therapy.[222–224, 228, 229] In this type of study, patients are simply considered users if they report continued use or nonusers if they do not. While there is some variation in the percentage of patients continuing to use CPAP in the different studies (called compliance), the results are remarkably similar: 64.7% to 78.3%,[225] 63%,[224] 64%,[228] 50%,[229] and 71% to

76%.[222] Compliance is lower in patients who are prescribed nasal CPAP for snoring (29%)[228] or mild disease. For patients with apnea/hypopnea indices between 15 and 30 events per hour, only 28% accepted this treatment.[229]

Several factors have been found to determine compliance rates. Interestingly, the majority of studies,[224, 225, 228] although not all,[229] have found that respiratory disturbance index is not an important determinant of use. Neither, somewhat unexpectedly, is the frequency of occurrence of the common nasal side effects.[222, 224] The factors that have been shown to determine use include the degree of sleepiness at presentation,[224, 228] with patients who are most sleepy having the highest usage of the equipment.[228] Similarly, the degree of symptomatic benefit experienced by patients using the equipment is an important determinant of its use.[222, 228] Other determinants of use that have been described are degree of desaturation with respiratory events in sleep and educational level. Some studies have shown that users of CPAP have larger degrees of desaturations during sleep.[225, 228, 229] The demonstration of such desaturations might lead to more persuasive reinforcement of use by physicians.[228] Educational level was found to be lower in nonusers in one study.[225]

An interesting aspect of these retrospective studies is the finding that there are patients who, after using the therapy, do not themselves note improvement[222, 228] nor do their relatives.[222] The explanation for this is unclear. Perhaps these patients had another sleep disorder and were misdiagnosed. More likely, however, is that the level of CPAP pressure that was prescribed was subtherapeutic. CPAP which is sufficient to abolish apneas may not be sufficient to abolish all arousals related to lesser forms of respiratory disturbance during sleep. Such patients may describe that they are still heard to snore even while using CPAP. Patients who do not report symptomatic benefit from use of CPAP should have a repeat sleep study performed while using CPAP to see if there are problems with inadequate pressure or the existence of another sleep disorder.

These findings from retrospective studies have been extended by the results of prospective studies. Studies using a counter to monitor how long the power was on have recorded average nightly "use" of 5.1 hours[230] and 6.1 hours.[231] The most complete prospective study is that reported recently by our group.[232] In this study a microprocessor was mounted in the CPAP device. Subjects were unaware of the presence of the monitor. The microprocessor was programmed to identify four events—power on, power off, mask on, mask off. The latter conditions were recognized by incorporating a pressure sensor and determining when the pressure rose, respectively, above or below a preset pressure threshold. Data stored on the microprocessor were downloaded every month and software determined the nightly use of CPAP. This study revealed that the average nightly use of CPAP was 4.88 hours. There was, however, a wide intrasubject variation in use. The pattern of use in four individual subjects is demonstrated in Figure 7. To begin to assess adequacy of therapy, we developed what we believe is a minimally acceptable criterion of use, i.e., 4

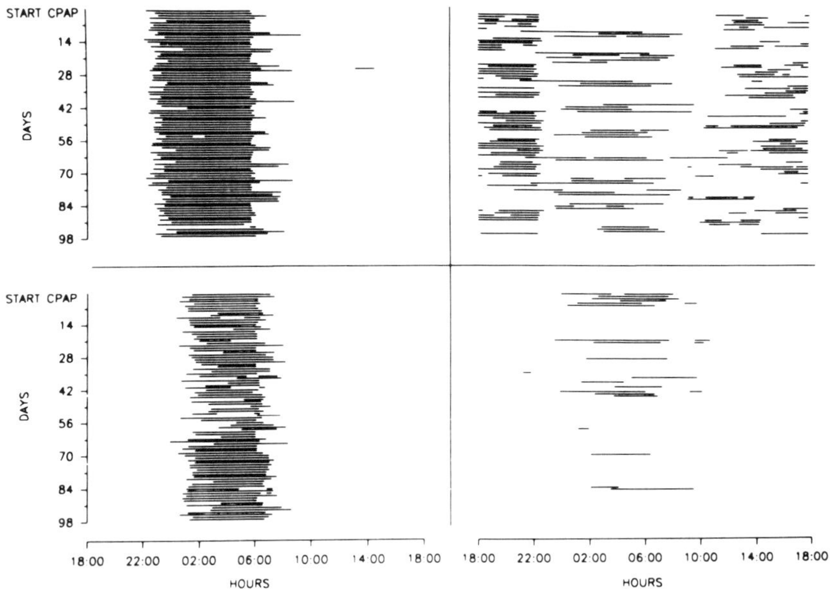

FIG 7.
Patterns of use of nasal continuous positive airway pressure (CPAP) in four different patients. Each graph shows time of day that CPAP was used *(solid line)* for each of 98 days from onset of CPAP therapy. The patients in the left panels were reasonably compliant with CPAP; the patient in the upper right panel was a shift-worker; and the patient in the lower right panel reported using CPAP nightly, but made only very intermittent use of the therapy. (From Kribbs NB, Pack AI, Kline LR, et al: Objective measurement of patterns of nasal CPAP use by patients with obstructive sleep apnea. *Am Rev Respir Dis* 1993; 147:887–895. Used by permission.)

hours of use per night for 5 out of 7 nights, i.e., 70% of the time. The 4-hour use is based on knowledge about normal sleep. We found that 19 of the 35 subjects studied did not meet this criterion for minimally acceptable use. We called these patients irregular users and the others regular users. However, 7 hours is a more normal period of sleep. If we use this as a criterion, only 2 of the 35 patients studied used CPAP for more than 7 hours per night on 70% of the nights tested. Both of these patients were women. The individual data are shown in Figure 8 for 4 hours of use and 7 hours of use for all subjects. Solid squares represent nights when the patient use exceeded the time period (4 hours, *top panel,* or 7 hours, *bottom panel*). The number of nights when even 4 hours of use was not obtained is readily apparent, and raises important concerns about how effective CPAP therapy is.

There were certain characteristics of regular users as compared to irregular users. These differences are similar to those found in retrospective studies of whether CPAP is used or not. We found that regular users reported

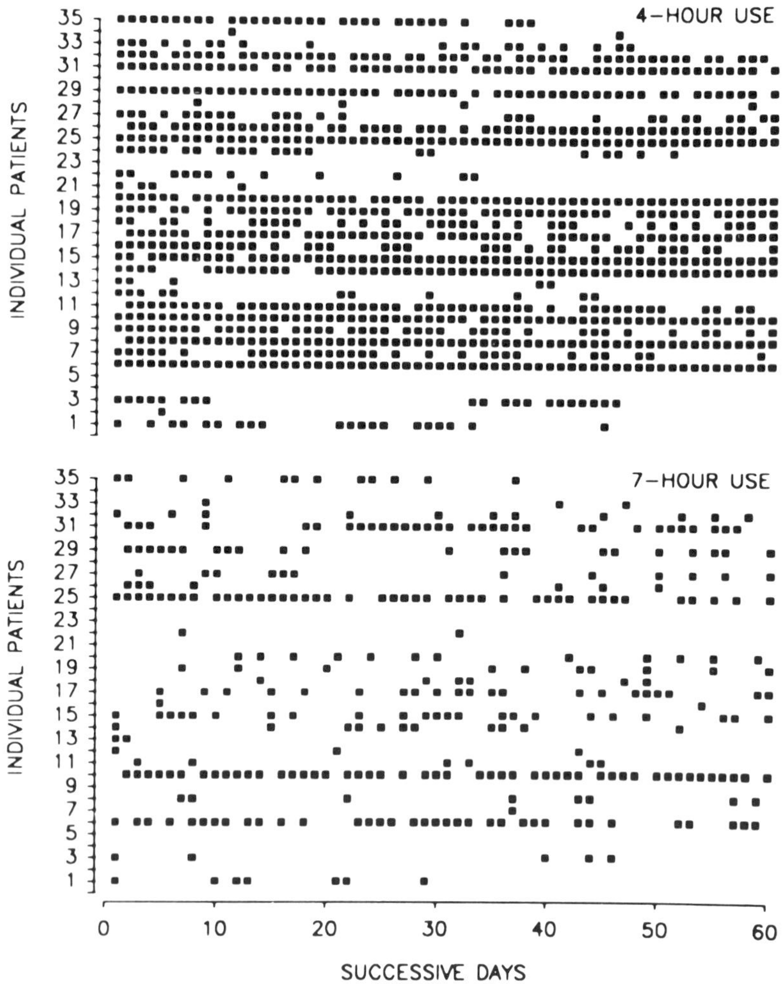

FIG 8.
Daily amount of continuous positive airway pressure (CPAP) use in 35 subjects (y axis) over first 60 days of use. In the top panel a *solid square* represents at least 4 hours of use; in the bottom panel a *square* represents at least 7 hours of use. The large number of patients who fail to use CPAP for these amounts of time are clearly seen. (From Kribbs NB, Pack AI, Kline LR, et al: Objective measurement of patterns of nasal CPAP use by patients with obstructive sleep apnea. *Am Rev Respir Dis* 1993; 147:887–895. Used by permission.)

more frequent excessive daytime sleepiness, larger improvements in energy level with treatment, more satisfaction with CPAP treatment, and more years of education. The respiratory disturbance index at diagnosis was no different between the two groups. Moreover, the frequency of nasal symptoms related to CPAP use was no different between the groups. However, eight out of the nine patients who complained of claustrophobia with use of CPAP were irregular users. Thus, claustrophobia may be a particularly difficult side effect for patients to deal with.

These data raise important concerns about how often use of CPAP is an effective long-term treatment for obstructive sleep apnea. There is no doubt that CPAP can abolish sleep-disordered breathing events in a sleep laboratory, but the goal of therapy should relate to long-term normalization of daytime function. At the present time, there is no simple methodology that can be used to assess this. The nightly use patterns that we have demonstrated would imply, however, that many patients are likely to be functioning at suboptimal levels on many days in their lives. There is a need to establish new goals for therapeutic outcome and to develop appropriate methodology to assess efficacy.

The somewhat disappointing nightly use patterns with CPAP raise questions about whether this can be improved. One approach is to have a program with frequent patient contact to reinforce use. While many sleep centers employ this approach, there is a paucity of data on its effectiveness. The only published study found no benefit from this intervention[231]; but the number of subjects was extremely small (six with reinforcement, four without) and the group with regular reinforcement had an average 1 hour extra use per night. Thus, more studies on this aspect are needed.

Another approach to improving use is modification of the CPAP machine and/or attachments. Development of intranasal soft catheters or pillows reduces the complaints related to leaking of air, e.g., eye irritation.[233] A number of different modifications of the CPAP machine are also now available. Some systems include a ramp feature, whereby no pressure is applied when the device is first worn and the pressure then ramps up to the prescribed level over a 30- to 45-minute period. The concept is that there will be less difficulty with CPAP use if the pressure is applied during sleep. There are, however, no studies that show improved CPAP use with this approach. A major change in CPAP is the use of a bilevel pressure system, often called BiPAP. Here, the inspiratory and expiratory pressure can be set independently. Inspiratory pressure assists inspiration, whereas expiratory pressure retards expiratory airflow and leads to hyperinflation. Thus, reduction of expiratory pressure could lead to less hyperinflation and potentially increased utilization of the device. Recent data, however, do not support this contention. When patients were randomly assigned to groups using either CPAP or BiPAP, there was no difference in nightly average use over a study period of several months.[234] Given the design of the study, this is hardly surprising, since the expiratory pressure with BiPAP was, on average, 3.0 cm H_2O less than the CPAP level. At the present time, we do not know the relative roles of inspiratory pressure

(IPAP) and expiratory pressure (EPAP) in preventing collapse during sleep. Thus, current algorithms to adjust the pressures independently are empiric and lead to little difference on average between the EPAP pressure with BiPAP and the CPAP pressure.[235] Such small differences make it unlikely that switching from CPAP to BiPAP will make a major difference in use. There are, however, in practice, certain patients who can tolerate BiPAP but cannot use CPAP. The characteristics of such patients are not well defined. It is likely that they are patients who need higher levels of pressure and/or have side effects such as chest pain related to hyperinflation. More extensive use of BiPAP needs to be based on understanding the relative role of IPAP and EPAP in abolishing apneas so that a more rational approach to setting these pressures is developed.

Intraoral Devices

Because of concerns about patterns of use of CPAP, other approaches to treatment are being pursued. A second nonsurgical mechanical approach is use of an intraoral device. The two most commonly used are the tongue-retaining device[198, 236] and the mandibular positioning device.[237, 241] The tongue-retaining device operates by placing the tongue into a cup or a bubble positioned between the front teeth. The tongue is then held there by surface adhesion. The concept is, therefore, to prevent backward motion of the tongue during sleep that could occlude the airway. This presupposes that backward motion of the tongue plays the major role in occlusion. The device does reduce the respiratory disturbance index, at least in some patients, to acceptable levels.[198] It seems to work best in those with mild to moderate apnea or positional apneas.[198] There are no data about relief of sleepiness or long-term usage patterns. Thus, at the present time, the tongue-retaining device is an unproved therapy.

The mandibular positioning device has been somewhat more extensively studied.[237–241] There are different designs.[237–241] The basic concept is that the device is worn during sleep and moves the mandible forward and brings the tongue passively with it. In the recent report by Clark et al.,[241] the device that was used consisted of two separate upper and lower full-coverage clear acrylic appliances that snapped onto the teeth. The appliances were connected by two rod and tube devices that allowed variable protrusion of the mandible. Successful treatment with this device required a relatively large forward motion of the mandible. Typically the jaw had to be advanced about 75% of the maximum possible protrusion.[241] There are reports of the effect of wearing such devices on the respiratory disturbance index during sleep.[240, 241] The response to this form of therapy is highly variable in individual patients.[240, 241] There are some individuals with high levels of respiratory disturbance during sleep whose respiration is normalized while wearing the device. Other patients, however, do not show any improvement and may even become worse. The reason for this variable response is currently unknown. Thus, all patients cannot be treated by use of an intraoral device. Current information would suggest that if this device is used, there should be an adjustment period to determine the degree of protrusion. This initial adjustment should be based on self-report or on report by the bed partner about the persistence of snoring. After the adjustment period, a repeat polysomnogram should be performed to determine whether this treatment is likely to prove effective. If the respiratory disturbance index using the device is still greater than 15 events/hr, then alternative treatment modalities should be sought.

A number of patients will not benefit from this form of therapy because of lack of effectiveness in obliterating apneas. Others will not benefit because of problems with long-term use. There are, however, no comparable data about use patterns such as those we have for CPAP. There is an indication of satisfactory long-term use for 36 months based on self-report in 52% of patients initiating this form of therapy.[241] The therapy is, moreover, not without its side effects. The forward protrusion of the mandible could result in changes in the temporomandibular joint with dysfunction of the joint. Transient episodes of pain in this joint associated with use of the device have been described.[241] Long-term changes in bite might also occur because of forward pressure on the mandibular teeth and backward pressure on the maxillary teeth. There are insufficient long-term data to assess the likelihood and severity of these various potential side effects.

Surgical Treatment

Surgical approaches for mechanical treatment of obstructive apnea have also been used. These have evolved over the last 2 decades as the lack of effectiveness or the side effects of earlier surgical treatments became recognized. The different surgical approaches that have been employed are now described.

Nasal Surgery and Removal of Tonsils and Adenoids.—The first role to be considered for surgical treatment of obstructive sleep apnea is correction of an obvious upper airway anatomical problem. Patients with obstructive sleep apnea might have a deviated nasal septum. Surgical correction of the deviated septum can improve the degree of respiratory disturbance during sleep, but is not usually completely curative.[242–244] Nevertheless, patients with a significant nasal septal deviation should have it surgically corrected. This not only improves their respiratory disturbance index during sleep, but also makes it easier for such patients to subsequently use nasal CPAP.[244]

Another not uncommon anatomical abnormality in patients with sleep apnea is enlargement of tonsils and adenoids. This can be a cause of obstructive sleep apnea in children.[245–247] There are case reports of cure of obstructive sleep apnea in children following tonsillectomy[248–249] and of correction of daytime CO_2 retention.[250] In adults, enlarged tonsils may also precipitate apnea. There are case reports of severe sleep apnea with cor pulmonale following acute tonsillitis in adults[251] and, as in children, tonsillectomy can be curative.[242, 251–254] The results of tonsillectomy in adults are, however, not uniformly successful.[254, 255] Moser and Rajagopal[254] and Aubert-Tulkins et al.[255] have reported small series of patients who had tonsillectomy performed for sleep apnea and have summarized the previous literature. All series are unfortunately small. Tonsillectomy is successful in returning the respiratory disturbance during sleep to normal in about one half of patients with sleep apnea and enlarged tonsils. Thus patients with enlarged tonsils and sleep apnea should have their tonsils removed. They should be cautioned, however, that the surgery might not be successful. All such patients should have polysomnograms performed before and after surgery.

Tracheostomy.—The initial treatment for obstructive sleep apnea that could be employed in all patients was tracheostomy.[256] The concept is simple—bypass the obstruction. The tracheostomy tube that is used is fenestrated. The tracheostomy stoma is kept capped during the day to allow speech, but opened at night to permit respiration, even when the upper airway is collapsed. Tracheostomy can relieve hypersomnolence[170, 257] and normalize hypercapnia in certain of the patients exhibiting these symptoms.[257] It can also lead to a reduction in blood pressure[169, 170] and eliminate, or reduce, the frequency of arrhythmias associated with the disease.[257, 258] While effective, this therapy is not without its adverse effects.[170, 257] These occur in three major areas: First, there are local problems at the site of the stoma in the form of recurrent local infections and/or local granulation tissue.[170, 257] Second, recurrent purulent bronchitis may occur[257]; this is presumably related to loss of upper airway protective mechanisms. Finally, there are psychosocial consequences that can be major.[170, 257] Depression following the surgery is relatively common but can be transient. Loss of employment has been described.[257] There is an important change in body self-image.

These adverse consequences have resulted in tracheostomy being used very infrequently for treatment of the disease. It is still used in patients who are very sick as a result of OSA. Often these patients are morbidly obese. They may have obvious right-sided failure, significant arrhythmias, and hypercapnia. Such patients may need suction-assisted lipectomy of the subcutaneous tissue in the neck to facilitate placement of the tracheostomy.[259] In morbidly obese patients, it may be feasible to reverse the tracheostomy after a period, if the patients lose sufficient weight.[257] This decision should be based on showing first that acutely plugging the tracheostomy during sleep does not result in an immediate return of significant sleep-disordered breathing. If this is successful, it should then be shown that sleeping with the tracheostomy plugged for a period of a few weeks does not result in return of symptoms and significant sleep apnea. If this also is successful, the tracheostomy can be reversed.

Uvulopalatopharyngoplasty.—Of the various surgical treatments used for all patients with obstructive sleep apnea, uvulopalatopharyngoplasty (UPPP) has been the most widely employed. The operation was introduced by Fujita et al. in 1981.[253] In this surgical procedure, there is removal of the uvula, a portion of the soft palate, and redundant tissues from the posterior pharyngeal wall. Although relatively widely employed after its introduction in 1981, concerns about the success of the surgery have led to its much less frequent use.

Initially the surgery was considered a success, if the apnea index declined by 50%.[253] This can no longer be considered an acceptable criterion for surgery. Patients who by this definition are "successfully" treated but still have an apnea index of greater than 20 events per hour (i.e., their pretreatment apnea index was >40 events per hour) have an increased risk of mortality.[117] Thus, definitions of success with this form of therapy have been liberal.

Even with this liberal definition of "success," success rates are poor. The success rate in various published series varies between 0 and 90% (for summary and reviews of published results, see Rodenstein[260] and Shepard[261]) with the average being in the 50% to 60% range.[261] While the varying success may reflect differences in the nature of the patients being operated on, there are no obvious predictors of success. With respect to severity of disease, one study has found that patients with more severe disease do better.[262] Others have found the opposite, i.e., that patients with milder disease do better,[263–265] while other studies have found no effect of preoperative severity on success rates.[266–268] Likewise, the degree of obesity does not seem predictive of outcome. Studies have reported better results in more obese subjects,[266] better results in less obese subjects,[269] or no difference with respect to degree of obesity.[262, 267, 268, 270, 271] Part of the explanation for these different results may be different surgical techniques.[270]

In several of the published reports, however, a few patients who by any definition are cured by this surgery, i.e., their postoperative respiratory disturbance during sleep is in the normal range. This has prompted attempts to try to identify such patients preoperatively. The most obvious likely predictor is the location of the airway obstruction during sleep. Certain patients obstruct in the retropalatal region, while others obstruct at the base of the tongue (retroglossal or hypopharyngeal).[57, 272, 273] The site of obstruction tends to be reproducible within an individual patient.[57, 272, 273] Intuitively, it would seem that patients who obstruct in the retropalatal region should have better results with UPPP. The first attempts to identify such patients were based on measurements made in wakefulness. Sher et al.[274] used a Mueller maneuver with direct visualization of the airway through a fiberoptic nasopharyngoscope to determine at what level patients obstructed. They found that the level of obstruction (retropalatal) was a good predictor of outcome. Others[275, 276] using this approach have not obtained results as favorable. These different results may be in part related to differences in interpretation, since the technique is qualitative and dependent on the impressions of the observer. More quantitative techniques have also been employed based on imaging of the upper airway.[275, 277, 280] These have shown the somewhat expected results. The success rate of UPPP is greater in patients with larger soft palates as revealed by lateral cephalograms,[277, 278] and in those with smaller upper airways,[279, 280] particularly when the narrowest part of the airway is within 20 mm of the hard palate rather than more distal.[280] While success rates differ, dependent on the site of obstruction, these techniques are not sufficiently predictive that a good surgical outcome can be reasonably guaranteed. We do know, however, that a poorer outcome occurs in patients where the minimum size of the airway is behind the tongue.[280]

An important consideration in these studies is whether the site of collapse in sleep is related to the narrowing present in wakefulness. Recent studies with ultrafast MRI suggest that this is not so.[54] Thus, attempts have been made to more directly assess the airway during normal or sedative-induced sleep before performing UPPP.[281, 282] Studies using differential pressure measurements to locate the site of collapse[281] or direct visualization[282] have shown that retropalatal obstructers do better with UPPP. The results are, however, relatively disappointing. In the small study of Hudgel et al.,[281] only 4 of 7 patients who obstructed in the retropalatal region had apnea/hypopnea indices of less than 20 events per hour following surgery. Thus, at the present time, UPPP is a potential treatment for obstructive sleep apnea. Patients are described who seem to be cured by the surgery. The problem is that these patients cannot be reliably identified prior to surgery. Thus, even with careful selection, success rates are unacceptably low. Moreover, deaths from this surgery have been described.[283, 284] Complications such as nasal regurgitation, which is usually self-limited and resolves in 4 to 8 weeks, and more permanent pharyngeal stricture also occur.[283, 285] Thus, UPPP on its own cannot at this time be recommended for treatment of obstructive sleep apnea.

Mandibular/Maxillary Surgery.—The disappointment with UPPP, following an initial enthusiasm, has led surgeons to consider new approaches to the surgical management of the disease.[286] Of the new surgical treatments proposed, the most extensive results are from the Stanford group of Riley, Powell, and Guilleminault. These investigators have utilized two new surgical techniques which are now combined into a staged surgical approach.[287] The first component of the approach includes mandibular osteotomy with hyoid mytotomy/suspension.[287–290] With this surgery, there is advancement of the mandible with simultaneous advancement of the hyoid. The second component of the approach, which has been shown to be as effective as CPAP in reducing the respiratory disturbance index,[291] is mandibular and maxillary osteotomy with advancement of both.[287, 291, 292]

In current practice, the Stanford group performs a staged approach with the first stage being based on the perceived level of obstruction in wakefulness.[287] Each patient is classified into one of the three types according to the site of obstruction: type I, oropharynx; type II, oropharynx/hypopharynx; and type III, hypopharynx. This classification is based on findings on the physical examination, direct fiberoptic pharyngoscopy including Mueller maneuver, and lateral cephalometrics. The overall approach that they employ is shown in the flow diagram in Figure 9.

Results of this surgery have been reported for 306 consecutively treated patients.[287] The definition of success that is employed is more rigid than

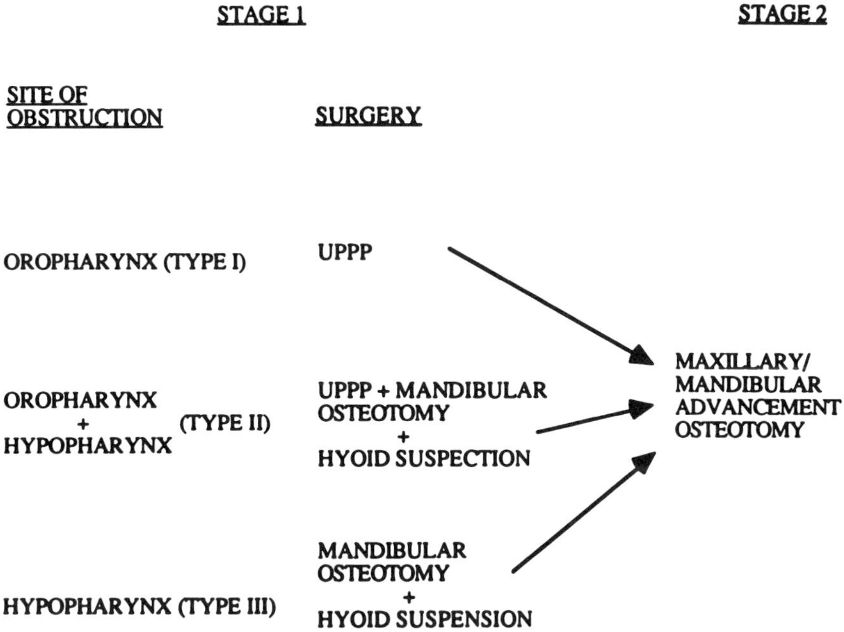

FIG 9.
Staged surgical approach used by Riley et al.[287] For further details, see text.

with earlier studies with UPPP. Surgery is defined as successful if the RDI is equivalent to that using CPAP, or if the postoperative RDI is less than 20 events per hour with at least a 50% reduction. The success rates are shown in Table 1. Overall, in phase 1 of the surgery, 61% of the operations were successful. The success rate was lowest (42%) in those patients with the most severe sleep apnea (i.e., RDI >60 events per hour). The success rate of phase 2 surgery, i.e., mandibular/maxillary osteotomy with advancement, was higher, i.e., 97%. However, only 24 of the 94 patients who failed phase 1 surgery elected to have the more extensive phase 2 surgery. Some of the patients who had stage 2 surgery in the Stanford series had failed UPPP at other institutions.

These results are encouraging. No deaths were reported and the side effects of the surgery were largely transient. The mean length of stay was a short 2.1 days for phase 1 and only 2.4 days for the more extensive phase 2 surgery. At present such surgery should only be done, however, in major medical centers with the relevant expertise. Confirmation of the Stanford results are needed before the approach can be widely advocated. Moreover, there is a need for longer-term follow-up to ensure that success is long lasting. Nevertheless, this approach seems the most promising at this time with respect to surgical treatment of obstructive sleep apnea.

Alternative Surgical Approaches.—Other surgical approaches have also been used. These include intrapalatine resection, which is a full-thick-

TABLE 1.
Success Rates in Two-Stage Surgical Approach of Riley, Powell, and Guilleminault*

Phase	Type of Obstruction	Surgery Groups	Total No. of Patients	Success (%)/No. of Patients
One	I	UPPP	10	80/8
	II	UPPP + mandibular osteotomy/hyoid advancement	233	60/133
	III	Mandibular osteotomy/hyoid advancement	6	66/4
		Totals	239	61/145
Two		Unsuccessful phase I	24	100/24
		Skeletal deformity (without UPPP)	7	100/7
		Unsuccessful UPPP (outside referral—severe OSA)	60	97/58
		Totals	91	97/89

*From Riley RW, Powell NB, Guilleminault C: Obstructive sleep apnea syndrome: A review of 306 consecutively treated surgical patients. *Otolaryngol Head Neck Surg* 1993; 108:117–125. Used by permission.

ness resection of the proximal part of the soft palate,[293] and reduction of tongue volume,[294] which can now be achieved by a laser approach. There are, however, few data about the outcomes of these surgical approaches, and they need to be considered experimental at this time.

Staged Approach to Therapy

This discussion of the various treatment approaches indicates that therapy for obstructive sleep apnea is evolving. Although some differences in the therapeutic approach to be employed will be necessitated by special features of individual patients, at present one would advocate a three-stage approach (Fig 10). This is a personal view about how to approach management of the average patient with sleep apnea, but currently there are no definitive data as to its efficacy.

In my view, nasal CPAP remains the treatment of choice. There are the most convincing data about its effectiveness in abolishing apneas and other respiratory disturbances during sleep and in improving sleepiness. All patients starting on this therapy should have its use monitored. The pattern of

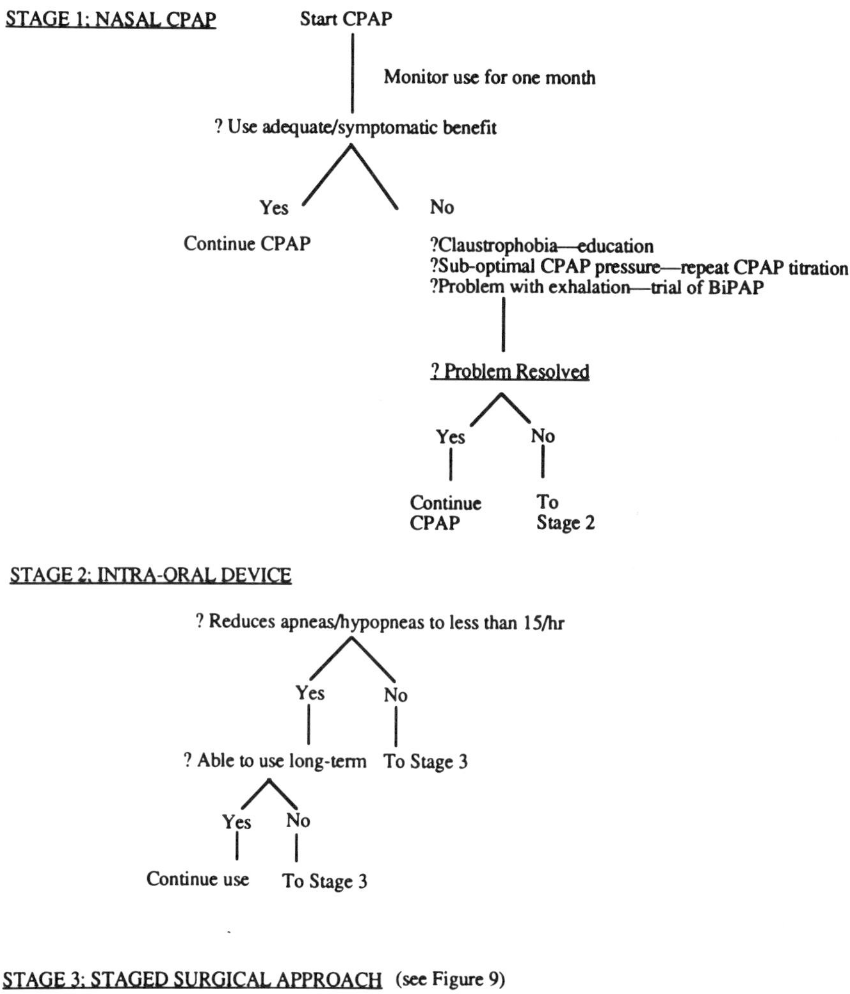

FIG 10.
Proposed staged approach to therapy of obstructive sleep apnea: The first stage is use of nasal continuous positive airway pressure (CPAP); the second stage is use of an intraoral device; and the third stage is surgery. For further details, see text.

use during the first month of treatment is highly predictive of later use.[232] At the end of this month, the physician should carefully assess the pattern of use of CPAP and the benefit of therapy. Patients not using the therapy sufficiently, for example less than a total of 120 hours over a 1-month period (i.e., less than 4 hours on average per night), should be assessed carefully. They should be questioned about claustrophobia and failure to obtain symptomatic benefit, since both of these have been identified as predictors of nonuse.[232] Patients with claustrophobia should be given special education, although at this time there are no data about whether this can be effective. Patients who report no symptomatic benefit should, in my view, be restudied with their CPAP in place. There is the distinct possibility that their CPAP pressure is suboptimal and that sleep-related respiratory events are still occurring. Those patients who cannot tolerate CPAP because of difficulty exhaling or who find the pressure difficult to tolerate should be given a trial with bilevel therapy (BiPAP).

In the majority of patients, CPAP therapy should be continued with close observation for the next 2 months or so. Attempts should be made to reinforce use in those patients experiencing difficulties. If, however, after that period, patients are still not using the therapy sufficiently, e.g., less than 120 hours of total use per month, they should be considered CPAP failures and move to the second stage.

In my view, the next stage of therapy should be the use of an intraoral device. The data for its efficacy are somewhat less compelling than are those for CPAP. Nevertheless, information is growing, and intraoral devices can be effective in certain patients. What we do not know, however, is how to reliably identify such patients, and what the long-term patterns of use of this device are. There is a need to develop systems to monitor use, similar to the ones we have currently for CPAP. Failure of the intraoral device might also occur due to two major factors. First, the device may not correct the respiratory disturbance during sleep to acceptable levels.[240, 241] Second, patients may not be able to tolerate its use nightly.

If patients also become therapeutic failures with the intraoral device, then surgery should be considered. The most promising approach is that described by the Stanford group.[287] It is still, however, a somewhat new approach and currently should only be done in major centers.

This synthesis of available information into a proposed staged approach is a personal opinion. Although there are data about individual components of the approach, there are no data about the efficacy of the overall plan. There is a real lack of data from controlled clinical trials for treatment of this extremely common disease.

Conclusion

Obstructive sleep apnea is an extremely common condition. Its medical impact is only beginning to be recognized. It is a disease which, because of the increased risk of driving accidents, puts not only the patient at risk but others on the highway as well. This places an extra burden on physicians to recognize the disease at an early point and to particularly ensure that patients with severe, untreated sleep apnea are not engaged in driving trucks, buses, and trains, or piloting aircraft. Given the high prevalence of the disease, new, more cost-effective approaches to diagnosis need to evolve. Although effective treatments are available, these are not without problems, and there is clearly a need for new approaches. Effective treatment of obstructive sleep apnea will not only improve the quality of life and increase the productivity of the patient, but it would also seem to reduce mortality and remove a correctable risk factor for acute vascular events.

Acknowledgments

I am grateful to Drs. Richard J. Schwab, Richard O. Davies, Leszek K. Kubin, and David F. Dinges for helpful discussions, and to Daniel C. Barrett for preparation of the manuscript. Original research reported was supported in part by NIH SCOR grant HL-42236.

References

1. Young T, Palta M, Dempsey J, et al: The occurrence of sleep-disordered breathing among middle-aged adults. *N Engl J Med* 1993; 328:1230–1235.
2. Phillipson EA: Sleep apnea—A major public health problem (editorial). *N Engl J Med* 1993; 328:1271–1273.
3. Johns MW: A new method for measuring daytime sleepiness: The Epworth Sleepiness Scale. *Sleep* 1991; 14:540–545.
4. Kapuniai LE, Andrew DJ, Crowell DH, et al: Identifying sleep apnea from self-reports. *Sleep* 1988; 11:430–436.
5. Viner S, Szalai JP, Hoffstein V: Are history and physical examination a good screening test for sleep apnea? *Ann Intern Med* 1991; 115:356–359.
6. Maislin G, Kribbs NB, Pack AI, et al: A survey screen for likelihood ratio prediction of apnea. *Sleep Res* 1993; 22:369.
7. White DP: Central sleep apnea, in Kryger MH, Roth T, Dement WC (eds): *Principles and Practice of Sleep Medicine.* Philadelphia, WB Saunders, 1989, pp 513–524.
8. Bradley TD, Phillipson EA: Central sleep apnea. *Clin Chest Med* 1992; 13:493–505.
9. Guilleminault C, van den Hoed J, Mitler M: Clinical overview of the sleep apnea syndromes, in Guilleminault C, Dement W (eds): *Sleep Apnea Syndromes.* New York, Alan R. Liss, 1978, pp 1–12.
10. Carskadon MA, Dement WC: Respiration during sleep in the aged human. *J Gerontol* 1981; 36:420–423.
11. Ancoli-Israel S, Kripke DF, Mason W, et al: Sleep apnea and periodic movements in an aging sample. *J Gerontol* 1985; 40:419–425.
12. Berry DT, Webb WB, Block AJ: Sleep apnea syndrome. A critical review of the apnea index as a diagnostic criterion. *Chest* 1984; 86:529–531.
13. Knight H, Millman RP, Gur RC, et al: Clinical significance of sleep apnea in the elderly. *Am Rev Respir Dis* 1987; 136:845–850.
14. Gould GA, Whyte KF, Rhind GB, et al: The sleep hypopnea syndrome. *Am Rev Respir Dis* 1988; 137:895–898.
15. Guilleminault C, Stoohs R, Duncan S: Snoring. I. Daytime sleepiness in regular heavy snorers. *Chest* 1991; 99:40–48.
16. Guilleminault C, Stoohs R, Clerk A, et al: From obstructive sleep apnea syndrome to upper airway resistance syndrome: Consistency of daytime sleepiness. *Sleep* 1992; 15:S13–S16.
17. Wittig RM, Romaker A, Zorick FJ, et al: Night-to-night consistency of apneas during sleep. *Am Rev Respir Dis* 1984; 129:244–246.

18. Bliwise DL, Carsakdon MA, Dement WC: Nightly variation of periodic leg movements in sleep in middle aged and elderly individuals. *Arch Gerontol Geriatr* 1988; 7:273–279.
19. Mosko SS, Dickel MH, Ashurst J: Night-to-night variability in sleep apnea and sleep-related periodic leg movements in the elderly. *Sleep* 1988; 11:340–348.
20. Meyer TJ, Eveloff SE, Kline LR, et al: One negative polysomnogram does not exclude obstructive sleep apnea. *Chest* 1993; 103:756–760.
21. Davies SF, Iber C: Obstructive sleep apnea associated with adult-acquired micrognathia from rheumatoid arthritis. *Am Rev Respir Dis* 1983; 127:245–247.
22. Mezon BJ, West P, MaClean JP, et al: Sleep apnea in acromegaly. *Am J Med* 1980; 69:615–618.
23. Grunstein RR, Ho KY, Sullivan CE: Sleep apnea in acromegaly. *Ann Intern Med* 1991; 115:527–532.
24. Marcus CL, Keens TG, Bautista DB, et al: Obstructive sleep apnea in children with Down syndrome. *Pediatrics* 1991; 88:132–139.
25. Davies RJ, Ali NJ, Stradling JR: Neck circumference and other clinical features in the diagnosis of the obstructive sleep apnoea syndrome. *Thorax* 1992; 47:101–105.
26. Davies RJ, Stradling JR: The relationship between neck circumference, radiographic pharyngeal anatomy, and the obstructive sleep apnoea syndrome. *Eur Respir J* 1990; 3:509–514.
27. Bohlman ME, Haponik EF, Smith PL, et al: CT demonstration of pharyngeal narrowing in adult obstructive sleep apnea. *AJR Am J Roentgenol* 1983; 140:543–548.
28. Kuna ST, Bedi DG, Ryckman C: Effect of nasal airway positive pressure on upper airway size and configuration. *Am Rev Respir Dis* 1988; 138:969–975.
29. Rivlin J, Hoffstein V, Kalbfleisch J, et al: Upper airway morphology in patients with idiopathic obstructive sleep apnea. *Am Rev Respir Dis* 1984; 129:355–360.
30. Suratt PM, Dee P, Atkinson RL, et al: Fluoroscopic and computed tomographic features of the pharyngeal airway in obstructive sleep apnea. *Am Rev Respir Dis* 1983; 127:487–492.
31. Haponik EF, Smith PL, Bohlman ME, et al: Computerized tomography in obstructive sleep apnea. Correlation of airway size with physiology during sleep and wakefulness. *Am Rev Respir Dis* 1983; 127:221–226.
32. Stauffer JL, Zwillich CW, Cadieux RJ, et al: Pharyngeal size and resistance in obstructive sleep apnea. *Am Rev Respir Dis* 1987; 136:623–627.
33. Rodenstein DO, Dooms G, Thomas Y, et al: Pharyngeal shape and dimensions in healthy subjects, snorers, and patients with obstructive sleep apnoea. *Thorax* 1990; 45:722–727.
34. Schwab RJ, Gefter WB, Hoffman EA, et al: Dynamic upper airway imaging during respiration in normal subjects and patients with sleep disordered breathing. *Am Rev Respir Dis* (in press).
35. Horner RL, Sheat SA, McIvor J, et al: Pharyngeal size and shape during wakefulness and sleep in patients with obstructive sleep apnoea. *Q J Med* 1989; 72:719–735.
36. Horner RL, Mohiaddin RH, Lowell DG, et al: Sites and sizes of fat deposits

around the pharynx in obese patients with obstructive sleep apnoea and weight matched controls. *Eur Respir J* 1989; 2:613–622.

37. Shelton KE, Gay SB, Hollowell DE, et al: Mandible enclosure of upper airway and weight in obstructive sleep apnea. *Am Rev Respir Dis* 1993; 148:195–200.
38. Schwab RJ, Gupta KB, Hoffman EA, et al: Differences in upper airway soft tissue anatomy in normal subjects and patients with sleep disordered breathing. *Am Rev Respir Dis* 1993; 147:A947.
39. Lowe AA, Gionhaku N, Takeuchi K, et al: Three-dimensional CT reconstructions of tongue and airway in adult subjects with obstructive sleep apnea. *Am J Orthod Dentofacial Orthop* 1986; 90:364–374.
40. Ryan CF, Lowe AA, Li D, et al: Three-dimensional upper airway computed tomography in obstructive sleep apnea. A prospective study in patients treated by uvulopalatopharyngoplasty. *Am Rev Respir Dis* 1991; 144:428–432.
41. deberry-Borowiecki B, Kukwa A, Blanks RH: Cephalometric analysis for diagnosis and treatment of obstructive sleep apnea. *Laryngoscope* 1988; 98:226–234.
42. Lyberg T, Krogstad O, Djupesland G: Cephalometric analysis in patients with obstructive sleep apnoea syndrome: II. Soft tissue morphology. *J Laryngol Otol* 1989; 103:293–297.
43. Ryan CF, Lowe AA, Li D, et al: Magnetic resonance imaging of the upper airway in obstructive sleep apnea before and after chronic nasal continuous positive airway pressure therapy. *Am Rev Respir Dis* 1991; 144:939–944.
44. Brown IG, Bradley TD, Phillipson EA, et al: Pharyngeal compliance in snoring subjects with and without obstructive sleep apnea. *Am Rev Respir Dis* 1985; 132:211–215.
45. Issa FG, Sullivan CE: Upper airway closing pressures in obstructive sleep apnea. *J Appl Physiol* 1984; 57:520–527.
46. Suratt PM, McTier RF, Wilhoit SC: Collapsibility of the nasopharyngeal airway in obstructive sleep apnea. *Am Rev Respir Dis* 1985; 132:967–971.
47. Suratt PM, Wilhoit SC, Cooper K: Induction of airway collapse with subatmospheric pressure in awake patients with sleep apnea. *J Appl Physiol* 1984; 57:140–146.
48. Schwartz AR, Smith PL, Wise RA, et al: Induction of upper airway occlusion in sleeping individuals with subatmospheric nasal pressure. *J Appl Physiol* 1988; 64:535–542.
49. Smith PL, Wise RA, Gold AR, et al: Upper airway pressure-flow relationships in obstructive sleep apnea. *J Appl Physiol* 1988; 64:789–795.
50. Schwab RJ, Gefter WB, Pack AI, et al: Dynamic imaging of the upper airway during respiration in normal subjects. *J Appl Physiol* 1993; 74:1504–1514.
51. Mezzanotte WS, Tangel DJ, White DP: Waking genioglossal electromyogram in sleep apnea patients versus normal controls (a neuromuscular compensatory mechanism). *J Clin Invest* 1992; 89:1571–1579.
52. Sanders MH, Moore SE: Inspiratory and expiratory partitioning of airway resistance during sleep in patients with sleep apnea. *Am Rev Respir Dis* 1983; 127:554–558.
53. Sanders MH, Rogers RM, Pennock BE: Prolonged expiratory phase in sleep apnea. A unifying hypothesis. *Am Rev Respir Dis* 1985; 131:401–408.
54. Suto Y, Matsuo T, Kato T, et al: Evaluation of the pharyngeal airway in pa-

tients with sleep apnea: value of ultrafast MR imaging. *AJR Am J Roentgenol* 1993; 160:311–314.

55. Wiegand DA, Latz B, Zwillich CW, et al: Upper airway resistance and geniohyoid muscle activity in normal men during wakefulness and sleep. *J Appl Physiol* 1990; 69:1252–1261.
56. Skatrud JB, Dempsey JA: Airway resistance and respiratory muscle function in snorers during NREM sleep. *J Appl Physiol* 1985; 59:328–335.
57. Hudgel DW: Variable site of airway narrowing among obstructive sleep apnea patients. *J Appl Physiol* 1986; 61:1403–1409.
58. Remmers JE, deGroot WJ, Sauerland EK, et al: Pathogenesis of upper airway occlusion during sleep. *J Appl Physiol* 1978; 44:931–938.
59. Onal E, Lopata M, O'Connor T: Pathogenesis of apneas in hypersomnia-sleep apnea syndrome. *Am Rev Respir Dis* 1982; 125:167–174.
60. Hendricks JC, Kovalski RJ, Kline LR: Phasic respiratory muscle patterns and sleep-disordered breathing during rapid eye movement sleep in the English bulldog. *Am Rev Respir Dis* 1991; 144:1112–1120.
61. Hendricks JC, Petrof B, Panckeri K, et al: Compensatory hyperactivity of an upper airway dilator in bulldogs. *Am Rev Respir Dis* 1992; 145:A211.
62. Hwang JC, St John WM, Bartlett D Jr: Afferent pathways for hypoglossal and phrenic responses to changes in upper airway pressure. *Respir Physiol* 1984; 55:341–354.
63. Mathew OP, Abu-Osba YK, Thach BT: Genioglossus muscle responses to upper airway pressure changes: afferent pathways. *J Appl Physiol* 1982; 52:445–450.
64. Mathew OP, Abu-osba YK, Thach BT: Influence of upper airway pressure changes on genioglossus muscle respiratory activity. *J Appl Physiol* 1982; 52:438–444.
65. Van Lunteren E, Van de Graaff WB, Parker DM, et al: Nasal and laryngeal reflex responses to negative upper airway pressure. *J Appl Physiol* 1984; 56:746–752.
66. Mathew OP: Upper airway negative-pressure effects on respiratory activity of upper airway muscles. *J Appl Physiol* 1984; 56:500–505.
67. Horner RL, Innes JA, Murphy K, et al: Evidence for reflex upper airway dilator muscle activation by sudden negative airway pressure in man. *J Physiol (Lond)* 1991; 436:15–29.
68. Leiter JC, Daubenspeck JA: Selective reflex activation of the genioglossus in humans. *J Appl Physiol* 1990; 68:2581–2587.
69. Horner RL, Innes JA, Morrell M, et al: The effect of sleep on reflex pharyngeal dilator muscle activation by negative airway pressure stimuli in man. *Am Rev Respir Dis* 1992; 145:A212.
70. Wheatley JR, White DP: Influence of sleep on genioglossus (GG) EMG reflex response to negative pressure in normal subjects. *Am Rev Respir Dis* 1992; 145:A212.
71. Baghdoyan HA, Rodrigo-Angulo ML, McCarley RW, et al: A neuroanatomical gradient in the pontine tegmentum for the cholinoceptive induction of desynchronized sleep signs. *Brain Res* 1987; 414:245–261.
72. Jones BE: Paradoxical sleep and its chemical/structural substrates in the brain. *Neuroscience* 1991; 40:637–656.
73. Lydic R, Baghdoyan HA: Cholinoceptive pontine reticular mechanisms cause state-dependent respiratory changes in the cat. *Neurosci Lett* 1989; 102:211–216.

74. Lydic R, Baghdoyan HA, Wertz R, et al: Cholinergic reticular mechanisms influence state-dependent ventilatory response to hypercapnia. *Am J Physiol* 1991; 261:R738–R746.
75. Lydic R, Baghdoyan HA, Zwillich CW: State-dependent hypotonia in posterior cricoarytenoid muscles of the larynx caused by cholinoceptive reticular mechanisms. *FASEB J* 1989; 3:1625–1631.
76. Kimura H, Kubin L, Davies RO, et al: Cholinergic stimulation of the pons depresses respiration in decerebrate cats. *J Appl Physiol* 1990; 69:2280–2289.
77. Taguchi O, Kubin L, Pack AI: Evocation of postural atonia and respiratory depression by pontine carbachol in the decerebrate rat. *Brain Res* 1992; 595:107–115.
78. Morales FR, Engelhardt JK, Soja PJ, et al: Motoneuron properties during motor inhibition produced by microinjection of carbachol into the pontine reticular formation of the decerebrate cat. *J Neurophysiol* 1987; 57:1118–1129.
79. Morales FR, Chase MH: Postsynaptic control of lumbar motoneuron excitability during active sleep in the chronic cat. *Brain Res* 1981; 225:279–295.
80. Morales FR, Boxer P, Chase MH: Behavioral state-specific inhibitory postsynaptic potentials impinge on cat lumbar motoneurons during active sleep. *Exp Neurol* 1987; 98:418–435.
81. Morales FR, Chase MH: Repetitive synaptic potentials responsible for inhibition of spinal cord motoneurons during active sleep. *Exp Neurol* 1982; 78:471–476.
82. Chase MH, Soja PJ, Morales FR: Evidence that glycine mediates the postsynaptic potentials that inhibit lumbar motoneurons during the atonia of active sleep. *J Neurosci* 1989; 9:743–751.
83. Kubin L, Kimura H, Tojima H, et al: Suppression of hypoglossal motoneurons during the carbachol-induced atonia of REM sleep is not caused by fast synaptic inhibition. *Brain Res* 1993; 611:300–312.
84. Manaker S, Tischler LJ, Morrison AR: Raphespinal and reticulospinal axon collaterals to the hypoglossal nucleus in the rat. *J Comp Neurol* 1992; 322:68–78.
85. Jacobs BL, Azmitia EC: Structure and function of the brain serotonin system. *Physiol Rev* 1992; 72:165–229.
86. Kubin L, Tojima H, Davies RO, et al: Serotonergic excitatory drive to hypoglossal motoneurons in the decerebrate cat. *Neurosci Lett* 1992; 139:243–248.
87. Berger AJ, Bayliss DA, Viana F: Modulation of neonatal rat hypoglossal motoneuron excitability by serontonin. *Neurosci Lett* 1992; 143:164–168.
88. Bayliss DA, Viana F, Berger AJ: Mechanisms underlying excitatory effects of thyrotropin-releasing hormone on rat hypoglossal motoneurons *in vitro*. *J Neurophysiol* 1992; 68:1733–1745.
89. Schmidt HS: L-tryptophan in the treatment of impaired respiration during sleep. *Bull Eur Physiol Respir* 1982; 19:625–629.
90. Hanzel DA, Proia NG, Hudgel DW: Response of obstructive sleep apnea to fluoxetine and protriptyline. *Chest* 1991; 100:416–421.
91. ATS Consensus Conference. Indications and standards for cardiopulmonary sleep studies. *Am Rev Respir Dis* 1989; 139:559–568.
92. Iber C, O'Brien C, Schluter J, et al: Single night studies in obstructive sleep apnea. *Sleep* 1991; 14:383–385.
93. Jamieson AO: Split-night studies: A new standard? Forcing the examination of outcome. *Sleep* 1991; 14:381–382.

94. Sanders MH, Black J, Costantino JP, et al: Diagnosis of sleep-disordered breathing in half-night polysomnography. *Am Rev Respir Dis* 1991; 144:1256–1261.
95. Sanders MH, Kern NB, Costantino JP, et al: Adequacy of prescribing positive airway pressure therapy by mask for sleep apnea on the basis of a partial-night trial. *Am Rev Respir Dis* 1993; 147:1169–1174.
96. Stradling JR: Sleep studies for sleep-related breathing disorders (Consensus Report). *J Sleep Res* 1992; 1:265–273.
97. Thorpy M (chairperson): Role of unattended monitoring. Position Statement. American Sleep Disorders Association, Rochester, Minn, 1993.
98. George CF, Millar TW, Kryger MH: Identification and quantification of apneas by computer-based analysis of oxygen saturation. *Am Rev Respir Dis* 1988; 137:1238–1240.
99. Allan MA, Fitzpatrick MF, Molloy J, et al: Correlation between oximetry and polysomnography in patients with sleep apnea/hypopnea syndrome. *Am Rev Respir Dis* 1990; 141:A858.
100. Williams AJ, Yu G, Santigo S, et al: Screening for sleep apnea using pulse oximetry and a clinical score. *Chest* 1991; 100:631–635.
101. Douglas NJ, Thomas S, Jan MA: Clinical value of polysomnography. *Lancet* 1992; 339:347–350.
102. Gyulay S, Olson LG, Hensley MJ, et al: A comparison of clinical assessment and home oximetry in the diagnosis of obstructive sleep apnea. *Am Rev Respir Dis* 1993; 147:50–53.
103. Sèriés F, Marc I, Cornier Y, et al: Nocturnal home oximetry in patients with suspected sleep apnea hypopnea syndrome. *Ann Intern Med* 1993; 119:449–453.
104. Slutsky AS, Strohl KP: Quantification of oxygen saturation during episodic hypoxemia. *Am Rev Respir Dis* 1980; 121:893–895.
105. Lavie P: Incidence of sleep apnea in a presumably healthy working population: a significant relationship with excessive daytime sleepiness. *Sleep* 1983; 6:312–318.
106. Gislason T, Almqvist M, Eriksson G, et al: Prevalence of sleep apnea syndrome among Swedish men—an epidemiological study. *J Clin Epidemiol* 1988; 41:571–576.
107. Stradling JR, Crosby JH: Predictors and prevalence of obstructive sleep apnoea and snoring in 1001 middle aged men. *Thorax* 1991; 46:85–90.
108. Gislason T, Taube A: Prevalence of sleep apnea syndrome—Estimation by two stage sampling. *Ups J Med Sci* 1987; 92:193–203.
109. Gislason T, Benediktdóttier D, Björnsson JD, et al: Snoring, hypertension and the sleep apnea syndrome. *Chest* 1993; 103:1147–1151.
110. Block AJ, Boysen PG, Wynne JW, et al: Sleep apnea, hypopnea and oxygen desaturation in normal subjects. A strong male predominance. *N Engl J Med* 1979; 300:513–517.
111. Guilleminault C, Quera-Salva MA, Partinen M, et al: Women and the obstructive sleep apnea syndrome. *Chest* 1988; 93:104–109.
112. Ambrogetti A, Olson LG, Saunders NA: Differences in the symptoms of men and women with obstructive sleep apnoea. *Aust N Z J Med* 1991; 21:863–866.
113. Stradling JR, Crosby JH, Payne CD: Self reported snoring and daytime sleepiness in men aged 35–65 years. *Thorax* 1991; 46:807–810.

114. Gonzalez-Rothi RJ, Foresman GE, Block AJ: Do patients with sleep apnea die in their sleep? *Chest* 1988; 94:531–538.
115. Partinen M, Jamieson A, Guilleminault C: Long-term outcome for obstructive sleep apnea syndrome patients. Mortality. *Chest* 1988; 94:1200–1204.
116. Partinen M, Guilleminault C: Daytime sleepiness and vascular morbidity at seven-year follow-up in obstructive sleep apnea patients. *Chest* 1990; 97:27–32.
117. He J, Kryger MH, Zorick FJ, et al: Mortality and apnea index in obstructive sleep apnea. Experience in 385 male patients. *Chest* 1988; 94:9–14.
118. Seppälä T, Partinen M, Penttilä A, et al: Sudden death and sleeping history among Finnish men. *J Intern Med* 1991; 229:23–28.
119. Findley LJ, Levinson MP, Bonnie RJ: Driving performance and automobile accidents in patients with sleep apnea. *Clin Chest Med* 1992; 13:427–435.
120. Kribbs NB, Getsy JE, Dinges DF: Investigation and management of daytime sleepiness in sleep apnea, in Saunders NA, Sullivan CE (eds): *Sleep and Breathing,* vol. 2. New York, Marcel Dekker, 1993.
121. George CF, Nickerson PW, Hanley PJ, et al: Sleep apnoea patients have more automobile accidents. *Lancet* 1987; 2:447.
122. Findley LJ, Unverzagt ME, Suratt PM: Automobile accidents involving patients with obstructive sleep apnea. *Am Rev Respir Dis* 1988; 138:337–340.
123. Findley LJ, Fabrizio M, Thommi G, et al: Severity of sleep apnea and automobile crashes. *N Engl J Med* 1989; 320:868–869.
124. Haraldsson PO, Carenfelt C, Laurell H, et al: Driving vigilance simulator test. *Acta Otolaryngol (Stockh)* 1990; 110:136–140.
125. Findley LJ, Fabrizio MJ, Knight H, et al: Driving simulator performance in patients with sleep apnea. *Am Rev Respir Dis* 1989; 140:529–530.
126. Findley LJ, Weiss JW, Jabour ER: Drivers with untreated sleep apnea. A cause of death and serious injury. *Arch Intern Med* 1991; 151:1451–1452.
127. Parsons M: Fits and other causes of loss of consciousness while driving. *Q J Med* 1986; 58:295–303.
128. The People of the State of Illinois v. Errol Wilson. Supreme Court of Illinois 1991. III. Lesux 28, April 18, 1991.
129. Shepard JW Jr: Cardiopulmonary consequences of obstructive sleep apnea. *Mayo Clin Proc* 1990; 65:1250–1259.
130. Bradley TD: Right and left ventricular functional impairment and sleep apnea. *Clin Chest Med* 1992; 13:459–479.
131. Shepard JW Jr: Hypertension, cardiac arrhythmias, myocardial infarction, and stroke in relation to obstructive sleep apnea. *Clin Chest Med* 1992; 13:437–458.
132. Waller PC, Bhopal RS: Is snoring a cause of vascular disease? An epidemiological review. *Lancet* 1989; 1:143–146.
133. Levinson PD, Millman RP: Causes and consequences of blood pressure alterations in obstructive sleep apnea. *Arch Intern Med* 1991; 151:455–462.
134. Hoffstein V, Chan CK, Slutsky AS: Sleep apnea and systemic hypertension: A causal association review. *Am J Med* 1991; 91:190–196.
135. Mancia G, Zanchetti A: Cardiovascular regulation during sleep, in Orem J (ed): *Physiology of Sleep.* New York, Academic Press, 1980.
136. Bristow JD, Honour AJ, Pickering TG, et al: Cardiovascular and respiratory changes during sleep in normal and hypertensive subjects. *Cardiovasc Res* 1969; 3:476–485.

137. Snyder F, Hobson SA, Morrison DF, et al: Changes in respiration, heart rate and systolic blood pressure in human sleep. *J Appl Physiol* 1964; 19:417–422.
138. Khatri IM, Freis ED: Hemodynamic changes during sleep. *J Appl Physiol* 1967; 22:867–873.
139. Guilleminault C, Pool P, Motta J, et al: Sinus arrest during REM sleep in young adults. *N Engl J Med* 1984; 311:1006–1010.
140. Coccagna G, Mantovani M, Brignani F, et al: Laboratory note. Arterial pressure changes during spontaneous sleep in man. *Electroencephalogr Clin Neurophysiol* 1971; 31:277–281.
141. Littler WA: Sleep and blood pressure: Further observations. *Am Heart J* 1979; 97:35–37.
142. Coccagna G, Mantovani M, Brignani F, et al: Continuous recording of the pulmonary and systemic arterial pressure during sleep in syndromes of hypersomnia with periodic breathing. *Bull Physiopathol Respir* 1972; 8:1159–1172.
143. Schroeder JS, Motta J, Guilleminault C: Hemodynamic studies in sleep, in Guilleminault C, Dement WC (eds): *Sleep Apnea Syndromes.* New York, Alan R. Liss, 1978.
144. Shepard JW Jr: Gas exchange and hemodynamics during sleep. *Med Clin North Am* 1985; 69:1243–1264.
145. Tilkian AG, Guilleminault C, Schroeder JS, et al: Hemodynamics in sleep-induced apnea. Studies during wakefulness and sleep. *Ann Intern Med* 1976; 85:714–719.
146. Zwillich C, Devlin T, White D, et al: Bradycardia during sleep apnea. Characteristics and mechanism. *J Clin Invest* 1982; 69:1286–1292.
147. Buda AJ, Schroeder JS, Guilleminault C: Abnormalities of pulmonary artery wedge pressures in sleep-induced apnea. *Int J Cardiol* 1981; 1:67–74.
148. Guilleminault C, Motta J, Mihm F, et al: Obstructive sleep apnea and cardiac index. *Chest* 1986; 89:331–334.
149. Podszus T, Mayer J, Penzel T, et al: Nocturnal hemodynamics in patients with sleep apnea. *Eur J Respir Dis Suppl* 1986; 146:435–442.
150. Guilleminault C, Suzuki M: Sleep-related hemodynamics and hypertension with partial or complete upper airway obstruction during sleep. *Sleep* 1992; 15:S20–S24.
151. Stoohs R, Guilleminault C: Cardiovascular changes associated with obstructive sleep apnea syndrome. *J Appl Physiol* 1992; 72:583–589.
152. Guilleminault C, Connolly SJ, Winkle RA: Cardiac arrhythmia and conduction disturbances during sleep in 400 patients with sleep apnea syndrome. *Am J Cardiol* 1983; 52:490–494.
153. Shepard JW Jr, Garrison MW, Grither DA, et al: Relationship of ventricular ectopy to oxyhemoglobin desaturation in patients with obstructive sleep apnea. *Chest* 1985; 88:335–340.
154. Miller WP: Cardiac arrhythmias and conduction disturbances in the sleep apnea syndrome. Prevalence and significance. *Am J Med* 1982; 73:317–321.
155. Shiomi T, Guilleminault C, Stoohs R, et al: Leftward shift of the intraventricular septum and pulsus paradoxus in obstructive sleep apnea syndrome. *Chest* 1991; 100:894–902.
156. Ringler J, Basner RC, Shannon R, et al: Hypoxemia alone does not explain blood pressure elevations after obstructive apneas. *J Appl Physiol* 1990; 69:2143–2148.

157. Hedner J, Ejnell H, Sellgren J, et al: Is high and fluctuating muscle nerve sympathetic activity in the sleep apnoea syndrome of pathogenetic importance for the development of hypertension? *J Hypertens Suppl* 1988; 6:S529–S531.
158. Kales A, Bixler EO, Cadieux RJ, et al: Sleep apnoea in a hypertensive population. *Lancet* 1984; 2:1005–1008.
159. Fletcher EC, DeBehnke RD, Lovoi MS, et al: Undiagnosed sleep apnea in patients with essential hypertension. *Ann Intern Med* 1985; 103:190–195.
160. Williams AJ, Houston D, Finberg S, et al: Sleep apnea syndrome and essential hypertension. *Am J Cardiol* 1985; 55:1019–1022.
161. McGinty D, Beahm E, Stern N, et al: Nocturnal hypotension in older men with sleep-related breathing disorders. *Chest* 1988; 94:305–311.
162. Lavie P, Ben-Yosef R, Rubin AE: Prevalence of sleep apnea syndrome among patients with essential hypertension. *Am Heart J* 1984; 108:373–376.
163. Warley ARH, Mitchell JH, Stradling JR: Prevalence of nocturnal hypoxaemia amongst men with mild to moderate hypertension. *Q J Med* 1988; 68:637–644.
164. Hirshkowitz M, Karacan I, Gurakar A, et al: Hypertension, erectile dysfunction, and occult sleep apnea. *Sleep* 1989; 12:223–232.
165. Millman RP, Redline S, Carlisle CC, et al: Daytime hypertension in obstructive sleep apnea. Prevalence and contributing risk factors. *Chest* 1991; 99:861–866.
166. Ali NJ, Davies RJO, Fleetham JA, et al: The acute effects of continuous positive airway pressure and oxygen administration on blood pressure during obstructive sleep apnea. *Chest* 1992; 101:1526–1532.
167. Sforza E, Capecchi V, Lugaresi E: Haemodynamic effects of short-term nasal continuous positive airway pressure therapy in sleep apnoea syndrome: Monitoring by a finger arterial pressure device. *Eur Respir J* 1992; 5:858–863.
168. Guilleminault C, Eldridge FL, Dement WC: Une anomalie du systeme nerveux peut elle etre responsable de troubles hemodynamiques. *Presse Med* 1975; 4:1343–1348.
169. Motta J, Guilleminault C, Schroeder JS, et al: Tracheostomy and hemodynamic changes in sleep-induced apnea. *Ann Intern Med* 1978; 89: 454–458.
170. Guilleminault C, Simmons FB, Motta J, et al: Obstructive sleep apnea syndrome and tracheostomy: Long-term follow-up experience. *Arch Intern Med* 1981; 141:985–988.
171. Jennum P, Wildschiødtz G, Christensen NJ, et al: Blood pressure, catecholamines, and pancreatic polypeptide in obstructive sleep apnea with and without nasal continuous positive airway pressure (nCPAP) treatment. *Am J Hypertens* 1989; 2:847–852.
172. Hoffstein V, Rubinstein L, Mateika S, et al: Determinants of blood pressure in snorers. *Lancet* 1988; 2:992–994.
173. Stradling JR, Crosby JH: Relation between systemic hypertension and sleep hypoxaemia or snoring: Analysis in 748 men drawn from general practice. *BMJ* 1990; 300:75–78.
174. Muller JE, Ludmer PL, Willich SN, et al: Circadian variation in the frequency of sudden cardiac death. *Circulation* 1987; 75:131–138.
175. Willich SN, Levy D, Rocco MB, et al: Circadian variation in the incidence of

sudden cardiac death in the Framingham Heart Study population. *Am J Cardiol* 1987; 60:801–806.
176. Muller JE, Stone PH, Turi ZG, et al: Circadian variation in the frequency of onset of acute myocardial infarction. *N Engl J Med* 1985; 313:1315–1322.
177. Marshall J: Diurnal variation in occurrence of strokes. *Stroke* 1977; 8:230–231.
178. Palomaki H, Partinen M, Jurela S, et al: Snoring as a risk factor for sleep-related brain infarction. *Stroke* 1989; 20:1311–1315.
179. Marler JR Price TR, Clark GL, et al: Morning increase in onset of ischemic stroke. *Stroke* 1989; 20:473–476.
180. Mitler MM, Hajdukovic RM, Shafor R, et al: When people die. Causes of death versus time of death. *Am J Med* 1987; 82:266–274.
181. Koskenvuo M, Kaprio J, Telakivi T, et al: Snoring as a risk factor for ischaemic heart disease and stroke in men. *Br Med J* 1987; 294:16–19.
182. Partinen M, Palomaki H: Snoring and cerebral infarction. *Lancet* 1985; 2:1325–1326.
183. D'Alessandro R, Magelli C, Gamberini G, et al: Snoring every night as a risk factor for myocardial infarction: A case-control study. *BMJ* 1990; 300:1557–1558.
184. Hung J, Whitford EG, Parsons RW: Association of sleep apnoea with myocardial infarction in men. *Lancet* 1990; 336:261–264.
185. Rajagopal KR, Abbrecht PH, Derderian SS, et al: Obstructive sleep apnea in hypothyroidism. *Ann Intern Med* 1984; 101:491–494.
186. Grunstein RR, Sullivan CE: Sleep apnea and hypothyroidism: Mechanisms and management. *Am J Med* 1988; 85:775–779.
187. Smith PL, Gold AR, Meyers DA, et al: Weight loss in mildly to moderately obese patients with obstructive sleep apnea. *Ann Intern Med* 1985; 103:850–855.
188. Rubinstein I, Colapinto N, Rotstein LE, et al: Improvement in upper airway function after weight loss in patients with obstructive sleep apnea. *Am Rev Respir Dis* 1988; 138:1192–1195.
189. Pasquali R, Colella P, Cirignotta F, et al: Treatment of obese patients with obstructive sleep apnea syndrome (OSAS): Effect of weight loss and interference of otorhinolaryngoiatric pathology. *Int J Obes* 1990; 14:207–217.
190. Sugerman HJ, Fairman RP, Baron PL, et al: Gastric surgery for respiratory insufficiency of obesity. *Chest* 1986; 90:81–86.
191. Schwartz AR, Gold AR, Schubert N, et al: Effect of weight loss on upper airway collapsibility in obstructive sleep apnea. *Am Rev Respir Dis* 1991; 144:494–498.
192. Krol RC, Knuth SL, Bartlett D Jr: Selective reduction of genioglossal muscle activity by alcohol in normal human subjects. *Am Rev Respir Dis* 1984; 129:247–250.
193. Robinson RW, White DP, Zwillich CW: Moderate alcohol ingestion increases upper airway resistance in normal subjects. *Am Rev Respir Dis* 1985; 132:1238–1241.
194. Mitler MM, Dawson A, Henriksen SJ, et al: Bedtime ethanol increases resistance of upper airways and produces sleep apneas in asymptomatic snorers. *Alcoholism Clin Exp Res* 1988; 12:801–805.
195. Issa FG, Sullivan CE: Alcohol, snoring and sleep apnea. *J Neurol Neurosurg Psychiatry* 1982; 45:353–359.
196. Phillips BA, Okeson J, Paesani D, et al: Effect of sleep position on sleep apnea and parafunctional activity. *Chest* 1986; 90:424–429.

197. McEvoy RD, Sharp DJ, Thornton AT: The effects of posture on obstructive sleep apnea. *Am Rev Respir Dis* 1986; 133:662–666.
198. Cartwright RD, Diaz F, Ristanovic R: Comparing two treatments for positional sleep apnea: TRD and posture alarm. *Sleep Res* 1990; 19:202.
199. Tojima H, Kunitomo F, Kimura H, et al: Effects of acetazolamide in patients with the sleep apnoea syndrome. *Thorax* 1988; 43:113–119.
200. Gothe B, Strohl KP, Levin S, et al: Nicotine: A different approach to the treatment of obstructive sleep apnea. *Chest* 1985; 87:11–17.
201. Remmers JE, Anch AM, deGroot WJ, et al: Oropharyngeal muscle tone in obstructive sleep apnea before and after strychnine. *Sleep* 1980; 3:447–453.
202. Zwillich CW, Natalino MR, Sutton FD, et al: Effects of progesterone on chemosensitivity in normal men. *J Lab Clin Med* 1978; 92:262–269.
203. Bayliss DA, Millhorn DE: Central neural mechanisms of progesterone action: Application to the respiratory system. *J Appl Physiol* 1992; 73:393–404.
204. Bayliss DA, Cidlowski JA, Millhorn DE: The stimulation of respiration by progesterone in ovariectomized cat is mediated by an estrogen-dependent hypothalamic mechanism requiring gene expression. *Endocrinology* 1990; 126:519–527.
205. Lyons HA, Huang CT: Therapeutic use of progesterone in alveolar hypoventilation associated with obesity. *Am J Med* 1968; 44:881–888.
206. Sutton FD Jr, Zwillich CW, Creagh CE, et al: Progesterone for outpatient treatment of Pickwickian syndrome. *Ann Intern Med* 1975; 83:476–479.
207. Bayliss DA, Millhorn DE: Chronic estrogen exposure maintains elevated levels of progesterone receptor mRNA in guinea pig hypothalamus. *Brain Res Mol Brain Res* 1991; 10:167–172.
208. Schwab RJ, Getsy JE, Pack AI: Central nervous system failure, including sleep disorders, in Carlson RW, Geheb MA (eds): *The Principles and Practice of Medical Intensive Care.* Philadelphia, WB Saunders Co, 1993; 773–786.
209. Strohl KP, Hensley MJ, Saunders NA, et al: Progesterone administration and progressive sleep apneas. *JAMA* 1981; 245:1230–1232.
210. Rajagopal KR, Abbrecht PH, Jabbari B: Effects of medroxyprogesterone acetate in obstructive sleep apnea. *Chest* 1986; 90:815–821.
211. Cook WR, Benich JJ, Wooter SA: Indices of severity of obstructive sleep apnea syndrome do not change during medroxyprogesterone acetate therapy. *Chest* 1989; 96:262–266.
212. Millman RP. Medroxyprotesterone and obstructive sleep apnea. *Chest* 1989; 96:225–226.
213. Bonora M, St. John WM, Bledsoe TA: Differential elevation by protriptyline and depression by diazepam of upper airway respiratory motor activity. *Am Rev Respir Dis* 1985; 131:41–45.
214. Clark RW, Schmidt HS, Schaal SF, et al: Sleep apnea: Treatment with protriptyline. *Neurology* 1979; 29:1287–1292.
215. Brownell LG, West P, Sweatman P, et al: Protriptyline in obstructive sleep apnea: A double-blind trial. *N Engl J Med* 1982; 307:1037–1042.
216. Conway WA, Zorick F, Piccione P, et al: Protriptyline in the treatment of sleep apnoea. *Thorax* 1982; 37:49–53.
217. Smith PL, Haponik EF, Allen RP, et al: The effects of protriptyline in sleep-disordered breathing. *Am Rev Respir Dis* 1983; 127:8–13.
218. Stepanski EJ, Conway WA, Young DK, et al: A double-blind trial of protriptyline in the treatment of sleep apnea syndrome. *Henry Ford Hosp Med J* 1988; 36:5–8.
219. Findley LJ, Wilhoit SC, Suratt PM: Apnea duration and hypoxemia during

REM sleep in patients with obstructive sleep apnea. *Chest* 1985; 87:432–436.
220. Sullivan CE, Issa FG, Berthon-Jones M, et al: Reversal of obstructive sleep apnoea by continuous positive airway pressure applied through the nares. *Lancet* 1981; 1:862–865.
221. Kribbs NB, Pack AI, Kline LR, et al: Effects of one night without nasal CPAP treatment on sleep and sleepiness in patients with obstructive sleep apnea. *Am Rev Respir Dis* 1993; 147:1162–1168.
222. Hoffstein V, Viner S, Mateika S, et al: Treatment of obstructive sleep apnea with nasal continuous positive airway pressure. Patient compliance, perception of benefits, and side effects. *Am Rev Respir Dis* 1992; 145:841–845.
223. Sanders H, Gruendl CA, Rogers RM: Patient compliance with nasal CPAP therapy for sleep apnea. *Chest* 1986; 90:330–333.
224. Waldhorn RE, Herrick TW, Nguyen MC, et al: Long-term compliance with nasal continuous positive airway pressure therapy of obstructive sleep apnea. *Chest* 1990; 97:33–38.
225. Nino-Murcia G, McCann CC, Bliwise DL, et al: Compliance and side effects in sleep apnea patients treated with nasal continuous positive airway pressure. *West J Med* 1989; 150:165–169.
226. Jarjour NN, Wilson P: Pneumocephalus associated with nasal continuous positive airway pressure in a patient with sleep apnea syndrome. *Chest* 1989; 96:1425–1426.
227. Bamford CR, Quan SF: Bacterial meningitis—A possible complication of nasal continuous positive airway pressure therapy in a patient with obstructive sleep apnea syndrome and a mucocele. *Sleep* 1993; 16:31–32.
228. Rolfe I, Olson LG, Saunders NA: Long-term acceptance of continuous positive airway pressure in obstructive sleep apnea. *Am Rev Respir Dis* 1991; 144:1130–1133.
229. Rauscher H, Popp W, Wanke T, et al: Acceptance of CPAP therapy for sleep apnea. *Chest* 1991; 100:1019–1023.
230. Krieger J, Kurtz D: Objective measurement of compliance with nasal CPAP treatment for obstructive sleep apnoea syndrome. *Eur Respir J* 1988; 1:436–438.
231. Fletcher EC, Luckett RA: The effect of positive reinforcement on hourly compliance in nasal continuous positive airway pressure users with obstructive sleep apnea. *Am Rev Respir Dis* 1991; 143:936–941.
232. Kribbs NB, Pack AI, Kline LR, et al: Objective measurement of patterns of nasal CPAP use by patients with obstructive sleep apnea. *Am Rev Respir Dis* 1993; 147:887–895.
233. Harris C, Daniels B, Herold D, et al: Comparison of cannula and mask systems for administration of nasal continuous positive airway pressure for treatment of obstructive sleep apnea. *Sleep Res* 1990; 19:233.
234. Reeves-Hoche MK, Hudgel D, Meck R, et al: BiPAP vs. CPAP: patient compliance in the treatment of obstructive sleep apnea, six month data in a two-year study. *Am Rev Respir Dis* 1993; 147:A251.
235. Sanders MH, Kern N: Obstructive sleep apnea treated by independently adjusted inspiratory and expiratory positive airway pressures via nasal mask. Physiologic and clinical implications. *Chest* 1990; 98:317–324.
236. Cartwright RD, Samelson CF: The effects of a nonsurgical treatment for obstructive sleep apnea. *JAMA* 1982; 248:705–709.
237. Soll BA, George PT: Treatment of obstructive sleep apnea with a nocturnal airway-patency appliance. *N Engl J Med* 1985; 313:386–387.

238. George PT: A modified functional appliance for treatment of obstructive sleep apnea. *J Clin Orthod* 1987; 21:171–175.
239. Clark GT, Nakano M: Dental appliances for the treatment of obstructive sleep apnea (review). *J Am Dent Assoc* 1989; 118:611–619.
240. Schmidt-Nowara WW, Meade TE, Hays MB: Treatment of snoring and obstructive sleep apnea with a dental orthosis. *Chest* 1991; 99:1378–1385.
241. Clark GT, Arand D, Chung E, et al: Effect of anterior mandibular positioning on obstructive sleep apnea. *Am Rev Respir Dis* 1993; 147:624–629.
242. Rubin A-H, Eliaschar I, Joachim Z, et al: Effects of nasal surgery and tonsillectomy on sleep apnea. *Bull Eur Physiopathol Respir* 1983; 19:612–615.
243. Heimer D, Scharf SM, Lieberman A, et al: Sleep apnea syndrome treated by repair of deviated nasal septum. *Chest* 1983; 84:184–185.
244. Dayal VS, Phillipson EA: Nasal surgery in the management of sleep apnea. *Ann Otol Rhinol Laryngol* 1985; 94:550–554.
245. Guilleminault C, Eldridge FL, Simmons FB, et al: Sleep apnea in eight children. *Pediatrics* 1976; 58:23–30.
246. Brouillette RT, Fernbach SK, Hunt CE: Obstructive sleep apnea in infants and children. *J Pediatr* 1982; 100:31–40.
247. Mangat D, Orr WC, Smith RO: Sleep apnea, hypersomnolence, and upper airway obstruction secondary to adenotonsillar enlargement. *Arch Otolaryngol* 1977; 103:383–386.
248. Stool SE, Eavey RD, Stein NL, et al: The "chubby puffer" syndrome. Upper airway obstruction and obesity, with intermittent somnolence and cardiorespiratory embarrassment. *Clin Pediatr* 1977; 16:43–50.
249. Eliaschar I, Lavie P, Halperin E, et al: Sleep apneic episodes as indications for adenotonsillectomy. *Arch Otolaryngol* 1980; 106:492–496.
250. Lind MG, Lundell BPW: Tonsillar hyperplasia in children. A cause of obstructive sleep apneas, CO_2 retention, and retarded growth. *Arch Otolaryngol* 1982; 108:650–654.
251. Randall CS, Braman SS, Millman RP: Rapid development of cor pulmonale following acute tonsillitis in adults. *Chest* 1989; 95:462–463.
252. Orr WC, Martin RJ: Obstructive sleep apnea associated with tonsillar hypertrophy in adults. *Arch Intern Med* 1981; 141:990–992.
253. Fujita S, Conway W, Zorick F: Surgical correction of anatomic abnormalities in obstructive sleep apnea syndrome: Uvulopalatopharyngoplasty. *Otolaryngol Head Neck Surg* 1981; 89:923–934.
254. Moser RJ, Rajagopal KR: Obstructive sleep apnea in adults with tonsillar hypertrophy. *Arch Intern Med* 1987; 147:1265–1267.
255. Aubert-Tulkins G, Hamoir M, Van den Eeckhaut JVD, et al: Failure of tonsil and nose surgery in adults with long-standing severe sleep apnea syndrome. *Arch Intern Med* 1989; 149:2118–2121.
256. Kuhlo W, Doll E, Franck MD: Ezfolgreiche Behandlung einea Pickwick Syndroms durch eine Dauertrachealkantile. *Dtsch Med Wochenschr* 1969: 94:1280–1290.
257. Conway WA, Victor LD, Magilligan DJ Jr, et al: Adverse effects of tracheostomy for sleep apnea. *JAMA* 1981; 246:347–350.
258. Tilkian AG, Guilleminault C, Schroeder JS, et al: Sleep-induced apnea syndrome. Prevalence of cardiac arrhythmias and their reversal after tracheostomy. *Am J Med* 1977; 63:348–358.
259. Fedok FG, Houck JR, Manders EK: Suction-assisted lipectomy in the management of obstructive sleep apnea. *Arch Otolaryngol Head Neck Surg* 1990; 116:968–970.

260. Rodenstein DO: Assessment of uvulopalatopharyngoplasty for the treatment of sleep apnea syndrome. *Sleep* 1992; 15:S56–S62.
261. Shepard JW Jr, Olsen KD: Uvulopalatopharyngoplasty for treatment of obstructive sleep apnea. *Mayo Clin Proc* 1990; 65:1260–1267.
262. Caldarelli DD, Cartwright R, Lilic JK: Severity of sleep apnea as a predictor of successful treatment by palatopharyngoplasty. *Laryngoscope* 1986; 96:945–947.
263. Guilleminault C, Hayes B, Smith L, et al: Palatopharyngoplasty and obstructive sleep apnea syndrome. *Bull Eur Physiopathol Respir* 1983; 19:595–599.
264. deBerry-Borowiecki B, Kukwa AA, Blanks RHI: Indications for palatopharyngoplasty. *Arch Otolaryngol* 1985; 111:659–663.
265. Gislason T, Lindholm CE, Almqvist M, et al: Uvulopalatopharyngoplasty in the sleep apnea syndrome. Predictors of results. *Arch Otolaryngol Head Neck Surg* 1988; 114:45–51.
266. Fujita S, Conway WA, Zorick FJ, et al: Evaluation of the effectiveness of uvulopalatopharyngoplasty. *Laryngoscope* 1985; 95:70–74.
267. Katsantonis GP, Walsh JK, Schweitzer PK, et al: Further evaluation of uvulopalatopharyngoplasty in the treatment of obstructive sleep apnea syndrome. *Otolaryngol Head Neck Surg* 1985; 93:244–250.
268. Harmon JD, Chaudhary BA: Uvulopalatopharyngoplasty and obstructive sleep apnea. *South Med J* 1986; 79:197–200.
269. Simmons FB, Guilleminault C, Miles LE: The palatopharyngoplasty operation for snoring and sleep apnea: an interim report. *Otolaryngol Head Neck Surg* 1984; 92:375–380.
270. Kimmelman CP, Levine SB, Shore ET, et al: Uvulopalatopharyngoplasty: A comparison of two techniques. *Laryngoscope* 1985; 95:1488–1490.
271. Dickson RI, Blokmanis A: Treatment of obstructive sleep apnea by uvulopalatopharyngoplasty. *Laryngoscope* 1987; 97:1054–1059.
272. Chaban R, Cole D, Hoffstein V: Site of upper airway obstruction in patients with idiopathic obstructive sleep apnea. *Laryngoscope* 1988; 98:641–647.
273. Shepard JW Jr, Thawley SE: Localization of upper airway collapse during sleep in patients with obstructive sleep apnea. *Am Rev Respir Dis* 1990; 141:1350–1355.
274. Sher AE, Thorpy MJ, Shprintzern RJ, et al: Predictive value of Muller maneuver in selection of patients for uvulopalatopharyngoplasty. *Laryngoscope* 1985; 95:1483–1487.
275. Crumley RL, Stein M, Gamsu G, et al: Determination of obstructive site in obstructive sleep apnea. *Laryngoscope* 1987; 97:301–308.
276. Katsantonis GP, Maas CS, Walsh JK: The predictive efficacy of the Muller maneuver in uvulopalatopharyngoplasty. *Laryngoscope* 1989; 99:677–680.
277. Hegstrom T, Emmons LL, Hoddes E, et al: Obstructive sleep apnea syndrome: preoperative radiologic evaluation. *AJR Am J Roentegenol* 1988; 150:67–69.
278. Ryan CFP, Dickson RI, Lowe AA, et al: Upper airway measurements predict response to uvulopalatopharyngoplasty in obstructive sleep apnea. *Laryngoscope* 1990; 100:248–253.
279. Ryan CF, Lowe AA, Li D, et al: Three-dimensional upper airway computed tomography in obstructive sleep apnea. A prospective study in patients treated by uvulopalatopharyngoplasty. *Am Rev Respir Dis* 1991; 144:428–432.

280. Shepard JW Jr, Thawley SE: Evaluation of the upper airway by computerized tomography in patinets undergoing uvulopalatopharyngoplasty for obstructive sleep apnea. *Am Rev Respir Dis* 1989; 140:711–716.
281. Hudgel DW, Harasick T, Katz RL, et al: Uvulopalatopharyngoplasty in obstructive apnea. Value of preoperative localization of site of upper airway narrowing during sleep. *Am Rev Respir Dis* 1991; 143:942–946.
282. Launois SH, Feroah TR, Campbell WN, et al: Site of pharyngeal narrowing predicts outcome of surgery for obstructive sleep apnea. *Am Rev Respir Dis* 1993; 147:182–189.
283. Fairbanks DNF: Uvulopalatopharyngoplasty complications and avoidance strategies. *Otolaryngol Head Neck Surg* 1990; 102:239–245.
284. Sanders H, Johnson JT, Keller FA, et al: The acute effects of uvulopalatopharyngoplasty on breathing during sleep in sleep apnea patients. *Sleep* 1988; 11:75–89.
285. Harmon JD, Morgan W, Chaudhary B: Sleep apnea: morbidity and mortality of surgical treatment. *South Med J* 1989; 82:161–164.
286. Crampette L, Carlander B, Mondain M, et al: Surgical alternatives to uvulopalatopharyngoplasty in sleep apnea syndrome. *Sleep* 1992; 15:S63–S68.
287. Riley RW, Powell NB, Guilleminault C: Obstructive sleep apnea syndrome: a review of 306 consecutively treated surgical patients. *Otolaryngol Head Neck Surg* 1993; 108:117–125.
288. Riley R, Guilleminault C, Powell N, et al: Mandibular osteotomy and hyoid bone advancement for obstructive sleep apnea: a case report. *Sleep* 1984; 7:79–82.
289. Riley RW, Powell NB, Guilleminault C: Inferior sagittal osteotomy of the mandible with hyoid myotomy-suspension: a new procedure for obstructive sleep apnea. *Otolaryngol Head Neck Surg* 1986; 94:589–593.
290. Riley RW, Powell NB, Guilleminault C: Inferior mandibular osteotomy and hyoid myotomy suspension for obstructive sleep apnea: a review of 55 patients. *J Oral Maxillofac Surg* 1989; 47:159–164.
291. Riley RW, Powell NB, Guilleminault C: Maxillofacial surgery and nasal CPAP. A comparison of treatment for obstructive sleep apnea syndrome. *Chest* 1990; 98:1421–1425.
292. Riley RW, Powell NB, Guilleminault C: Maxillary, mandibular, and hyoid advancement for treatment of obstructive sleep apnea: a review of 40 patients. *J Oral Maxillofac Surg* 1990; 48:20–26.
293. Crestinu JM: Intrapalative resection (IPR) in the treatment of sleep apnea and snoring. *Plast Reconstr Surg* 1991; 87:467–469.
294. Mixter RC, Ewanowski SJ, Carson LV: Central tongue reduction for macroglossia. *Plast Reconstr Surg* 1993; 91:1159–1162.

Medical Management of Prostatic Diseases

Peter N. Schlegel, M.D.

Assistant Professor of Urology, James Buchanan Brady Foundation, Department of Urology, The New York Hospital-Cornell Medical Center, New York; Staff Scientist, The Population Council, Center for Biomedical Research, New York, New York

Prostatic diseases are nearly universal in elderly men, one of the largest growing segments of our population. Anatomic evidence indicates that benign prostatic hyperplasia (BPH) and hypertrophy affect more than 40% of men 50 to 60 years of age, and the prevalence of this disease increases to greater than 80% of men older than 80 years of age[1] (Fig 1). Recent advances in medical treatments and other alternative therapies for BPH have advanced the promise of new treatments for this very common medical condition that are less invasive than the commonly used surgical procedures such as transurethral prostatectomy. With the propagation of these treatments and the promise of improved treatment opportunities for men with BPH, there comes an increased requirement for all physicians to understand BPH and other diseases that may affect the prostate.

During the past 5 years, the use of prostate specific antigen (PSA), a new and highly specific tumor marker,[2] has become widespread; this provides physicians with the opportunity to diagnose prostate cancer at an earlier stage. Earlier diagnosis carries both the opportunity to cure a higher proportion of men with this disease and the risk of detecting men with latent disease who do not need invasive therapy. The development of medical hormonal treatments allow an alternative and less invasive opportunity for the palliative treatment of metastatic prostate cancer. The impact of these advances to the treatment of prostatic diseases as they apply to the internist will be presented in this chapter.

Benign Prostatic Hypertrophy

Overview and Treatment Options

The disease of benign prostatic growth is commonly referred to as BPH, meaning benign prostatic hypertrophy or hyperplasia. Histologically, both hyperplasia and hypertrophy of epithelial cells in the prostate are seen. Pathologically, enlargement of the transitional zone of the prostate results in compression of the urethral space by a hyperplastic adenoma and ob-

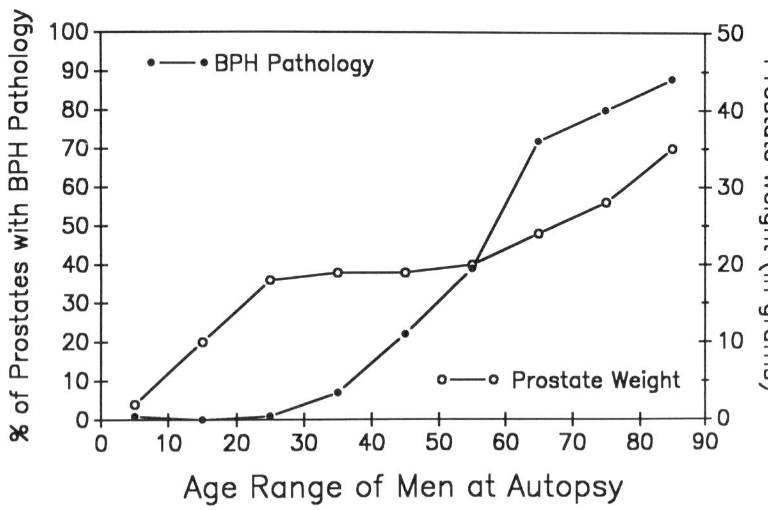

FIG 1.
Prevalence of histologic and clinical (palpable) benign prostatic hypertrophy with aging in 8,454 men. (Adapted from Berry SJ, Coffey DS, Walsh PC, et al: *J Urol* 1984; 132:474–479.)

struction to urinary outflow if the prostatic capsule is not compliant. The growth of the prostatic adenoma is a histologically heterogeneous process, dependent on the presence of androgens (predominantly the male hormones testosterone and dihydrotestosterone). The adenoma consists of both glandular and fibromuscular components. The muscular tone of the prostatic capsule and adenoma is, at least in part, related to the presence of α-adrenergic receptors. The contribution of both hormonal factors and α-adrenergic tone to the development and maintenance of prostate-related bladder outlet obstruction allow for the potential of pharmacologic management of this disease.[3]

Obstruction of the bladder outlet may result in hydronephrosis, predisposition to urinary tract infection, formation of stones, or renal failure, but the most common presentation of BPH is the development of voiding symptoms. Prostatism is the symptom complex of decreased force of urinary flow, hesitancy in initiating urination, terminal dribbling, and sense of incomplete voiding. In addition, irritative voiding symptoms (urinary frequency, nocturia, and dysuria) may reflect BPH. Voiding symptoms may also relate to bladder dysfunction (including flaccid neurogenic bladder and bladder instability). The presence of any factors that may predispose the patient to neurogenic bladder dysfunction must be carefully assessed in the patient with BPH especially, diabetes, other neuropathy, stroke, or spinal cord injury. Indeed, up to 40% of patients with symptoms of prostatism may actually have a neurogenic cause for voiding dysfunction, and the clinician caring for such patients should be aware of the relationship between bladder dysfunction and voiding symptoms.[4] Further evaluation with urodynamic testing is indicated if suspicion of neurologic dysfunction is clinically present.

Patient Evaluation

Global evaluation of voiding symptoms with the quantification of a symptom score is becoming more popular and allows a more meaningful evaluation of BPH symptoms. The American Urological Society (AUA) symptom score questionnaire is presented in Table 1. This quantitative summary score of prostatism symptoms can be used to categorize patients as having mild, moderate, and severe obstructive symptoms. The classification of symptoms is of importance, because treatment outcomes are affected by the classification of initial symptoms. In addition, with the growing use of guidelines for medical care,[5] it is possible that reimbursement for treatments may be affected by the symptom score. For example, in patients with mild symptoms (AUA symptom score < 7), watchful waiting may be the most appropriate intervention. Although all options should be presented to patients, it is foreseeable that third-party payers may no longer cover some expensive treatment options, if the predicted outcome of treatment is marginal for that symptom score category. Additional standardized questionnaires that may improve the clinician's ability to determine the importance of the patient's symptoms to his quality of life are the AUA bother score and quality of life assessment (Tables 2 and 3). A history of prostate cancer in first-degree relatives of the patient (brother, father) increases the risk of concomitant asymptomatic cancer in an enlarged prostate and should be obtained from the patient.[6]

Physical examination should detect the presence of a distended bladder as well as assess the size and consistency of the prostate. Any asymmetry of the prostate or other structural abnormalities (including the presence of a classic prostatic nodule) should lead to further evaluation of the prostate for appropriate individuals.

Laboratory evaluation should include a urinalysis and blood urea nitrogen (BUN) creatinine. Although not required in the BPH management guidelines, determination of a serum PSA level prior to rectal examination is essential for any man who will undergo medical therapy or watchful waiting for BPH. Any prostatic irregularity on physical examination or PSA elevation should be followed with transrectal ultrasound-guided biopsies of the prostate. It must be remembered that 10% to 20% of all men who previously underwent transurethral resection of the prostate (TURP) were found to have prostatic cancer[7, 8]; it is expected that a similar proportion of men who are treated medically for presumed BPH will have prostate cancer detectable in their prostate. Failure to perform a prudent evaluation for the possibility of prostate cancer may constitute negligent management of a patient with BPH.

The absolute level of PSA elevation that should prompt further evaluation for the presence of prostate cancer is controversial and still evolving.[9] Most experts would agree that men with a life expectancy greater

TABLE 1.
Urinary Symptoms*†

	Not at all	Less Than 1 Time in 5	Less Than Half the Time	About Half the Time	More Than Half the Time	Almost Always
1. Over the past month or so, how often have you had a sensation of incomplete emptying of your bladder?	0	1	2	3	4	5
2. Over the past month or so, how often have you had to urinate again less than 2 hours after you finished urinating?	0	1	2	3	4	5
3. Over the past month or so, how often have you stopped and started again several times when you urinated?	0	1	2	3	4	5
4. Over the past month or so, how often have you found it difficult to postpone urination?	0	1	2	3	4	5
5. Over the past month or so, how often have you had a weak urinary stream?	0	1	2	3	4	5

*From Barry MJ, Fowler FJ Jr, O'Leary MP, et al: The American Urological Association symptom index for benign prostatic hyperplasia. *J Urol* 1993; 148:1549–1557. Used by permission.

†Patient questionnaire for evaluation of symptoms of prostatism, based on American Urological Society symptom score evaluation. Responses from section A (A1–A7) are added together, and the sum score indicates the degree of symptomatology.

Continued.

TABLE 1. (cont.).

6. Over the past month or so, how often have you had to push or strain to begin urination?	0	1	2	3	4	5
7. Over the past month, how many times did you most typically get up to urinate from the time you went to bed until the time you got up in the morning?	No times 0	One time 1	Two times 2	Three times 3	Four times 4	Five or more 5

than 6 to 8 years and a serum PSA greater than 10 ng/mL or a prostatic abnormality on physical examination should undergo transrectal ultrasound (TRUS)–guided biopsy. Transrectal ultrasound allows for the precise placement of a biopsy needle into prostatic tissue. In addition, abnormalities of prostatic tissues, such as hypoechoic areas, which may suggest a possibility of local cancer growth, can be identified with TRUS. Therefore, TRUS is an important part of any prostate biopsy. For men with a PSA between 4 and 10 ng/mL, the size of the prostate is taken into account, since the overall "leak" of the protein PSA into serum is related to the volume of prostatic adenoma present. A new, derived, value of the PSA referred to as PSA density (PSAD) is obtained by dividing the serum PSA by the volume of the prostate (usually determined with transrectal ultrasound). I recommend biopsy for all men with a serum PSA of 4 to 10 ng/mL and a PSAD greater than 0.1.[10] There are a number of controversies regarding the optimal biopsy evaluation of men with suspected prostate cancer. At a minimum, suspicious (hypoechoic) lesions on TRUS within the prostate should be biopsied, and probably it is optimal to perform six (sextant) sampling biopsies of the prostate. With this approach, a maximal number of localized cancers are found, with a minimal risk of detecting clinically insignificant "latent" cancers.

Prostate cancers are highly prevalent in older men with BPH, and many of these tumors may not be detected during treatment with medical management. Therefore, it is incumbent on the physician caring for these patients to consider and initiate evaluation for the incidental presence of prostate cancer in men with a 6- to 8-year life expectancy who are being medically treated for BPH.

Additional testing for a man with symptoms of prostatism has not been standardized at present. For most men, uroflowmetry should be per-

TABLE 2.
Problems Due to Symptoms*†

	No Problem	Very Small Problem	Small Problem	Medium Problem	Big Problem
1. Over the past month, how much has the sensation of not emptying your bladder been a problem for you?	0	1	2	3	4
2. Over the past month, how much has frequent urination during the day been a problem for you?	0	1	2	3	4
3. Over the past month, how much has getting up at night to urinate been a problem for you?	0	1	2	3	4
4. Over the past month, how much has stopping and starting when you urinate been a problem for you?	0	1	2	3	4
5. Over the past month, how much has a need to urinate with little warning been a problem for you?	0	1	2	3	4
6. Over the past month, how much has impaired size and force of urinary stream been a problem for you?	0	1	2	3	4
7. Over the past month, how much has having to push or strain to begin urination been a problem for you?	0	1	2	3	4

*From Barry MJ, Fowler FJ Jr, O'Leary MP, et al: The American Urological Association symptom index for benign prostatic hyperplasia. *J Urol* 1992; 148:1549–1557. Used by permission.

†American Urological Association Bother Score = Sum of questions B1–B7.

TABLE 3.
Quality of Life Due to Urinary Problems*†

1. Over the past month, how much physical discomfort did any urinary symptoms cause you?
   0 None 1 Only a little 2 Some 3 A lot
2. Over the past month, how much did you worry about your health because of any urinary problems?
   0 None 1 Only a little 2 Some 3 A lot
3. Overall, how bothersome has any trouble with urination been during the past month?
   0 Not at all bothersome 1 Bothers me a little 2 Bothers me some
   3 Bothers me a lot
4. If you were to spend the rest of your life with your urinary condition just the way it is now, how would you feel about that?
   0 Delighted
   1 Pleased
   2 Mostly satisfied
   3 Mixed (about equally satisfied and dissatisfied)
   4 Mostly dissatisfied
   5 Unhappy
   6 Terrible
5. Over the past month, how much of the time has any urinary problem kept you from doing the kinds of things you would usually do?
   0 None of the time
   1 A little of the time
   2 Some of the time
   3 Most of the time
   4 All of the time

*From Barry MJ, Fowler FJ Jr, O'Leary MP, et al: The American Urological Association symptom index for benign prostatic hyperplasia. *J Urol* 1992; 148:1549–1557. Used by permission.
†Patient questionnaire on effect of prostatism symptoms on quality of life. Each question is evaluated individually.

formed, but the evaluation of maximum or mean flow rates must be carefully assessed relative to the voided volume. If a man voids less than 100 mL, maximum flow rates will clearly be less than what would be expected for a voided volume of 400 mL. In general, voided volumes of less than 150 mL are highly unreliable.[11]

Pressure/flow urodynamics with simultaneous videourographic studies (contrast study of the bladder with pressure measurement) provide definitive proof and delineation of the prostatic component of bladder outlet obstruction due to BPH.[12–14] Although this type of study is critical to evaluate bladder function for individuals with complex voiding dysfunction, it is not indicated for routine evaluation of a man with symptoms of prostatism.

Transabdominal ultrasound evaluation provides evaluation of hydronephrosis and incidental renal anomalies, including tumors. In addition, transabdominal ultrasound is a noninvasive means to evaluate residual urinary volume. Intravesical extension of BPH can also be visualized, which is of value, since this component of BPH may not be as easily managed with medical therapy. Transabdominal ultrasound has some value in estimating the volume of the prostate gland. Magnetic resonance imaging and transrectal ultrasonography provide highly accurate estimates of prostatic volume, but their routine use in evaluation of BPH should be avoided because of their high cost and limited benefit.

Cystoscopic evaluation of the bladder may further delineate the degree of bladder outlet obstruction, but it is clearly more invasive and less specific than pressure/flow studies in demonstrating obstruction. Cystoscopy has its greatest value in detecting coexisting bladder conditions, such as diverticula, stones, or bladder tumors. It is a mandatory evaluation for all patients with hematuria, suspicion of urethral stricture disease, stones, or other structural bladder abnormalities.

The presence of hematuria, either by history or on microscopic urinalysis, should prompt evaluation with urinary cytologies and intravenous urography (IVP) or retrograde urographic studies to rule out a transitional cell carcinoma. Cystoscopic evaluation is always indicated for hematuria, and computed tomography should be performed for any patient with an abnormal IVP. Urinary cytologies should also be obtained for any patient with predominantly irritative voiding symptoms, to rule out the presence of carcinoma in situ.

Treatment Options

Medical management of BPH is an accepted and worthwhile alternative to surgical or other interventional treatment of this disease. However, surgical treatment remains the standard of therapy, because it provides optimal improvements in urinary flow, symptomatology, and quality of life for men with BPH. However, surgery (and other interventional alternatives such as balloon dilation, prostatic coils, and hyperthermia) is invasive and associated with periprocedural complications and retreatment rates (Table 4). In addition, a retrospective study suggests long-term cardiovascular morbidity associated with TURP.[15] An overview of some of the risks and benefits of the options for treatment of men with moderate symptoms of prostatism is presented in Table 4.

The presence of different histologic components of prostatic hyperplasia (glandular and fibromuscular) along with the two different pharmacologic approaches to treatment of BPH (hormonal and α-blockers) which theoretically treat different components (static or bulk and dynamic, respectively) of BPH, have made a rational approach to treatment of the individual patient possible. Theoretically, one could biopsy the prostate adenoma of a patient prior to treatment and then choose the individual therapy most likely to be effective. Unfortunately, this approach has yet to be shown to be effective in a prospective manner, and it may be limited by the remarkable diversity of this disease within an individual man's prostate gland. In addition, a significant improvement in symptoms of BPH may occur from placebo effect alone.[16] This placebo effect may limit the importance of an exact determination of the "best" treatment for an individual patient.

α-*Adrenergic Blockade*

The average component of smooth muscle tissue in prostatic enlargement from BPH is 40%. This finding, in conjunction with the demonstration by Raz,[17] Caine,[18] and Shapiro and colleagues[19] that human prostate contains a relative abundance of α-receptors, has led to the treatment of BPH symptoms with α-adrenergic antagonists. The treatment of BPH with α-adrenergic blockers should decrease resistance along the prostatic urethra by relaxing the smooth muscle component of the prostate. Indeed, Shapiro and colleagues[19] have demonstrated a relationship between the increase in urinary flow rate of patients treated with α-selective blockers and the percent-area density of smooth muscle in 26 patients, although only a small number of random prostatic biopsies were performed. This relationship between smooth muscle content and clinical response supports this proposed mechanism of the development of bladder outlet obstruction being mediated by increased prostatic smooth muscle tone.

α-Blockers that have been evaluated for the therapy of BPH are presented in Table 5. Phenoxybenzamine was the first α-blocker shown to be effective in the treatment of BPH, as published by Caine et al. in 1976.[20] Unfortunately, many of the early studies of α-blockers were uncontrolled and used nonselective blockers. Nevertheless, 27 of the reported 30 clinical trials of α-blockers were effective for the treatment of BPH.[21]

α-Blockers may be subgrouped according to receptor subtype selectivity and duration of serum elimination half-lives (Table 5). Phenoxybenzamine is a nonselective α-blocker; it antagonizes both α_1- and α_2- adrenoreceptors. Prazosin, alfuzosin, YM617, indoramin, terazosin and doxazosin are selective α_1-antagonists. Phenoxybenzamine, prazosin, terazosin and doxazosin are commercially available in the United States, but none of these agents is currently approved for the indication of treatment of BPH. The major advantage of the use of selective α_1-antagonists is that the incidence and severity of adverse effects associated with the use of these agents are fewer than those with nonselective α-blockers.

The most common adverse effects associated with selective α_1-blockers are dizziness, lightheadedness, and asthenia.[22] The postural hypotension that may occur with these agents is usually limited by initiating therapy with a lower, bedtime dose of medication, and subsequently incrementally increasing the dosage. Phenoxybenzamine has had limited use recently and is not recommended for long-term use because of the demonstration of mutagenicity in Ames test and mouse-lymphoma assays.

The overall proportion of patients who have demonstrated improvement in urinary symptoms on treatment with α-blockers ranges from 75% to

TABLE 4.
Risks, Complications and Treatment Efficacy of Some Interventions for Men With Moderate Symptoms of Prostatism*†

	Balance Sheet (Applies to Male Patient With Moderate Symptoms)					
		Surgical Options			Conservative Options	
	Balloon Dilation	TUIP	Open Surgery	TURP	Watchful Waiting	Alpha Blocker
Chance for improvement of symptoms	57%	80%	98%	88%	42%	74%
Degree of symptom improvement (1% reduction in symptom score)	51%	73%	79%	85%	≤32%	51%
Morbidity/complication associated with surgical or medical treatment assume that about 20% of all compl. are significant.	4.5%	14.0%	21.7%	16.1%	1–5 Complications from progression of BPH	16.4%
Chance of dying within 30–90 days of treatment	0.7%–12.4%	1%	0.9%–5.3%	1.5%	.8 Chance of death ≤90 d for 67 yo men	
Risk of total incontinence of urine	? None reported	0.1%	0.4%	0.8%	0%	0%

Need for operative treatment for surgical complications in the future	? None reported	2.9%	4.2%	3.3%	0%	0%
Need for BPH treatment in the future	20.1%	8.1%	0.4%	3.4%	26.4%	50% probability ≥10 but ≤26%
Loss of worktime (days)	4	7–21	21–28	7—21	1	3.5
Hospital stay (days)	1	1–3	5–10	3–5	0	0
Cost of treatment in $	4,200	7,500	11,800	8,500	2,300	2,800–3,900 5–10 mg qd of diff. drugs
Risk of retrograde ejaculation (% of pts)?		39	71.5	68	0	6.7
Risk of impotence	(See watchful waiting, no long follow-up available)	12.6	19.0	15.7		About 2% (1/50) men your age become impotent per year. Long-term data on alpha blocker treatment are not available
Pain associated with treatment						
Injectable drugs (days)	0–1	0–2	2–4	0–2	0	0
Oral drugs (days)	1–2	2–3	7–10	2–4	0	0

*Data from Roehrborn CA, McConnell JD: Data from Agency for Health Care Policy and Research. BPH Guideline Panel, 1991.

†Table is a balance sheet apply to men with moderate symptoms. TUIP = transurethral incision of the prostate; TURP = transurethral resection of the prostate; BPH = benign prostatic hyperplasia.

TABLE 5.
Selective and Nonselective α-Blockers That Have Been Evaluated for the Treatment of Benign Prostatic Hyperplasia

Nonselective α-blockers
Phenoxybenzamine
Selective α_2-blockers
Prazosin
YM617
Alfuzosin
Indoramin
Selective long-acting α_1-blockers
Terazosin
Doxazosin

82% to 93% respectively for nonselective, selective α_1- and long acting selective α_1-blockers. A 49% improvement in Boyarsky symptom scores has been reported for patients treated with the long-acting selective α_1-blocker, terazosin. The mean improvement in maximum urinary flow rate is approximately 44% for patients treated with terazosin. These improvements have been shown to be statistically better than improvements in symptom scores and flow rates for men treated with placebo. One major question in the use of α_1-blockers for BPH is its durability. Tachyphylaxis has been demonstrated to be a problem in the use of α_1-blockers for treatment of hypertension. Since the duration of effect for any pharmacologic therapy of BPH is thought to continue only while treatment is ongoing, long-term efficacy of α_1-blocker therapy will be needed to demonstrate the efficacy of this modality for treatment of BPH.

Our experience with α_1-antagonist therapy is greatest in the use of the terazosin. We usually initiate therapy with a 1 mg dose, given at bedtime. Additional daily doses of 1 mg are administered each morning for 3 more days, followed by 2 mg/day for a total of 2 weeks. The dosage is then increased to 5 mg/day. Additional increases in daily dosage to 10 mg/day may improve efficacy, but the proportion of patients who experience side effects increases with this increase in dosage, and it is uncommonly necessary. In one study, 1.3% of patients treated with 10 mg/day of terazosin experienced syncope.[22]

Treatment with α_1-blockers is the preferred therapy for the acute treatment of symptoms of BPH, including acute urinary retention, in patients who are poor surgical candidates. It remains unknown whether α_1-blockers are more effective than hormonal therapy for men with BPH and whether the benefits of α_1-antagonist therapy are durable. Since α-adrenergic antagonists may also have an effect directly on the bladder, relief of symptoms is possible even if no direct effect occurs on the prostate. Since patients are primarily interested in relief of symptoms, and α-blockers may affect bladder-based irritative symptoms, some additional benefits of pharmacologic treatment with selective α_1-blockers may be achieved relative to that obtained for patients treated with hormonal therapy alone. Finally, the apparently increased side effects of treatment with α_1-blockers must be taken into account, and steps taken to minimize these effects.

Hormonal Therapy

While α-adrenergic blockade attempts to alleviate bladder outlet obstruction and prostatism by relieving the dynamic component of BPH, hormonal manipulation reduces prostatic size, thereby decreasing the mechanical component of obstruction of urinary outflow. Stromal and epithelial hyperplasia in BPH is related to aging and testicular hormones. Prolactin, androstenedione, and estrogen all play minor roles in induction and maintenance of BPH; however, androgens are clearly the major hormonal factor related to BPH. Leydig cells within the testes produce 95% of all testosterone, the major circulating androgen present in men.[23] Testosterone is predominantly bound to serum binding proteins. In its free form, testosterone enters androgen-dependent cells and is irreversibly reduced to 5α-dihydrotestosterone (DHT), catalyzed by the enzyme 5α-reductase. The effects of androgens at the level of the prostate cell are mediated by its intracellular binding to the androgen receptor. Testosterone and DHT can both bind to androgen receptors, but the intracellular effect of DHT is seven- to tenfold greater than that of testosterone.[24] In addition, androgens are converted to estrogens by the enzyme aromatase. Estrogens act synergistically with androgens in animal models to support growth of prostatic hyperplasia, possibly by inhibiting epithelial cell death.

Androgens are proposed to affect the number of cells in the prostate gland. Although there is no demonstrable increase in cell growth in patients with BPH, the increase in cell number in the prostatic adenoma may be caused by a decrease in cell death.[24] It has been hypothesized that estrogens may inhibit cell death and, thereby, promote prostatic growth. Hormonal therapy may be effected by (1) preventing androgen production at the testicular level, (2) blocking testosterone conversion to the highly potent androgen, DHT, (3) blocking the effects of testosterone at the androgen receptor level, or (4) inhibiting conversion of androgens to estrogens. These mechanisms of action are schematically illustrated at the cellular level in Figure 2.

The first recorded attempt to hormonal manipulation for BPH was reported by White in 1895. He published a series that included 111 men with urinary outflow obstruction treated by castration.[25] Of those surviving the procedure, 87% showed a rapid decrease in prostatic volume. Other attempts at complete androgen deprivation for BPH have been limited by the side effects (loss of libido) and the irreversible nature of this treatment. Decrease in prostatic size of approximately 25% is possible with inhibition of

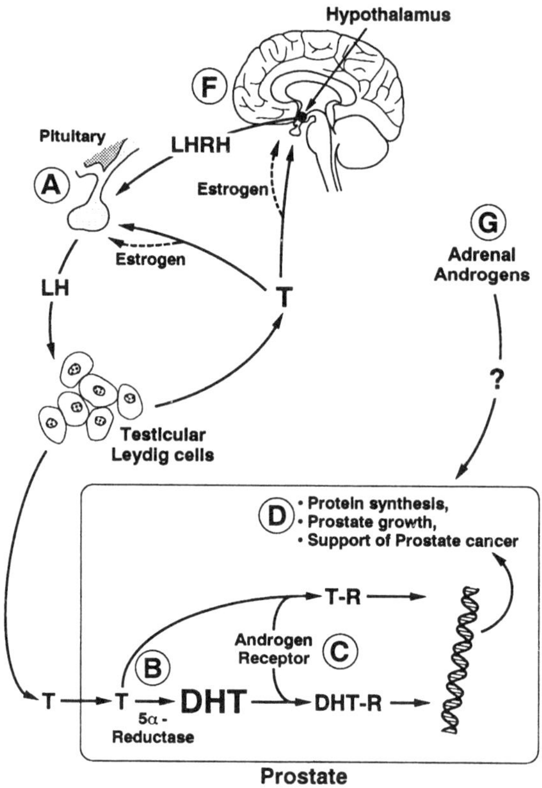

FIG 2.
Schematic illustration of mechanisms for blockade of androgen action on prostatic cell function. A = inhibition of LH release (gonadotropin-releasing hormone [GnRH] agonists: leuprolide acetate, buserelin acetate, nafarelin acetate, goserelin acetate, estrogens (DES), estramustine, medroxyprogesterone acetate (weak), cyproterone acetate (weak), megesterol (weak); B = 5α-reductase inhibitors (finasteride); C = androgen receptor blockade/inhibition of androgen-receptor translocation (flutamide, anandron, casodex, cyproterone acetate, medroxyprogesterone acetate, megesterol (weak); D = direct inhibition of prostatic growth (estramustine, ? estrogens, ? ketoconazole); F = central inhibition of GnRH release (? estrogens); G = inhibition of adrenal (and testicular) hormone synthesis (ketoconazole, spironolactone, aminoglutethimide).

testicular production of androgens,[26] including castration, but trials have been inadequately controlled to adequately delineate its effectiveness. Given its irreversible nature, surgical castration is hardly an acceptable treatment for most men with BPH. However, the development of gonadotropin-releasing hormone (GnRH) agonists that provide a "medical castration" by inhibition of pituitary production of luteinizing hormone (LH), and subsequently, testicular production of testosterone are now available. Nafarelin acetate,[26] buserelin[27] and leuprolide acetate[28] are all GnRH agonists that produce castrate levels of testosterone with prolonged use and have been used for treatment of men with BPH. Peters and Walsh treated nine men with decreased peak urine flow rates (<15 mL/sec) due to BPH for a period of 6 months.[26] A mean decrease in prostatic size of 24% was achieved, and three of nine men had a clinically significant improvement in symptoms of bladder outlet obstruction. There was no improvement in residual urinary volumes. Keane and associates treated 20 patients with BPH using buserelin and found no improvement in flow rate.[27] Schlegel and Brendler[28] treated six men with urinary retention and severe medical problems which precluded their consideration as surgical candidates. A mean 30% reduction in prostatic volume was achieved on leuprolide acetate, and all patients were able to void spontaneously, but acceptable voiding patterns were only achieved for two men.

The use of GnRH agonists for BPH is currently limited to men with severe medical problems who are willing to accept its side effects (hot flashes, loss of libido, fluid retention). Cotreatment with an androgen receptor blocker, such as flutamide, is suggested to avoid the "flare" response seen in the first month of treatment and allow the earliest response to treatment.

Treatment with antiandrogens alone avoids some of the side effects of GnRH agonists, since it interferes with androgen action at the cellular level, allowing the maintenance of serum testosterone levels. Flutamide competes with testosterone and DHT for binding to the androgen receptor. Since flutamide does not effectively cross the blood-brain barrier, libido is usually maintained on flutamide monotherapy. Long-term treatment with flutamide only results in an increase in LH levels from an inhibition of testosterone (T) feedback at the cellular level of the pituitary, with a subsequent increase in serum T levels. Eventually, the increased serum T levels result in enhanced aromatization of T to estrogens, with gynecomastia. In addition, the increased T overcomes the competitive blockade of androgen receptors by flutamide, with only partial inhibition of androgen action at the cellular level. Therefore, long-term treatment with flutamide alone has little benefit, because of the compensatory increase in T production. Stone et al. in an uncontrolled series of patients treated with flutamide reported a 27% shrinkage in prostate size in 64 evaluable patients with a minimal change in urinary flow rate, but a 44% reduction in residual urine.[29] Caine et al. reported no evidence of flutamide effect on residual urine or prostatic size in 30 patients with clinical BPH when compared with a placebo-treated control group.[30] Cyproterone acetate, a synthetic steroid with antiandrogenic activity at the androgen receptor level, also has been reported to have clinical activity in treating men with BPH.[31]

Megestrol acetate is another progestational antiandrogen, like cyproterone acetate, that blocks the androgen receptor and also centrally inhibits LH release, which results in decreased testosterone biosynthesis. Hence, megestrol acetate has effects on both androgen production and action. Geller and associates treated 61 patients with clinical BPH and decreased urine flow rates.[32] Statistically significant improvements in urine flow rates were seen on treatment, but the magnitude of improvement in flow rates was only 30%, and 70% of men experienced complete loss of libido and erection. Clinical symptoms of BPH were unaffected.

The most widely accepted hormonal therapy for BPH is the use of the oral drug, finasteride (Proscar, MK906, Merck & Co., Piscataway, NJ). Finasteride is Food and Drug Administration–approved for the treatment of BPH. Finasteride is a specific inhibitor of the enzyme 5α-reductase. Daily treatment with finasteride results in a prompt decrease in prostatic intracellular levels of DHT, and a subsequent decrease in serum DHT levels. Intraprostatic DHT levels decrease by 80% with a 5 mg/day dosage level, and serum DHT levels decrease by 70%.[33] Serum testosterone levels increase by an average of 10%, but stay within the physiological range for most patients.

A decrease in mean prostate size of approximately 20% is achieved within 3 months and a further decrease of approximately 22% is achieved after 12 months.[16] Overall improvements in urinary flow rates of only 1.3–1.6 mL/sec were achieved in the international and North American studies on finasteride within 1 year. Although these changes are statistically significant when compared with changes in placebo-treated patients they are not dramatic or clinically significant. Between 25% and 30% of all patients achieved an increase in peak urinary flow rates greater than 3 mL/sec. Only 18% of placebo-treated patients achieved this degree of symptom improvement. Mean changes in total symptom scores from baseline were significantly better in finasteride-treated patients than in controls after 3 to 6 months, although the magnitude of difference was small (1 to 2 points on a maximum scale of 36).[16] In contrast, mean improvement in urinary flow after TURP is usually approximately 8 mL/sec, and symptom score improvement is usually approximately 5 to 10 points.

The moderate improvement in urinary symptoms and flow rates was clearly influenced by the patient selection in the finasteride trials sponsored by Merck. The greatest differences in subjective or objective improvements seen in treated patients vs. controls were obtained for patients with the most severe symptoms; however, the treatment group was heavily weighted toward patients with mild obstructive urinary symptoms. Therefore, Merck's data on treatment results with their own drug may underestimate its effects, since most patients with mild symptoms are best managed with watchful waiting, and most patients to be treated will have greater symptomatology.

The greatest advantage of finasteride therapy is its remarkably low incidence of side effects. Impotence occurred in 3.7% of men treated with finasteride vs. 1.1% of placebo-treated patients. Similarly, 2% to 3% of men reported decreased libido and decreased ejaculate volumes.[16] These complaints appear to be minimal relative to the side effects of surgical treatment (see Table 2)[34] and justify the widespread use of this drug in patients with troublesome symptoms of BPH. Since finasteride has only been in testing in humans for the past 6 to 7 years, long-term follow-up will be needed to confirm the safety of this drug over the years. It is important to remember that, as a hormonally active agent that can cross the placenta, finasteride should not be handled by pregnant women. In experimental studies, the development of hypospadias was noted in 3% to 100% of the male offspring of pregnant female rats treated with this agent.[35]

Finasteride is administered in a daily dose of 5 mg per day, given orally. The maximum effects of finasteride may not be seen for up to 6 months, although the hormonal effects are prompt, and the majority of the decrease in prostatic size is obtained within 3 months.

Prostate specific antigen levels decrease by an average of about 50% in men who are being treated with 5 mg of finasteride per day. The serum PSA drops to a baseline level within 3 months of treatment.[36] Men who do not have a significant decrease in serum PSA on finasteride may be considered at risk for having coexistent prostate cancer present in their prostate gland. Appropriate management is to obtain a serum DHT level to confirm that the patient is compliant with taking the medication. If serum DHT levels are suppressed, then TRUS and biopsy are indicated. It has been suggested that the depression of serum PSA levels contributed by benign prostatic tissue allows the clinician to more easily detect the presence of prostate cancer. There is no single recognizable pattern of change in PSA levels among the men who have been found to have prostate cancer during treatment with finasteride.[16]

My present approach to the detection of prostate cancer in men who have started treatment with finasteride is to obtain a serum PSA before treatment and 3 months after initiating treatment. Men in whom PSA is not significantly suppressed are further evaluated with serum DHT and possibly TRUS-guided biopsies. Men who demonstrate an increase greater than 0.75 ng/mL/year increase in serum PSA are also further evaluated with TRUS and biopsy. This is the same rate of increase in serum PSA that should result in further evaluation for men who are being followed with watchful waiting.[36] Further clinical information regarding guidelines for detection of prostate cancer in men being treated with finasteride should be available in the next several years.

The use of finasteride as a 5α-reductase inhibitor is slightly limited by its ability to inhibit only one of the two isoenzymes of 5α-reductase that catalyze conversion of testosterone to DHT. Jenkins et al. have presented genetic, biochemical, and pharmacologic evidence for at least two 5α-reductase enzyme activities recently. Although finasteride blocks the major form of this enzyme, dihydrotestosterone levels in serum and tissue are not completely ablated. With the development of new inhibitors that block both Type 1 and Type 2 5α-reductase, there may be a more effective clinical result in terms of prostate shrinkage and possibly its clinical effects on BPH.

In summary, treatment of men with moderate to severe symptoms of BPH can be initiated with the oral agent, finasteride. Approximately 30% of men are expected to have clinically significant improvement in BPH symptoms and urinary flow rates, although these changes in urinary flow rates are somewhat less than what would be expected after TURP.

Combined Therapy

The most rational approach to medical treatment of BPH is the combined treatment of both static and dynamic components of this disease using hormonal agents combined with α-receptor blocking agents. Unfortunately, there is very limited information available regarding treatment of patients with this combination therapy. Lepor and Machi[37] recently conducted an open-label study comparing terazosin, the α-blocker, with terazosin and flutamide. Terazosin provided a 56% decrease in Boyarsky symptom scores and a 38% increase in peak urinary flow rates. Subsequent addition of flutamide to terazosin for an additional 5 months resulted in a further reduction of 8% in the total symptom score. Twenty-five percent of subjects exhibited moderate symptom improvement following the addition of the androgen receptor blocker. There was no statistically significant difference in outcomes between patients treated with the α-blocker plus flutamide. However, relatively few patients were enrolled in this study, limiting its power to detect small differences in urinary flow rate or symptomatic improvement. Moreover, flutamide is not the most effective long-term hormonal agent available for treatment of BPH.

Lepor has initiated a randomized, multicenter placebo-controlled study to compare four treatment regimens; placebo; α-blocker (terazosin) alone; androgen suppression (finasteride) alone; and combined α_1-blocker and androgen suppression. If properly performed and presented, this study may provide definitive information on the combined medical therapy of BPH in the 1,200 men whom Lepor plans to treat under this protocol.

Prostate Cancer

Overview

Recent advances in the detection of early-stage prostate cancer with PSA and the approval of GnRH agonists (that provide medical castration) have revolutionized our approaches to the diagnosis and treatment of prostate cancer. Prostate cancer is a highly prevalent disease, with an incidence of approximately 132,000 cases in 1992.[38] The incidence of prostate cancer has nearly doubled over the past decade, and it is now the most common cancer among men. Given the general aging of our population, it is likely that prostate cancer will remain the most common cancer among men in the United States for many years. In this section, we will emphasize the management options that are most commonly applicable for internists managing patients with prostate cancer, but an overview of management of this disease is required for greater understanding of the role of medical management.

Treatment by Stage

Stage A

Stage A prostate cancer is defined by the incidental detection of a cancer in a gland not previously suspected on clinical grounds, usually during TURP or open (retropubic or suprapubic) prostatectomy. Stage A is subdivided into Stage A1 and A2 disease, with these separations based on some general expectations of the clinical behavior of this disease. In general, stage A1 disease (less than 5% of the BPH specimen involved with cancer, and a Gleason's sum score of less than 7) is slowly progressive and, indeed, many men with stage A1 disease will have no cancer remaining in their gland after TURP. For stage A1 disease, if the post-TURP PSA is less than 1.0 ng/mL, observation alone is recommended, based on the volume of cancer present in radical prostatectomy specimens for stage A1 patients. If the PSA is greater than 10 ng/mL, these men should be managed as if stage B disease were present. For post-TURP PSA levels between 1 and 10 ng/mL, the options of definitive treatment or observation are possible.[39] In general, repeat biopsies of the prostate gland are of little additional value. The patient's age and general medical status are of the greatest importance; overall 8-year progression rates for stage A1 prostate cancer are approximately 16%.[40] Therefore, it is most important to consider the patient's overall health status prior to initiating treatment for stage A1 disease.

Stage A2 prostate cancer is clinically indistinguishable from stage B disease. The only difference appears to be that the transitional (middle) zone of the prostate is involved with A2 disease, whereas the peripheral zone is more commonly involved for B disease. Since prostate cancer is a multifocal process, the site of origination of disease is relatively unimportant. Indeed, since many A2 cancers were able to grow significantly without detection on physical examination, many men with A2 disease may have had greater progression of their disease than men with B disease, prior to its detection. The widespread use of PSA and TRUS may allow much earlier detection of what would have been A2 disease and may minimize the number of patients who have stage A detection completely.

Stage AX/BO (Also Called Stage T_{1c})

There are no standard criteria for definition of the staging of a man with prostate cancer with a palpably normal gland, detected solely on the basis of an elevated PSA. Since prostate cancer is a slowly progressive disease and its presence in autopsy studies is so much higher than its clinical presentation, there is some concern that men with latent or clinically insignificant cancers will be found with overaggressive application of PSA as a tool to detect prostate cancer. Early reports suggest that less than 5% of cancers found on evaluation of an elevated PSA alone will have clinically insignificant cancer (less than 0.2 mL cancer volume) at radical prostatectomy.[40] Since many cancers are now being found at a curable stage, rather than with locally extensive or metastatic spread, the use of PSA appears to have shifted the stage at detection with great benefit to the patient, although definitive data are not yet available. In general, men with stage AX/BO disease should be managed as though they have B disease.

Stage B

Stage B prostate cancer is defined by the presence of cancer in a palpably abnormal prostate gland. The disease has been subdivided into B1 nodule, B1, and B2 (or B1-3), based on the extent of involvement of the palpable nodule. These subdivisions have allowed some predictions to be made regarding the actual pathological stage of disease, which is commonly "upstaged" from the clinical (palpable) stage of disease. It is possible that the use of PSA, and/or PSAD may provide additional information regarding the true extent of cancer within the prostate. The curability of men with local treatment appears to decrease when the PSAD increases. Metastatic evaluation with bone scan, enzymatic acid phosphatase determination, and liver function tests are indicated. Computed tomographic scan evaluation is necessary for men with a PSA greater than 50 ng/mL, and it is occasionally helpful for men with lower PSA levels.

The most important factor for determining appropriate treatment of men with stage B prostate cancer is the life expectancy of the patient. For men with a less than 6- to 8-year life expectancy, observation alone may be of value. Unfortunately, our ability to detect cancer growth in the window of curability is very limited; it is unreliable to assume that a man who is a candidate for cure can be followed for a period with treatment initiated *when* the cancer begins to grow but *before* it becomes locally extensive or metastatic. My personal anecdotal experience with patients who were managed with this approach to cancer of the prostate is disastrous. Most men who are followed with what was clearly clinical stage B disease have progressed to clinical stage C before that progression was clinically detectable.

Curative options for men with stage B disease include radiation or radical prostatectomy. Radiation may be delivered either as external beam or interstitial (brachytherapy) treatment or combined treatment. Perioperative morbidity is avoided with radiation, since an open operation is not performed. However, 38% to 90% of men with prostate cancer will still have cancer present in their prostate gland after definitive radiotherapy with external beam[42] or interstitial treatment,[43] respectively. At least 20% of these men will be shown to have disease progression within 5 years.[44] Advances in the improved placement of radioactive seeds (with TRUS and computed tomographic guidance) have theoretical potential to improve cure rates with radiation. Preliminary data suggest that curative treatment with radiation should result in serum PSA levels that progressively decrease to less than 1.0 ng/mL.

Radical prostatectomy has the potential to cure patients with localized prostate cancer. If cancer is confined to the prostate, and the entire prostate gland, seminal vesicles, and attached fascias are removed, then the patient should be cured. Statistically, disease-free survival is only 85% at 15 years after radical prostatectomy.[45] This is because the surgical margins that can be achieved with radical prostatectomy are limited to a few millimeters outside of the prostate gland. The margins with a retropubic approach are significantly better than those with a perineal approach, and simultaneous sampling of obturator nodes is possible during retropubic prostatectomy, making this approach the procedure of choice. Improvements in preservation of sexual function, urinary continence, and decrease in blood loss have improved the acceptability of radical prostatectomy.

Regardless of the treatment modality for stage B prostate cancer, multiple retrospective studies have shown that approximately 50% of all patients will die of diseases other than prostate cancer within 15 years.

Stage C

Stage C disease is characterized by the local extension of cancer beyond the prostate gland into local structures, including the pelvic (musculature) sidewalls. This extension is usually detected on physical examination, but may be confirmed with computed tomography or magnetic resonance imaging. A high proportion of men with clinical stage C disease already have microscopic spread of tumor to local lymph nodes in the pelvis, a marker of diffuse metastatic disease. Therefore, the use of local curative radiotherapy is somewhat limited. Symptomatic obstruction of urinary outflow may be treated with hormonal therapy or radiotherapy. Surgery is generally not indicated, as few patients will have negative surgical margins, and the risk of local recurrence is excessively high.

Stage D

Stage D disease implies the metastatic spread of cancer beyond the prostate gland. It may be subdivided into D0 disease, characterized by elevated serum enzymatic acid phosphatase levels, in the absence of demonstrable metastases, D1 disease, characterized by metastatic tumor in local lymph nodes, or D2 disease, with metastases beyond the obturator nodes, usually involving bone metastases. The standard treatment of stage D prostate cancer is delayed hormonal therapy, administered when there are symptomatic metastases or local growth of prostate cancer causing obstructive uropathy. Often, patients will ask why treatment should be delayed if the hormonal therapy is effective in affecting prostate cancer growth. Although hormonal therapy does kill androgen-dependent prostate cancer cells, a cohort of androgen-independent tumors coexists in essentially all cancers. The androgen-independent clones will continue to grow and metastasize despite hormonal therapy. The overall result is that there is no evidence that early hormonal therapy will influence life expectancy for patients with stage D prostate cancer.[46, 47] These data are predominantly derived from the Veteran's Administration (VA) studies where patients were treated at the time of diagnosis of stage D disease, or after symptomatic metastatic spread was present (which is actually late treatment vs. late late treatment of prostate cancer). Since there are adverse effects of hormonal therapy (hot flashes, impotence, decreased libido, cardiovascular side effects), and there is no survival benefit, we recommend instituting hormonal therapy only when symptoms of prostate cancer are present (urinary symptoms or bone pain from metastases). The management of the patient with microscopic spread to local lymph nodes (found on pathological evaluation of the specimen after radical prostatectomy) is controversial. Some animal data suggest that very early hormonal therapy after surgical debulking may prolong survival with a Dunning tumor model.[47] In addition, a retrospective study of patients with D1 disease, found during radical prostatectomy, may have better survival if treated with early orchiectomy.[48] This post-radical prostatectomy data from the Mayo Clinic was subsequently reevaluated relative to tumor ploidy status, and the improvement in survival (and time to progression of disease) was more related to ploidy status than to early hormonal therapy.[49] This study was retrospective, and it remains unknown what treatment biases may have entered into the decision to treat or not treat with hormones. Since the data are only retrospective, and no other center has confirmed these findings, the best evidence that we have is that no therapy (watchful waiting, radical prostatectomy, hormonal therapy, or radiotherapy) provides any survival benefit for patients with stage D1 prostate cancer. Indeed, even at the Mayo Clinic, routine, early hormonal therapy is not instituted after radical prostatectomy for stage D patients with diploid tumors.[50]

Hormonal Therapy

Chemoprevention of Prostate Cancer With 5α-Reductase Inhibitors

The National Cancer Institute has recently embarked on a long-term study of 18,000 men with finasteride as a potential agent to prevent the development of prostate cancer. The rationale behind this study is the finding that men who are at higher risk for the development of prostate cancer (American blacks, whites) tend to have higher serum DHT levels than men with lower risk for development of prostate cancer (Asian men).[51] It is hypothesized that the lower tissue DHT levels, which may be reflected in lower serum DHT levels, results in a milieu less likely to result in the development of prostate cancer. Unfortunately, it is not known whether the lower serum DHT levels truly reflect lower intraprostatic DHT levels, or whether an increased volume of prostate and other androgen-dependent cells in men at higher risk for prostate cancer results in the production of higher serum DHT levels. In addition, the age of men to be treated must be very early and follow-up extensive to actually demonstrate any effect of prevention of this slow-growing cancer. No results are to be expected in the near future on this approach to chemoprevention of prostate cancer.

Stage B/C

It has been proposed that preoperative hormonal therapy, instituted for men with localized prostate cancer, may improve local control and "downstage" the cancer prior to surgical treatment. Since androgen-dependent tumor cells will die and overall prostate cancer volume will shrink, there is some theoretical support for this concept of prostate cancer management.

However, extracapsular cancers are highly unlikely to "move" back within the capsule of the prostate. Although little published data exist since the early unsuccessful studies of Scott and Boyd,[52] preliminary reports of this increasing practice of "down-staging" suggest that it may improve negative margin rates after radical prostatectomy, but has not altered survival or improved local control.[53, 54] Given the lack of solid theoretical support for this practice and the lack of data suggesting any improvement in local control or survival, its use should be condemned as a means to attempt to widen the indications for radical prostatectomy.

For the patient with a localized tumor in whom surgical therapy is delayed for a month or two because of overriding medical concerns, use of preoperative hormonal therapy may help to delay further progression of disease. The most poorly differentiated tumor cells, which are most likely to metastasize, are also the cells least likely to be androgen sensitive. Therefore, long-term preoperative hormonal treatment should be avoided, and there are no data to support the routine use of this practice.

In rare cases of patients with very large (>150 g) prostate glands, a decrease in overall prostate size, achieved with hormonal therapy, may be beneficial prior to surgical prostatectomy or radiotherapy. Very large prostates can be technically difficult to remove (as are very small prostate glands), and hormonal down-*sizing* may make radical prostatectomy technically easier. My limited anecdotal experience with this preoperative hormonal therapy is that some patients may respond with a dramatic decrease in prostatic cancer volume, relative to what would have been predicted preoperatively, but that there is little difference in the technical ease of radical prostatectomy after treatment. Given the lack of data on the safety of delay of treatment, widespread use of preoperative hormonal therapy is not standard practice. Prior to external beam radiotherapy, prostate downsizing may decrease scatter to the rectum or other adjacent pelvic organs, decreasing the potential side effects of radiation. If hormonal therapy is used prior to radiation, a 3-month course of treatment appears to optimally provide a decrease in prostatic size, without an undue delay in treatment.

Stage D

Rationale.—In 1941, Huggins and Hodges reasoned that since normal prostatic epithelium is androgen dependent, prostatic cancer should be similarly androgen dependent.[55] Indeed, many studies have suggested that hormonal therapy is effective in alleviating symptoms of metastatic cancer in 80% of all men with this disease and prolongs survival, relative to untreated symptomatic patients. Early treatment (as discussed earlier) does not further prolong survival. In 1979, Labrie reintroduced the concept of androgen ablation for cure.[56] He suggested that the adrenal production of androgens, that persists after orchiectomy, may allow for persistent tumor survival. Although this concept of "total androgen ablation" remains controversial, there are no reliable data to indicate that any hormonal therapy is curative for prostate cancer. The consensus remains that androgen ablation is not curative, but that hormonal therapy can play an important role in alleviating bony metastatic pain, improving symptoms secondary to tumor compression, and, in selected patients, increasing survival.

Role of 5α-Reductase Inhibitors.—Since 5α-reductase inhibitors decrease the intracellular levels of DHT, the most potent androgen needed for cell growth, it has been proposed that men with prostate cancer may benefit from early treatment with a 5α-reductase inhibitor, such as finasteride. One published study has evaluated the effect of finasteride treatment on prostate cancer, as evaluated by serum PSA levels. Measurement of serum PSA levels is an inaccurate method to evaluate disease status, if one is attempting to compare prostate cancer volume before and after any hormonal treatment, since PSA production is an androgen-dependent process. Simply decreasing intracellular levels of DHT may decrease serum PSA without affecting cancer volume or metastatic ability. Presti et al.[57] published the results of a double-blind study of patients with stage D prostate cancer finasteride. Over a 6-week period of treatment, only 8 of 13 treated men were evaluable for follow-up serum PSA levels. Overall PSA levels increased less in the finasteride-treated group than in the control group. However, all men with bone metastases prior to treatment had increased serum PSA levels despite finasteride therapy. Given the known effect of finasteride on serum PSA production from BPH, it is possible that the decrease in PSA seen in the finasteride group, relative to control patients, was at least in part due to a decrease in PSA production from benign prostate tissue, not an antitumor effect.

The use of finasteride is without documented benefit for men with prostate cancer. Since finasteride treatment may be instituted in place of truly effective hormonal therapy, it should be emphasized that there is no role for the use of finasteride in the treatment of men with prostate cancer.

Testicular Androgen Ablation.—Although surgical castration is psychologically difficult to accept for both physicians and patients alike, bilateral orchiectomy is the standard of therapy for permanent androgen deprivation. After bilateral orchiectomy, the source of the majority of the powerful circulating androgen, testosterone, is removed. Indeed, serum T levels decrease within hours and prompt symptomatic relief is achieved for most patients within days. This manipulation decreases prostatic DHT levels to less than 20% of pretreatment values in most patients, is associated with few side effects except for loss of libido and impotence, and leaves no question as to the reliability of therapeutic compliance. Clearly, surgical castration is the most cost-effective treatment for ablation of testicular androgen production.

Oral administration of estrogens reduces the pituitary release of luteinizing hormone, thereby removing the central stimulation for the testes to produce androgens. Castrate levels of testosterone are achieved in 14 to 21 days with doses of 3 mg/day or more of diethylstilbestrol. In addition, the major serum protein carrier for testosterone, testosterone-binding globulin (TeBG), is increased, further decreasing the free or "bio-available" circulating T. There is also the possibility that estrogens may have direct cytotoxic effects on prostate cancer cells, although this has never been fully substantiated. Although no surgical procedure is needed, daily administration of the drug is necessary, and side effects are minimized with administration three times per day. Side effects of estrogen therapy include nausea, vomiting, headaches, fluid retention, gynecomastia, loss of libido and potency, and a significant increase in serious cardiovascular events (myocardial infarction, stroke, and deep venous thrombosis). The cardiovascular toxicity for patients receiving this therapy is three times greater than age-matched populations not on estrogen therapy. At 1 mg diethyl stilbesterol (DES) per day, inconsistent reduction of T levels is achieved and similar clinical results are achieved, although the VA study suggested a trend toward earlier death with this lower estrogen dose level.[46] Although DES itself is inexpensive, the overall treatment costs are far greater than orchiectomy when cardiovascular toxicity is taken into account. Given the alternative options currently available, estrogen treatment probably has only a historical role in the contemporary management of men with prostate cancer. Estramustine is an estrogenic agent with the added benefit of providing a nitrogen mustard moiety to effect a cytotoxic action on prostate cancer. However, a European Oncology Research Treatment Council (EORTC) prospective trial of men with prostate cancer randomized to treatment with estrogen (3 mg/day) or estramustine (280 mg/day for 8 weeks followed by 140 mg/day) failed to show any significant difference between these treatments with respect to response of metastases, response of primary tumor, distant progression, and overall survival or death of prostate cancer.

GnRH agonists have provided the most recent major advance in the hormonal treatment of prostate cancer. These analogues of native GnRH have a substituted sixth D-amino acid (instead of glycine) and a deleted tenth amino acid instead of the native decapeptide. These structural changes result in a substantial increase in affinity for the GnRH receptor in the pituitary. Tonic stimulation of these receptors (instead of the normal pulsatile release of GnRH from the hypothalamus) results in an abrupt increase in LH release, followed by a long-term decrease in both GnRH receptors and GnRH responsiveness, decreased LH release, and a decrease in gonadal LH receptor sites. The clinical effects are that a "flare effect" of increased serum testosterone occurs within 1 week of treatment, followed by achievement of castrate levels of serum T within 21 to 28 days. The flare effect may result in tumor growth and increased cancer-related pain, if it is not blocked by anti-androgens. In the initial studies of leuprolide acetate, the flare was severe enough to halt treatment for 7% of all patients.[68] The cost of monthly depot administration of leuprolide acetate or goserelin acetate, the two GnRH agonists Food and Drug Administration approved for use in men with prostate cancer, is approximately $6,000 to $7,000 per year. This is a high cost for men on permanent therapy, just to avoid the psychological concerns that a patient may have to surgical castration. The side effects of loss of libido, and impotence, are the same with castration or GnRH agonists.

Treatment of men with leuprolide acetate has essentially equivalent results when compared with DES in terms of time to first progression of disease and actuarial survival.[58] The common side effects of GnRH analog treatment are certainly less severe than those of DES and include profuse flushing, occasional irritation at the injection site, and impotence. Cardiovascular side effects were few. Fluid retention is common and may cause an increase in weight of 1 to 2 kg. Initially, leuprolide acetate and goserelin (the two GnRH analogs approved for use in the United States) were administered with daily (1 mg) subcutaneous injections. Depot injections (7.5 mg of leuprolide, 3.6 mg of goserelin) given monthly are now used, and multimonth injections may be available in the near future. In summary, monthly administration of GnRH agonists are as effective as DES and their toxicity profile is significantly better.[58]

Antiandrogens are a class of compounds that peripherally inhibit the action of DHT by interfering with binding of hormone to the androgen receptor with subsequent effects to block receptor binding to DNA or receptor regulatory functions. They may be broadly classified into either steroidal or nonsteroidal agents. The steroidal agents include cyproterone acetate, medroxyprogesterone acetate, and megestrol, a progestational agent with central as well as peripheral effects. Although pure antiandrogens increase LH release, progestational agents also have central effects that decrease LH release, thereby decreasing testicular T production. All steroidal antiandrogens competitively inhibit androgen binding to the cytosolic androgen receptors. In addition, progestational agents inhibit the enzyme 5α-reductase. In general, all antiandrogens should be used only in conjunction with a GnRH agonist or castration (to block adrenal steroid action), because central escape from megestrol control and the competitive inhibition seen with other agents is inadequate to effectively decrease androgen action because of increased circulating serum androgens. Five-year survival of randomized patients in an EORTC trial receiving DES, medroxyprogesterone acetate (MPA), or cyproterone acetate (CPA) showed significantly better survival for patients treated with CPA or DES; progression rate was better only for patients treated with DES.

Nonsteroidal antiandrogens such as flutamide have few central effects but have potent peripheral effects. Since no central effects occur, serum T levels may increase 1.5–2× initial values, and this may limit the effectiveness of these competitive androgen receptor blockers. Some animal studies have also questioned the effectiveness of androgen blockade with flutamide, even in the presence of normal serum T levels. Side effects of flutamide are related to aromatization of high serum T levels when used as monotherapy (gynecomastia, 25% to 50%), carrier (lactose) effects (diarrhea, 10% to 15%), or drug effects (liver dysfunction, 2% to 10%; flushing, 15% to 30%). Flutamide is available in 125-mg capsules, and the usual dosage is two capsules three times a day.

Other nonsteroidal antiandrogens are anandron (RU 23908, Roussel Pharmaceuticals, Germany) and casodex (ICI America). Anandron has a longer serum half-life, but toxicity includes visual difficulties with dark adaptation, alcohol intolerance, and occasional cases of severe interstitial pneumonitis. Casodex was originally thought to not pass through the blood-brain barrier, which would decrease the compensatory increase in serum androgen levels, because pituitary feedback from testosterone would be preserved. However, clinical trials suggest little difference between this agent and other antiandrogens. Casodex does have the advantages of a long serum half-life and minimal side effects that may make it a superior clinical agent. All of the aforementioned antiandrogens should be used clinically only in conjunction with a GnRH agonist or castration.

Other agents that inhibit steroid synthesis include ketoconazole, aminoglutethimide, and spironolactone. They act by inhibiting multiple enzymes important for steroid biosynthesis. Ketoconazole inhibits the cytochrome P450 enzymes 17-20 desmolase and 17 hydroxylase. After an oral dose of 400 mg of ketoconazole, a rapid decrease in serum testosterone is seen because of inhibition of both testicular and adrenal androgen production. Ketoconazole is most useful in the treatment of men who have not previously received antiandrogen therapy and who present with disseminated intravascular coagulopathy (DIC) or acute spinal cord compression. These patients are not good candidates for orchiectomy, but a rapid clinical response is needed. Ketoconazole is also useful as an adjunct to the use of GnRH agonists to prevent the flare response or suppress adrenal androgen synthesis.

Use of ketoconazole is not without drawbacks. Dosing of ketoconazole must be performed every 8 hours to ensure its activity. Severe, but reversible, hepatic toxicity occurs in 1:8,000 to 1:16,000 patients. Nausea is seen in approximately 20% of all patients. Other side effects include asthenia and glucocorticoid insufficiency, as well as dry skin and mucous membranes.

Ketoconazole has some promise for clinically hormone-resistant prostate cancers, since it has in vitro activity against cytochrome P450-dependent intracellular activities. Newer analogs of ketoconazole have more specific sites of action, decreased side effects and a longer duration of action.

Total Androgen Blockade.—Early enthusiasm on the concomitant use of combined GnRH agonist and antiandrogen treatments were fueled by the exuberant uncontrolled trials of Labrie and co-investigators,[55] suggesting that a remarkably low rate of tumor progression occurred in patients treated with total androgen blockade. In order to best evaluate the potential benefit of total androgen blockade, one must separate the studies that include a possibly detrimental flare effect from unblocked GnRH agonist therapy with those that include blockade of adrenal androgen action. The true role of total androgen blockade remains highly controversial, although numerous studies have investigated its role in management of stage D prostate cancer patients.

The intergroup study reported 617 patients with demonstrated metastatic disease. There was a significant survival benefit for the patients treated with leuprolide acetate and flutamide (34.9 months) vs. patients treated with leuprolide acetate alone. Patients with minimal disease and good performance demonstrated a marked benefit to combined treatment.

The difference in this subgroup of patients for time to progression and survival was 34 months and 20 months, respectively.[59] Since the control group experienced a significant clinical flare to GnRH agonist treatment was not blocked, this study did not indicate whether the benefit of therapy existed from blockade of adrenal androgens, or blockade of the GnRH agonist flare effect.

The International Anandron Trial also reported benefits to combination therapy with castration and anandron vs. castration and placebo. Time to progression was delayed by approximately 6 months and time to death was 7 months longer in the combination-treated group.[60]

However, EORTC studies[61] (goserelin plus flutamide vs. orchiectomy), as well as studies from Denmark[62] (goserelin plus flutamide vs. orchiectomy), France[63] (goserelin plus flutamide vs. goserelin), Italy[63, 64] (goserelin vs. goserelin plus cyproterone acetate) and (goserelin vs. goserelin plus flutamide) have failed to confirm a survival benefit for total androgen blockade. Therefore, many experts support the recommendation that orchiectomy alone or long-term monotherapy is appropriate therapy for men with symptomatic metastatic prostate cancer.[65] For men who refuse orchiectomy and are candidates for hormonal manipulation of prostate cancer, I usually add the oral antiandrogen flutamide (750 mg three times per day), starting 2 to 3 days prior to GnRH agonist treatment to block the flare effect and determine whether the patient will tolerate this oral antiandrogen. The flutamide is stopped when the second monthly injection of GnRH agonist is given. Given the present available data, this treatment regimen minimizes long-term side effects and reduces prostate cancer treatment costs by more than $2,000 per year with no demonstrable limitation of treatment efficacy.

Nonhormonal Therapy for Androgen-Independent Prostate Cancer

The response of symptomatic prostate cancer to androgen ablation is dramatic, but biochemical and/or clinical disease progression occurs in a median of 12 of 18 months. The median survival for patients treated with nonhormonal approaches is only 6.3 months.[66] Novel approaches to the treatment of androgen-independent prostate cancer include bone-seeking radiopharmaceuticals and the growth-factor blocker, suramin. The use of bone-seeking radiopharmaceuticals has previously been limited to imaging of prostate cancer metastases. β-Emitting agents limit radiation exposure to several millimeters, reducing toxicity to normal tissues. Rhenium-186 hydroxyethylidene diphosphonate (186-ReHEDP) and Samarium-153 phosphonic acid (1,2-ethyanediyl bis[nitrilobis (methylene)]) tetrakis-monohydrate (Sm-153-EDTMP are two metal diphosphonates that have been used for this treatment with imaging and therapeutic potential.[67] The isotope deposits primarily in the area of the osteoblast, the most common pathologic change seen from metastatic prostate cancer in bone. An 89% correlation of imaged sites (compared to standard 99m-technetium-methylene diphosphonate bone scanning) was obtained.[68] Median duration of response was approximately 6 weeks after an average single injection of 186-ReHEDP, suggesting the need for a repetitive dose schedule. Sixty-seven percent of patients treated at Memorial Sloan-Kettering Cancer Center with a 35-mCi dose regimen have shown significant reduction in pain intensity, but 22% showed a flare in pain that resolved within 1 week. Reversible myelosuppression was mild. No consistent changes in PSA or acid phosphatase were noted.[69] Similar effectiveness is now available through the use of Stroutium-89, which has recently been approved by the Food and Drug Administration for treatment of diffuse symptomatic metastatic prostate cancer attributable to bony metastases.

Use of suramin, typically as a continuous infusion with hydrocortisone support, has resulted in a measurable tumor regression of more than 50% in 19% of patients, with PSA decrease of greater than 50% in 47% of cases. An improvement in pain was noted by 70% of patients in one study. Toxicity includes adrenal suppression, a polyradiculopathy that can progress to a Guillain-Barré syndrome, coagulopathy, and vortex keratopathy, as well as severe infections.[70, 71]

Etidronate sodium (Didronel, Norwich Eaton Pharmaceuticals, Norwich, NY) has also been used to control pain in men with osseous metastases from advanced prostate cancer. This agent acts on bone to inhibit the formation, growth, and dissolution of hydroxyapatite crystals and their amorphous precursors by chemisorption to calcium phosphate surfaces. Usual oral dosage is 5 to 10 mg/kg/day, and subjective responses are obtained in up to 40% of patients with a minimum of side effects.

Summary

A variety of new pharmacologic agents has allowed expanded therapeutic options for men with benign prostatic hypertrophy as well as men with prostate cancer. Appropriate implementation of these agents requires an understanding of their mechanisms of action, as well as awareness of the underlying pathological processes. Medical therapy of BPH is less invasive than standard surgical intervention, but it carries the risks of missing clinically significant prostate cancers. In addition, medical treatment of BPH is less effective than prostatectomy; however, since symptomatic relief is usually the end point of treatment for BPH, medical therapy is successful for many men without the risks of surgery.

The GnRH agonists (and GnRH antagonists to be developed) allow medical hormonal therapy to be implemented for men with symptomatic prostate cancer without the psychological effects of castration. Oral antiandrogens allow for a prompt blockade of androgen action on prostate cancer during GnRH agonist use, and they may improve longevity for some men with prostate cancer. The widespread use of these agents should be tempered by their relatively high costs with long-term use.

References

1. Berry SJ, Coffey DS, Walsh PC, et al: The development of human benign prostatic hyperplasia with age. *J Urol* 1984; 132:474–479.
2. Oesterling JE: Prostate specific antigen: A critical assessment of the most useful tumor marker for adenocarcinoma of the prostate. *J Urol* 1991; 145:907.
3. McConnell JD: The pathophysiology of benign prostatic hyperplasia. *J Androl* 1991; 12:356–363.
4. Kirby RS: The clinical assessment of benign prostatic hyperplasia. *Cancer* 1992; 70:284–290.
5. Barry MJ, Fowler FJ Jr, O'Leary MP, et al: The American Urological Association symptom index for benign prostatic hyperplasia. *J Urol* 1992; 148:1549–1557.
6. Steinberg GD, Carter BS, Beaty TH, et al: Family history and the risk of prostate cancer. *Prostate* 1990; 17:337–347.
7. Emmett JL, Barber KW Jr, Jackman RJ: Transrectal biopsy to detect prostatic carcinoma: A review and report of 203 cases. *Trans Am Assoc Genitourin Surg* 1961; 53:460.
8. Armenian HK, Lilienfeld AM, Diamond EL, et al: Relation between benign prostatic hyperplasia and cancer of the prostate. *Lancet* 1974; 2:115–117.
9. Oesterling JE: Prostate-specific antigen: Improving its ability to diagnose early prostate cancer. *JAMA* 1992; 267:2236–2238.
10. Benson MC, Whang IS, Pantuck A, et al: Prostate specific antigen density: A means of distinguishing benign prostatic hypertrophy and prostate cancer. *J Urol* 1992; 147:815–816.
11. Jorgensen JB, Jensen KM, Bille-Brahe NE, et al: Uroflowmetry in asymptomatic elderly males. *Br J Urol* 1986; 58:390–395.
12. Barry MJ, Mulley AG Jr, Fowler FJ, et al: Watchful waiting vs immediate transurethral resection for symptomatic prostatism. *JAMA* 1988; 259:3010–3017.
13. Fowler FJ Jr, Wennberg JE, Timothy RP, et al: Symptom status and quality of life following prostatectomy. *JAMA* 1988; 259:3018–3022.
14. Roehrborn CA, McConnell JD: Data from Agency for Health Care Policy and Research. BPH Guideline Panel, 1991.
15. Wennberg JE, Roos N, Sola L, et al: Use of claims data systems to evaluate health care outcomes: Mortality and reoperation following prostatectomy. *JAMA* 1987; 257:933–936.
16. Gormley GJ, Stoner E, Bruskewitz RC, et al and the Finasteride Study Group: *New Engl J Med* 1992; 327:1185–1191.
17. Raz S, Ziegler M, Caine M: Pharmacological receptors in the prostate. *Br J Urol* 1973; 45:663–667.
18. Caine M, Raz S, Zeigler M: Adrenergic and cholinergic receptors in the human prostate, prostatic capsule and bladder neck. *Br J Urol* 1975; 47:193–202.
19. Shapiro E, Hartanto V, Lepor H: The response to alpha blockade in benign prostatic hyperplasia is related to the percent area density of prostate smooth muscle. *Prostate,* 1992; 21:297–307.
20. Caine M, Pfau A, Perlberg S: The use of alpha-adrenergic blockers in benign prostatic obstruction. *Br J Urol* 1976; 48:255–263.
21. Lepor H: The role of alpha blockade in the therapy of benign prostatic hyperplasia, in Lepor H, Lawson RK (eds): *Prostatic Diseases.* Philadelphia, WB Saunders Co, 1993.
22. Lepor H, Auerbach S, Puras-Baez A, et al: A randomized, placebo-controlled

multicenter study of the efficacy and safety of terazosin in the treatment of benign prostatic hyperplasia. *J Urol* 1992; 148:1467–1474.

23. Lipsett MB. Steroid secretion by the testis in man, in James VH et al (eds): *The Endocrine Function of the Human Testis,* vol 2, New York, Academic Press, 1974.
24. Coffey DS. The molecular biology, endocrinology, and physiology of the prostate and seminal vesicles, in Walsh PC, Retik AB, Stamey TA et al (eds): *Campbell's Urology,* ed 6, vol 1, Philadelphia, WB Saunders, 1992, pp 221–266.
25. White JW: The results of double castration in hypertrophy of the prostate. *Ann Surg* 1895; 22:1–80.
26. Peters CA, Walsh PC: The effect of nafarelin acetate, a luteinizing-hormone-releasing hormone agonist, on benign prostatic hyperplasia. *N Engl J Med* 1987; 317:599–604.
27. Keane PF, Timoney AG, Kiely E, et al: Response of the benign hypertrophied prostate to treatment with an LHRH analogue. *Br J Urol* 1988; 62:162–165.
28. Schlegel PN, Brendler CB: Management of urinary retention due to benign prostatic hyperplasia using luteinizing hormone-releasing hormone agonist. *Urology* 1989; 34:69–72.
29. Stone NN, Ray PS, Smith JA, et al: A double-blind randomized controlled study of the effect of flutamide on benign prostatic hypertrophy: Clinical efficacy. *J Urol* 1989; 141:240A.
30. Caine M, Perlberg S, Gordon R: The treatment of benign prostatic hypertrophy with flutamide (SCH 13521): A placebo controlled study. *J Urol* 1975; 114:564–568.
31. Scott WW, Wade JC: Medical treatment of benign prostatic hyperplasia with cyproterone acetate. *J Urol* 1969; 101:81.
32. Geller J, Nelson CG, Albert JK, et al: Effect of megestrol acetate on uroflow rates in patients with benign prostatic hypertrophy. *Urology* 1979; 14:5.
33. McConnell JD, et al: Finasteride, an inhibitor of 5 alpha-reductase, suppress prostatic dihydrotestosterone in men with benign prostatic hyperplasia. *J Clin Endocrinol Metab* 1992; 74:505–508.
34. Brendler C, Schlegel P, Dowd J et al: Surgical treatment for benign prostatic hyperplasia. *Cancer* 1992; 70:371–373.
35. Clark RL, Antonello JM, Grossman SJ, et al: External genitalia abnormalities in male rats exposed in utero to finasteride, a 5 alpha-reductase inhibitor. *Tertology* 1990; 42:91–100.
36. Carter HB, Pearson JD, Metter EJ, et al: Longitudinal evaluation of prostate-specific antigen levels in men with and without prostate disease. *JAMA* 1992; 267:2215–2220.
37. Lepor H, Machi G: The relative efficacy of terazosin versus terazosin and flutamide for the treatment of symptomatic BPH. *Prostate* 1992; 20:89–95.
38. Prostate Cancer Trends-United States, 1980-1988. *MMWR* 1992; 41:401–404.
39. Larsen MP, Carter HB, Epstein JI: Can stage A1 tumor extent be predicted by transurethral resection tumor volume, per cent or grade? A study of 64 stage A1 radical prostatectomies with comparison to prostates removed for stages A2 and B disease. *J Urol* 1991; 146:1059–1063.
40. Epstein JI, Paull G, Eggleston JC, et al: Prognosis of untreated stage A1 prostatic carcinoma: A study of 94 cases with extended followup. *J Urol* 1986; 136:837–839.
41. Andriole GL, Ponas SH, Catalona WJ: The implication of focal well differenti-

ated prostate cancer in men with elevated serum PSA and palpably normal prostates (abstract 920) *J Urol* 1992; 147:442A.
42. Dugan TC, Shipley WU, Young RH, et al: Biopsy after external beam radiation therapy for adenocarcinoma of the prostate: Correlation with original histological grade and current prostate specific antigen levels. *J Urol* 1991; 146:1313–1316.
43. Waehre H, Amellem O, Stenwig AE, et al: Deoxyribonucleic acid cytometry and histological findings before and after ^{125}Iodine implantation of primary prostate cancer. *J Urol* 1992; 148:838–842.
44. Scardino PT, Frankel JM, Wheeler TM, et al: The prognostic significance of post-irradiation biopsy results in patients with prostatic cancer. *J Urol* 1986; 135:510.
45. Walsh PC, Jewett HJ: Radical surgery for prostatic cancer. *Cancer* 1980; 45:1906.
46. Veterans Administration Cooperative Urological Research Group: Treatment and survival of patients with cancer of the prostate. *Surg Gynecol Obstet* 1967; 124:1011.
47. Carter HB, Isaacs JT: Overview of hormonal therapy for prostate cancer. *Prog Clin Biol Res* 1990; 350:129–140.
48. Zincke H, Utz DC, Myers RP, et al: Bilateral pelvic lymphadenectomy and radical retropubic prostatectomy for adenocarcinoma of prostate with regional lymph node involvement. Urology 1982; 19:238.
49. Myers RP, Larson-Keller JJ, Bergstralh EJ, et al: Hormonal treatment at time of radical retropubic prostatectomy for stage D1 prostate cancer: Results of long-term followup. *J Urol* 1992; 147:910–915.
50. Oesterling JE: Meet the professors. Presentation at the 90th Annual meeting of the New York Section of the American Urological Association, Berlin, Germany, October 17–24, 1992.
51. Ross RK, Bernstein L, Lobo RA, et al: 5-Alpha reductase activity and risk of prostate cancer among Japanese and US white and black males. *Lancet* 1992; 339:887–889.
52. Scott WW, Boyd HL: Combined hormone control therapy and radical prostatectomy in the treatment of selected cases of advanced carcinoma of the prostate: A retrospective study based upon 25 years of experience. *J Urol* 1969; 101:86.
53. Vapnek JM, Carroll PR: Neoadjuvant hormonal downsizing of clinical stage C carcinoma of the prostate. *J Urol* 1992; 147:247A.
54. Macfarlane MT, Abi-Aad A, Stein A, et al: Neoadjuvant hormonal deprivation in patients with locally advanced prostate cancer. *J Urol* 1992; 147:246A.
55. Huggins C, Hodges CV: Studies on prostatic cancer; Effect of castration, of estrogen and of androgen injection on serum phosphatases in metastatic carcinoma of the prostate. *Cancer Res* 1941; 1:293.
56. Labrie F, Dupont A, Belanger A, et al: New hormonal therapy in prostatic carcinoma: Combined treatment with LHRH agonist and an antiandrogen. Clin Invest Med 1982; 5:267–275.
57. Presti JC Jr, Fair WR, Andriole G, et al: Multicenter, randomized double-blind, placebo controlled study to investigate the effect of finasteride (MK-906) on stage D prostate cancer. *J Urol* 1992; 148:1201–1204.
58. Leuprolide study group: Leuprolide versus diethylstilbestrol for metastatic prostate cancer. *N Engl J Med* 1984; 311:1281–1286.
59. Crawford ED, Eisenberger MA, McLeod DG, et al: A controlled trial of leupro-

lide with and without flutamide in prostatic carcinoma. *N Engl J Med* 1989; 321:419–424.
60. The Canadian Anandron Study Group: Total androgen ablation in the treatment of metastatic prostatic cancer. *Semin Urol* 1990; 8:159–165.
61. Denis L, Smith PH, Carneiro deMoura JL, et al: Orchiectomy vs. zoladex plus flutamide in patients with metastatic prostate cancer. *Eur Urol* 1990; 18(suppl 3):34–40.
62. Iverson P and Danish Prostatic Cancer Group: Zoladex plus flutamide vs. orchidectomy for advanced prostatic cancer. *Eur Urol* 1990; 18(suppl 3):41–44.
63. Fourcade RO, Cario G, Coloby P, et al: Total androgen blockade with zoladex plus flutamide vs. zoladex alone in advanced prostatic carcinoma: Interim report of a multicenter, double-blind, placebo-controlled study. *Eur Urol* 1990; 18(suppl 3):45–47.
64. Boccardo F, Decensi A, Guarneri D, et al: Zoladex with or without flutamide in the treatment of locally advanced or metastatic prostate cancer: Interim analysis of an ongoing PONCAP study. *Eur Urol* 1990; 18(suppl 3):48–53.
65. Walsh PC: Editorial comment. *J Urol* 1992; 147:290.
66. Petrylak DP, Scher H, Li Z, et al: Prognostic factors for survival of patients treated with single-agent chemotherapy for bidimensionally measurable hormone refractory metastatic prostate cancer. *Proc Am Assoc Cancer Res* 1990; 31:225.
67. Scher HI, Curley T, Yeh S, et al: Therapeutic alternatives for hormone-refractory prostatic cancer. *Semin Urol* 1992; 10:55–64.
68. Maxon HR, Deutsch EA, Thomas SR, et al: Re-186(Sn)HEDP for treatment of multiple metastatic foci in bone: Human biodistribution and dosimetric studies. *Radiology* 1988; 166:501–507.
69. Curley T, Scher H, Thaler H, et al: Rhenium[Re-186-HEDP] for palliation of painful bone metastases from prostatic cancer (abstract 1231). *Proc Am Soc Clin Oncol* 1991; 10:347.
70. Scher HI, Heston WDW: Suramin as an archetypical compound in the development of growth factor antagonists for inhibition of genitourinary tumors, in Lawson R, Lepor H (eds): *Genitourinary Oncology*. New York, Martinus Nijhoff, 1992, pp 131–151.
71. Stein CA, LaRocca R, Myers C: Suramin: An old compound with new biology. *Principles Practice Oncol* 1990; pp 1–12.

Medical Management of Hyperlipidemic States

Mary J. Malloy, M.D.

Clinical Professor of Medicine and Pediatrics, Cardiovascular Research Institute, University of California, San Francisco, School of Medicine, San Francisco, California

John P. Kane, M.D., Ph.D.

Professor of Medicine, Professor of Biochemistry and Biophysics, Cardiovascular Research Institute, University of California, San Francisco, School of Medicine, San Francisco, California

The rationale for treatment of hyperlipidemia rests on the etiologic roles of lipoproteins in atherogenesis and in the initiation of acute pancreatitis. Abundant evidence now supports the concept that intervention with diet and, if necessary, drugs can not only inhibit the progression of coronary atherosclerosis, but also can lead to measurable reversal of existing lesions and to a reduction in occlusive events. Likewise, control of hypertriglyceridemia clearly reduces the risk of acute pancreatitis. The advent of potent new hypolipidemic agents and the development of synergistic combined drug regimens affords the clinician the means to achieve normal or even "ideal" levels of plasma lipoproteins in the majority of compliant patients. Whereas such intervention could, under long-term scrutiny, be found to have some adverse effects, it is already apparent that a major net benefit will be realized from large reductions in death and morbidity from coronary heart disease (CHD), because it is the leading cause of death in the United States and much of Europe.

Atherosclerosis is a truly multifactorial disease. Recent advances in understanding of the process by which arteriosclerotic lesions are initiated and develop allow for the construction of a pathophysiologic model that provides the basis for rational choice of intervention strategies. This contemporary model identifies known and emerging mechanisms of atherogenesis in addition to hyperlipidemia, per se, suggesting new potential venues of preventive or ameliorative treatment. As our understanding of the mechanistic basis of atherosclerosis develops, additional risk factors will surely emerge. Such factors are reflected now only in the natural history of coronary disease within kindreds. Thus, one of the most important elements in clinical decision making with respect to the initiation of therapy is the appearance of premature coronary disease in the patient or close relatives.

Advances in Internal Medicine®, vol 39

The objective of this review is to present a contemporary view of the pathogenesis of lipoprotein-related disease and of lipoprotein metabolism so as to provide a mechanistic basis for the clinical management of lipid disorders.

Relationship of Lipoproteins to Atherogenesis

Hypercholesterolemia has been associated with increased risk of coronary atherosclerosis in virtually all large-scale epidemiologic studies in the United States and Europe.[1] In the Framingham Study[2] and the Multiple Risk Factor Intervention Trial (MRFIT)[3] in which over 300,000 men were screened, this relationship was found to confer at least additive incremental risk when combined with other significant risk factors such as cigarette smoking and hypertension. When population means for serum cholesterol level and death from coronary heart disease in seven large Asiatic and European populations were studied, a generally linear positive relationship of risk was found.[4] In these studies, risk of coronary disease among individuals with total serum cholesterol levels around 160 mg/dl was about one fifth to one eighth of that among individuals with serum cholesterol levels around 230 mg/dl and continued to mount in individuals and populations with higher total cholesterol levels. Furthermore, elevated serum cholesterol levels in early adulthood have been shown to be predictive of coronary disease in mid-life.[5] Low-density lipoprotein (LDL) cholesterol levels correlate better with coronary risk than total serum cholesterol levels, particularly in women where higher levels of high-density lipoprotein (HDL) cholesterol tend to weaken the relationship. These studies lead to the conclusion that serum LDL levels are closely allied to the etiology of coronary disease and that the optimum level of total serum cholesterol for the human species lies in the vicinity of 150 to 160 mg/dl. Some studies have suggested that remnant lipoprotein particles that are metabolic precursors of LDL (Fig 1) may also be atherogenic.[6] Increased serum levels of the Lp(a) lipoproteins, known to be structurally related to LDL, have been found to be significantly linked to risk of coronary disease in a number of studies,[7, 8] probably representing both a direct atherogenic role in the artery wall and impairment of thrombolysis.

The relationship of levels of triglyceride-rich lipoproteins to coronary disease has been less clear in epidemiologic studies to date. Premature coronary disease is often observed to cosegregate with hypertriglyceridemia in kindreds in which no other recognized risk factors are found, suggesting that triglyceride-rich elements of the very low-density lipoprotein (VLDL) cascade (Fig 1) may indeed be atherogenic. The recent discovery of triglyceride-containing lipoproteins in human atherosclerotic lesions lends strong support to this hypothesis (Rapp J, Kane J: Personal communication, September, 1993). Failure to detect a relationship in some epidemiologic studies may be due to part to the contribution of chylomicrons containing triglycerides of dietary origin to the total triglyceride level in a sig-

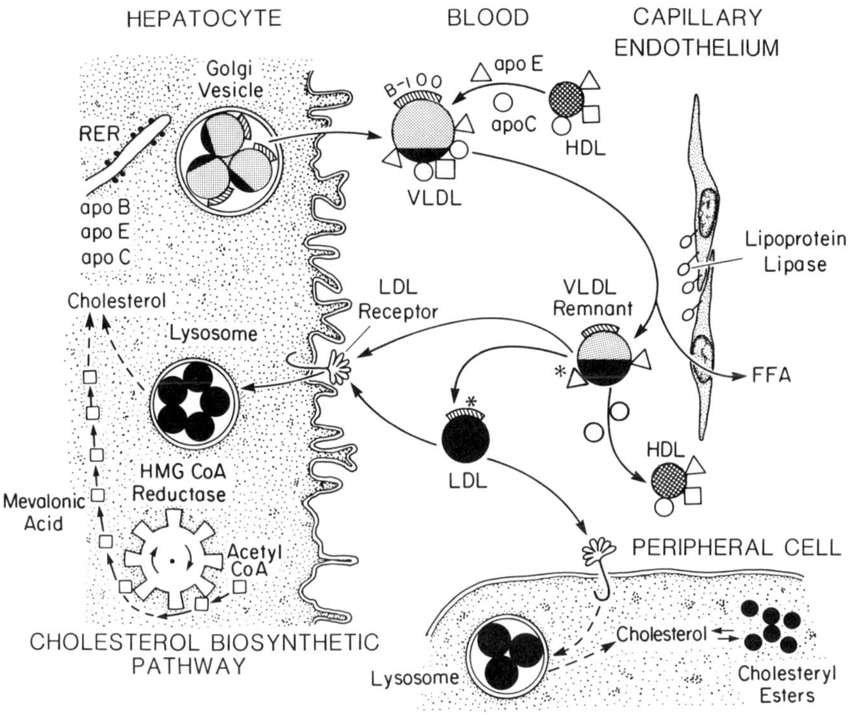

FIG 1.
Metabolism of lipoproteins of hepatic origin. *Black areas* denote cholesteryl esters; *stippled areas,* triglycerides; *cross hatched areas,* high density lipoprotein (HDL) particles; * denotes a functional ligand for LDL receptor; *triangles* indicate apolipoprotein E; and *open circles and squares* represent C apolipoproteins. RER = rough endoplasmic reticulum; apo = apolipoprotein; VLDL = very low-density lipoprotein; HDL = high-density lipoproteins; LDL = low-density lipoproteins; FFA = free fatty acid.

nificant number of patients, thus diluting the number of those with valid increases in VLDL. In fact, many studies have shown a positive relationship of coronary risk to serum triglyceride levels in univariate analysis. However, on multiple logistic regression analysis in which total cholesterol level and HDL cholesterol level are included, the significance of the relationship to triglycerides is markedly diminished or eliminated. This treatment of the data is inappropriate because triglycerides are not an independent physical element, separated from other components of the lipoprotein system. Clearly, a portion of plasma cholesterol is carried in VLDL particles and indeed is probably their most atherogenic component. Subtraction of the risk attributable to the total cholesterol level would then include the cholesterol contained in VLDL. Furthermore, as will be described, HDL cholesterol levels are systematically decreased as triglyceride levels increase in plasma, compounding the error of the analysis. Lastly, it is now understood that the distribution of subspecies of VLDL may vary greatly among individuals. It is likely that individuals with smaller, more dense VLDL particles or those that differ from normal in some other qualitative respect may be at increased risk. Thus, clinical experience leads us to the position that hypertriglyceridemia is indeed a major risk factor for atherogenesis, requiring dietary and pharmacologic intervention.

High Density Lipoproteins and the Risk of Coronary Heart Disease

Whereas lipoproteins of the apo B-100 cascade appear to act as the etiologic agents of atherogenesis, a number of epidemiologic studies have found an inverse relationship between plasma levels of high-density lipoproteins and the risk of coronary atherosclerosis.[9–11] In the Framingham study, the risk for men in the lowest quintile (HDL cholesterol level <35 mg/dl) was more than four times as great as for those in the highest quintile (>54 mg/dl). A steep inverse dependence of risk on HDL cholesterol levels was also observed among women, those in the uppermost quintile (HDL cholesterol >69 mg/dl) having less than one third the risk of those in the lowest quintile (HDL cholesterol <45 mg/dl).[12] Though some studies have not supported this finding,[13–16] the preponderance of evidence is supportive of it.[17–22] Because triglyceride levels in plasma have a major impact on HDL cholesterol levels via an exchange of triglycerides for cholesteryl esters, some of the correlation of low levels of HDL cholesterol with increased risk may be due to atherogenic effects of triglyceride-rich lipoproteins.

There are several known metabolic roles of HDL that could have a protective function against atherogenesis. The acquisition of cholesterol from peripheral tissues by HDL with subsequent delivery to liver (Fig 2) provides a major mechanism for recovery of sterol from the atheroma. Thus, the rate of progression of arterial lesions probably reflects, in part, the relative rates of deposition of cholesterol carried in LDL and other apo B-100-containing lipoproteins and cholesterol retrieval via the centripetal transport pathway. Other mechanisms by which HDL could protect the artery include inhibition of the oxidation of LDL,[23, 24] modification of the distribution of LDL particle species, and direct effects on endothelium.[25, 26]

Abnormally low levels of HDL cholesterol must be regarded as a significant risk factor for coronary heart disease, especially the very low levels that can be encountered in familial hypoalphalipoproteinemia. The presence of low HDL cholesterol levels is a rational basis for decreasing the threshold level for treatment of hypercholesterolemia, especially if the patient has a significant family history of premature coronary disease. It is also an impetus to achieve optimal LDL cholesterol levels, circa 100 mg/dl. Whereas there has yet been no clear demonstration that elevation of HDL cholesterol levels, per se, is an effective intervention, this may prove to be the case. It should be noted that the drug regimens that have been associated with regression of coronary disease, especially those that include nia-

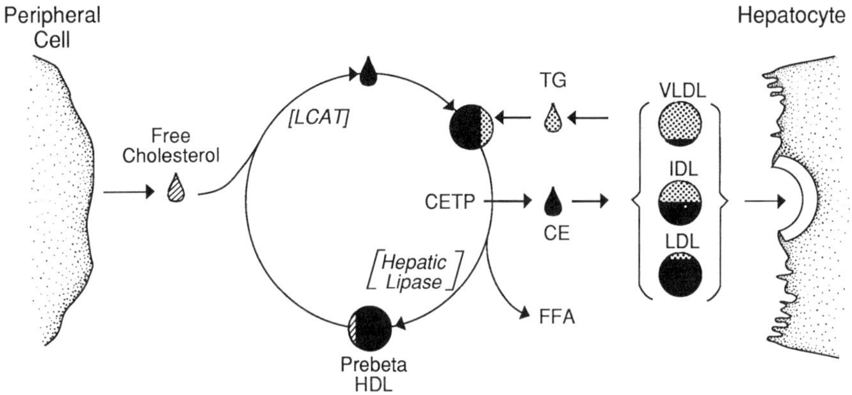

FIG 2.
The role of prebeta high-density lipoprotein (HDL) in reverse cholesterol transport. *Black areas* denote cholesteryl esters; *stippled areas,* triglycerides; *hatched areas,* free cholesterol. LCAT = lecithin-cholesterol acyl transferase; CETP = cholesteryl ester transfer protein; TG = triglycerides; CE = cholesteryl esters; FFA = free fatty acid; VLDL = very low-density lipoprotein; IDL = intermediate-density lipoproteins; LDL = low-density lipoproteins.

cin, tend to increase HDL cholesterol levels. Thus, niacin should be considered as the drug of choice in individuals with hypoalphalipoproteinemia unless otherwise contraindicated. Clinical experience has demonstrated that the HDL effect is exerted at relatively low doses (1.5-2.5 g/day).

Family History—A Risk Factor for Coronary Disease

In addition to abnormalities of lipoproteins, epidemiologic studies have conclusively implicated a number of other risk factors including cigarette smoking, arterial hypertension, and sedentary life style.[2, 3] Over 20 years ago, it was established that first degree relatives of patients with coronary disease are at increased risk.[27, 28] A 3.5-fold risk was observed for brothers of affected probands in a study in North Finland.[29, 30] The importance of early appearance of coronary disease was demonstrated by a risk increment of seven- to elevenfold, if the disease presented in the proband before 45 years of age. Vertical risk associations have also been demonstrated.[31] Certainly some of this familial association is attributable to common inheritance of traits for lipoprotein abnormalities or hypertension etc. and even to commonality of environment, for instance, diet or smoking. However, multivariate analysis of data from the Tecumseh study clearly shows significant residual risk attributable to familial association, independent of known risk factors.[32] The unaccountable risk residual has been estimated to be as great as the sum of all risk factors that are currently recognized. Thus, family history and the course of disease in the patient, per se, are the only means available of assessing some of the determinants of risk at this time and therefore are important elements in the clinical evaluation of all patients.

Relationship of Lipemia to Pancreatitis

Pancreatitis has long been associated with severe hypertriglyceridemia.[33, 34] Early investigators arrived at the conclusion that pancreatitis caused a secondary lipemia because the lipemia tends to clear as pancreatitis resolves. Extensive clinical observation has since demonstrated that this clearing of lipemia is due to inanition and that the lipemia, if untreated, tends to recur in the absence of pancreatitis.[35] In many patients, recurrent attacks of pancreatitis occur as triglyceride levels increase beyond 2000 mg/dl, suggesting a threshold effect. It is probable that the attacks are precipitated by the hydrolysis of triglycerides and phospholipids in blood by pancreatic lipase and phospholipase A_2, respectively. These enzymes release free fatty acids and lysolecithins in the pancreatic capillary bed as they act on the mass of substrate chylomicrons and VLDL present in plasma. The free fatty acids and lysolecithins stimulate thrombogenesis and are lytic to cell membranes, causing the local liberation of pancreatic enzymes that initiate a self-propagating chemical pancreatitis. Clinical experience has unequivocally demonstrated that most recurrences of pancreatitis associated with hyperlipemia can be prevented if triglyceride levels are brought under control.

Mechanisms of Atherogenesis

The development of the atherosclerotic plaque is a highly complex process involving the participation of a number of macromolecular and cellular elements. Several recent reviews describe the multilateral interaction of these elements.[36–38] The process appears to depend on the central initiatory role of atherogenic lipoproteins.[39–41] These apparently include LDL, IDL (intermediate-density lipoproteins, which are lipolytic remnants of VLDL), some VLDL, and the Lp(a) lipoproteins. The earliest visible lesions are composed of lipid-filled foam cells formed from macrophages and smooth muscle cells by endocytosis of lipoproteins. Because LDL receptors are down-regulated by high levels of intracellular cholesterol, the uptake depends on other species of receptors collectively termed scavenger receptors. There are probably at least three molecular species of scavenger receptors, two of which have been cloned.[42, 43] It is probable that chemical modification of lipoproteins is required for endocytosis via these receptors. The most important mechanism of modification appears to be oxidation by free radical mediated mechanisms originating with molecular oxygen.[44] Oxidation begins with lipoprotein lipids and then propagates to covalent modification of the protein moieties. Formation of oxidized LDL has been demonstrated in vivo and oxidized LDL particles have been found in atherosclerotic plaques.[45, 46] Minimally modified LDL exhibits important properties vis á vis lesion formation even before the extent of modification is sufficient to promote uptake by scavenger receptors. It is capable of eliciting the production of a protein chemoattractant for monocytes and monocyte colony stimulating factor.[47] Oxidized lipoproteins are also toxic to endothelium and appear to be capable of eliciting an autoimmune response. The importance of lipoprotein oxidation in atherogenesis is suggested by the observation that the antioxidant probucol significantly mitigates the atherosclerotic process in homozygous LDL receptor–deficient rabbits.[48] Smoking appears to enhance the oxidative modification of lipoproteins.[49]

Cellular proliferation, principally involving smooth muscle cells, is a major element in the development of complex lesions[41] and may be the principal mechanism underlying restenosis after angioplasty or surgical revascularization. Platelet-derived growth factor, originating from platelets adhering to regions where endothelium is damaged or absent, is an important element in this process, but a complex matrix of cytokine release probably involves all the cellular elements of the plaque.[41] One consequence of the proliferative phase of atherogenesis is the deposition of collagen, leading to the classical fibrous lesion. Clinical events are precipitated by the expanding plaque in two ways. The lesion may expand slowly enough to the point of occlusion of a vessel such that growth of collateral vessels precludes infarction. Stable angina may occur in such patients. In other instances, the inflammatory activity of macrophages, probably involving the secretion of collagenase, may weaken the collagen scaffolding underlying the endothelium leading to rupture or fissuring of the plaque.[36, 37, 50] An acute fissure exposes the subintima to platelets, initiating a platelet thrombus with subsequent propagation of a fibrin thrombus that may produce a sudden occlusive event.

Lipoproteins appear to play significant roles in several of these processes. Reduction of the circulating levels of atherogenic lipoproteins in plasma would be expected to reduce the burden of oxidized lipoprotein confronting macrophages and transformed smooth muscle cells. Antioxidant protection of lipoprotein lipids should also retard atherogenesis. If the antithrombolytic effect of the Lp(a) lipoprotein is pathologically important, reduction of Lp(a) levels in plasma would be expected to improve the outcome in the presence of plaque rupture as well as retarding the development of the lesions themselves. Lastly, the accumulation of lipids in atheromata may be viewed as the net result of processes that deliver cholesterol to the foam cells and the natural processes of retrieval of cholesterol from peripheral cells. The latter, dependent upon certain molecular species of HDL, might be influenced by interventions that impact on HDL. Still further effects might be mediated by enhancement of the antioxidant properties of HDL.[23, 51]

Lipoprotein Metabolism

A working knowledge of the major processes in lipid transport and metabolism provides a framework for the understanding of lipoprotein disorders and for the selection of appropriate treatment modalities.[7, 52] The endogenous transport of triglycerides begins with the secretion of VLDL by liver (Fig 1). These particles contain one copy of apo B-100, a few copies of apo E, and three molecular species of C apolipoproteins. A further complement of apo E and C apolipoproteins is transferred to VLDL from HDL. Triglyceride secretion is increased materially when caloric intake exceeds the body's energy requirement or when alcohol is being metabolized. Exogenous estrogen also increases hepatic secretion of VLDL. A large fraction of VLDL triglycerides is hydrolyzed by lipoprotein lipase (LPL) which resides on capillary endothelium in tissues such as skeletal and cardiac muscle and in adipose tissue. A small apolipoprotein, Apo CII, is a necessary cofactor for LPL as is heparin. As triglycerides are removed, the particle diameter decreases. C apolipoproteins and some apo E dissociate from the lipoprotein complex. The resultant VLDL remnant particle (IDL) retains the apolipoprotein B-100 molecule originally secreted with the particle from liver, and several copies of apolipoprotein E. About half of IDL particles are endocytosed by liver by a process that requires the apo E as ligand. The particles that are not endocytosed lose most of the remaining triglycerides to form yet smaller, cholesteryl-ester-rich lipoproteins (LDL) that contain only one apolipoprotein, apo B-100. Hepatic lipase is required for the efficient removal of triglycerides from IDL. Low-density lipoproteins serve to deliver cholesterol to all nucleated cells via endocytosis by the LDL receptor. Apo B-100 serves as the receptor ligand in this process (see Fig 1).

Chylomicrons are triglyceride-rich lipoproteins that originate in the intestine and carry triglycerides of dietary origin in the blood. They are analogous in structure to VLDL but their B-apoprotein moiety, B-48, is a truncated version of apo B-100, corresponding to the amino terminal 48% of the apo B-100 sequence. Chylomicron triglycerides are hydrolyzed by LPL even more efficiently than are those of VLDL, rapidly producing remnant particles that are quantitatively removed by endocytosis in the liver, yielding no particle analogous to LDL. Apo E is the ligand required for this process.

The Lp(a) lipoprotein appears to be formed in plasma from lipoproteins of the endogenous cascade, chiefly LDL. It is distinguished by the attachment of a high molecular weight protein (Lp[a]) to the apo B-100 protein. The Lp(a) protein, containing a variable number of Kringle structures (disulfide stabilized loop structures characteristic of many proteins involved in clotting and thrombolysis), is the product of a gene apparently derived in evolution from the gene for plasminogen. Many different isoforms exist, representing a wide range of molecular weights. The Lp(a) protein is capable of occupying the binding sites for plasminogen on endothelium and on fibrin, interfering with fibrinolysis.

The content of cholesterol in many body cells appears to regulate the expression of LDL receptors as well as de novo production of cholesterol via the pathway for sterol biosynthesis. HMGCoA reductase catalyzes the first committed step (and one of the rate limiting steps) in that pathway.

Retrieval of surplus cholesterol from peripheral cells and its subsequent transport to liver appears to proceed by several pathways. The major pathway involves the desorption of unesterified cholesterol from cell membranes and its uptake by the newly discovered 65-kd prebeta HDL species (Fig 2). The free cholesterol is then esterified by lecithin-cholesterol acyl transferase (LCAT) forming larger HDL species of alpha mobility. Cholesteryl esters are then transferred from these complexes to the cores of chylomicrons, VLDL, IDL, and LDL with the participation of cholesteryl ester transfer protein (CETP). Ultimate transfer of cholesteryl ester to liver occurs as the acceptor lipoproteins undergo endocytosis. Cholesterol can be secreted into bile directly or can be transformed into bile acids.

The content of cholesteryl esters in HDL, that contributes the bulk of total HDL cholesterol, is strongly influenced by the level of triglycerides in plasma. High triglyceride levels result in exchange of triglycerides for cholesteryl esters in the cores of the HDL particles. This may have significant impact on the function of HDL and invariably produces a decrease in measurable HDL cholesterol levels.

Genetic Disorders of Lipoprotein Metabolism

Accumulation of Triglyceride-Rich Lipoproteins in Plasma.—The chylomicronemia syndrome, in which chylomicron particles accumulate in blood, often with VLDL, results from genetic defects in lipoprotein lipase or its cofactor, apo C-II.[53] Patients with these defects have very high levels of plasma triglycerides, especially after ingesting fat, and are prone to develop acute pancreatitis. The hypertriglyceridemia is aggravated by caloric surplus and by the administration of exogenous estrogens. The ingestion of alcohol, even in moderate amounts, raises levels of triglycerides greatly in these patients.

Endogenous lipemia is a common phenotype of obscure etiology in which VLDL are the predominant lipoproteins. When VLDL saturate lipoprotein lipase, chylomicrons may also be retained in plasma, a phenotype termed mixed lipemia.

Accumulation of Remnant Particles in Plasma.—Apolipoprotein E, the requisite ligand for hepatic endocytosis of remnant particles formed from VLDL and chylomicrons, occurs in several common allelic variants. Whereas the apo E3 and apo E4 proteins function normally as ligands in hepatic endocytosis, the apo E2 protein does not. Individuals homozygous for apo E2 or less common ligand-defective mutations may accumulate large amounts of IDL and chylomicron remnants if other determinants of hyperlipidemia are present, a condition termed *dysbetalipoproteinemia*.[54] This disorder is associated with increased risk of peripheral vascular disease and coronary disease. Remnant-like particles rich in triglycerides may also accumulate in the plasma of individuals with the rare genetic deficiency of hepatic lipase.

Accumulation of LDL in Plasma.—A number of molecular defects in the structure of the LDL receptor or its synthesis and processing are now recognized[55] as causes of the disorder termed *familial hypercholesterolemia* (FH). In the heterozygous state, total cholesterol levels are usually in the 300 to 400 mg/dl range, though other heritable factors can cause them to be either lower or higher. In these patients tendinous xanthomas occur frequently and premature coronary disease is common. Approximately one in 500 individuals in the U.S. is heterozygous for FH. In homozygotes, serum cholesterol levels vary from 600 to over 1000 mg/dl. These patients often have clinically apparent coronary disease in childhood and are resistant to therapy with drugs that act by inducing expression of receptors.

Just as defective receptors impair the endocytosis of LDL, so also do defects in the ligand domain of apo B-100, a condition termed *ligand defective apo B.* A mutation at amino acid residue 3500 of the protein occurs with an incidence of approximately 1 in 1000 individuals of Western European descent.[56] Because the ligand domain of apo B-100 appears to be structurally complex and at least one additional ligand-defective apo B mutation is now known,[57] it is likely that others will be identified.

Variable Accumulation of VLDL and LDL in Plasma.—The genetic defect(s) underlying this phenotype known as *familial combined hyperlipoproteinemia* are as yet unknown. However it is clearly the most prevalent of the recognized phenotypic disorders of lipoproteins, perhaps occurring as frequently as 1 in 200 individuals. Evidence has been adduced from kinetic studies that the secretion of VLDL is increased about twofold above normal. Elevated levels of either VLDL or LDL may predominate, but in the most common presentation both are elevated. It is transmitted as a codominant trait and is associated with an increased risk of coronary disease. Xanthomas are uncommon in these patients.

Deficiency of HDL.—In many kindreds, low levels of HDL cholesterol and the major HDL apolipoprotein, apo AI, occur in the absence of hypertriglyceridemia. This phenotype, termed *familial hypoalphalipoproteinemia* often appears to behave as a codominant trait and is associated with increased risk of coronary disease. The genetic basis for this phenotype is not yet known. It is probable that a number of defects will be found to cause primary deficiency of HDL.[58] In a very rare disorder, Tangier disease, HDL levels are almost undetectable. Patients may have neuropathies and frequently have enlarged, orange pigmented tonsils.[59] Atherosclerosis occurs in these patients but is not strikingly premature, perhaps reflecting their extremely low levels of LDL cholesterol.

Compound Genetic States.—Because of the relatively high prevalence of many of the mutations known to affect lipoprotein metabolism, their simultaneous occurrence can be anticipated in clinical practice. The combination of FH and familial combined hyperlipidemia appears to cause severe hyperlipidemia. Likewise, compound states including FH with primary hypoalphalipoproteinemia or high levels of Lp(a) tend to be associated with an exceptionally high risk of coronary disease.

Clinical Differentiation of Lipoprotein Disorders

Normally the clinician must determine a patient's lipoprotein phenotype with a limited repertory of laboratory determinations, his clinical observations, and the patient's family history. Perhaps nine tenths of clinical diagnoses can be made without further biochemical data. The laboratory tests that are most useful are the total plasma cholesterol and triglyceride levels and the HDL cholesterol level. Triglyceride levels are only interpretable after a fast of at least ten hours. Lipoprotein electrophoresis is useful in certain cases and immunoassay for Lp(a) will be a necessary determination when reliability of commercially available methods is established.

If the triglyceride level is not over 400 mg/dl, the LDL cholesterol can be estimated by the Friedewald formula, using the total triglycerides, total and HDL cholesterol levels.[60] VLDL cholesterol is estimated as one-fifth of the total triglycerides. Subtracting VLDL cholesterol and HDL cholesterol from the total yields a reasonable estimate of LDL cholesterol.

Three general lipoprotein phenotypic patterns are encountered:

1. *Predominant hypertriglyceridemia.* In this case, triglycerides substantially exceed the total cholesterol level. From Figure 1, it can be deduced that the abnormality must be an excess of VLDL, chylomicrons, or both. This phenotype encompasses the defects in removal of triglyceride-rich lipoproteins, the phase of familial combined hyperlipidemia in which VLDL predominates, and endogenous lipemia. Eruptive cutaneous xanthomas are seen with severely elevated triglycerides resulting from any cause. Secondary causes of this pattern include the hypertriglyceridemia of uncontrolled diabetes, nephrosis, renal failure, lipodystrophy, and lipemia associated with monoclonal gammopathy. Obesity, alcohol abuse or, in women, exogenous estrogens and pregnancy may amplify any of the primary or secondary forms of lipemia.
2. *Isolated hypercholesterolemia.* The total and LDL cholesterol levels are elevated in the absence of hypertriglyceridemia. Measurement of HDL cholesterol allows the clinician to identify those patients, usually women, who have HDL cholesterol levels so high that they increase total cholesterol levels significantly. The phenotypic pattern of isolated hypercholesterolemia includes familial hypercholesterolemia, ligand-defective apo B-100, and the hypercholesterolemic phase of familial combined hyperlipidemia. The presence of tendon xanthomas suggests familial hypercholesterolemia or ligand-defective apo B-100. Secondary hypercholesterolemia may occur with hypothyroidism, early nephrosis, cholestasis, monoclonal gammopathies, and anorexia nervosa.
3. *Combined hypercholesterolemia and hypertriglyceridemia.* In this pattern, total serum cholesterol and triglyceride levels are elevated to ap-

proximately the same degree. The primary genetic disorders that can present with this pattern are familial combined hyperlipidemia and familial dysbetalipoproteinemia. These can be differentiated in two ways. On electrophoresis, bands of beta (LDL) and prebeta (VLDL) lipoproteins can be seen to be clearly separated in the case of familial combined hyperlipidemia, whereas the remnant particles of dysbetalipoproteinemia yield a single "broad beta" band. The diagnosis of dysbetalipoproteinemia can be confirmed by the demonstration of homozygosity for apo E-2, a determination available in research laboratories. A few less common mutations that impair receptor ligand function of apo E may be indistinguishable from the predominate normal form (apo E-3) by isoelectric focusing. The presence of tuberous xanthomas on extensor surfaces or planar xanthomas of the palmer creases is suggestive of dysbetalipoproteinemia. Secondary hyperlipidemia associated with nephrosis or monoclonal gammopathy can mimic this phenotype.

The Decision to Treat

Elevated levels of LDL, Lp(a), and VLDL, and low levels of HDL cholesterol are associated with risk for coronary artery disease. The National Institutes of Health Consensus Development Conference has recently proposed guidelines concerning measurement of triglycerides and HDL-cholesterol. A level of HDL cholesterol below 35 mg/dl is considered a major risk factor for CHD and determines follow-up for primary prevention in persons without CHD. Current National Cholesterol Education Program (NCEP) guidelines state that a desirable LDL cholesterol level for an asymptomatic patient with two or more risk factors is <130 mg/dl and 100 mg/dl or less for a patient with CHD.[61] The authors suggest that more aggressive reduction of LDL cholesterol may be indicated to increase the chance of stabilization or reversal of lesions. A treatment goal for high-risk patients as well as those with known atherosclerotic heart disease might more appropriately be 90 to 100 mg/dl. It is also becoming evident that elevated levels of VLDL triglycerides or Lp(a) and low HDL cholesterol levels should be considered in the decision to treat and in the establishment of treatment goals. Other factors that contribute to risk include: age, male sex, postmenopausal status in women, diabetes mellitus, hypertension, smoking (active or passive), weight >30% above "ideal," evidence of atherosclerosis in peripheral or cerebral arteries, family history of atherosclerosis before age 65, and the presence of other diseases such as nephrosis, or chronic use of medications that adversely affect plasma lipoproteins. These include steroids, some beta-blockers, and diuretics.

All adults should know their cholesterol and triglyceride levels. Those whose initial lipid levels are increased should be further evaluated and followed along the general guidelines of the NCEP. Children should be screened for lipoprotein abnormalities when a parent is known to be affected, when there is a family history of premature CHD, or when the child has another health problem or treatment that could cause secondary hyperlipidemia or contribute to risk of CHD.[62] At least two fasting (10 hr) blood specimens should be obtained for measurement of cholesterol, triglycerides, and HDL cholesterol (if triglycerides are less than 400 mg/dl), and calculation of LDL cholesterol in patients with known disease or two or more risk factors for CHD. Fasting levels of triglycerides in excess of 150 mg/dl may be significant as a risk for CHD and those greater than 800 mg/dl could pose a risk for pancreatitis. Although a first attack of pancreatitis associated with hypertriglyceridemia usually does not occur until levels of triglycerides reach 2000 mg/dl or more, the LPL-dependent clearance mechanism becomes saturated when triglycerides are in the 700 to 800 mg/dl range, increasing the risk of pancreatitis with any further oral fat intake.

Reduced levels of HDL cholesterol in the presence of hypertriglyceridemia must be interpreted in the context of the known inverse logarithmic relationship of these two lipid values. When triglycerides are elevated above 400 mg/dl, the HDL cholesterol levels are uninformative.[63]

Secondary causes of hyperlipidemia, including those related to drug treatment, must be identified and management then directed to the primary problem. As patients with renal failure or transplant are living longer, more are succumbing to CHD, presumably at least partly due to their hyperlipidemia. Although treatment of secondary hyperlipidemia has not been adequately studied, such patients should be treated in the hope of retarding the progression of their vascular disease. Unrecognized hypothyroidism is a relatively frequent cause of modest hypercholesterolemia and may contribute to partial failure of diet and drug regimens in treatment of a genetic hypercholesterolemia. Exogenous estrogen administration can increase levels of triglycerides. This effect may be particularly dramatic in women with genetic hypertriglyceridemic states, increasing their risk of pancreatitis.

Age, at either extreme, is not necessarily a contraindication to drug treatment. With the exception of children with severe hyperlipidemia secondary to nephrosis, only those with genetic hyperlipidemia should be given drug therapy, and relatively few of these should receive medication before the late teenage years.[62] Special considerations in the decision to treat children with drugs include the presence of compound genetic lipoprotein states, other health problems and treatments, age at onset of symptomatic CHD in the affected parent or grandparent, etc. Elderly patients should be offered diet and drug therapy, if their individual assessment of risk to benefit so warrants. Those with symptomatic CHD should be treated more aggressively. Left ventricular hypertrophy on ECG or echocardiography has now been recognized as an important risk factor for CHD in the elderly[10, 64] and may also be an indication for drug therapy in an otherwise asymptomatic patient. Intervention trials in older persons are currently under way and should result in the development of better guidelines for treatment.

Despite popular misconceptions, the most frequent cause of death in women is coronary heart disease. Results of the only intervention trial reported to date that included significant numbers of women indicate that women respond to lipid-lowering intervention as well or better than men with respect to regression of plaque dimensions.[65] Women with genetic hyperlipidemias, hypoalphalipoproteinemia, or with other risk factors including a positive family history for early CHD are candidates for treatment.

Diet Modification

Dietary changes are always the first step in management of hyperlipidemia and may be the only treatment needed for patients with mild to moderate hypercholesterolemia or with hypertriglyceridemia.[66] Referral to a registered dietitian is very helpful in the adaptation and implementation of diet therapy. The American Heart Association diet is a judicious choice for most adults. Further reduction in risk of CHD can be achieved by the Step II diet recommended by the NCEP Expert Panel. General guidelines of this diet include a daily cholesterol intake of 200 mg or less with no more than 7% of total calories as saturated fat. Calories should be restricted so as to achieve and maintain ideal body weight. Weight control is particularly important for the hypertriglyceridemic patient and small reductions in weight may reduce levels of triglycerides appreciably. The physician should be aware that if a patient is actively losing weight, levels of LDL and VLDL will be lower than can be maintained once caloric balance is stabilized, even on a diet of ideal composition. Exercise programs are, of course, an important adjunct to dietary treatment if compatible with the patient's cardiovascular status. Dietary triglycerides (total fat) should be reduced in all patients but particularly those with hypertriglyceridemia. Alcohol should be restricted or eliminated in hypertriglyceridemic patients so as to decrease VLDL secretion. Omega-3 fatty acids found in cold water marine fish are of some use in selected patients with severe hypertriglyceridemia, but generally are of no value in reducing levels of LDL. They may also significantly reduce levels of HDL in some individuals. Polyunsaturated fats should be used minimally because of potential carcinogenicity and their propensity to decrease HDL cholesterol. Use of monounsaturates is preferable and their moderate use usually results in small increases of HDL cholesterol compared with HDL levels observed in persons who eat diets extremely low in total fat. Patients with familial chylomicronemia or other severe forms of hypertriglyceridemia who present with triglycerides over 1000 mg/dl can often be successfully managed by acute elimination of all fat from the diet for about 72 hr, followed by greatly reduced fat intake (10 to 15 g total fat daily). If signs or symptoms of incipient pancreatitis are present, all oral intake should be eliminated and the patient will require hospitalization for intravenous fluids and other supportive care as needed. Once the acute episode is controlled, oral fat must be introduced gradually and total fat limited to 10 g, then 15 g daily. Most of these patients can avoid pancreatitis and keep their triglycerides under 700 to 800 mg/dl if their fat intake does not exceed 15 to 20 g daily.

Contemporary nutritional research suggests that intake of natural antioxidants including ascorbic acid, beta carotene, and tocopherol may be important in preventing free radical mediated oxidative processes such as the oxidation of LDL. Optimal levels of intake for this purpose are yet to be determined. Certain types of dietary fiber, notably the bran found in oats, rice, and some other foods appear to have a limited ability to lower levels of LDL cholesterol.

Drug Treatment

If diet, exercise, and treatment of underlying secondary causes of hyperlipidemia have failed to achieve desired goals, drug therapy may be indicated. The effectiveness of drug treatment is enhanced by continued dietary modification. Drug treatment should be commenced immediately in adult patients with the severe genetic hyperlipidemias (other than primary chylomicronemia) and in hyperlipidemic patients with symptomatic CHD. The choice of agent should be based on its mechanism of action, the patient's specific lipoprotein phenotype, the side effect profile, treatment goals, the patient's age, other drug treatment, and cost.[67] No drugs should be given to pregnant or lactating women, and fibrates and reductase inhibitors should also be avoided in women who are likely to become pregnant. Table 1 summarizes the suggested agent(s) for each primary lipoprotein disorder.

Bile Acid Binding Resins.—These agents, used in the treatment of hypercholesterolemia, sequester bile acids in the intestine, decreasing their reabsorption. There is increased bile acid production from cholesterol via 7-alpha-hydroxylation resulting in the induction of LDL receptors in liver. This leads to lower levels of plasma LDL in spite of the increased synthesis of cholesterol in liver via the mevalonate pathway that also results from resin treatment.[68]

Colestipol and cholestyramine are the two resins in current use. They lower levels of LDL as much as 25% in most hypercholesterolemic disorders. They are given in daily doses up to 30 g and 24 g, respectively. Starting daily doses are 5 g or 4 g, and doses should be increased by 5 g or 4 g increments over a few weeks to increase tolerability. The patient should be instructed to mix the resin with water, dilute juice (for calorie control), or soft food and take it with meals. Although twice-daily dosage is preferred for convenience, these drugs are more effective if given with each meal. If a lower dose suffices and it is only taken once daily, it should be taken in the morning. There are essentially no important systemic side effects. Common intestinal side effects include constipation, indigestion, mild abdominal discomfort, nausea, and a bloated feeling. Individually adjusted doses of psyllium, added to the resin mixture, usually relieves these symptoms. Dry skin has been described with long-term treatment. There is a theoretical risk of cholelithiasis, especially in obese patients, because the resins change the composition of bile micelles. In patients with bowel disease or cholestasis, malabsorption of fat or fat-soluble vitamins and hy-

TABLE 1.
Suggested Agents for Treatment of Primary Lipoprotein Disorders*

Lipoprotein Disorder	Lipoprotein(s) Elevated	Drugs of Choice	Combined Therapy
Familial hypercholesterolemia	LDL-(cholesterol)	Resin, niacin, RI	Resin + niacin Resin + RI Niacin + RI Resin + RI + niacin
Familial combined hypercholesterolemia	LDL-(cholesterol) and/or VLDL (triglycerides)	Niacin, RI	Niacin + resin Niacin + RI
Dysbetalipoproteinemia	IDL-(cholesterol and triglycerides)	Niacin, fibrate*	Niacin + fibrate Niacin + RI
Primary hypertriglyceridemia	VLDL (triglycerides)		
	-moderate	Niacin	
	-severe	Niacin, fibrate	Niacin + fibrate
Primary chylomicronemia	Chylomicrons (triglycerides)	(Diet only)	

*LDL = low-density lipoprotein; VLDL = very low-density lipoprotein; IDL = intermediate-density lipoprotein; RI = Reductase inhibitor; fibrate = fibric acid derivative.

poprothrombinemia may occur when resins are given. Because they may bind other drugs, all medications (except niacin) should be given at least 1 hour before or 2 hours after the resin. A resin, given as a single agent, is contraindicated in patients with hypertriglyceridemia since it often increases levels of VLDL.

Niacin (Nicotinic Acid).—This B vitamin decreases levels of LDL-cholesterol and triglyceride-rich lipoproteins and is the only agent that may remarkably increase levels of HDL-cholesterol. It is also the only drug that appears to reduce levels of the Lp(a) lipoprotein. The amide (niacinamide) has no effect on lipoproteins. The primary effect of niacin is probably the inhibition of secretion of VLDL from the liver, indirectly leading to decreased production of LDL.[69] Removal of VLDL triglyceride via the LPL pathway is enhanced and cholesterogenesis is inhibited.[70] There is also increased excretion of cholesterol in bile. Inhibition of HDL catabolism appears to occur with a resultant increase in levels of HDL-cholesterol and apo A-I. Niacin may effect thrombogenesis by inducing a decrease in circulating levels of fibrinogen and an increase in release of tissue plasminogen activator.

Niacin is given two or three times daily with meals and its absorption is not affected by concomitant use of a resin. The starting dose is 100 mg three times daily with, or just after, a meal. Dosage is increased slowly by 100 mg to 200 mg daily increments. Mild to moderate hypercholesterolemia and moderate hypertriglyceridemia may respond appreciably to as little as 1 to 3 g daily. More severe hypertriglyceridemia and the severe genetic hypercholesterolemic states may require up to 6 g daily. Doses exceeding 6.5 g daily should be avoided. Niacin is a useful agent in combined drug therapy regimens and often the dose can then be kept under 3 g daily even in extreme hyperlipidemic states.

Transient cutaneous flushing and pruritus are common side effects initially, when dosage is increased, or if the drug is resumed after several missed doses. Aspirin (0.3 g) taken 20 to 30 minutes beforehand or a morning dose of ibuprofen will mitigate this prostaglandin-mediated phenomenon. Tachyphylaxis to these side effects usually occurs after a few days or weeks at a given dose. The three-times daily dosage is recommended to enhance this effect. However, niacin should not be given more frequently than three times daily. Gastric irritation, usually relieved by antacids, may occur. Antacids containing aluminum should be avoided because aluminum nicotinate is absorbed very slowly, potentially causing the toxicity associated with sustained release preparations of niacin. Niacin should be given with caution, or avoided, in patients who have active peptic ulcer disease. Uric acid levels may increase during niacin therapy, but unless the patient has had gout, this rarely requires discontinuance of the drug. Occasionally, it is necessary to treat with allopurinol if gout develops in a patient who requires niacin to control severe hyperlipidemia. Impairment of glucose tolerance may occur but is usually reversible when the drug is stopped. Niacin should be given with special caution and frequent monitoring to patients with type II diabetes. Reversible toxic amblyopia, evident as distorted distance vision, and acanthosis nigricans have occurred rarely. Arrhythmias and hypotension have developed rarely during niacin therapy, but have been observed at very low dosage. Moderate increases (up to threefold) in transaminase activity without symptoms are frequently observed and are not an indication for discontinuing niacin. They are probably the result of enzyme induction. Severe hepatic toxicity is rare with regular niacin. However, time-release preparations of niacin should be avoided because of the catastrophic liver failure that has, rarely, been associated with their use even at very low dosage levels. Several types of sustained release niacin have been associated with this phenomenon suggesting that it could occur with all such preparations. Niacin should not be given to patients with hepatic parenchymal disease.

Transaminase levels, blood glucose, and uric acid should be measured at baseline and about 6 weeks after commencing treatment. A liver panel should be done no less frequently than every 4 to 5 months thereafter, assuming transaminase levels remain stable and there are no symptoms suggestive of liver toxicity. Glucose and uric acid should be measured about every 6 to 8 months.

HMGCoA Reductase Inhibitors.—These drugs inhibit the rate-limiting enzyme in cholesterol biosynthesis.[71] By decreasing intracellular levels, they induce increased expression of LDL receptors.[72, 73] This results in increased endocytosis and catabolism of LDL, thereby lowering levels of cholesterol in serum. They are the most potent agents used in the treatment of hypercholesterolemia. Although they may induce modest reductions in levels of VLDL, they are not indicated for the treatment of hypertriglyceridemia. Levels of HDL-cholesterol may be modestly increased, but there is no indication for their use when hypoalphalipoproteinemia is the only lipoprotein abnormality.

Three drugs in this class are now available in the United States. Lovastatin, the first to be released, has about the same potency as pravastatin on a mass basis, whereas simvastatin is about twice as potent. These agents may be given once or twice daily. Although lovastatin and simvastatin may be slightly better absorbed with food, they appear in practice to be just as effective when given at other times. Since production of cholesterol is increased at night, there is a theoretical advantage to take the reductase inhibitor with dinner or at bedtime. Starting doses of lovastatin and pravastatin are 10 to 20 mg daily, and of simvastatin, 5 to 10 mg daily. Patients with genetic hypercholesterolemia will require higher dosages and the starting dose could reflect this. Maximum daily doses are: lovastatin 80 mg; pravastatin 40 mg; simvastatin 40 mg.

These drugs have no common short-term side effects. Minor gastroenteric symptoms, headache, insomnia, rashes, and fatigue have been reported. Modest elevations of transaminases and skeletal muscle creatine kinase (CK) may occur without symptoms. Levels of CK may be particularly high in patients who exercise heavily. The important serious side effects, chemical hepatitis and a myopathic syndrome, are rare. With hepatitis, malaise and nausea may be initial complaints. With the myopathy, muscle symptoms may include tenderness, cramping, pain, or only weakness. If recognized early, these problems are reversible when the drug is discontinued. Myopathy can progress to rhabdomyolysis with myoglobinuria and eventual renal shutdown if treatment is not stopped. A dermatomyositis-like syndrome has been described rarely in patients receiving lovastatin.

Measurement of liver function and CK should be made before treatment commences and about 4 to 6 weeks after. If levels are stable, the interval can be increased to 8, then 12 weeks. Creatine kinase levels probably do not need to be measured more than once a year if the patient remains asymptomatic. The risk of developing the myopathic syndrome is prominent when a reductase inhibitor is taken with certain other drugs including cyclosporine, fibric acid derivatives, and erythromycin. In the case of cyclosporine, greatly reduced dosage of the reductase inhibitor should be used and the patient, in all instances, monitored very closely. In general, the combinations of reductase inhibitor with fibric acid derivatives or erythromycin should be avoided. Concomitant use with niacin may incur a slightly increased risk of myopathy and hepatic dysfunction. Therefore, more frequent monitoring of liver and muscle enzymes is indicated. These drugs should be avoided or used with great caution in a patient with a history of liver disease.

Fibric Acid Derivatives.—These agents appear to increase clearance of triglyceride-rich lipoproteins by enhancing the activity of lipoprotein lipase[74] and may also decrease synthesis of VLDL. They often reduce levels of triglycerides, have variable effects on LDL-cholesterol, and may increase HDL-cholesterol to a modest degree.[75] The fibrates are useful in the treatment of severe hypertriglyceridemia and in dysbetalipoproteinemia. Many patients with combined hyperlipidemia have increased levels of LDL-cholesterol when a fibrate is given to reduce triglycerides, requiring the addition of another agent or substitution of other hypolipidemic drugs. The most commonly used fibrate in this country is gemfibrozil. Recent review of data from the Helsinki Heart Study follow-up extension and the ancillary study to that trial resulted in the recommendation that gemfibrozil should not be used in patients with combined hyperlipidemia who have a history or symptoms of atherosclerotic heart disease. These studies were difficult to interpret because of the small sample size and other problems leaving the impact of gemfibrozil treatment on secondary prevention incompletely known at this time.

Gemfibrozil and the first generation fibric acid derivative, clofibrate, are available in the United States. The usual dose of gemfibrozil is 600 mg once or twice daily. Clofibrate is rarely used because it was associated in a large trial with an increase in overall mortality and an increased incidence of gastrointestinal cancers.

Common side effects of fibrate therapy include nausea, abdominal pain and flatulence. Rarely, leukopenia, anemia, hypokalemia, myalgias or overt myositis, headache, increased incidence of gallstones, increased liver enzymes, and arrhythmias have been described. Metabolites of these drugs are excreted by the kidneys. They should be avoided in patients with renal insufficiency and nephrosis because of the increased risk of toxic effects. Doses of Coumadin and indanedione anticoagulants should be reduced when treatment with a fibrate is initiated since their activity may be potentiated.

Antioxidants.—The only potent antioxidant currently available is probucol, a drug that has been marketed for many years for its moderate cholesterol-lowering effect. The potential clinical significance of its antioxidant property was only recently recognized when the importance of lipoprotein oxidation emerged. No clinical trials have yet been completed that could establish its effectiveness in preventing coronary disease in humans. However, there was a significant impact on atherosclerosis in rabbits homozygous for familial hypercholesterolemia who were given probucol.[48] Also some beneficial effect was described in a limited number of humans with that disease.[76, 77] Until results of two current trials are reported, the use of this drug is based upon hypothesis. Marked reductions of HDL-cholesterol are observed during treatment with probucol. It appears, however, that the transfer of cholesteryl esters from HDL to acceptor lipoproteins mediated by cholesteryl ester transfer protein is enhanced. Thus, the decreased levels of HDL cholesterol could reflect chiefly the increased efficiency of centripital transport. In practice, there seems to be no compound toxicity when probucol is used with resins, niacin, or HMGCoA reductase inhibitors.[78] When used with fibrates, probucol produces extremely low levels of HDL cholesterol.

The usual dose of probucol is 500 mg twice daily. Side effects include an increased QT interval; therefore it should be avoided if a patient has a preexisting prolonged QT interval, a predisposition to ventricular arrhythmia, or is taking other agents known to prolong the interval such as digitalis, quinidine, or erythromycin. Increased levels of bilirubin, alkaline phosphatase, transaminases, CK, uric acid, and glucose have been reported. Thrombocytopenia and neuropathy have been reported rarely. Nausea, diarrhea, and abdominal discomfort are more frequent side effects.

Drug Combination Therapy

In all instances, a single agent should be used first. If the desired levels of lipoproteins are not achieved, combined drug treatment should be considered. There are three categories of patients in whom combined therapy is frequently employed: (1) in persons with hypercholesterolemia in whom significantly elevated levels of VLDL occur during treatment with a resin; (2) persons who have combined elevations of LDL and VLDL at the outset; and (3) in individuals with a severe hyperlipidemia that does not respond fully to a single agent. The use of drug combination therapy frequently allows doses of the constituent agents to be lower and hence better tolerated. Very little, if any, increase in drug side effects is observed if only recommended combinations are used and the dosage levels are not excessive.

The increased levels of VLDL observed in some patients who take a resin for hypercholesterolemia are usually easily controlled by adding niacin. These drugs can be taken together with meals since absorption of niacin is not affected by the resin.

Niacin, with either a reductase inhibitor or a resin, is often needed to normalize levels of LDL and VLDL in patients with combined hyperlipidemia, particularly those in whom elevation of VLDL is prominent. The niacin dosage that is required varies but often can be kept under 3.0 g daily. Since niacin lowers levels of LDL as well as VLDL, the previous dose of resin or reductase inhibitor can sometimes be decreased with this combination. Liver function and CK activity should be monitored at least every 3 months when the reductase inhibitor-niacin combination is used, especially when either drug is used in higher dosage. However, in practice, no increase in liver toxicity or myositis has been observed in patients who have been followed as long as five years on this combination in the authors' clinic.

In patients with severe hypertriglyceridemia, niacin can be given with gemfibrozil for further reduction of triglycerides. In the case of severe hypercholesterolemia, binary or ternary combinations of the LDL-lowering agents (resin, niacin, reductase inhibitor) are used.[79–82] Lovastatin is the only reductase inhibitor that has been studied in combined regimens, but it is expected that the others will behave similarly.

Possible Untoward Consequences of Lipid-Lowering Therapy

Virtually all epidemiologic surveys have found the risk of coronary heart disease to increase monotonically with increasing levels of LDL cholesterol. A conference on low levels of cholesterol in serum and their association with mortality suggested that levels below 160 mg/dl may be associated weakly with increased risk of noncoronary disease.[83] Wasting illnesses in general result in very low LDL levels and the correlation between deaths from certain respiratory and digestive disorders and low levels of serum cholesterol would be expected to reflect this effect. A large number of the deaths attributable to digestive disease occur in patients with cirrhosis. The low levels of lipoproteins in these patients are clearly due to failure of hepatic parenchymal cells, the source of all apo B-100 containing lipoproteins. This is perhaps best illustrated in China, where hepatitis B is prevalent. The majority of cases of noncoronary mortality associated with low serum cholesterol levels are due to hepatic failure from chronic hepatitis B infection. Increased uptake of LDL by malignant cells is also known to decrease levels of LDL in plasma. Two studies have shown a small increase in risk of hemorrhagic stroke when serum cholesterol levels are below 130 mg/dl.[84, 85] In one, the effect was confined to hypertensive patients. The results of clinical trials are equivocal as to whether a discernible increase in noncoronary death might result from lipid-lowering intervention. Such a relationship is very weak if the trials employing fibric acid derivatives are excluded,[86, 87] suggesting that lipid lowering per se does not significantly increase risk for most noncoronary causes of death.[88–92] In the MRFIT Study, a proportionate hazards analysis adjusting for covariance indicated that in fact the lowest net death rate occurs at a serum cholesterol level of 122 mg/dl.[93]

Populations such as Japan, in which many individuals have serum cholesterol levels below 160 mg/dl, do not have an increased incidence of the noncoronary causes of death under consideration. In fact, the Japanese have a significantly longer life expectancy than do people in the United States or other industrialized nations. About 45% of deaths in the United States and Europe are attributable to cardiovascular disease, predominantly coronary artery disease. This fact is of great importance in resolving the question of the relative benefit of lipid-lowering therapy. Projection of a significant reduction in fatal occlusive coronary events into the age range where coronary disease predominates would be expected to far outweigh the marginal increases that might occur in other causes of death. However, in view of the relationship of hemorrhagic stroke with very low levels of plasma cholesterol (<130 mg/dl), the therapeutic goal for patients with known coronary artery disease should be a total cholesterol level of 150–160 mg/dl (LDL cholesterol level 90–100 mg/dl) until that relationship is better understood.

Evidence of Regression of Coronary Lesions

To date, three trials employing paired quantitative angiography and hypolipidemic therapy have been published. Each of these found a correlation between reduction in LDL cholesterol and regression. The Familial Atherosclerosis Treatment Study (FATS) trial included 120 men with CHD and elevated levels of apo B in plasma.[94] The men were managed with diet and drug therapy. They were assigned randomly to one of three treatment groups: 40 mg lovastatin plus 30 g colestipol daily; 4 g niacin plus 30 g colestipol, or conventional treatment with placebo (or colestipol for those whose LDL cholesterol level was increased). By multivariate analysis, significant net regression of lesions correlated independently with reductions in levels of apo B or LDL cholesterol and in systolic blood pressure. There was also a significant relationship of regression with increased levels of HDL cholesterol. The incidence of cardiovascular events, including death, myocardial infarction, and need for revascularization, was reduced significantly among the men who received intensive lipid-lowering treatment during the 2½-year, double-blind study. The SCOR trial (Specialized Center of Research in Atherosclerosis) studied 72 asymptomatic women and men with heterozygous FH.[65] A total of 457 lesions were measured before and after a 26-month period in these patients who were assigned randomly to one of two treatment groups: diet or diet plus 15 g colestipol daily; or diet plus combined drug regimens that included up to 30 g colestipol with up to 7.5 g niacin daily or up to 60 mg lovastatin in binary or ternary combinations with colestipol and niacin. The primary outcome variable, within-patient change in percent area stenosis, correlated with on-trial levels of LDL. There was significant regression of lesions in the more intensively treated patients. In contrast, lesions in the control group showed net progression. When analyzed separately, lesions in the women behaved similarly, suggesting that the benefit of treatment applies to women and men alike. Seventy-four men with CHD and only modestly elevated serum cholesterol levels were followed for 39 months in the STARS (St. Thomas' Atherosclerosis Regression Study) trial.[95] The treatment groups included usual care, diet therapy, and diet plus cholestyramine. Dietary treatment slowed overall progression and increased the likelihood of regression of lesions. Diet plus resin was additionally associated with net regression, whereas all angiographic criteria worsened in the patients who received usual care. Net regression of lesions correlated with both reduction of LDL cholesterol levels and increased levels of HDL cholesterol. Both intervention groups had improvement in severity of angina, but angina symptoms were not changed significantly in the usual care group. Of the 14 patients who had clinical cardiovascular events during the study, 10 were in the usual care group.

Two trials examined the effect of various interventions on coronary lesions by consensus panel. In the Cholesterol Lowering Atherosclerosis Study (CLAS II) coronary lesions were compared visually on baseline and follow-up angiograms at 2 and 4 years in men who had undergone surgical revascularization of the coronary arteries.[96] Among the 103 men who continued to 4 years in the trial, apparent regression of CHD was three times more frequent in the men who were treated with colestipol and niacin than in control subjects. Regression correlated with reduction in LDL-cholesterol and increased HDL-cholesterol levels. In the Progress on the Surgical Control of the Hyperlipidemias (POSCH) trial,[88] 838 patients with symptomatic CHD (760 men; 78 women) were followed for 9.7 years. They were randomly assigned to a surgical group that underwent partial ileal bypass or to a control group. All patients followed the AHA phase II diet. There was significantly less progression of coronary lesions and fewer new coronary events in the surgery group. Although it did not reach significance, overall mortality and mortality related to CHD were reduced in the surgically treated patients. These findings correlated with decreased levels of LDL cholesterol and increased levels of HDL cholesterol. In a small study, extreme diet and lifestyle changes were associated with reduction in coronary lesion size in 22 patients relative to 19 controls as measured by quantitative angiography.[97]

The finding in these studies that reduction in plasma levels of LDL indeed correlated with regression of existing coronary disease has conclusively validated the lipid hypothesis. Further, correlation of regression in several of the studies with increases in HDL-cholesterol suggests that strategies of intervention directed at the triglyceride-HDL axis may be effective as well. Because the lipid-lowering treatment was effective in patients with a variety of disorders, including familial hypercholesterolemia, familial combined hyperlipidemia and milder hyperlipidemic states, it appears that it is the impact on the levels of atherogenic lipoproteins per se that is important. Likewise, a similar outcome occurred regardless of treatment modality, indicating that the degree of perturbation of levels of atherogenic lipoproteins was the determining factor.

A corollary of these results is that a maximum impact on atherosclerotic lesions can be expected as the levels of LDL, HDL, and probably other lipoproteins (VLDL, Lp(a), IDL) approach the optimum. The observation is well established that lipid-optimizing therapy can not only retard the progression of atherosclerotic lesions but can induce measurable regression. This underscores the dynamic nature of atherogenesis and the ability of restorative mechanisms to stabilize and repair arterial damage if exposure to offending lipoproteins is reduced. Thus, the clinician should not be discouraged from initiating treatment even in the presence of advanced coronary disease.

References

1. McGee D, Gordon T: The results of the Framingham Study applied to four other US-based epidemiologic studies of cardiovascular disease, in Kannel WD, Gordon T (eds): *The Framingham Study: An Epidemiological Investigation of Cardiovascular Disease,* U.S. Department of Health, Education and Welfare, 1976.
2. Kannel WB, Castelli SP, Gordon T, et al: Serum cholesterol, lipoproteins and the risk of coronary heart disease: The Framingham Study. *Ann Intern Med* 1971; 74:1–12.
3. Kannel WB, Neaton JD, Wentworth D, et al: Overall and coronary heart diseae mortality rates in relation to major risk factors in 325,348 men screened for the MRFIT. *Am Heart J* 1986; 112:825–836.
4. Keys A, Menotti A, Karvonen M-J, et al: The diet and 15-year death rate in the Seven Countries Study. *Am J Epidemiol* 1986; 124:908–915.
5. Klag MJ, Ford DE, Mead LA, et al: Serum cholesterol in young men and subsequent cardiovascular disease. *N Engl J Med* 1993; 328:313–318.
6. Gofman JW, de Lalla O, F. G, et al: The serum lipoprotein treatment system in health, metabolic disease, atherosclerosis and coronary artery disease. *Plasma* 1954; 2:413.
7. Kane JP, Havel RJ: Disorders of the biogenesis and secretion of lipoproteins containing the B-apolipoproteins, in Scriver CR, Beaudet AL, Sly WS et al (eds): The Metabolic Basis of Inherited Disease, ed 6. New York, McGraw-Hill, 1989, pp 1139–1164.
8. Uttermann G: The mysteries of lipoprotein(a). *Science* 1989; 246:904–910.
9. Rhoads GG, Gulbrandssen CL, Kagan A: Serum lipoproteins and coronary heart disease in a population study of Hawaii Japanese men. *N Engl J Med* 1976; 294:293–298.
10. Gordon T, Castelli WP, Hjortland MC, et al: Predicting coronary heart disease in middle-aged and older persons. The Framingham Study. *JAMA* 1977; 238:497–499.
11. Miller NE, Thelle DS, Forde OH, et al: The Tromso heart study: High-density

lipoprotein and coronary heart disease: a prospective case-control study. *Lancet* 1977; i:964–968.
12. Gordon T, Hjortland M, Kannel W, et al: High density lipoprotein as a protective factor against coronary heart disease: The Framingham Study. *Am J Med* 1977; 66:707–714.
13. Wiklund O, Wilhelmsen L, Elmfeldt D: Alpha-lipoprotein cholesterol concentration in relation to subsequent myocardial infarction in hypercholesterolemic men. *Atherosclerosis* 1980; 37:47–53.
14. Keys A, Karvonen MJ, Punsar Sea: HDL serum cholesterol and 24-year mortality of men in Finland. *Int J Epidemiol* 1984; 13:428–435.
15. Pocock SJ, Shaper AG, Phillips AN, et al: High density lipoprotein cholesterol is not a major risk factor for ischemic heart disease in British men. *Br Med J* 1986; 292:515–519.
16. Levy RI, Klimov AN: High density lipoprotein cholesterol (HDL-C) and mortality in USSR and US middle-age men: The Collaborative US-USSR Mortality Follow-Up Study. *Circulation* 1987; 76(suppl IV):167.
17. Brunner D, Weisbort J, Mashulam N: Relation of serum total cholesterol and high-density lipoprotein cholesterol percentage to the incidence of definite coronary events. Twenty-year follow-up of the Donolo-Tel-Aviv prospective coronary artery disease study. *Am J Cardiol* 1987; 59:1271–1276.
18. Livshits G, Weisbort J, Meshulam N, et al: Multivariate analysis of the twenty-year follow-up of the Donolo-Tel-Aviv prospective coronary artery disease study and the usefulness of high density lipoprotein cholesterol percentage. *Am J Cardiol* 1989; 63:676–681.
19. Goldbourt U, Medalie JH: High density lipoprotein cholesterol and incidence of coronary heart disease—The Israeli schemic heart disease study. *Am J Epidemiol* 1979; 109:296–308.
20. Assmann G, Schulte M: The PROCAM Trial—Prospective Cardiovascular Muenster Trial, Hedingen/Zuerich, Panscientia Verlag, 1986.
21. Enger SC, Hjerman T, Foss OP: High density lipoprotein cholesterol and myocardial infarction and sudden coronary death: A prospective care-control study in middle-aged men of the Oslo study. *Artery* 1979; 5:170–181.
22. Goldbourt U, Holtzman E, Neufeld HN: Total and high density lipoprotein cholesterol in the serum and risk of mortality: Evidence of the threshold effect. *Br Med J* 1985; 290:1239–1243.
23. Kunitake ST, Jarvis MR, Hamilton RL, et al: Binding of transition metals by apolipoprotein A-I-containing plasma lipoproteins: Inhibition of oxidation of low density lipoproteins. *Proc Natl Acad Sci USA* 1992; 89:6993–6997.
24. Parthasarathy S, Barnett J, Fong LG: High-density lipoprotein inhibits the oxidative modification of low-density lipoprotein. *Biochim Biophys Acta* 1990; 1044:275–283.
25. Darbon JM, Tournier JF, Tauber JP, et al: Possible role of protein phosphorylation in the mitogenic effect of high density lipoproteins on cultured vascular endothelial cells. *J Biol Chem* 1986; 261:8002–8008.
26. Spector AA, Scanu AM, Kaduse TL, et al: Effect of human plasma lipoproteins on prostacyclin production by cultured endothelial cells. *J Lipid Res* 1985; 26:288–299.
27. Goldbourt U, Neufeld HN: Genetic aspects of arteriosclerosis. *Arteriosclerosis* 1986; 6:351–373.
28. Slack J, Evans KA: The increased risk of death from ischaemic heart disease in the first degree relatives of 121 men and 96 women with ischaemic heart disease. *J Med Genet* 1966; 3:239–257.

29. Rissanen AM: Familial aggregation of coronary heart disease in a high incidence area (North Karelia, Finland). *Br Heart J* 1979; 42:294–303.
30. Rissanen AM: Familial occurrence of coronary heart disease: Effect of age at diagnosis. *Am J Cardiol* 1979; 44:60–66.
31. Scholtz RI, Rosenmann RH, Brand RI: The relationship of reported family history to the incidence of coronary heart disease in the Western Collaborative Group Study. *Am J Epidemiol* 1975; 102:350–356.
32. Neufeld HN, Goldbourt U: Coronary heart disease: genetic aspects. *Circulation* 1983; 67:943–954.
33. Havel RJ, Goldstein JL, Brown MS: Lipoproteins and lipid transport, in Bondy PK, Rosenberg LE (ed): *Metabolic Control and Disease,* ed 8, Philadelphia, WB Saunders Co, 1980, pp 393–494.
34. Brunzell RJ, Bierman EL: Chylomicronemia syndrome. *Med Clin North Am* 1982; 66:455–468.
35. Brunzell JD, Schrott HG: Interaction of familial and secondary causes of hypertriglyceridemia: Role in pancreatitis. *Trans Assoc Am Physicians* 1973; 86:245–254.
36. Fuster V, Badimon L, Badimon JJ, et al: Mechanisms of disease: The pathogenesis of coronary artery disease and the acute coronary syndromes (Part 1). *N Engl J Med* 1992; 326:242–250.
37. Fuster V, Badimon L, Badimon JJ, et al: Mechanisms of disease: The pathogenesis of coronary artery disease and the acute coronary syndromes (Part 2). *N Engl J Med* 1992; 326:310–318.
38. Schwartz CJ, Valente AJ, Sprague EA, et al: The pathogenesis of atherosclerosis: An overview. *Clin Cardiol* 1991; 14-I-1.
39. Steinberg D: Lipoproteins and atherosclerosis: A look back and a look ahead. *Arteriosclerosis* 1983; 3:283–301.
40. Mahley RW: Development of accelerated atherosclerosis: Concepts derived from cell biology and animal model studies. *Arch Pathol Lab Med* 1983; 107:393–399.
41. Ross R: The pathogenesis of atherosclerosis—An update. *N Engl J Med* 1986; 314:488–500.
42. Kodama T, Reddy P, Kishimoto C, et al: Purification and characterization of a bovine acetyl low density lipoprotein receptor. *Proc Natl Acad Sci USA* 1988; 85:9238–9242.
43. Kodama TK, Freeman M, Rohrer L, et al: Type I macrophage scavenger receptor contains alpha-helical and collagen-like coiled coils. *Nature* 1990; 343:531–535.
44. Steinberg D, Parthasarathy S, Carew T, et al: Beyond cholesterol. Modifications of low density lipoprotein that increase its atherogenicity. *N Engl J Med* 1989; 320:915–924.
45. Palinski W, Rosenfeld ME, Yla-Herttuala S, et al: Low density lipoprotein undergoes oxidation modification in vivo. *Proc Natl Acad Sci USA* 1989; 86:1372–1376.
46. Yla-Herttuala S, Palinski W, Rosenfeld ME, et al: Evidence for the presence of oxidatively modified low density lipoprotein in atherosclerotic lesions of rabbit and man. *J Clin Invest* 1989; 84:1086–1095.
47. Cushing SD, Berliner JA, Valente AJ, et al: Minimally modified low density lipoprotein induces monocyte chemotactic protein I in human endothelial cells and smooth muscle cells. *Proc Natl Acad Sci USA* 1990; 87:5134–5138.
48. Kita T, Nagano Y, Yokode M, et al: Probucol prevents the progression of atherosclerosis in Watanabe heritable hyperlipidemic rabbit, an animal model for familial hypercholesterolemia. *Proc Natl Acad Sci USA* 1987; 84:5928–5931.

49. Yokode M, Kita T, Arai H, et al: Cholesteryl ester accumulation in macrophages incubated with low density lipoprotein pretreated with cigarette smoke extract. *Proc Natl Acad Sci USA* 1988; 85:2344–2348.
50. Forrester JS, Litvack F, Grundfest W: Initiating events of acute coronary arterial occlusion. *Ann Rev Med* 1991; 42:35–45.
51. Parthasarathy S, Fong LG, Steinberg D: Inhibitory effect of high density lipoprotein (HDL) on oxidative modification of low density lipoprotein. *Circulation* 1987; 76(suppl IV):479.
52. Havel RJ, Kane JP: Introduction: Structure and metabolism of plasma lipoproteins, in Scriver CR, Beaudet AL, Sly WS, et al (eds): *The Metabolic Basis of Inherited Disease.* New York, McGraw-Hill, 1989, pp 1129–1138.
53. Brunzell JD: Familial lipoprotein lipase deficiency and other causes of the chylomicronemia syndrome, in Scriver CR, Beaudet AL, Sly WS, et al (eds): *The Metabolic Basis of Inherited Disease,* ed 6. New York, McGraw-Hill, 1989, pp 1165–1180.
54. Mahley RW, Rall SC Jr: Type III hyperlipoproteinemia (dysbetalipoproteinemia): The role of apolipoprotein E in normal and abnormal lipoprotein metabolism, in Scriver CR, Beaudet AL, Sly WS, et al (eds): *The Metabolic Basis of Inherited Disease.* New York, McGraw Hill, 1989, pp 1195–1213.
55. Goldstein JL, Brown MS: Familial hypercholesterolemia, in Scriver CR, Beaudet AL, Sly WS, et al (eds): *The Metabolic Basis of Inherited Disease,* ed 6. New York, McGraw Hill, 1989, pp 1215–1250.
56. Soria LF, Ludwig EH, Clarke HRG, et al: Association between a specific apolipoprotein B mutation and familial defective apolipoprotein B-100. *Proc Natl Acad Sci USA* 1989; 86:587–591.
57. Pullinger C, Malloy MJ, Frost P, et al: Unpublished data.
58. Malloy MJ, Kane JP: Hypolipidemia. *Med Clin North Am* 1982; 66:469–484.
59. Assmann G, Schmitz G, Brewer HB Jr: Familial high density lipoprotein deficiency: Tangier disease, in Scriver CR, Baudet AL, Sly WS, et al (eds): *The Metabolic Basis of Inherited Disease,* ed 6. New York, McGraw Hill, 1989, pp 1267–1282.
60. Kane JP, Malloy MJ: Disorders of lipoprotein metabolism, in Greenspan FS, Forsham PH (eds): *Basic and Clinical Endocrinology,* ed 3. Los Altos, Calif, Lange Medical Publications, 1990, pp 663–693.
61. Summary of the Second Report of the National Cholesterol Education Program (NCEP) Expert Panel on Detection, Evaluation and Treatment of High Blood Cholesterol in Adults (Adult Treatment Panel II). *JAMA* 1993; 269:3015–3023.
62. Malloy MJ: Disorders of lipoprotein metabolism, in Eichenwald HF, Stroder J (eds): *Pediatric Therapy,* ed 3. Chicago, Mosby 1993, pp 210–216.
63. Myers LH, Phillips NR, Havel RJ: Mathematical evaluation of methods for estimation of the concentration of the major lipid components of human serum lipoproteins. *J Lab Clin Med* 1976; 88:491–505.
64. Castelli WP, Wilson PW, Levy D, et al: Cardiovascular risk factors in the elderly. *Am J Cardiol* 1989; 63:12H–9H.
65. Kane JP, Malloy MJ, Ports TA, et al: Regression of coronary atherosclerosis during treatment of familial hypercholesterolemia with combined drug regimens. *JAMA* 1990; 264:3007–3012.
66. Connor WE, Connor S: The dietary treatment of hyperlipidemia. *Med Clin North Am* 1982; 66:485–518.
67. Malloy MJ, Kane JP. Agents used in hyperlipidemia, in Katzung B (ed): *Basic and Clinical Pharmacology,* ed 5. Norwalk, Conn, Appleton & Lange, 1992, pp 477–490.

68. Kane JP, Havel RJ: Treatment of hypercholesterolemia. *Ann Rev Med* 1986; 37:427–435.
69. Grundy SM, Mok HYI, Zech L, et al: Influence of nicotinic acid on metabolism of triglycerides and cholesterol in man. *J Lipid Res* 1981; 22:24.
70. Miettinen TA: Effect of nicotinic acid on catabolism and synthesis of cholesterol in man. *Clin Chim Acta* 1968; 20:43–51.
71. Alberts AW, Chen J, Kuron G: A highly potent competitive inhibitor of hydroxymethylglutaryl-coenzyme: A reductase and a cholesterol lowering agent. *Proc Natl Acad Sci* 1980; 77:3957–3961.
72. Bilheimer DW, Grundy SM, Brown MD, et al: Mevinolin and colestipol stimulate receptor-mediated clearance of low density lipoprotein from plasma in familial hypercholesterolemia heterozygotes. *Proc Natl Acad Sci USA* 1983; 80:4124–4128.
73. Grundy SM, Vega GL: Influence of mevinolin on metabolism of low density lipoproteins in primary moderate hypercholesterolemia. *J Lipid Res* 1985; 26:1464–1475.
74. Boberg J, Boberg M, Gross R: The effect of treatment with clofibrate on hepatic triglyceride and lipoprotein lipase activities of post-heparin plasma in male patients with hyperlipidemia. *Atherosclerosis* 1977; 27:499.
75. Lewis JE: Long term use of genfibrozil (Lopid) in the treatment of dyslipidemia. *Angiology* 1982; 33:603.
76. Baker SG, Joeffe BI, Mendelsohn D, Seftel HC: Treatment of homozygous familial hypercholesterolemia with probucol. *S Afr Med J* 1982; 62:7–11.
77. Yamamoto AY, Matsuzawa B, Kishino B, et al: Effects of probucol on homozygous cases of familial hypercholesterolemia. *Atherosclerosis* 1983; 48: 157–166.
78. Witztum JL, Simmons D, Steinberg D: Intensive combination drug therapy of familial hypercholesterolemia with lovastatin, probucol, and colestipol hydrochloride. *Circulation* 1989; 79:16–28.
79. Malloy MJ, Kane JP, Kunitake ST, et al: Complementarity of colestipol, niacin, and lovastatin in treatment of severe familial hypercholesterolemia. *Ann Intern Med* 1987; 107:616–623.
80. Illingworth DR: Mevinolin plus cholestyramine therapy for severe heterozygous familial hypercholesterolemia. *Ann Intern Med* 1984; 101:598–604.
81. Grundy SM, Vega GL, Bilheimer DW: Influence of combined therapy with mevinolin and interruption of bile acid reabsorption of low density lipoproteins in heterozygous familial hypercholesterolemia. *Ann Intern Med* 1985; 103:339–343.
82. Kane JP, Tun P, Malloy MJ, et al: Normalization of low density lipoprotein levels in heterozygous familial hypercholesterolemia with a combined drug regimen. *N Engl J Med* 1981; 304:251–258.
83. Jacobs D, Blackburn H, Higgins M: Report of the conference on low blood cholesterol: Mortality associations. *Circulation* 1992; 86:1046–1060.
84. Ueshima H, Lida M, Shimamoto T, et al: Eight-year follow-up study of farming villages in Akita, Japan. *Prev Med* 1980; 9:722–740.
85. Iso H, Jacobs DR, Wentworth D, et al: Serum cholesterol levels and six-year mortality from stroke in 350,977 men screened for the MRFIT. *N Engl J Med* 1989; 320:904–910.
86. Frick MH, Elo MO, Haapa K: Helsinki Heart Study: Primary prevention trial with gemfibrozil in middle aged men with dyslipidemia: Safety of treatment, changes in risk factors, and incidence of coronary heart disease. *N Engl J Med* 1987; 317:1237–1245.

87. Committee of Principal Investigators: WHO Cooperative Trial on primary prevention of ischaemic heart disease using clofibrate to lower serum cholesterol: mortality follow-up. *Lancet* 1980; 2:379–385.
88. Buchwald H, Varco RL, Matts JP: Effect of partial ileal bypass surgery on mortality and morbidity from coronary heart disease in patients with hypercholesterolemia: Report of the program on the Surgical Control of the Hyperlipidemias (POSCH). *N Engl J Med* 1990; 323:946–955.
89. Hjermann I, Velve Byre K, Holme I, et al: Effect of diet and smoking intervention on the incidence of coronary heart disease: Report from the Oslo Study Group of a randomized trial in healthy men. *Lancet* 1981; 2:1303–1310.
90. Multiple Risk Factor Intervention Trial Research Group: Coronary heart disease death, nonfatal acute myocardial infarction and other clinical outcomes in the Multiple Risk Factor Intervention Trial. *Am J Cardiol* 1986; 58:1–13.
91. Multiple Risk Factor Intervention Trial Research Group: Mortality rates after 10.5 years for participants in the Multiple Risk Factor Intervention Trial: Findings related to a prior hypothesis of the trial. *JAMA* 1990; 263:1795–1801.
92. World Health Organization European Collaborative Trial of Multifactorial Prevention of Coronary Heart Disease: Final report on the 6-year results. *Lancet* 1986; 1:1869–1872.
93. Neaton JD, Blackburn H, Jacobs D: Serum cholesterol level and mortality findings for men screened in the Multiple Risk Factor Intervention Trial. *Arch Intern Med* 1992; 152:1490.
94. Brown G, Albers JJ, Fisher LD, et al: Regression of coronary artery disease as a result of intensive lipid-lowering therapy in men with high levels of apolipoprotein B. *N Engl J Med* 1990; 323:1289–1298.
95. Watts GF, Lewis B, Brunt JN, et al: Effects on coronary artery disease of lipid-lowering diet, or diet plus cholestyramine in the St. Thomas Atherosclerosis Regression Study. *Lancet* 1992; 339:563–569.
96. Cashin-Hemphill J, Mack WJ, Pogoda JM, et al: Beneficial effects of colestipol-niacin or coronary atherosclerosis. A 4-year follow-up. *JAMA* 1990; 264:3013–3017.
97. Ornish D, Brown SE, Scherwitz LJ, et al: Can lifestyle changes reverse coronary heart disease? *Lancet* 1990; 336:129–133.

Hypertension and Diabetic Vascular Complications

Pamela W. Anderson, M.D.

Assistant Professor of Medicine, University of Southern California School of Medicine, Los Angeles, California

Willa A. Hsueh, M.D.

Professor of Medicine, University of Southern California School of Medicine, Los Angeles, California

Background

Nearly 16 million people in the United States (6% of the population) have diabetes mellitus. Of these patients, 90% to 95% have non-insulin-dependent diabetes mellitus (NIDDM) or Type II diabetes.[1] By ages 65 to 74, as many as 17% of white Americans,[2] 25% of black Americans,[2] 33% or more of Hispanic Americans,[3] and up to 50% of Pima Indians[4] will develop impaired glucose tolerance or diabetes mellitus. Both genetic and environmental factors contribute to their development.

The major vascular complications of diabetes fall into two basic categories: microvascular (retinopathy and nephropathy) and macrovascular (cardiovascular, cerebrovascular, and peripheral vascular) disease. The impact of hyperglycemia on the development of the microvascular and macrovascular complications is distinctly different. The occurrence and extent of microvascular complications is generally related to the duration and magnitude of hyperglycemia experienced by the patient.[5] However, other factors in addition to hyperglycemia may affect the development of microvascular disease, since it does not occur in all diabetics. Background diabetic retinopathy can be detected in 80% to 90% of people who have had insulin-dependent diabetes mellitus (IDDM) for 20 years or more,[6] and clinically evident nephropathy occurs in up to 30% to 50% of IDDM and NIDDM patients.[7] In contrast, the occurrence and extent of macrovascular complications do not bear a close relationship to the duration and extent of hyperglycemia. Macrovascular complications, while not unique to diabetes, are more likely to occur in diabetic patients compared with nondiabetic patients, tend to occur at an early age, and tend to be more extensive.[8] In addition, macrovascular complications cause excessive morbidity and mortality in diabetic patients as compared to nondiabetic patients. For example, 35% to 66% of the mortality in diabetic patients is due to cardiovascular disease, compared to 23% mortality in nondiabetic patients.[9–11] Cerebrovascular accidents (CVAs) are increased sixfold in diabetic patients as compared to nondiabetic patients.[12] In addition, peripheral vascular disease contributes to the markedly increased incidence of gangrene and lower extremity amputations among diabetics.[13] It is also important to note that patients with impaired glucose tolerance who are not yet frankly diabetic, also have an increased risk of macrovascular disease compared to normal individuals, suggesting that the atherosclerotic "clock" is running even prior to the development of diabetes.[14]

The incidence of hypertension is also increased in the diabetic compared to the nondiabetic population. Approximately 50% of patients with diabetes have hypertension, compared with 25% of patients without diabetes.[15] Diabetic nephropathy is an important contributor to hypertension in IDDM, while hypertension in NIDDM is likely to be essential.[16] The presence of hypertension dramatically exacerbates all diabetic vascular complications. Loss of renal function is accelerated in the presence of untreated hypertension, and the risk of additional visual loss is increased.[17, 18] Hypertension also affects outcome in macrovascular disease, as high blood pressure is the major risk factor in predicting CVAs in diabetic patients and is a major risk factor for coronary artery disease as well.[12, 19]

Though the mechanisms may be different, diabetes and hypertension both damage the vessel wall, ultimately leading to the development of vascular complications. Understanding the interaction of these commonly occurring diseases at a cellular level in the vessel will be important in elucidating the mechanisms of vascular damage and in recognizing early markers of vascular complications. This approach is critical to the ultimate definition of prevention and treatment modalities.

Effects of Diabetes and Hypertension on Vascular Biology

Normal Endothelial Cell Function.—Endothelial cells and vascular smooth muscle cells are the two major components of the vessel wall. In normal vessels, endothelial cells provide a mechanical barrier to plasma and formed elements in the blood. By shielding the collagen in the subendothelial space, they prevent hemostasis. In addition, they synthesize a number of factors that affect hemostasis, including prostacyclin and lipooxygenase products, endothelial-derived relaxing factor, von Willebrand factor, and tissue type plasminogen activator (t-PA) (Table 1[20]). Endothelial cells also produce a variety of factors which can act in a paracrine fashion to alter vascular tone (see Table 1[21]). These include angiotensin-converting enzyme (which produces the vasoconstrictor angiotensin II), and endothelin (a powerful peptide vasoconstrictor).[22, 23] These vasoconstrictor substances are balanced by the endothelial production of vasodilating agents such as endothelial-derived relaxing factor (EDRF), vasodilating

TABLE 1.
Functions of the Endothelium*

Hemostasis
Prostacyclin
Endothelial-derived relaxing factor (EDRF)
13-HODE (13-hydroxy-9,11-octodecadienoic acid)
15-HETE (15-hydroxy-5,8,13-eicosatentraenoic acid)
von Willebrand factor
Tissue type plasminogen activator (t-PA)
Vascular Tone
Angiotensin-converting enzyme (ACE)
Prostaglandins
Endothelin
EDRF
Endothelium-derived hyperpolarizing factor
Histamine
Growth Promoters
Platelet-derived growth factor (PDGF)
Basic fibroblast growth factor (bFGF)
Interleukin 1 (IL-1)
Insulin-like growth factor (IGF-1)
Endothelin
Angiotensin II (AII)
Thrombospondin
Growth Inhibitors
Heparins
Adenosine
Prostaglandin E_1
EDRF
Transforming growth factor beta ($TGF\text{-}\beta_1$)

*Listed are the functions of the endothelium and individual factors that may influence them.

prostaglandins, and histamines.[24, 25] Substances produced by the endothelium also influence vascular smooth muscle cell growth (see Table 1). These include growth factors, inflammatory substances, coagulation factors, and adhesion molecules.[21] In general, vasoconstricting substances tend to promote growth of vascular smooth muscle cells, while vasodilators tend to inhibit smooth muscle growth.[26] Thus, the endothelium, far from being an inert vascular lining, plays an important role in regulating vascular tone, vascular remodeling, cellular growth, and hemostasis.

Endothelial Dysfunction in Diabetes Mellitus.—In vivo and in vitro assessments of endothelial cell function suggest that marked alterations occur in diabetes mellitus (Table 2), which tend to promote clotting, vasoconstriction, and vascular smooth muscle cell growth. Diabetic patients are hypercoaguable and demonstrate enhanced platelet aggregation, possibly due to increased circulating levels of von Willebrand factor (a marker for endothelial cell damage), decreased levels of tissue type plasminogen activator (t-PA),[27] and enhanced platelet thromboxane formation.[28] Enhanced vasoconstriction may also be related to hyperglycemia. Vascular segments from diabetic animals and vascular segments incubated in high glucose in vitro demonstrate impaired endothelium-dependent relaxation.[29] Hyperglycemia also activates protein kinase C in the endothelial cell, stimulating the production of vasoconstrictor prostaglandins, and lowering the generation of nitric oxide, thus decreasing vascular relaxation.[30] Elevated glucose also enhances secretion of endothelin from cultured aortic endothelial cells,[31] which may contribute to the hypertension. Hyperglycemia contributes to structural changes in the endothelial cell as well, including generalized basement membrane thickening, enhancement of endothelial collagen type IV and fibronectin production, and increased activity of enzymes involved in collagen synthesis.[32, 33] Glucose toxicity may worsen the endothelial damage by inhibiting replication or accelerating endothelial demise.[34] In addition, other metabolic derangements that occur in diabetes (such as hypertriglyceridemia, enhanced oxidation, and glyco-

TABLE 2.
Effects of Diabetes and Hypertension on the Vessel

Function	Effect
Diabetes	
Hemostasis	Increased coaguability, increased platelet aggregation.
Vascular tone	Relaxation diminished. Increased vasoconstriction. Increased release of vasoactive peptides.
Growth	Endothelial cell replication delayed, cell death accelerated. Generalized basement membrane thickening. Acceleration of vascular smooth muscle growth.
Transport	Increased leakage of small and large proteins.
Hypertension	
Hemostasis	Increase in leukocyte adherence, macrophage accumulation.
Vascular tone	Relaxation diminished. Increased vasoconstriction.
Growth	Endothelial shape change and increase in number. VSMCs undergo hypertrophy and polyploidy and accumulate.
Transport	Permeability decreased.

sylation) have all been shown to disturb normal endothelial cell function.[35, 36] Hyperglycemia also contributes to abnormal vascular smooth muscle cell (VSMC) growth in the diabetic vessel. VSMCs from diabetic animals have been shown to have enhanced rates of growth in culture, compared with VSMCs from nondiabetic animals, reflecting the pathological stimulation that these cells experience in vivo.[37]

Endothelial Dysfunction in Hypertension.—Humans and animals with hypertension also exhibit endothelial dysfunction (see Table 2), although the specific mechanisms differ somewhat from those found in diabetes. Hypertension primarily affects blood vessels by altering shear stress, defined as the frictional force on the intimal surface, which is proportional to blood velocity and viscosity. Even modestly elevated shear stress has been shown to induce structural changes in the vasculature, alterations in endothelial cell metabolism, and even endothelial cell detachment.[38] Specific morphological changes seen in hypertension include changes in endothelial cell shape and number.[39] Hypertension also increases leukocyte adherence, with increased accumulation of macrophages in the subendothelial space.[40, 41] Secretion of cytokines by macrophages may further affect endothelial cell structure and function. Endothelial cell production of vasoactive substances, ions, and ion channels/transport is altered.[38, 42] Patients with essential hypertension display functional vascular changes, such as a decreased vascular response to acetylcholine (an endothelium-dependent vasodilator), but normal responses to sodium nitroprusside, a direct smooth muscle vasodilator.[43] Endothelial abnormalities can develop when hypertension is induced in animal models, and antihypertensive treatment can normalize endothelial-dependent relaxation.[39] Changes in VSMCs in hypertension consist primarily of an increase in cell mass (hypertrophy), accompanied by polyploidy, resulting in a thickening of the arterial wall. In some animal models of hypertension, thickening occurs as a result of hyperplasia without hypertrophy or polyploidy.[44]

Effects of Endothelial Cell Damage on Smooth Muscle.—Temporally, abnormalities in endothelial integrity and function are followed by abnormalities in growth and/or extracellular matrix production in the smooth muscle cells directly beneath the affected endothelium. Vascular smooth muscle cell growth and extracellular matrix production have been demonstrated to play critical pathophysiologic roles in the development of the vascular and renal complications of diabetes. When abnormal growth occurs in vascular smooth muscle cells in large vessels, it results in the formation of atherosclerotic plaques, but when it occurs in mesangial cells in the renal glomerulus, it leads to glomerulosclerosis. Because of differences in milieu, however, endothelial cells from different locations are likely to function and respond to stress differently and affect their neighboring vascular smooth muscle cells differently. Thus, in retinal vessels, pericytes (the vascular smooth muscle and mesangial cell equivalent) disappear or "drop-out."[6] It is likely that the endothelial cell and smooth muscle cell function as a unit under normal circumstances, each producing a wide variety of substances that affect the growth, contractility, and synthetic capability of the other. With damage or death of the endothelial cell, the partner smooth muscle cell is unable to maintain normal function and the hallmark abnormalities appear, i.e., either abnormal smooth muscle cell growth and excessive matrix production or death.

Atherosclerosis

There are a variety of risk factors which may contribute to the development of atherosclerosis in diabetes. These include (1) hypertension, (2) hyperglycemia, (3) platelet and clotting abnormalities, (4) altered circulating lipids, and (5) hyperinsulinemia and/or insulin resistance. Most of these factors are independent risk factors for coronary artery disease and are more common in the diabetic patient. This probably accounts for the increased incidence of atherosclerosis in diabetics, since the presence of multiple atherosclerotic risk factors markedly increases the risk of atherosclerotic coronary artery disease.[45]

Although hyperglycemia does not correlate with the development of atherosclerosis, it may lead to the development of advanced glycosylation end-products (AGEs). Hyperglycemia first causes nonenzymatic attachment of glucose molecules (glycation) to proteins (via the Amadori reaction), and then, by a series of slowly occurring, irreversible chemical reactions, AGEs are produced, some of which are capable of forming covalent bonds with amino groups on other proteins. If AGEs form on long-lived molecules, like collagen, the effect they exert can also be long-lived. Experimental data have shown that AGE formation on collagens and matrix proteins tends to decrease endothelial cell adhesion and replication[46–48] and increase lipoproteins and immune complex adhesion,[49] both of which are seen early in atherosclerosis. Accumulation of AGEs in the extracellular matrix may also blunt the effect of vasodilatory (EDRF) and antimitogenic factors (nitric oxide),[35, 50] leading to vasoconstriction and cellular proliferation. In addition, endothelial cells (as well as mesangial cells, macrophages, and monocytes) have specific AGE receptors. Binding to receptors by ligand induces tissue factor activity, which ultimately causes alterations in coagulation, as well as increased endothelin production,[46] which may cause further vasoconstriction. Therefore, the presence of AGEs may accelerate the development of atherosclerosis in the diabetic patient.

Platelet abnormalities are central to the formation of fibrous atherosclerotic plaques by vascular smooth muscle cells. Platelets contain a variety of growth factors such as platelet-derived growth factor (PDGF), epidermal growth factor (EGF), insulin-like growth factor-1 (IGF-1), and transforming growth factor-β (TGF-β), which may directly affect vascular smooth muscle cell growth.[51] Also, platelets from diabetic subjects tend to aggregate more readily than do platelets from nondiabetics, and they exert greater mitogenic effects on vascular smooth muscle than do platelets from normal subjects.[52, 53] It has been noted that platelets from patients with diabetes produced more thromboxane A_2 than did platelets from nondiabetics;[54] however, studies also showed normal plasma and urinary thromboxane of platelet origin in diabetic patients shortly before developing microvascular complications. This suggests that platelets may not play a primary role in the development of complications.[55] The enhanced platelet aggregation may be due, in part, to the hypomagnesemia that commonly accompanies diabetes, since abnormal aggregation can be induced in NIDDM patients with a low magnesium diet, and platelet aggregation abnormalities can be partially corrected with the administration of oral magnesium supplements.[56]

The frequency of dyslipidemia is increased up to twofold in diabetic populations[57] and may contribute significantly to atherosclerosis. Abnormalities involve all classes of lipoproteins, but most commonly consist of elevated triglycerides and very-low-density lipoproteins (VLDL), with near normal low-density lipoprotein (LDL) levels, and low high-density lipoprotein (HDL) levels. Diabetics may have an increase in oxidized and/or glycated LDL. These modifications decrease their metabolic clearance and enhance their toxicity to endothelial cells. Oxidized LDL stimulates the formation of foam cells, which are typically seen in the development of atherosclerosis. Oxidized LDL also has procoagulant effects.[58, 59] Glycation of LDL enhances the accumulation of subendothelial LDL, LDL oxidation, LDL uptake by macrophages, as well as platelet aggregation,[60] all of which may accelerate the atherosclerotic process.

Hyperinsulinemia and/or insulin resistance may further predispose the diabetic patient to atherosclerosis. Early in their disease, NIDDM patients are hyperinsulinemic and demonstrate defects in peripheral tissue glucose uptake in response to insulin.[61] Several studies have found higher insulin responses to oral glucose in subjects at greater risk of cardiovascular disease.[62–68] Of these, three prospective studies demonstrate that hyperinsulinemia precedes coronary artery disease.[65–68] In Caucasian male government workers followed for 5 to 10 years, the incidence of coronary artery disease was significantly greater in subjects with higher fasting or 2-hour glucose-stimulated insulin levels.[65] In another study of Caucasian men and women, 1-hour glucose-stimulated insulin levels were significantly related to the 6-year incidence of, and 12-year mortality from, coronary artery disease in men, but not in women.[68] A meta-analysis of these prospective studies found that the hyperinsulinemic, insulin-resistant groups had other risk factors for atherosclerosis, including high triglycerides, lower HDL-cholesterol, higher total cholesterol, and an increased frequency of hypertension.[69] In 12% of white American hypertensive patients and in some hypertensive families, these risk factors co-cluster.[70] However, while the highest incidence of NIDDM (and presumably hyperinsulinemia) has been identified in Pima Indians and Mexican-Americans, both populations have a lower incidence of hypertension and cardiovascular disease than the general population.[71, 72] Thus, insulin resistance and hyperinsulinemia do not co-cluster with other risk factors for atherosclerosis in all populations.

Hyperinsulinemia and/or insulin resistance may influence atherosclerosis by promoting growth of vascular smooth muscle, altering lipoproteins, and contributing to hypertension. Insulin has been shown to cause vascular smooth muscle cell growth in vitro[73] and high levels may contribute to the abnormal growth of vascular smooth muscle cells which make up the fibrous plaque, although its exact role in vivo is unknown. Elevated circulating VLDL is common in patients with NIDDM due to hyperinsulinemia and enhanced liver production as well as elevated plasma free fatty acid (FFA) levels.[74] This may increase macrophage uptake of VLDL and accumulation of intracellular lipid.[75] High-density lipoprotein cholesterol is decreased in patients with NIDDM, possibly due to hyperinsulinemia, so that total cholesterol levels, in general, remain unchanged. The administration of high physiologic doses of insulin to normotensive rats (but not dogs) causes a rise in blood pressure.[76, 77] In addition, two agents with different structures which enhance skeletal muscle insulin action, thiazolidinedione analogues (such as pioglitazone) and metformin, lower blood pressure in several hypertensive rat models.[78, 79] Insulin may also influence blood pressure through increased absorption of sodium by the kidney, enhanced sympathetic nervous system activity, and altered vascular structure.[80, 81]

Diabetic Nephropathy

Diabetic nephropathy is currently the most common cause of end-stage renal disease (ESRD) in the United States.[82] The incidence of ESRD due to diabetes is increasing, especially among ethnic groups, such as American Indians, Hispanic Americans, black Americans, and Asian Americans.[83] There is a strong association between the presence of nephropathy (as defined by the presence of proteinuria or microalbuminuria) and premature mortality from cardiovascular disease.[84] In nephropathy, the presence of hypertension has important therapeutic implications.

As is the case in atherosclerosis, diabetic glomerulosclerosis may result from altered interaction between the glomerular endothelium and mesangium. The glomerular endothelial cell is a long-lived cell which forms a fixed, though fenestrated barrier between the capillary lumen and the cells of the glomerular tuft. It is separated from its nearest neighbor, the mesangial cell, by only its basement membrane; therefore, the passage of material between these two cells is easily accomplished.[85] Since endothelial cells are capable of synthesizing many different substances, all of which have been shown to impact on mesangial cell growth, and some of which have been shown to alter mesangial cell synthesis of matrix components, abnormal function of the endothelial cell may result in abnormal mesangial cell growth and/or excessive matrix production, which are the morphological hallmarks of diabetic nephropathy. Also, mesangial cell growth may be stimulated by substances such as cytokines from activated macrophages, or from mesangial cells themselves.[86] In addition, growth-altering substances may gain access to the mesangial area through the fenestrated endothelial cell pores. The charge, size, and plasma concentration of the circulating substances, as well as glomerular pressures and flow rates, will determine the ease with which they enter the mesangium.[87] Once substances have entered the mesangial area, they may bind to the mesangial cell and/or undergo endocytosis and subsequent processing, thus potentially affecting mesangial function and growth.

Hypertension hastens the development of glomerulosclerosis due to the inability of the glomerular vasculature to normally autoregulate intraglomerular pressure. In the diabetic patient with hypertension, afferent arteriolar resistance fails to increase normally, allowing transmission of systemic hypertension into the glomerular capillary, which results in intraglomerular hypertension.[88] Glomerular capillary hypertension is associated with altered glomerular endothelial structure and function. It is possible that disordered endothelial function in the afferent arteriole, due to diabetes, hypertension, or both, further aggravates the altered afferent arteriolar resistance.

Diabetic nephropathy develops slowly over the course of 10 to 15 years. The first abnormalities seen are an increase in glomerular size and overall kidney size,[89] accompanied by glomerular hyperfiltration (defined as a glomerular filtration rate [GFR] in excess of 150 mL/min per 1.73 m^2), which reflects an imbalance between afferent and efferent arteriolar resistance. Increases in glucose, insulin, glucagon, growth hormone, atrial naturetic factor, ketone bodies, prostaglandins, dietary protein content, as well as increased activity of the renin-angiotensin system have been implicated in the etiology of the hyperfiltration.[90] After 1.5 to 6 years of disease, the next structural change is glomerular basement membrane thickening, the importance of which is not entirely clear, since there does not appear to be any correlation between basement membrane thickness and renal function.[91, 92] In addition, glomerular basement membrane thickness does not necessarily correlate with basement membrane thickening in other parts of the body.[93] Once urinary microalbuminuria (urinary albumin excretion 20–200 mg/day) is detected, incipient diabetic nephropathy is present. However, this is best thought of not as a prelude to nephropathy, but rather as the earliest clinically detectable stage of nephropathy.[94] Over 85% of patients with persistent microalbuminuria will progress to overt proteinuria.[95] The charge and size of the fenestrated glomerular endothelial pores are altered due to loss of heparan sulfate proteoglycan from the glomerular basement membrane, resulting in passage of albumin through the normally protein-proof pores.[96] After 5 to 15 years of diabetes in patients with IDDM, mesangial cell abnormalities usually appear.[97] The most common abnormality seen by light microscopy is diffuse intercapillary sclerosis due to expansion of the mesangial area. The mesangial expansion is primarily due to mesangial cell hypertrophy and increased accumulation of mesangial cell matrix. Matrix material consists of components similar to those found in basement membranes and is primarily a nonspecific, "polyclonal" increase in mesangial matrix components.[98] With mesangial expansion, overt persistent proteinuria (>0.5 g/24 hrs) develops and glomerular closure proceeds. Mesangial expansion appears to be directly responsible for glomerular capillary closure.[99] The reasons for the increase in the size of mesangial cells and the marked increase in mesangial matrix are unknown, although many factors have been noted to cause mesangial growth and matrix production in vitro.[100] Without intervention, the GFR falls by approximately 1 mL/min/month; thus, the estimated time from the first appearance of proteinuria to dialysis is 5 years without intervention.[7]

Currently, there is no known treatment that can completely halt or regress the mesangial lesions of diabetic nephropathy, although therapy with converting enzyme inhibitors and the institution of low-protein diets (0.6 g protein/kg body weight) have been shown to decrease the rate of decline of kidney function in humans.[101, 102] Even in patients receiving pancreas transplants who became euglycemic, normalization of morphologic lesions in the kidney did not occur, though glomerular and mesangial volume decreased 2 years posttransplant.[103] This demonstrated that even the establishment of euglycemia after a certain amount of damage has occurred to the kidney is insufficient to reverse the lesions. Until the causes for the expansion of the mesangium are known, the likelihood of regressing the abnormal growth is small.

Diabetic Retinopathy

Diabetic retinopathy is the major cause of blindness in adults in the United States. The incidence of retinopathy increases with duration of diabetes; twenty years after diagnosis, 80% of NIDDM and 90% of IDDM patients have background retinopathy.[104] Hyperglycemia and hypertension are two important factors in the development of retinopathy.[18, 105] A major target is the retinal capillary endothelial cell which plays a prominent and direct role in the structural abnormalities of diabetic retinopathy.

Based on prognosis, retinopathy has been classified as either the relatively benign nonproliferative ("background") retinopathy which consists of microaneurysms, dot-blot hemorrhages, and hard exudates, occurring in virtually all patients with diabetes, or the more ominous proliferative retinopathy, which involves neovascularization, bleeding, chronic scarring, retinal detachment, and possible blindness. In nonproliferative retinopathy, one of the earliest structural changes is vasodilation of the retinal capillaries, which is felt to be due to abnormal tissue oxygenation[106] and may reflect an endothelial cell reaction to hypoxia. The vasodilation is accompanied by retinal hyperperfusion.[107] In addition, capillary permeability increases early in the development of retinopathy.[107–109] At this stage, strict diabetic control can reduce capillary permeability towards normal.[110] Another important early change is pericyte degeneration. Pericytes are the mesenchymally derived cells whose counterparts in the vessel and glomerulus are the vascular smooth muscle cell and mesangial cell, respectively. Pericytes elaborate an inhibitory growth factor for endothelial cells.[111] Early loss of this inhibitory growth factor may allow the endothelial cell to mobilize or proliferate in an abnormal fashion. The reasons for pericyte dropout are unclear but may be due to impaired replication. In diabetic patients with proliferative retinopathy, serum and vitreous levels of growth hormones such as IGF-1 are not consistently elevated, so the local role of hormones and growth factors is also unclear.[112] More obvious structural changes in the retina follow, including chronic microaneurysm formation, pericyte degeneration, basement membrane thickening, and endothelial cell proliferation. In patients who develop proliferative retinopathy, neovascularization with leaky and fragile new capillaries appears. When new retinal vessels form, the endothelial cell first thickens and shows evidence of becoming more synthetically active, then the basement membrane breaks down, and endothelial cells migrate through the vessel walls forming new capillary loops.[113] Vision is compromised when these fragile new capillary loops bleed; retinal detachments can occur when there is chronic scarring and fibrous strands put traction on the retina.

The exact mechanism(s) by which diabetes cause(s) extensive vascular proliferation in the retina is unknown. Hyperglycemia appears to be a more important factor than hypertension in the development of retinopathy, since retinopathy commonly occurs in the absence of frank elevations in blood pressure.[6] Hypoxia and ischemia (possibly due to increased renal cell aggregation in damaged capillaries) are also major contributors to the retinal vessel changes in diabetes,[114, 115] although studies using inhibitors of platelet aggregation have not been useful in preventing the development of proliferative diabetic retinopathy.[116] The hormonal milieu is also felt to influence the development and progression of diabetic retinopathy, since pregnancy, puberty, and hypophysectomy have been reported to alter progression of retinopathy.[117–119]

Prognostic and Therapeutic Implications

Prevention and Early Recognition.—Currently, there is no "cure" for the microvascular complications of diabetes, although some therapies may either slow down their rate of appearance, their rate of progression, or ameliorate their negative consequences (Table 3). Therefore, for diabetic patients, prevention of microvascular complications is fundamental, and those at risk for the development of such complications should ideally be identified early. Although there are currently no clear-cut markers that allow the physician to identify which patients will develop complications before they occur, certain information may help the physician to identify those patients at greatest risk (Table 4).

Since macrovascular and microvascular complications are common and may lead to major medical consequences, it is crucial to anticipate the development of these complications, diagnose them as soon as possible, and start effective therapy in a timely fashion. For the diagnosis of nephropathy, the American Diabetes Association recommends that urinary microalbumin determinations be performed yearly on IDDM patients after puberty and on NIDDM patients after 6 years of known disease.[120] Corre-

TABLE 3.
Preventing Complications

Microvascular
- Strict blood sugar control (Most effective before complications appear)
  - Appropriate diet
  - Exercise
  - Intensive insulin therapy (or oral agents, if appropriate)
- Aggressive early intervention in hypertension
  - Compare to baseline BP ("relative" hypertension important)
  - Consider ACEI or calcium-channel blocker
  - Desireable BP unknown (130/85 mmHg?)
- Aggressive treatment of hyperlipidemia
  - Good blood sugar control
  - Dietary treatment
  - Exercise
  - Maintain ideal body weight
  - Be aware of relative contraindications in use of lipid-lowering drugs in diabetics

Macrovascular
- All of the above, plus:
  - After cardiovascular risk factors
    - Maintain ideal body weight
    - Regular exercise
    - Estrogen supplementation in post-menopausal women
    - Stop smoking

lation with biopsy studies suggest IDDM patients with elevated albumin excretion rates already have significant histologic abnormalities.[99] If urinary microalbumin excretion is elevated, the patient should be referred to a specialist in the treatment of diabetic renal disease, usually an endocrinologist or a nephrologist. Patients with diabetes of more than 5 years of duration or who are under the age of 30 should be examined at yearly intervals by an ophthalmologist (not an optometrist) for the presence of retinopathy. The importance of the ophthalmologic exam should not be underestimated, since laser therapy of diabetic retinopathy is quite effective unless extensive bleeding has already occurred.[121] Physicians should also attempt

TABLE 4.
Risk Factors for the Development of Microvascular Complications

- Nephropathy
  - Hyperglycemia
  - Presence of retinopathy
  - Hypertension
  - Long duration of diabetes and young age at diagnosis
  - Parental history of hypertension
  - Family history of diabetic nephropathy
  - High protein intake
  - Macrovascular disease
  - Race (whites < blacks < Hispanics < American Indians)
  - Poverty
  - Elevated Na^+-Li^+ countertransport
  - Retinopathy
- Hyperglycemia
  - Presence of nephropathy
  - Long duration of diabetes and young age at diagnosis
  - Hypertension
  - Male sex
  - Pregnancy
  - Race (whites < blacks < Hispanics < American Indians)
  - Puberty

to lower cardiovascular risk factors in patients by discouraging smoking and treating modifiable risk factors. There are as yet no recommendations for special evaluation of the heart in patients with diabetes. However, in view of the fact that significant coronary artery disease may frequently be "silent" in the diabetic patient and have a poorer prognosis,[122] earlier use of diagnostic modalities may be appropriate. For example, ECHO-documented left ventricular hypertrophy may serve as a marker of heart disease,[123] since cardiac enlargement is an independent risk factor for coronary artery disease.

Hyperglycemia.—Since the duration and magnitude of hyperglycemia correlate with the extent and rate of progression of microvascular complications, it is logical that strict glucose control would be essential in preventing microvascular complications. However, some studies have shown that blood glucose does not consistently correlate with the development or severity of complications. The results of the 10-year Diabetes Control and

Complications Trial (DCCT) sponsored by the National Institutes of Health (NIH) were presented at the annual American Diabetes Association meetings in June 1993.[124] IDDM patients with and without microvascular complications were randomized to either conventional insulin treatment ($\leq$2 shots of mixed insulin/day) or intensive insulin treatment ($\geq$3 injections/day or insulin pump therapy). The mean hemoglobin A_1C (HA_1C) was 8.9% in the conventional treatment group and 7.0% in the intensive treatment group (upper limit of normal in nondiabetics, 6%). Despite the fact that the intensively treated patients did not achieve normoglycemia, as reflected by a HA_1C above the upper limit of normal for nondiabetic patients, the intensively treated patients achieved an overall 35% to 70% reduction in the risk of retinopathy, a 45% reduction in the risk of progressing to severe retinopathy, and a 45% reduction in the need for laser intervention. Studies looking at the impact of intensive treatment on nephropathy showed a 35% overall risk reduction in the incidence of urinary microalbumin and a 56% risk reduction in the incidence of overt proteinuria in the intensively treated group. In addition, when macrovascular events (cardiovascular, cerebrovascular, or peripheral vascular) were examined, there were 21 events in the intensively treated group and 38 in the conventionally treated group. Although the number of total events is small, this represents a 44% reduction in risk of macrovascular events with intensive treatment. However, intensive insulin treatment was not totally benign. Intensively treated patients gained an average of 10 pounds more body weight during the study than conventionally treated patients. There were 180 catheter infections in 105 patients. Most significantly, there was a threefold increase in the number of episodes of hypoglycemia requiring the assistance of another person and a threefold increase in the number of hypoglycemic comas and seizures, when compared to the conventionally treated group. There was also a threefold increase in the number of traffic accidents due to hypoglycemia in the intensively treated group, although there was only one motor vehicle death. Overall, there was no difference in the number of hospitalizations in the intensively and conventionally treated groups. Also, despite the increased frequency of hypoglycemic reactions, the patients in the intensively treated and conventionally treated groups had no differences in their quality of life as assessed by questionnaires. Since the DCCT results have not yet been published and closely scrutinized by the entire medical community, the final opinion concerning the role of tight glucose control on the prevention or progression of diabetic complications cannot be made.

In other studies, tight or strict blood glucose control was more stringently defined as meaning an average blood sugar of $<$100–125 mg/dl.[125–128] This level of control generally was not achievable using conventional approaches (2 to 3 injections of intermediate and short-acting insulin per day); rather, intensive insulin therapy (4 to 5 shots per day, or use of an insulin pump) was necessary for this degree of control. Not all patients were able to achieve and maintain this kind of blood sugar control, especially in view of the fact that the frequency of symptomatic hypoglycemia usually increases, thus compromising the willingness of most patients to adhere to the regimen. While the data indicate that tight blood sugar control can improve albuminuria and reduce kidney size in patients with incipient nephropathy,[125–128] strict glucose control in patients with retinopathy can temporarily worsen the retinopathy in early stages, sometimes significantly.[125–128] Also, despite establishment of normoglycemia, diabetic retinopathy may progress for some time.[129]

Hypertension.—Given the adverse effect of hypertension on diabetic macrovascular and microvascular complications the early diagnosis and effective treatment of hypertension associated with diabetes mellitus should have a major impact on morbidity and mortality. Blood pressure should be carefully monitored and antihypertensive treatment instituted in a timely fashion. In adult IDDM patients, it is important to compare the blood pressure to previous baseline readings, as patients may be hypertensive relative to their baseline blood pressure, but not actually reach the level of 140/90 mm Hg.[130, 131] In IDDM patients, rising blood pressure almost invariably means the onset of nephropathy.[132] Several studies documenting the effectiveness of antihypertensive therapy in slowing down the progression of renal disease in so-called "normotensive" nephropathic patients have been helpful in underscoring the importance of monitoring relative changes in blood pressure and treating blood pressure to slow the progression of nephropathy.[17, 101, 133] As with nondiabetic patients, secondary causes of hypertension (pheochromocytoma, renovascular hypertension, primary or secondary aldosteronism) must be considered, and if there is clinical suspicion, must be ruled out.

Effective antihypertensive treatment has been shown to significantly decrease proteinuria. However, in short-term studies, angiotensin-converting enzyme inhibitors (ACEIs) and certain calcium channel antagonists (nicardipine, verapamil, and diltiazem) appear to have beneficial effects beyond those attributable to blood pressure control alone.[134] A recent meta-regression analysis examining the effects of various antihypertensive treatments on blood pressure, glomerular filtration rate, renal blood flow, and urinary protein excretion demonstrated that ACEIs had a unique ability to decrease proteinuria and preserve renal function, above and beyond their effect on blood pressure.[135] The as-yet unpublished study by the Collaborative Study Group on the effect of ACEIs in patients with diabetic nephropathy[136] showed a dramatic effect of captopril on the progression of diabetic nephropathy. Patients with proteinuria were placed on placebo or captopril, and the time to doubling of the serum creatinine was determined. When the serum creatinine was 1 mg/dl, treatment with ACEI reduced by 17% the risk of doubling of the serum creatinine. However, when the serum creatinine was 2 mg/dl, there was a 76% reduction in the risk of doubling the serum creatinine. In addition, there were eight deaths in the placebo group and only two deaths in the captopril group, suggesting that ACEI treatment can not only reduce proteinuria, but can also decrease overall mortality. However, while captopril has been shown to decrease proteinuria in both early and late nephropathy,[17, 137] it may also cause severe hyperkalemia and accelerate renal failure in patients with advanced renal disease.[138] These are generally reversible, if the drug is stopped in a timely fashion.

Lowering blood pressure may also slow the rate of progression of proliferative diabetic retinopathy in patients with retinal disease. The absolute level of blood pressure desirable in the diabetic, hypertensive patient with microvascular and macrovascular complications is unknown. One study examining the outcome of proliferative retinopathy has suggested that the best improvement was seen in the patients with diastolic blood pressures of $<$70 mm Hg.[18] While this might be feasible in a younger patient population, older patients with significant carotid, renal, and/or coronary atherosclerosis would be at risk of an adverse cardiovascular event if blood pressure were lowered too aggressively—the so-called, "J-shaped curve." Mogensen et al., who have pioneered many studies in hypertensive IDDM patients with nephropathy, suggest as a goal a mean arterial blood pressure of 100 mm Hg (approximately a BP of 130/85 mm Hg) in order to preserve renal function.[139] Other investigators feel that the patient's baseline blood pressure before the onset of hypertension (when it is known) should be the goal; however, few investigators are willing to state specific blood pressure goals, since the data to support those statements are lacking.

Just as in the nondiabetic patient, effective antihypertensive treatment reduces the risk of stroke and, to a lesser extent, myocardial infarction.[140] However, in treating the diabetic patient with hypertension, several goals must be kept in mind. An ideal antihypertensive agent is effective when given once a day, would have beneficial effect on lipids and electrolytes, would improve insulin sensitivity (or at least not worsen it), and would have a beneficial effect on the complications of diabetes in addition to its antihypertensive effect, including the improvement of nephropathy, retinopathy, coronary artery disease, and peripheral vascular disease. Clearly, there is no one agent that can meet all three criteria. Diuretics worsen insulin sensitivity, total cholesterol, and electrolytes. The β-blockers worsen lipids and insulin sensitivity and have no impact on kidney disease, but may help coronary artery disease.[139–142] ACEIs have a beneficial effect on insulin sensitivity and a possible beneficial effect on atherosclerosis (as demonstrated in the Watanabe rabbit, a model of LDL receptor deficiency). They have specific renal benefits for patients with diabetic nephropathy apart from antihypertensive effects, either due to their action to lower systemic as well as intraglomerular hypertension,[88] or due to the inhibition of the growth effects of angiotensin II.[143] On the other hand, ACEIs may worsen preexisting hyperkalemia as well as precipitate acute renal failure. Prazosin, an α-inhibitor, improves insulin sensitivity, lowers LDL cholesterol and triglycerides, and increases HDL cholesterol. Whether this lipid-improving antihypertensive drug has renal protective effects is unknown. The calcium-channel blockers vary with regard to their effects on diabetics. For example, the dihydropyridine calcium channel blockers, of which nifedipine is an example, differ from the nondihydropyridines (diltiazem and verapamil) in that nifedipine does not alter protein excretion in diabetic nephropathy, while diltiazem decreases protein excretion.[134] Otherwise, the calcium channel blockers are neutral with regard to insulin sensitivity, lipids, and electrolytes. Thus, the current recommendations for the hypertensive diabetic include reducing blood pressure as well as optimizing the risk factor profile for patients, which appears to be improved by treatment with agents such as ACEIs and calcium channel blockers. Although the Fifth Report of the Joint National Commission on Hypertension (JNC-V) recommended first-line therapy with diuretics and/or β-blockers for "uncomplicated" hypertension, hypertension associated with diabetes is generally "complicated" hypertension, therefore, diuretics are not appropriate starting agents.[144]

Hyperlipidemia.—In addition to control of hypertension, normalization of lipid abnormalities is a highly desirable goal, not only because an elevated serum cholesterol is an independent risk factor for cardiac disease, but because high lipids may exacerbate renal disease. In experimental animals, treatment with lovastatin lowered serum cholesterol levels 38% and lowered urinary albumin excretion 76%, with an 83% reduction in glomerulosclerosis.[145] The characteristic findings in NIDDM patients are hypertriglyceridemia and low HDL, both of which can improve with good blood sugar control.[146] Hypertriglyceridemia may be a stronger risk factor for coronary artery disease than total cholesterol in the diabetic.[147, 148] In diabetics, the makeup of lipoproteins may be altered to make them more atherogenic. For example, low-density lipoproteins (LDLs) may be oxidized and/or glycated.[58, 59] Desirable lipid levels for patients without coronary artery disease (including diabetics) have been defined by the updated National Cholesterol Education Program (NCEP-2). These guidelines include the following values: total cholesterol <200 mg/dl, LDL <130 mg/dl, triglycerides 150 mg/dl, and HDL >35 mg/dl.[149] In patients with coronary artery disease, desirable levels of LDL are lower (<100 mg/dl). In addition, the organizers of the recent Consensus Conferences on lipid abnormalities in diabetes will publish their recommendations within the year in the journal *Diabetes Care*. The first measures that should be employed in the treatment of abnormal lipids in the diabetic are adequate glucose control, since improved glycemic control in the presence of adequate insulin restores lipoprotein lipase activity to normal[150] and weight loss, since weight reduction can beneficially influence lipid abnormalities in diabetics.[151] Another important cornerstone of management is dietary treatment. In a nondiabetic diet, dietary restriction of cholesterol and saturated fat is recommended because of resulting favorable changes in lipids. Saturated fat and cholesterol-based calories are replaced by calories from carbohydrate. Therefore, the current recommendations for a "low cholesterol-low saturated fat" diabetic diet are fat <30% of calories, saturated fatty acids <10% of calories, polyunsaturated fatty acids 6% to 8%, and cholesterol <300 mg/day. This raises the carbohydrate contribution to 50% to 60% of daily calories, with ≤10% consisting of simple carbohydrates.[152] These recommendations are undergoing reevaluation, since the high (≤60%) carbohydrate contribution worsens triglycerides, VLDL, and HDL levels, and since high carbohydrate diets are somewhat unpalatable.[153, 154] Regular exercise is also an important nonpharmacologic adjunct, since it assists with weight loss and improves lipids.[155] However, it must be employed carefully in patients with proliferative retinopathy or significant cardiac disease, since exercise may worsen retinopathy or angina.[156] Assuming nondrug therapy of hyperlipidemia is unsuccessful, pharmacologic therapy can be tailored for the specific abnormalities noted. For the hypertriglyceridemia typical of diabetic patients, gemfibrozil is very effective in lowering triglycerides and is probably the drug of choice.[157] If the hypertriglyceridemia is accompanied by high LDL, an HMG-CoA reductase-blocking agent is usually recommended,[158] because it not only lowers LDL cholesterol, but has effects to lower triglycerides and may increase HDL cholesterol. While the combination of gemfibrozil and a first generation HMG-CoA reductase inhibitor has been documented to rarely cause myopathy, the use of second generation agents may reduce this risk.[159] The use of nicotinic acid is contraindicated in diabetic patients, since it significantly worsens glucose tolerance.[160] Probucol, despite its potential role to lower total and oxidized LDL, is also relatively contraindicated in diabetics since it also decreases HDL cholesterol.[161] Bile acid resins (cholestyramine or colestipol) may be useful, but they may increase triglyceride levels[162] and aggravate diabetic gastroparesis, and thus, are relatively contraindicated.

Some cardiac risk factors, such as a positive family history, cannot be altered. Others, such as smoking and obesity, can be changed for the better. In the postmenopausal female, estrogens can be used to partially reestablish the premenopausal state to reduce cardiac risk.[163] Even the risk factor of male sex can be altered, though the cost is high. For example, the use of GnRH agonists in the male to induce acute hypogonadism was associated with a 26% increase in HDL levels, which was reversed by the injection of testosterone.[164]

A View Toward the Future

Table 5 provides possible future treatments for diabetic complications.

Prognostic Indicators.—Currently, there are few proven prognostic indicators that will accurately predict which diabetic patients will develop vascular complications. Elevated plasma prorenin may be a predictor of nephropathy which is positive before the advent of albuminuria. Prorenin is the biosynthetic precursor of renin and may be elevated because of a renal defect in processing prorenin to renin in diabetics. Wilson and Luetscher have followed IDDM patients with elevated prorenin levels. After 4 years, the majority eventually developed diabetic nephropathy or retinopathy, while patients with normal plasma prorenin levels did not.[165] Theoretically, at the earliest stage of disease, intervention might be able to effect regression, or at least, to halt any further deterioration. Thus, the development of accurate markers or predictors of disease in patients is of major importance.

TABLE 5.
Possible Future Treatments for Diabetic Complications

Cure diabetes
  Identify insulin gene(s)
  Pancreas/kidney transplants
Identify patients at risk for complications
Improve insulin delivery
  Peritoneal or portal vein delivery of insulin
Insulin-sensitizing agents
  Pioglitazone
  Metformin
AGE inhibitors
  Aminoguanidine
Aldose reductase inhibitor
  Tolrestat
Anti-oxidants
  Vitamins C and E, probucol
Anti-platelet agents
  Aspirin and dipyridamole
Gene therapy of affected organ

Endothelial dysfunction may be an early indicator of macrovascular disease, since the endothelium is one of the first areas of injury during vascular insult. Endothelial-dependent relaxation is abnormal in patients with known vascular disease such as hypertension, increased circulating LDL cholesterol, and diabetes.[166] There are some markers known to be associated with endothelial cell dysfunction, such as elevated von Willebrand factor,[27] and perhaps Lp(a).[167] Whether these endothelial markers will be useful in accurately predicting those diabetics at risk for vascular disease needs to be investigated.

Control of Blood Glucose.—Currently, much research is focused on developing a cure for diabetes mellitus itself. Some investigators are interested in identifying an overall "diabetes gene," responsible for disease transmission. Advances have been made in identifying: (1) the glucokinase gene as being tightly linked with, or possibly causative of, maturity-onset diabetes of the young (MODY),[168] (2) a gene serving as a marker of NIDDM in black patients[169] and, (3) a gene associated with a predisposition for IDDM in white patients.[170] Other investigators are looking at immunological intervention[171] in early IDDM, and still others are attempting to perfect pancreas/islet cell transplantation[171, 173] in the hopes of establishing long-lasting euglycemia. While whole pancreas transplants are being performed with success, islet cell transplants are currently not feasible (in humans) for long-term control of diabetes.

When the results of the DCCT became known, it became clear that tight blood sugar control was effective in preventing and/or ameliorating the impact of microvascular complications. However, while intensive insulin therapy sounds simple, it cannot be overemphasized that patients on intensive insulin therapy should be managed by a team of professionals, including an endocrinologist experienced in the management of such patients and appropriate support personnel (diabetic nurse educators, dieticians, and psychologists). Close communication with patients on intensive insulin therapy should be established; during the DCCT, patients often called their physicians daily for advice on insulin therapy or to discuss problems. The risks and benefits of intensive insulin therapy should be discussed with each patient, and, if desired, the patient should be referred to the appropriate team for initial hospitalization and management.

One way of improving glucose control is by the more effective delivery of insulin. Implanted insulin pumps which deliver insulin peritoneally or directly into the portal vein have been found to result in a more rapid and consistent absorption of insulin, improved average plasma glucose with fewer glycemic excursions, and fewer incidences of hypoglycemia. Moreover, these patients have shown a reduction in VLDL and triglycerides and an increase in HDL cholesterol as compared with patients on intensive subcutaneous insulin therapy.[174, 175] Because the infused insulin is absorbed into the portal circulation, with immediate delivery to the liver (and subsequent first-pass clearance of insulin), the peritoneal insulin pump is a more physiologic way of administering insulin and results in lower circulating insulin levels compared to subcutaneous insulin therapy.

The recent development of "insulin-sensitizing" agents, such as the thiozolidinoliones (e.g., pioglitazone) and their derivatives, means that insulin resistance, which may play an important role in the development of some complications, may be ameliorated pharmacologically. In mammals, treatment with pioglitazone for 3 to 10 days decreased hyperglycemia and hyperinsulinemia, increased autophosphorylation of insulin receptors in response to insulin, increased muscle glucose transporter type 4 (GLUT 4), and significantly lowered total and LDL cholesterol in conjunction with insulin.[176–179] Results from human studies in NIDDM show that 8 of 11 subjects responded well to an analogue of pioglitazone (CS-045) with improvement of insulin resistance, reduction in insulinemia, lowering of hepatic glucose productions and improvement in both fasting and postprandial glycemia.[180] The hope is that thiozolidinolione derivatives will not only provide an alternative means of controlling blood sugar but may also decrease the frequency and severity of atherosclerosis.

Another agent enjoying a resurgence in interest is the biguanide metformin. While its close cousin, phenformin, was banned from many countries including the United States due to the frequent occurrence of lactic acidosis, the incidence of lactic acidosis with metformin is virtually nonexistent when the drug is taken appropriately.[181] Experiments in animals demonstrate that while metformin does not cause insulin release, it increases insulin-mediated glucose uptake, decreases glucose absorption by the gut, and decreases serum triglycerides. It also enhances fibrinolytic activity by decreasing the concentration of a fibrinolytic inhibitor. It does not cause weight gain and is felt to have antiatherogenic effects, probably due to its effects on lipids and insulin.[182] It has been used successfully in combination with sulfonylureas for the therapy of NIDDM[183] and offers theoretical advantages over sulfonylureas alone with very little danger of lactic acidosis.

Biochemical Reactions Associated With Hyperglycemia.—Since the duration and magnitude of hyperglycemia correlates with the extent and rate of progression of microvascular complications, and since diabetic complications can occur well after euglycemia has been restored, it has been proposed that irreversible changes in long-lived molecules are responsible for microvascular complications. Prime candidates for these long-lived molecules are AGEs. In experimental animals with diabetes, a pharmacologic agent that blocks AGE formation, aminoguanidine, has been tested. In the retina, it decreased acellular capillaries by 80% compared with untreated animals, with no change in blood sugar or blood pressure.[184] In the glomerulus, it prevented an increase in mesangial volume and decreased albumin excretion.[185] It has also been shown to inhibit oxidative modification of LDL-apo B in vitro.[186] Clinical trials in patients with diabetic nephropathy are currently underway and will clarify the safety and efficacy of aminoguanidine in human patients.

In addition to AGEs, excess sorbitol may cause or worsen diabetic complications. In those tissues containing the enzyme aldose reductase, excess glucose is converted to sorbitol via the polyol pathway. It is hypothesized that excess intracellular sorbitol (due to chronic hyperglycemia) initiates a cascade of events which eventually leads to a loss of functional and structural integrity.[187] Therefore, the use of an aldose reductase inhibitor should allow investigators to determine the role of the sorbitol pathway in each of the vascular complications. Although early studies using aldose reductase inhibitors in human patients with neuropathy were disappointing, in part due to toxicity from the drugs, recent results are more positive. In humans with neuropathy, tolrestat has been shown to improve nerve conduction velocities and vibration thresholds with a marked improvement in painful neuropathy, but with little improvement in paresthesias.[188] In streptozotocin-diabetic rats, increases in urinary albumin excretion could be either prevented or significantly reduced with tolrestat administration alone.[189] This agent also prevented some of the typical morphological findings accompanying diabetic retinopathy in rats.[190]

Control of Oxidation.—The important role of lipid abnormalities in general, and oxidized LDL in particular, in the development of vascular disease has been demonstrated.[58] Ongoing protocols in humans using water-soluble antioxidants such as vitamin C and lipid-soluble antioxidants such as vitamin E, β-carotene, and probucol will be helpful in determining whether they will be useful in preventing or ameliorating the sequelae of oxidized LDL.[191]

Platelet Abnormalities.—Functional abnormalities in platelets may play an important role in the etiology of vascular disease. Normalization of platelet abnormalities can influence the progression of atherosclerosis, nephropathy, and retinopathy as well as acute thrombosis. It has been shown in vitro that magnesium, vitamin E, and aspirin can reduce platelet aggregatability in diabetic patients as can glycemic control.[55, 192] Patients with retinopathy who have taken aspirin have shown no improvement in the magnitude or progression of their disease.[193, 194] However, short-term administration of aspirin to patients with diabetic nephropathy showed a reduction of proteinuria.[195] A small group of diabetic patients with nephropathy who were followed for 10 years while on aspirin showed some stabilization of renal function, probably due to reduced platelet hypersensitivity and reduced production of thromboxanes by renal tissue and platelets.[196] Long-term studies in diabetic rats receiving aspirin show that the initial increase in GFR, basement membrane thickening, and later fall in GFR were prevented compared with their diabetic counterparts who did not receive aspirin.[197] Currently, no firm recommendations for the use of aspirin or for magnesium replacement (in order to normalize platelet abnormalities) exist.

Gene Therapy.—Other strategies are being aimed directly at vascular disease itself. Gene therapy has the potential to make a significant impact on vascular disease. For example, while the use of systemic growth factor inhibitors to treat atherosclerosis may be expensive, impractical, and dangerous, the local delivery of growth factor inhibitors into the abnormal vessel wall via the use of genetically engineered cells (such as macrophages) or noncellular vectors (such as liposomes or stents) might be effective in preventing abnormal growth of vascular smooth muscle locally, without causing disabling systemic effects.

In summary, although treatment of the vascular complications of diabetes mellitus is currently limited, the future looks hopeful. The next decade should see the emergence of a number of modalities which will ameliorate and, it is hoped, eliminate the impact of vascular complications on the diabetic patient.

References

1. Harris MI, Hadden W, Knowler WC, et al: Prevalence of diabetes and impaired glucose levels in US population aged 20–74 years. *Diabetes* 1987; 36:523–34.
2. Harris MI: Noninsulin-dependent diabetes mellitus in Black and White Americans. *Diab Metab Rev* 1990; 6:71–90.
3. Harris MI: Epidemiologic correlates of NIDDM in Hispanics, whites and blacks in the US population. *Diabetes Care* 1991; 14(suppl 3):639–648.
4. Knowler WC, Bennett PH, Hamman RF, et al: Diabetes incidence and preva-

lence in Pima Indians: A 19-fold greater incidence than in Rochester, Minnesota. *Am J Epidemiol* 1978; 108:497–505.
5. Raskin P, Rosenstock J: Blood glucose control and diabetic complications. *Ann Int Med* 1986; 105:254–263.
6. Kornerup T: Studies in diabetic retinopathy: An investigation of 1,000 cases of diabetes. *Acta Med Scand* 1955; 153:81–101.
7. Selby JV, FitzSimmons SC, Newman JM, et al: The natural history and epidemiology of diabetic nephropathy. *JAMA* 1990; 263:1954–1960.
8. American Diabetes Association. Consensus statement: Role of cardiovascular risk factors in prevention and treatment of macrovascular disease in diabetes. *Diabetes Care* 1990; 13(suppl 1):53–59.
9. Centers for Disease Control. Trends in diabetes mortality. *Morbid Mortal Weekly Report* 1988; 37:769–773.
10. Brand FN, Abbott RD, Kannel WB: Diabetes, intermittent claudication and risk of cardiovascular events. The Framingham study. *Diabetes* 1989; 38:504–509.
11. Barrett-Connor E, Cohn BA, Wingard DL, et al: Why is diabetes mellitus a stronger risk factor for fatal ischemic heart disease in men than in women? *JAMA* 1991; 265:627–631.
12. Barrett-Connor E, Khaw KT: Diabetes mellitus: An independent risk factor for stroke? *Am J Epidemiology* 1988; 128:116–123.
13. Bild DE, Selby VJ, Sinnock P, et al: Lower-extremity amputation in people with diabetes: Epidemiology and prevention. *Diabetes Care* 1989; 12:24–29.
14. Haffner SM, Stern MP, Hazuda HP, et al: Cardiovascular risk factors in confirmed prediabetic individuals. Does the clock for coronary heart disease start ticking before the onset of clinical diabetes? *JAMA* 1990; 263:2893–2898.
15. Horan MJ: Diabetes and hypertension, in *Diabetes in America.* Washington, DC: US Government Printing Office, 1985:1–22, NIH publication No. 85-1468.
16. The Working Group on Hypertension in Diabetes. Statement on hypertension in diabetes mellitus. *Arch Int Med* 1987; 147:830–842.
17. Parving H-H, Andersen AR, Smidt UM, et al: Early aggressive antihypertensive treatment reduces rate of decline in kidney function in diabetic nephropathy. *Lancet* 1983; I:1175–1179.
18. Janka HU, Warram JH, Rand LI, et al: Risk factors for progression of background retinopathy in long-standing IDDM. *Diabetes* 1989; 38:460–464.
19. Weinberger MH: Cardiovascular risk factors and antihypertensive therapy. *Am J Med* 1988; 84(suppl 4A):24–29.
20. Botting R, Vane JR: Mediators and the anti-thrombotic properties of the vascular endothelium. *Ann Med* 1989; 21:31–38.
21. Vallance P, Calver A, Collier J: The vascular endothelium in diabetes and hypertension. *J Hypertens* 1992; 10(suppl 1):S25–S29.
22. Kifor I, Dzau VJ: Endothelial renin-angiotensin pathway: Evidence for intracellular synthesis and secretion of angiotensins. *Circ Res* 1987; 60:422–428.
23. Yanagisawa M, Kurihara H, Kimura S, et al: A novel potent vasoconstrictor peptide produced by vascular endothelial cells. *Nature* 1988; 332:411–415.
24. Furchgott RF, Zawadzki JV: The obligatory role of endothelial cells in the relaxation of arterial smooth muscle by acetylcholine. *Nature* 1980; 288:373–376.
25. Gryglewski RJ, Botting RM, Vane JR: Mediators produced by the endothelial cell. *Hypertension* 1988; 12:530–548.

26. Dzau VJ, Gibbons GH: Cell biology of vascular hypertrophy in systemic hypertension. *Am J Cardiol* 1988; 62:30G–35G.
27. Bensoussan D, Levy-Toledana S, Passa P, et al: Platelet hyperaggregation and increased plasma level of von Willebrand factor in diabetic patients with retinopathy. *Diabetologia* 1975; 11:307–312.
28. Colwell JA, Winocour PD, Halushka PV: Do platelets have anything to do with diabetic microvascular disease? *Diabetes* 1983; 32:14–19.
29. Meraji S, Jayakody L, Senaratne MP, et al: Endothelium-dependent relaxation in aorta from diabetic rats. *Diabetes* 1987; 36:978–981.
30. Tesfamariam B, Brown ML, Cohen RA: Elevated glucose impairs endothelium-dependent relaxation by activating protein kinase C. *J Clin Invest* 1991; 87:1643–1648.
31. Yamauchi T, Ohnaka K, Takayanagi R, et al: Enhanced secretion of endothelin-1 by elevated glucose levels from cultured bovine aortic endothelial cells. *FEBS Letts* 1990; 267:16–18.
32. Cagliero E, Maiello M, Boeri D, et al: Increased expression of basement membrane components in human endothelial cells cultured in high glucose. *J Clin Invest* 1988; 82:735–738.
33. Cagliero E, Roth T, Roy S, et al: Characteristics and mechanisms of high-glucose-induced overexpression of basement membrane components in cultured human endothelial cells. *Diabetes* 1991; 40:102–110.
34. Lorenzi M, Cagliero E, Toledo S: Glucose toxicity for human endothelial cells in culture: delayed replication, disturbed cell cycle, and accelerated death. *Diabetes* 1985; 34:621–627.
35. Brownlee M, Cerami A, Vlassara H: Advanced glycosylation end products in tissue and the biochemical basis of diabetic complications. *N Engl J Med* 1988; 318:1315–1321.
36. Rosenfeld ME, Khoo JC, Miller E, et al: Macrophage-derived foam cells freshly isolated from rabbit atherosclerotic lesions degrade modified lipoproteins, promote oxidation of low-density lipoproteins, and contain oxidation-specific lipid-protein adducts. *J Clin Invest* 1991; 87:90–99.
37. Alipui C, Tenner TE, Ramos K: Rabbit aortic smooth muscle culture. A model for the pharmacological study of diabetes-induced alterations in cell proliferation. *J Pharm Methods* 1991; 26:211–222.
38. Fry DL: Certain histological and chemical responses of the vascular interface to acutely induced mechanical stress in the aorta of the dog. *Circ Res* 1969; 24:93–97.
39. Haudenschild CC, Prescott MR, Chobanian AV: Effect of hypertension and its reversal on aortic intimal lesions in the rat. *Hypertension* 1980; 2:33–42.
40. Brecher P, Chan CT, Fanzblau C: Effects of hypertension and its reversal on aortic metabolism in the rat. *Circ Res* 1975; 36:553–562.
41. Huttner I, Boutet M, Rona G, et al: Studies of protein passage through arterial endothelium: III. Effect of blood pressure levels on the passage of fine structure protein tracers through rat arterial endothelium. *Lab Invest* 1973; 29:536–546.
42. Peach MJ, Loeb AL: Changes in vascular endothelium and its function in systemic arterial hypertension. *Am J Cardiol* 1987; 60:110I–115I.
43. Panza JA, Quyyumi AA, Brush JE Jr, et al: Abnormal endothelium-dependent vascular relaxation in patients with hypertension. *N Engl J Med* 1990; 323:22–27.
44. Chobanian AV: 1989 Corcoran Lecture: Adaptive and maladaptive re-

sponses of the arterial wall to hypertension. *Hypertension* 1990; 15:666–674.
45. Garcia MJ, McNamara PM, Gordon T, et al: Morbidity and mortality in diabetics in the Framingham population: sixteen year follow-up study. *Diabetes* 1974; 23:105–111.
46. Brownlee M: Glycation products and the pathogenesis of diabetic complications. *Diabetes Care* 1992; 15:1835–1843.
47. Haitglou CS, Tsilibary EC, Brownlee M, et al: Altered cellular interactions between endothelial cells and non-enzymatically glycosylated laminin/type IV collagen. *J Biol Chem* 1992; 267:12404–12407.
48. Crowley ST, Brownlee M, Edelstein D, et al: Effects of nonenzymatic glycosylation on mesangial matrix on proliferation of mesangial cells. *Diabetes* 1991; 40:540–547.
49. Brownlee M, Vlassara H, Cerami A: Nonenzymatic glycosylation products on collagen covalently trap low-density lipoproteins. *Diabetes* 1985; 34:938–941.
50. Hogan M, Cerami A, Bucala R: Advanced glycosylation end products block the antiproliferative effect of nitric oxide. *J Clin Invest* 1992; 90:1110–1115.
51. Assoian RK, Grotendorst GR, Miller DM, et al: Cellular transformation by coordinated action of three peptide growth factors from human platelets. *Nature* 1984; 309:804–806.
52. Davi G, Rini GB, Averna M, et al: Thromboxane B_2 formation and platelet sensitivity to prostacyclin in insulin-dependent and independent diabetics. *Thromb Res* 1982; 26:359–370.
53. Butkus A, Srinska VA, Schumacker OP: Thromboxane production and platelet aggregation in diabetic subjects with clinical complications. *Thromb Res* 1980; 19:211–223.
54. DeRubertis FR, Craven PA: Contribution of platelet thromboxane production to enhanced urinary excretion and glomerular production of thromboxane and to the pathogenesis of albuminuria in the streptozotocin-diabetic rat. *Metab Clin Exp* 1992; 41:90–96.
55. Alessandrini P, McRae J, Feman S, et al: Thromboxane biosynthesis and platelet functions in Type I diabetes mellitus. *N Engl J Med* 1988; 319:208–212.
56. Nadler JL, Malayan S, Luong H, et al: Intracellular free magnesium deficiency plays a key role in increased platelet reactivity in Type II diabetes mellitus. *Diabetes Care* 1992; 15:835–841.
57. Dunn FL: Management of hyperlipidemia in diabetes mellitus. *Endo Metab Clin NA* 1992; 21:395–414.
58. Quinn MT, Parthasarathy S, Fong LG, et al: Oxidatively modified low density lipoproteins: A potential role in recruitment and retention of monocyte/macrophages during atherogenesis. *Proc Natl Acad Sci* 1987; 84:2995–2998.
59. Lyons TJ: Oxidized low-density lipoproteins—A role in the pathogenesis of atherosclerosis in diabetes? *Diabetic Med* 1991; 8:411–419.
60. Lyons TJ, Patrick JS, Baynes JW, et al: Glycation of low density lipoprotein in patients with type I diabetes: Correlation with other parameters of glycaemic control. *Diabetologia* 1986; 29:685–689.
61. Rothman DL, Shulman RG, Shulman GI: ^{31}P nuclear magnetic resonance measurements of muscle glucose-6-phosphate. Evidence for reduced insulin-dependent muscle glucose transport or phosphorylation activity in non-insulin dependent diabetes mellitus. *J Clin Invest* 1992; 89:1069–1075.

62. Ferrannini E, Buzzigoli G, Bonadonna R, et al: Insulin resistance in essential hypertension. *N Engl J Med* 1987; 317:350–357.
63. Logan RL, Riemersma RA, Thomson M, et al: Risk factors for ischaemic heart disease in normal men aged 40: Edinburgh-Stockholm study. *Lancet* 1978; 1:949–954.
64. Hughes LO, Cruickshank JK, Wright J, et al: Disturbances of insulin and its action in British Asian and White male survivors of myocardial infarction. *Br Med J* 1989; 299:537–541.
65. Pyörälä K: Relationship of glucose tolerance and plasma insulin to incidence of coronary heart disease: Results from two population studies in Finland. *Diabetes Care* 1979; 2:131–141.
66. Pyörälä K, Savolainen E, Kaukola S, et al: Plasma insulin as coronary heart disease risk factor: relationship to other risk factors and predictive value during $9\frac{1}{2}$ year follow-up of the Helsinki Policemen Study population. *Acta Med Scand Suppl* 1985; 701:38–52.
67. Ducimentiere P, Eschwege E, Papoz L, et al: Relationship of plasma insulin levels to the incidence of myocardial infarction and coronary heart disease in a middle-aged population. *Diabetologia* 1980; 19:205–210.
68. Welborn TA, Wearne K. Coronary heart disease incidence and cardiovascular mortality in Busselton with reference to glucose and insulin concentrations. *Diabetes Care* 1979; 2:154–160.
69. Zavaroni I, Bonara E, Pagliara M, et al: Risk factors for coronary artery disease in healthy persons with hyper-insulinemia and normal glucose tolerance. *N Engl J Med* 1989; 320:702–706.
70. Williams RR, Hunt SC, Hopkins PN, et al: Familial dyslipidemic hypertension: Evidence from 58 Utah families for a syndrome present in approximately 12% of patients with essential hypertension. *JAMA* 1988; 259:3570–3586.
71. Nelson RG, Seivers ML, Knowler WC, et al: Low incidence of fatal coronary heart disease in Pima Indians despite high prevalence of diabetes. *Circ* 1990; 81:987–995.
72. Mitchell BD, Stern MP, Haffner SM, et al: Risk factors for cardiovascular mortality in Mexican Americans and non-Hispanic whites. San Antonio Heart Study. *Am J Epidemiol* 1990; 131:423–433.
73. Stout RW: Insulin as a mitogenic factor: Role in pathogenesis of cardiovascular disease. *Am J Med* 1991; 90(2A):62S–65S.
74. Reaven GM: Non-insulin-dependent diabetes mellitus, abnormal lipoprotein metabolism and atherosclerosis. *Metabolism* 1987; 36:1–8.
75. Bondjers G, Glukhova M, Hansson GK, et al: Hypertension and atherosclerosis: Cause and effect or two effects with one cause? *Circ* 1991; 84(suppl VI):VI-2–VI-16.
76. Meehan WP, Buchanan TA, Shargill NS, et al: High blood pressure research: insulin, obesity, and metabolic abnormalities of hypertension (abstract). *Circ* 1990; 82(suppl III):86.
77. Brands MW, Hildebrandt DA, Mizelle HL, et al: Sustained hyperinsulinemia increases arterial pressure in conscious rats. *Am J Physiol* 1991; 260:R764–R768.
78. Meehan WP, Buchanan T, Hsueh WA. Pioglitazone reduces blood pressure and improves insulin sensitivity in fructose-fed rats (abstract). *Clin Res* 1993; 43:21A.

79. Landin-Wilhelmsen K: Metformin and blood pressure. *J Clin Pharm Therap* 1992; 17:75–79.
80. Rocchini AP, Katch V, Kveselis D, et al: Insulin and renal sodium retention in obese adolescents. *Hypertension* 1989; 14:367–374.
81. Anderson EA, Hoffman RP, Balon TW, et al: Hyperinsulinemia produces both sympathetic neural activation and vasodilation in normal humans. *J Clin Invest* 1991; 87:2246–2252.
82. U.S. Renal Data System: *United States Renal Data System 1990 Annual Data Report*. Bethesda, Md, The National Institutes of Health, National Institute of Diabetes and Digestive and Kidney Diseases, 1990.
83. Cowie CC, Port FK, Wolfe RA, et al: Disparities in incidence of diabetic end-stage renal disease according to race and type of diabetes. *N Engl J Med* 1989; 321:1074–1079.
84. Haffner SM, Stern MP, Gruber MK, et al: Microalbuminuria. Potential marker for increased cardiovascular risk factors in nondiabetic subjects. *Arteriosclerosis* 1990; 10:727–731.
85. Mené P, Cinotti GA: Paracrine and autocrine functions of glomerular mesangial cells. *J Endocrinol Invest* 1989; 12:497–509.
86. Werber HI, Emancipator SN, Tykocinski ML, et al: The interleukin-1 gene is expressed by rat glomerular mesangial cells and is augmented in immune complex glomerulonephritis. *J Immunol* 1987; 138:3207–3212.
87. Keane WF, Raij L: Relationship among altered glomerular barrier permselectivity, angiotensin II and mesangial uptake of macromolecules. *Lab Invest* 1985; 52:599–604.
88. Zatz R, Brenner BM: Pathogenesis of diabetic microangiopathy: The hemodynamic view. *Am J Med* 1986; 80:443–451.
89. Osterby R, Gundersen HJG: Glomerular size and structure in diabetes mellitus. I. Early abnormalities. *Diabetologia* 1975; 11:225–233.
90. Mogensen CE. Natural history of renal function abnormalities in human diabetes mellitus. In Berrer BM, Stein JH (eds): *The Kidney in Diabetes Mellitus*, New York, Churchill-Livingstone, 1989, pp 19–49.
91. Ellis EN, Steffes MW, Goetz FC, et al: Glomerular filtration surface in type I diabetes mellitus. *Kidney Internat* 1986; 29:889–894.
92. Ellis EN, Mauer SM, Goetz FC, et al: Relationship of muscle capillary basement membrane to renal structure function in diabetes mellitus. *Diabetes* 1986; 35:421–425.
93. Steffes MW, Sutherland DE, Goetz FC, et al: Studies of kidney and muscle biopsy specimens from identical twins discordant for type I diabetes mellitus. *N Engl J Med* 1985; 312:1282–1287.
94. Lane PH, Steffes MW, Mauer SM: Relationship of mesangial and interstitial structure to renal function in insulin-dependent diabetes mellitus (abstract). *J Amer Soc Nephrol* 1991; 293.
95. Mogensen C, Chirstiansen CK: Predicting diabetic nephropathy in insulin-dependent patients. *N Engl J Med* 1984; 311:89–93.
96. Friedman S, Jones III HW, Golbetz HV, et al: Mechanisms of proteinuria in diabetic nephropathy II: A study of the size-selective glomerular filtration barrier. *Diabetes* 1983; 32(suppl 2):40–46.
97. Gellman DD, Pirani CL, Soothill JF, et al: Diabetic nephropathy: A clinical and pathological study based on renal biopsies. *Medicine* 1959; 38:321–340.

98. Steffes MW, Bilous RW, Sutherland DER, et al: Cell and matrix components of the glomerular mesangium in type I diabetes. *Diabetes* 1992; 41:679–684.
99. Mauer SM, Steffes MW, Ellis EN, et al: Structural-functional relationships in diabetic nephropathy. *J Clin Invest* 1984; 74:1143–1155.
100. Mené P, Simonson MS, Dunn MJ: Physiology of the mesangial cell. *Physiology Rev* 1989; 69:1347–1424.
101. Mathiesen ER, Hommel E, Giese J, et al: Efficacy of captopril in postponing nephropathy in normotensive insulin dependent diabetic patients with microalbuminuria, *Br Med J* 1991; 303:81–87.
102. Zeller K, Whittaker E, Sullivan L, et al: Effect of restricting dietary protein on the progression of renal failure in patients with insulin-dependent diabetes mellitus. *N Engl J Med* 1991; 324:78–84.
103. Bilous RW, Mauer SM, Sutherland DER, et al: The effect of pancreas transplantation on the glomerular structure of renal allografts in patients with insulin-dependent diabetes. *N Engl J Med* 1989; 321:80–85.
104. Herman WH, Teutsch SM, Sepe SJ, et al: An approach to the prevention of blindness in diabetes. *Diabetes Care* 1983; 6:608–613.
105. Chase HP, Jackson WE, Hoops SL, et al: Glucose control and the renal and retinal complications of insulin-dependent diabetes. *JAMA* 1989; 261:1155–1160.
106. Stephansson T, Lander MB III, Wolbarsht ML: Oxygenation and vasodilation in relation to diabetic and other proliferative retinopathies. *Ophthalmic Surg* 1983; 14:209–226.
107. Kohner EM, Hamilton AM, Saunders SJ, et al: The retinal blood flow in diabetes. *Diabetologia* 1975; 11:27–33.
108. Krupin T, Waltman SR, Oestrich C: Vitreous fluorophotometry in juvenile-onset diabetes mellitus. *Arch Ophthalmol* 1978; 96:812–814.
109. Ishibashi T, Tanaka K, Taniguchi Y: Disruption of blood-retinal barrier in experimental diabetic rats: An electron microscopic study. *Exp Eye Res* 1990; 30:401–410.
110. White NH, Waltman SR, Krupin T, et al: Reversal of abnormalities in ocular fluorophotometry in insulin-dependent diabetes after 5–9 months of improved metabolic control. *Diabetes* 1982; 31:80–85.
111. Orlidge A, D'Amore PA: Inhibition of capillary endothelial cell growth by pericytes and smooth muscle cells. *J Cell Biol* 1987; 105:1455–1462.
112. Grant M, Russell B, Fitzgerald C, et al: Insulin-like growth factors in vitreous: Studies in control and diabetic subjects with neovascularization. *Diabetes* 1986; 35:416–420.
113. Tapper D, Albert DM, Robinson NL, et al: Capillary endothelial cell migration: Stimulating activity of aqueous humor from patients with ocular cancers. *J Natl Cancer Instit* 1983; 71:501–505.
114. Juhan I, Vague P, Buonocore M, et al: Abnormalities of erythrocyte deformability and platelet aggregation in insulin-dependent diabetics corrected by insulin in vivo and in vitro. *Lancet* 1982; 1:535–537.
115. Ditzel J, Standl E: The problem of tissue oxygenation in diabetes mellitus. II. Evidence of disordered oxygen release from erythrocytes of diabetics. *Acta Med Scand* 1975; 578(suppl):4–58.
116. ETDRS Investigators. Effects of aspirin treatment on diabetic retinopathy. ETDRS report number 8. *Ophthalmology* 1991; 98:757–765.
117. Klein BEK, Moss SE, Klein R: The effect of pregnancy on progression of diabetic retinopathy. *Diabetes Care* 1990; 13:34–40.

118. Murphy RP, Nanda M, Plotnick L, et al: The relationship of puberty to diabetic retinopathy. *Arch Ophthalmol* 1990; 108:215–218.
119. Lundbaek K: Growth hormone's role in diabetic microangiopathy. *Diabetes* 1976; 25(suppl 2):845–849.
120. American Diabetes Association. Clinical Practice Recommendations: Standards of medical care for patients with diabetes mellitus. *Diabetes Care* 1992; 15(suppl 2):10–13.
121. Raskin P, Arauz-Pachero C: The treatment of diabetic retinopathy: A view for the internist. *Ann Int Med* 1992; 117:226–233.
122. Weiner DA, Ryan TJ, Parsons L, et al: Significance of silent myocardial ischemia during exercise testing in patients with diabetes mellitus: A report from the Coronary Artery Surgery Study (CASS) Registry. *Am J Cardiol* 1991; 68:729–734.
123. Frohlich E: The heart in hypertension: A 1991 overview. *Hypertension* 1991; 18(suppl III):III-62–III-68.
124. Report of the Diabetes Control and Complications Trial. American Diabetes Association Annual Meetings, Las Vegas, Nev, June 1993.
125. Dahl-Jorgensen: Near normoglycemia and late diabetic complications. The Oslo study. *Acta Endocrinolog* 1987; 115(suppl 284):7–38.
126. The Kroc Collaborative Study Group. Blood glucose control and the evolution of diabetic retinopathy and albuminuria. *N Engl J Med* 1984; 311:365–372.
127. Steno Study Group. Effect of 6 months of strict metabolic control on eye and kidney function in insulin-dependent diabetics with background retinopathy. *Lancet* 1982; I:121–123.
128. Feldt-Rasmussen B, Mathiesen ER, Hegedüs L, et al: Kidney function during 12 months of strict metabolic control in insulin-dependent diabetic patients with incipient nephropathy. *N Engl J Med* 1986; 314:665–670.
129. Peterson MR, Vine AK, University of Michigan Transplant Evaluation Committee: Progression of diabetic retinopathy after pancreas transplantation. *Ophthalmol* 1990; 97:496–502.
130. Mathiesen ER, Oxenboll B, Johansen K, et al: Incipient nephropathy in type I (insulin-dependent) diabetes. *Diabetologia* 1984; 26:406–410.
131. Christiansen CK, Mogensen CE: The course of incipient diabetic nephropathy: Studies on albumin excretion and blood pressure. *Diab Med* 1985; 2:97–102.
132. Rosenstock J, Raskin P: Early diabetic nephropathy: Assessment and potential therapeutic interventions. *Diab Care* 1986; 9:529–545.
133. Parving H-H, Hommel E, Nielsen MD, et al: Effect of captopril on blood pressure and kidney function in normotensive insulin-dependent diabetics with nephropathy. *Br Med J* 1989; 299:533–536.
134. Valentino VA, Wilson MD, Weart W, et al: A perspective on converting enzyme inhibitors and calcium channel antagonists in diabetic renal disease. *Arch Int Med* 1991; 151:2367–2372.
135. Kasiske BL, Kalil RSN, Ma JZ, et al: Effect of antihypertensive therapy on the kidney in patients with diabetes. A meta-regression analysis. *Ann Int Med* 1993; 118:129–138.
136. Collaborative Study Group. Angiotensin Converting Enzyme Inhibition Trial. Presented at the Third NIDDK Symposium on Kidney Disease of Diabetes Mellitus. Crystal City, Calif, April 1993.
137. Taguma Y, Kitamoto Y, Futaki G, et al: Effect of captopril on heavy proteinuria in azotemic diabetics. *N Engl J Med* 1985; 313:1617–1620.

138. Reams GP, Bauer JH: Decrease in proteinuria with ACE inhibition does not predict attentuation of progression of renal disease (abstract). *Clin Res* 1991; 39:247.
139. Mogensen CE, Hansen KW, Pedersen MM, et al: Renal factors influencing blood pressure threshhold and choice of treatment for hypertension in IDDM. *Diabetes Care* 14(suppl 4):13–26.
140. Weinberger MH: Cardiovascular risk factors and antihypertensive therapy. *Am J Med* 1988; 84(suppl 4A):24–29.
141. Berne C, Pollare T, Lithell H: Effects of antihypertensive treatment on insulin sensitivity with special reference to ACE inhibitors. *Diab Care* 1991; 14(suppl 4):39–47.
142. Stein PP, Black HR: Drug treatment of hypertension in patients with diabetes mellitus. *Diabetes Care* 1991; 14:425–448.
143. Anderson PW, Do YS, Hsueh WA: Angiotensin II causes mesangial cell hypertrophy. *Hypertension* 1993; 21:29–35.
144. Joint National Committee on Detection, Evaluation and Treatment of High Blood Pressure. The Fifth Report of the Joint National Committee on detection, evaluation and treatment of high blood pressure (JNC V). *Arch Int Med* 1993; 153:154–183.
145. O'Donnell MP, Kasiske BL, Katz SA, et al: Lovastatin but not enalapril reduces glomerular injury in Dahl salt-sensitive rats. *Hypertension* 1992; 20:651–658.
146. Goldberg RB: Lipid disorders in diabetes. *Diabetes Care* 1981; 4:561–572.
147. Fontbonne A, Eschwège E, Cambien F, et al: Hypertriglyceridemia as a risk factor of coronary heart disease mortality in subjects with impaired glucose tolerance of diabetes. *Diabetologia* 1989; 32:300–304.
148. McKeigue PM, Marmot MG, Syndercombe-Court YD, et al: Diabetes, hyperinsulinemia and coronary risk factors in Bangladeshis in East London. *Br Heart J* 1988; 60:390–396.
149. Expert Panel on Detection, Evaluation and Treatment of High Blood Cholesterol in Adults. Summary of the Second Report of the National Cholesterol Education Program on Detection, Evaluation and Treatment of High Blood Cholesterol in Adults. *JAMA* 1993; 269:3015–3023.
150. Pfeifer MA, Brunzell JD, Best JP, et al: The response of plasma triglyceride, cholesterol and lipoprotein lipase to treatment in non-insulin dependent diabetic subjects without familial hypertriglyceridemia. *Diabetes* 1983; 32:525–531.
151. Liu GC, Coulston AM, Lardinois CK, et al: Moderate weight loss and sulfonylurea treatment of non-insulin dependent diabetes mellitus. *Arch Int Med* 1985; 145:665–669.
152. American Diabetes Association. Nutritional recommendations and principles for individuals with diabetes mellitus: 1986. *Diabetes Care* 1987; 10:126–132.
153. Bierman EL, Hamlin JT III: The hyperlipemic effect of a low-fat, high-carbohydrate diet in diabetic subjects. *Diabetes* 1961; 10:432–437.
154. Coulson AM, Hollenbeck CB, Swislocki ALM, et al: Deleterious metabolic effects of high carbohydrate, sucrose-containing diets in patients with diabetes mellitus. *Am J Med* 1987; 82:213–220.
155. Kennedy L, Washe K, Hadden DR, et al: The effect of intensive dietary therapy on serum high-density lipoprotein cholesterol in patients with type 2 non-insulin dependent diabetes mellitus. A prospective study. *Diabetologia* 1982; 23:24–27.

156. American Diabetes Association. Clinical practice recommendations 1991–1992: Diabetes mellitus and exercise. *Diabetes Care* 1992; 15:36.
157. Garg A, Grundy SM: Gemfibrozil alone and in combination with lovastatin for treatment of hypertriglyceridemia in NIDDM. *Diabetes* 1989; 38:364–372.
158. Crouse JR: Hypertriglyceridemia: A contraindication to the use of bile acid binding resins. *Am J Med* 1987; 83:243–248.
159. Garg A, Grundy SM: Lovastatin for lowering cholesterol levels in non-insulin-dependent diabetes mellitus. *N Engl J Med* 1988; 318:81–86.
160. Pierce LR, Wysowski DK, Gross TP: Myopathy and rhabdomyolysis associated with lovastatin-gemfibrozil combination therapy. *JAMA* 1990; 264:71–75.
161. Miettinen TA, Taskinen M-R, Pelkonen R, et al: Glucose tolerance and plasma insulin in man during acute and chronic administration of nicotinic acid. *Acta Med Scand* 1969; 186:247–253.
162. Parthasarathy S, Young SG, Witztum JL, et al: Probucol inhibits oxidative modification of low density lipoprotein. *J Clin Invest* 1986; 77:641–644.
163. Crosignani PG: Effects of hormone replacement therapy. *Int J Fertil* 1992; 37(suppl 2):98–103.
164. Bagatell CJ, Knopp RH, Vale WW, et al: Physiologic testosterone levels in normal men suppress high-density lipoprotein cholesterol levels. *Ann Int Med* 1992; 116(12 pt 1):967–973.
165. Wilson DM, Luetscher JA: Plasma prorenin activity and complications in children with insulin dependent diabetes. *N Engl J Med* 1990; 323:1101–1106.
166. Kiowski W: Endothelial function in humans. Studies of forearm resistance vessels. *Hypertension* 1991; 18(suppl II):II-84–II-89.
167. Winocour PH, Bhatnagar D, Ishola M, et al: Lipoprotein (a) and microvascular disease in type I (insulin-dependent) diabetes. *Diab Med* 1991; 8:922–927.
168. Vionnet N, Stoffel M, Takeda J, et al: Nonsense mutation in the glucokinase gene causes early-onset non-insulin-dependent diabetes mellitus. *Nature* 1992; 356:721–722.
169. Chiu KC, Province MA, Permutt MA: Glucokinase gene is genetic marker for NIDDM in American blacks. *Diabetes* 1992; 41:843–849.
170. Todd JA, Bell JI, McDevitt HO: HLA-DQβ igene contributes to susceptibility and resistance to insulin-dependent diabetes mellitus. *Nature* 1987; 329:599–604.
171. Lipton R, LaPorte RE, Becker DJ, et al: Cyclosporin therapy for prevention and cure of IDDM. Epidemiological perspective of benefits and risks. *Diabetes Care* 1990; 13:776–784.
172. Robertson RP: Pancreas transplantation in humans with diabetes mellitus. *Diabetes* 1991; 40:1085–1089.
173. Scharp DW, Lacy PE, Santiago JV, et al: Insulin independence after islet transplantation into type I diabetic patient. *Diabetes* 1990; 39:515–518.
174. Duckworth WC, Saudek CD, Henry RR: Why intraperitoneal delivery of insulin with implantable pumps in NIDDM? *Diabetes* 1992; 41:657–661.
175. Shishko PI, Kovalev PA, Goncharov VG, et al: Comparison of peripheral and portal (via the umbilical vein) routes of insulin infusion in IDDM patients. *Diabetes* 1992; 41:1042–1049.
176. Sugiyama Y, Taketomi S, Shimura Y, et al: Effects of pioglitazone on glucose and lipid metabolism in Wistar fatty rats. *Arzneimittel Forschung* 1990; 40:263–267.

177. Kobayashi M, Iwanishi M, Egawa K, et al: Pioglitazone increases insulin sensitivity by activating insulin receptor kinase. *Diabetes* 1992; 41:476–483.
178. Hofmann C, Lorenz K, Colca JR: Glucose transport deficiency in diabetic animals is corrected by treatment with the oral antihyperglycemic agent pioglitazone. *Endocrinology* 1991; 129:1915–1925.
179. Colca JR, Dailey CR, Palazuk BJ, et al: Pioglitazone hydrochloride inhibits cholesterol absorption and lowers plasma cholesterol concentrations in cholesterol-fed rats. *Diabetes* 1991; 40:1669–1674.
180. Suter SL, Nolan JJ, Wallace P, et al: Metabolic effects of new oral hypoglycemic agent CS-045 in NIDDM subjects. *Diabetes Care* 1992; 15:193–203.
181. Cavallo-Perin P, Aluffi E, Estivi P, et al: The hyperlactemic effect of biguanides: A comparison between phenformin and metformin during a 6-month treatment. *Med Pharmacol Sci* 1989; 11:45–49.
182. Bailey CJ: Biguanides and NIDDM. *Diabetes Care* 1992; 15;755–772.
183. Hermann LS: Biguanides and sulfonylureas as combination therapy in NIDDM. *Diabetes Care* 1990; 13(suppl 3):37–41.
184. Hammes H-P, Martin S, Federlin K, et al: Aminoguanidine treatment inhibits the development of experimental diabetic retinopathy. *Proc Natl Acad Sci* 1991; 88:11555–11558.
185. Soules-Liparota T, Cooper M, Papazoglou D, et al: Retardation by aminoguanidine of development of albuminuria, mesangial expansion, and tissue fluorescence in streptozotocin-induced diabetic rat. *Diabetes* 1991; 40:1328–1335.
186. Picard S, Parthasarathy S, Fruebis J, et al: Aminoguanidine inhibits oxidative modification of low density lipoprotein and the subsequent increase in uptake by macrophage scavenger receptors. *Proc Natl Acad Sci* 1992; 89:6876–6880.
187. Burg MB, Kador PF: Sorbitol, osmoregulation, and the complications of diabetes. *J Clin Invest* 1988; 81:635–640.
188. Macleod AF, Boulton AJ, Owens DR, et al: A multicentre trial of the aldose-reductase inhibitor tolrestat, in patients with symptomatic diabetic peripheral neuropathy. *Diabete et Metabolisme* 1992; 18:14–20.
189. McCaleb ML, Sredy J, Millen J, et al: Prevention of urinary albumin excretion in 6-month streptozotocin-diabetic rats with the aldose reductase inhibitor tolrestat. *J Diab Complications* 1988; 2:16–18.
190. Robison WG Jr, Tillis TN, Laver N, et al: Diabetes-related histopathologies of the rat retina prevented with an aldose reductase inhibitor. *Exp Eye Res* 1990; 50:355–366.
191. Chishold GM III: Antioxidants and atherosclerosis: A current assessment. *Clin Cardiol* 1991; 14:I25–I30.
192. Janero DR: Therapeutic potential of vitamin E in the pathogenesis of spontaneous atherosclerosis. *Free Radical Biol Med* 1991; 11:129–144.
193. Early Treatment Diabetic Retinopathy Study Research Group. Effects of aspirin treatment on diabetic retinopathy. ETDRS report number 8. *Ophthalmol* 1991; 98:757–765.
194. The DAMAD Study Group. The effect of aspirin alone plus dipyridamole in early diabetic retinopathy. *Diabetes* 1989; 38:491–498.
195. Hopper AH, Tindall H, Davies JA: Administration of aspirin-dipyridamole reduces proteinuria in diabetic nephropathy. *Nephrol Dialy Transpl* 1989; 4:140–143.

196. Donadio JV Jr, Ilstrup DM, Holley KE, et al: Platelet-inhibitor treatment of diabetic nephropathy: A 10-year prospective study. *Mayo Clin Proc* 1988; 63:3–15.
197. Moel DI, Safirstein RL, McEvoy RC, et al: Effect of aspirin on experimental diabetic nephropathy. *J Lab Clin Med* 1987; 110:300–307.

Evaluation of the Hypothalamic-Pituitary-Adrenal Axis: Importance in Steroid Therapy, AIDS, and Other Stress Syndromes

John D. Baxter, M.D.

Professor of Medicine, Director, Metabolic Research Unit and the Department of Medicine, University of California, San Francisco School of Medicine, San Francisco, California

J. Blake Tyrrell, M.D.

Metabolic Research Unit and the Department of Medicine, University of California, San Francisco School of Medicine, San Francisco, California

The hypothalamic-pituitary-adrenal (HPA) axis is responsible for producing cortisol, the major glucocorticoid in man. The major components of the axis (Fig 1) involve corticotropin-releasing hormone (CRH) and vasopressin (antidiuretic hormone [ADH]) of hypothalamic origin that drive the release of corticotropin (adrenocorticotropic hormone [ACTH]) from the anterior pituitary (adenohypophysis).[1–4] Adrenocorticotropic hormone stimulates the synthesis and secretion of cortisol from the adrenal cortex. Cortisol maintains cardiovascular integrity, especially in response to stress, and it mediates numerous influences on intermediary metabolism, such as the conservation of glucose at the expense of other substrate.[1–3]

Hypofunction of the axis results in cortisol deficiency with the consequent symptoms of adrenal glucocorticoid insufficiency and a potential danger of cardiovascular collapse, particularly in response to stress.[1–12] Hypofunction of the axis is most commonly observed following the withdrawal of glucocorticoid therapy.[6, 13–15] Although classical Addison's disease, primary adrenocortical failure, is a relatively rare disease, its incidence has recently increased due to the increase in the number of cases of the acquired immune deficiency syndrome (AIDS) and tuberculosis.[12, 16–21] It may also be more common than previously thought in pa-

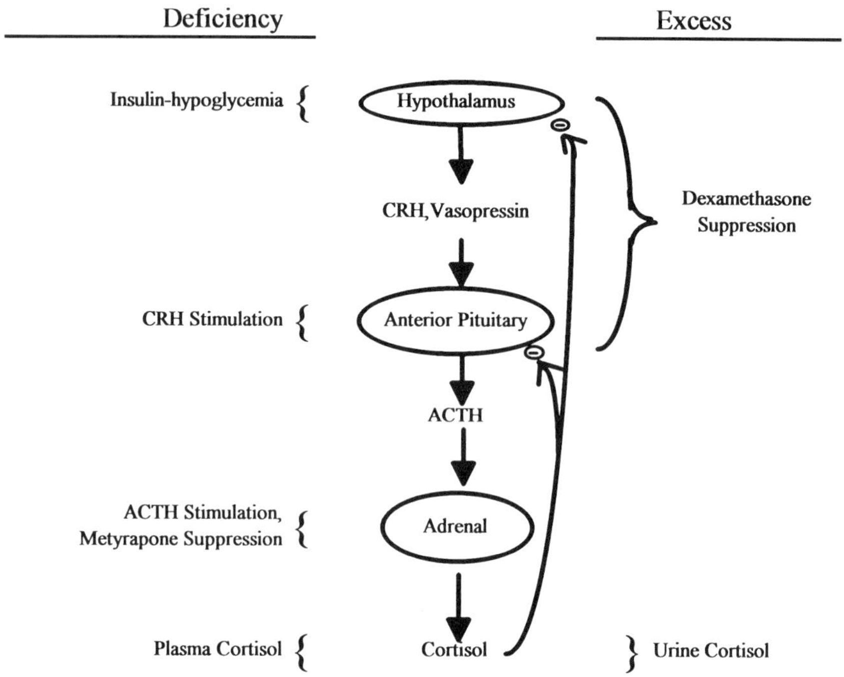

FIG 1.
Schematic representation of the hypothalamic-pituitary-adrenal (HPA) axis with the hormones released and the feedback inhibition by cortisol. Shown also are tests for evaluation of glucocorticoid excess *(left)* and deficiency *(right)*. *Brackets* indicate the site of action of the agent used for the test for the site of analysis. *CRH* = corticotropin-releasing hormone; ACTH = adrenocorticotropic hormone.

tients susceptible to adrenal hemorrhage[12, 22, 23] as well as in the intensive care unit setting.[5, 24–28] Thus, there is a large and increasing need to look for adrenal hypofunction.

Hyperfunction of the axis leads to cortisol excess, as is seen with spontaneous Cushing's syndrome, which is a rare condition. However, it occurs frequently with psychiatric problems, alcoholism, and ill patients with a lot of stress that are observed more commonly.[2, 3, 11, 27–37] The question arises frequently as to whether these patients have spontaneous Cushing's syndrome.[11] Thus, whereas circumstances in which glucocorticoid excess should be specifically treated are uncommon, the need to exclude the diagnosis of spontaneous Cushing's syndrome is relatively common.

Over the past few years, a lot of new information has been accumulated about both the hypofunctioning and the hyperfunctioning of the axis in various states and about how to evaluate them. In this chapter we review the disorders of the HPA axis, especially with respect to recent information, and we also review the approaches to diagnosis of hyperfunction and hypofunction. We emphasize situations that most commonly confront the nonspecialist in endocrinology, and we limit discussions of evaluation of both spontaneous Cushing's syndrome and adrenal insufficiency to the initial diagnosis. For more comprehensive discussions of the additional workup of such patients, particularly for distinguishing between the various causes of spontaneous Cushing's syndrome, the reader is referred to other sources.[2–4, 11]

The Hypothalamic-Pituitary-Adrenal Axis

The HPA axis is driven by the central nervous system (CNS). Input from the brain and spontaneous rhythms in the hypothalamus cause the release of CRH and vasopressin from the median eminence of the hypothalamus. CRH and vasopressin are released in a circadian fashion, i.e., in a pattern that repeats itself every 24 hours.[1–4, 11] Corticotropin-releasing hormone is produced in the paraventricular nuclei of the hypothalamus and in other parts of the CNS.[1, 38] Vasopressin is produced by magnocellular neurons of the supraoptic nuclei and also by neurons of the paraventricular nuclei.[3, 38] The neurons of the supraoptic nuclei terminate in the posterior pituitary and probably are not involved in regulation of ACTH. The neurons of the paraventricular nuclei release both CRH and vasopressin into the capillary vessels of the portal system that drains into the anterior pituitary and delivers these hormones for stimulation of ACTH. These hormones then bind to receptors specific for each hormone on the surface of corticotroph (ACTH-producing) cells in the anterior pituitary. CRH-binding activates adenyl cyclase, and vasopressin binding activates phosphoinositide hydrolysis with consequent effects on calcium ion mobilization and protein kinase C activation.[1, 39] Both of these processes stimulate ACTH release. In addition, CRH-induced ACTH secretion is potentiated by angiotensin II and inhibited by oxytocin.[1, 2] Adrenocorticotropic hormone is derived from a larger precursor protein, proopiomelanocortin (POMC).[2, 3] Corticotropin-releasing hormone and vasopressin stimulation also increase the production of POMC mRNA with consequent enhancement of POMC and ACTH synthesis.[1, 3] Corticotropin-releasing hormone also affects corticotroph function more generally. With long-term stimulation, there is corticotroph hyperplasia, whereas with suppressed CRH release, there is corticotroph atrophy.[1, 2]

The relative roles of CRH and vasopressin are still being deciphered.[1, 38, 39] In general, CRH alone is more potent than arginine vasopressin (AVP) alone, and the effects of CRH and AVP are synergistic.[1, 38, 39] Maximal responses require both hormones, and responses are blunted in the absence of either hormone.[1, 38, 39] Clinical disorders that destroy CRH production are likely to also impair hypothalamic release of vasopressin. Some stimuli, such as hypoglycemia, stimulate the release of both CRH and vasopressin, whereas others, such as exercise, stimulate the release of only vasopressin,[1, 40] implying that the two hormones have different but overlapping roles.[1, 39, 40]

The spontaneous rhythms of CRH and vasopressin release can be overridden by other influences on the CNS, dominantly stressful influences. Thus, severe anxiety, illness, trauma, and alcohol all can increase the stimulus to ACTH release.[1–4, 11, 27–37] These influences result in the long-term overstimulation of the axis with psychiatric problems, alcoholism, and illness.

The axis is also suppressed by glucocorticoids.[6, 10, 13–15] Cortisol feedback inhibits ACTH release through direct actions on both the corticotrophs and on the hypothalamus to block CRH release. The suppression involves both rapid influences that inhibit ACTH release within minutes and more delayed effects that suppress both ACTH synthesis and overall corticotroph function. Glucocorticoid suppression of the HPA axis is elicited both by endogenous cortisol and exogenously administered glucocorticoids. As discussed below, glucocorticoid suppression of the HPA axis with glucocorticoid therapy is a major medical problem.

The release of cortisol from the adrenal occurs in episodic pulses. These vary in magnitude and in frequency and result in rapid fluctuations in the plasma cortisol so that determinations taken within minutes can vary considerably.[2, 3, 41, 42] The number of pulses varies according to a circadian rhythm with an increasing number occurring in the early morning with a peak around 8:00 A.M., after which they decline considerably in number, so that cortisol in plasma can be nearly undetectable by late afternoon to early evening.

The daily production of cortisol is about 10 mg per 24 hours.[41, 43] This estimate is much lower than those obtained earlier.[2] It is of interest that the common glucocorticoid replacement doses were based on the earlier data, and the revised estimates, combined with clinical impressions that some patients receiving traditional replacement cortisol doses become cushingoid, have led to the suggestion that the replacement doses that are ordinarily given are too high.[43] Nevertheless, the overall experience with the previously used replacement doses has been favorable, and the currently available information does not provide a clear answer as to whether there should be any change. Until clearer data become available, we are continuing to utilize previously recommended regimens and recommend adjusting the dosages based on clinical assessment.

The activity of the HPA axis increases in stress.[2, 3, 27, 29, 31, 32] The major danger for the patient with Addison's disease is that stress can result in cardiovascular collapse. This is the reason for the poor prognosis of patients with Addison's disease in the era before the availability of glucocorticoids. When the first mineralocorticoid (deoxycorticosterone) became available, the prognosis of Addison's disease did not improve much, a finding that illustrates that it is the glucocorticoid component of the adrenal cortical secretions that is the most important for coping with the stresses.[2]

Whereas it is clear that glucocorticoids are required for coping with stress, it is not clear whether the increased levels of glucocorticoids that occur with stress are actually needed in these circumstances, and there are no good data on the issue in humans. However, a study in monkeys that were adrenalectomized and given either replacement or supraphysiologic doses of glucocorticoids before and after surgery revealed that the animals that had received the replacement doses had a better survival rate than did those that received higher doses of glucocorticoid.[44] Therefore, we cannot know that we need the higher dose of glucocorticoid. Whereas we continue to recommend administering higher doses of glucocorticoids for the patients with Addison's disease who are under stress, it is not clear that this is the best course.

The stimulation of the HPA axis and the total levels of cortisol that result is proportional overall to the severity of the illness/stress.[27, 28] In fact, in the patient without Addison's disease in the intensive care unit (ICU) setting, the basal level of cortisol correlates inversely with survival.[27, 28]

Abnormalities of the Hypothalamic-Pituitary-Adrenal Axis

Table 1 shows the various causes of both hypofunction and hyperfunction of the HPA axis, as well as the activities of the individual components of the axis that vary according to the nature of the primary disorder causing the abnormality. The table is organized according to the components that are deranged and depicts only endogenous components that are affected.

Hyperfunction

The most common causes of axis hyperfunction are excessive CNS stimulation secondary to stress, psychiatric problems, or excessive ethanol intake.[27, 29–37] The axis can also be excessively active in anorexia nervosa.[45] With stress, the activity to a point can be considered normal. The axis is usually excessively active with severe depression or anxiety.[29, 31–37] Typically, this has been correlated with nonsuppressed cerebrospinal fluid (CSF) CRH levels, potentially reflecting CRH hypersecretion in the etiology of the cortisol hypersecretion.[32, 46, 47] However, some patients without frank elevations of plasma cortisol levels can have low CSF CRH levels.[48] An unanswered question is whether the excessive activity of the axis in these disorders either aggravates or ameliorates the psychiatric problem. Not all psychiatric disorders are affected; for example the axis appears not to be activated excessively in many patients with schizophrenia.[49] The ethanol induced hyperactivity is related both to the amount and duration of use.[30, 50] It also occurs with withdrawal of ethanol.[30, 50]

The pituitary and adrenal are hyperactive with ACTH-producing pituitary tumors. Pituitary microadenomas account for about 60% to 70% of reported patients with spontaneous Cushing's syndrome, however, in many patients with the ectopic ACTH syndrome, the diagnosis is never established.[2, 4, 11, 51] The ACTH hypersecretion results in an increased number of pulses of cortisol release, with major increases during times of few releases in normals.[2, 52] Thus, the plasma cortisol levels tend to be more

TABLE 1.
Abnormalities of Hypothalamic-Pituitary-Adrenal Axis Function*

Abnormality	Effect on†		
	CRH	ACTH	Cortisol
Hyperfunction			
Hypothalamus, pituitary and adrenal			
Stress due to illness, trauma, surgery, etc.	↑	↑	↑
Psychiatric problems	↑	↑	↑
Alcoholism	↑	↑	↑
Pituitary and adrenal			
ACTH-producing pituitary tumors	↓	↑	↑
Ectopic CRH-producing tumors	↑	↑	↑
"Idiopathic" corticotroph hyperplasia	?	↑	↑
Adrenal			
Adrenal cortisol-producing tumors	↓	↓	↑
Ectopic ACTH-producing tumors	↓	↑	↑

Compensatory hyperfunction			
Congenital blocks in adrenal steroid biosynthesis (congenital adrenal hyperplasia)	↑	↑	↓→
Administration of blockers of adrenal steroid biosynthesis	↑	↑	↓→
Congenital glucocorticoid resistance	↑	↑	↑
Acquired glucocorticoid resistance	↑	↑	↑
Hypofunction			
Hypothalamus, pituitary and adrenal			
Glucocorticoid therapy	↓	↓	↓
After surgery for spontaneous Cushing's syndrome	↓	↓	↓
Pituitary and adrenal			
Panhypopituitarism	↑	↓	↓
Isolated ACTH deficiency	↑	↓	↓
Adrenal			
Addison's disease	↑	↑	↓
Congenital blocks in adrenal steroid biosynthesis	↑	↑	↓

*CRH = corticotropin-releasing hormone; ACTH = adrenocorticotropic hormone.
†Arrows refer to increased (up), decreased (down) or normal levels of activities of the various factors.

consistently higher during the late afternoon and evening than with normal subjects. With these tumors, the pituitary tumor is overactive; the cortisol excess suppresses the activity of both the normal corticotroph cells of the anterior pituitary and of the CRH-producing cells of the hypothalamus, but it suppresses the tumor cells only to a limited extent, such that ACTH hypersecretion persists.[2, 53]

Corticotropin-releasing hormone–producing tumors are exceedingly rare,[1] but they result in corticotroph hyperplasia and cortisol excess with suppression of CNS-CRH release.[1] There are rare reports of Cushing's syndrome caused by "idiopathic" corticotroph hyperplasia.[51] However, whether these are caused by CRH-producing tumors or are caused by one of the conditions that are described above is not clear. It is also not known whether problems such as ethanol abuse and psychiatric illness that stimulate the HPA axis result in corticotroph hyperplasia, although in principle, this is plausible. With corticotroph hyperplasia secondary to ectopic CRH hypersecretion, there presumably is cortisol-induced suppression of hypothalamic CRH release.

The adrenal is hyperactive in the ectopic ACTH syndrome and with cortisol producing adrenal tumors.[2–4, 11] With ectopic ACTH production, the cortisol excess suppresses both the hypothalamus and pituitary. This is also true with cortisol-producing adrenal tumors, but, in addition, the normal adrenal tissue is suppressed. More rarely, there is primary hyperplasia of the adrenal due to unknown causes, with adrenal hyperactivity and suppressed ACTH levels.[2–4, 11, 54]

Hypofunction

Primary Adrenocortical Insufficiency

Primary adrenal insufficiency (Addison's disease) is caused by destruction of the adrenal cortex. As cortisol production decreases, the lack of negative feedback increases the secretion of CRH and ACTH. The incidence of primary adrenocortical insufficiency is not known. As alluded to above, it appears to be increasing because of an increase in the incidence of AIDS and tuberculosis,[12, 16–21] both of which can lead to adrenal destruction. Moreover, its incidence caused by adrenal hemorrhage and in the intensive care unit setting may be generally underestimated.

Estimates of the incidence of overt adrenal insufficiency in patients with AIDS vary, but most estimates fall in the range of 5% or less.[5, 12, 16, 18, 55–57] However, pathologic adrenal abnormalities and more subtle abnormalities are seen in a much higher percentage (38%–88%).[5, 16, 18, 55–57]

At the time of its initial description, the most common cause of Addison's disease was tuberculous destruction of the adrenal.[2, 5, 12] With the gradual control of tuberculosis, this cause decreased substantially. The next major cause was the unusual syndrome of autoimmune destruction of the adrenal, which can be part of the polyglandular syndrome of autoimmune destruction, which can also affect the thyroid, gonads, parietal cells of the stomach, pancreatic islets, and parathyroids.[12, 16, 19–21] The incidence of tuberculosis is currently increasing because of the prevalence of AIDS and the emergence of antibiotic-resistant strains.[19–21]

Adrenal hemorrhage has been known for a long time to be a cause of adrenal insufficiency, and the original Waterhouse-Friderichsen syndrome was associated with bilateral adrenal hemorrhage.[2, 5, 12, 22, 23] However, this has generally been considered to be a rare cause of the disorder. More recent series do not provide precise numbers, but suggest that the problem may be more common than previously appreciated.[12, 22, 23] The patients who are most susceptible are those with complicated major medical illnesses in the setting of sepsis, anticoagulant therapy, or spontaneous coagulopathy.

The setting in which the question of the incidence of the disorder is the most important is with the severely ill patient, for example, those admitted to the intensive care unit. Failure to treat the patient with Addison's disease in these cases will frequently lead to cardiovascular collapse and death. The literature in this case is confusing. Based on earlier studies, it was suggested that the incidence of adrenal insufficiency in patients in the intensive care unit is high.[5, 24–26, 28] This view was more recently challenged in a study in which 70 selected patients were evaluated using the rapid ACTH test (discussed later), and only one case of de novo adrenal insufficiency was detected.[27] This patient's stimulated cortisol was 14 μg/dL and her hypotension responded to hydrocortisone.* A second patient was found to have adrenal insufficiency secondary to glucocorticoid therapy that was not elicited by the initial history. This patient had a stimulated cortisol of 13.6 μg/dL and required glucocorticoid replacement to ameliorate hypotension. The 70 patients that were examined were selected from 300 patients, and 92 patients were excluded because they were taking glucocorticoids. Since a significant proportion of these patients probably had secondary adrenal insufficiency (albeit many with secondary insufficiency), even this study may not exclude the possibility that the incidence of adrenal insufficiency in the intensive care unit is actually quite high.

Primary adrenal insufficiency also occurs in patients with congenital defects in adrenal steroid synthesis, of which the most common is deficiency of P450c21 (21α-hydroxylase). However, in patients with milder enzyme defects, adrenal cortical production can be normal due to the activation of the hypothalamus and pituitary with adrenal hyperplasia and production of enough steroids to overcome the block. Also, with a defect of P450c17 (17α-hydroxylase syndrome), there is compensatory increased production of corticosterone that can act as a glucocorticoid and overcome the block. Interestingly, 21-hydroxylase deficiency is one of the most common genetic diseases with an incidence of about 1 in 12,000 in the general population.[58]

*Plasma cortisol levels are indicated at μg/dL. Because nM/L is also commonly used, conversions are provided in Table 2.

TABLE 2.
Cortisol Conversion

μg/dL	nMol/L	nMOL/L	μg/dL
5	150	100	3.5
10	290	200	6.9
15	430	300	10.4
20	580	400	13.8
25	720	500	17.3
30	870	600	20.8
35	1010	700	24.2
40	1160	800	27.7

Secondary Adrenal Insufficiency

Secondary adrenocortical insufficiency is caused by inadequate ACTH that in turn can be caused by lesions of the pituitary that impair the ability of the corticotrophs to release ACTH, or hypothalamic lesions that impair release of CRH and vasopressin with secondary atrophy of adrenal cortical function.[1–4, 11] Deficiency of ACTH selectively impairs the cortisol-producing adrenal fasciculata and reticularis, and it only rarely is associated with impairment of the aldosterone-producing adrenal glomerulosa.

The most common cause for hypofunction of the HPA axis is glucocorticoid therapy that suppresses the axis at both hypothalamic and pituitary levels.[2, 3, 13, 14, 59] A similar but less common situation develops after corrective surgery for spontaneous Cushing's syndrome.[53] In spite of the introduction of a number of newer therapeutic modalities for suppression of inflammatory and immunologic responses, glucocorticoids continue to be used extensively in therapy. Suppression is most commonly observed with systemically administered glucocorticoids, and it is much less common with locally administered steroids.[13] Nevertheless, suppression can be observed when steroids are given topically, by intraarticular injection, or by inhalation.[5, 13, 14, 60]

The degree of suppression with glucocorticoid therapy is overall proportional to the total amount of glucocorticoid that is administered (dose times number of times administered).[6, 61–67] However, there is enormous variability in the extent of suppression in different individuals, and this makes it difficult to predict in individual cases.[6, 61–67] Whereas therapy with moderate to large doses of glucocorticoids for only a few days will in general profoundly suppress the axis, this suppression is rapidly reversible and does not persist. By contrast, when larger doses of glucocorticoid (e.g., 60 mg of prednisone per day) are given for longer periods of time (for example, over 1 year), there will be profound and longstanding suppression of the

HPA axis. Thus, if glucocorticoid therapy is discontinued, the patient will be unable to generate adequate quantities of cortisol and will exhibit glucocorticoid insufficiency.

Recovery of a profoundly suppressed HPA axis can require a long time. It was previously thought that such recovery will occur in most patients by 1 year,[53, 59] and this is probably true for most cases of suppression caused by glucocorticoid therapy.[53, 59, 66, 67] Further, the degree of suppression and recovery is roughly correlated with both the dose and the time of suppression.[53, 59, 66, 67] However, we have observed patients with ACTH-producing pituitary microadenomas with spontaneous Cushing's syndrome in whom as many as 2 years have been required for axis recovery following resection of the microadenoma. This has also been confirmed in other studies,[62, 63] in which the authors attributed the more delayed return to the fact that a number of patients received glucocorticoids for replacement for a longer period than did patients in the earlier studies.[62] Thus, all patients who have been exposed to large doses of exogenously administered or endogenously produced glucocorticoids for a significant period are candidates for potential HPA axis suppression, and when the clinical situation dictates, these patients should be evaluated for HPA axis suppression and/or receiving appropriate replacement glucocorticoid. Of course, this only becomes a problem when the glucocorticoid therapy is withdrawn.

More uncommon causes of secondary adrenal insufficiency are tumors and other infiltrative and invasive disorders of the hypothalamus and pituitary that lead to decreased CRH and/or ACTH secretion and cause secondary adrenocortical atrophy. Isolated ACTH deficiency is a rare cause of secondary hypoadrenalism which in some cases in caused by an autoimmune process.[68–70]

Glucocorticoid Resistance

In principle, hormone resistance in the presence of ordinarily adequate levels of glucocorticoids could also lead to a hormone deficiency syndrome. Given the extensive regulation of the sensitivity to hormones that is observed in other systems such as with insulin, it is surprising that there is so little evidence for the role of hormone resistance with glucocorticoids or glucocorticoid therapy. However, this probably occurs in several settings that are relevant for evaluating the HPA axis.

The most convincing syndrome includes the rare cases of glucocorticoid resistance that have in some instances been shown to be due to defects in the glucocorticoid receptor.[71–75] The resistance in these cases is partial, and the patients compensate by increased cortisol production. This can sometimes lead to a mineralocorticoid-excess syndrome,[72] caused by the mineralocorticoid actions of the excess cortisol and in other instances to hirsuitism[75] or isosexual precocity,[71] due to adrenal androgen hypersecretion. Addisonian problems have not, to our knowledge, been described in these patients.

A syndrome of glucocorticoid resistance is seen after withdrawal of glucocorticoids. The syndrome, termed the "steroid withdrawal syndrome,"[2, 13, 53, 65] has been observed most commonly following surgery for spontaneous Cushing's syndrome but also can be observed after withdrawal of glucocorticoid therapy. These patients complain of classical symptoms of adrenal insufficiency that are not relieved by the usual replacement doses of glucocorticoids, but are relieved by administering higher than replacement doses.[2, 13, 53, 65] Ultimately, the problem disappears. This observation implies that the patients are reversibly glucocorticoid resistant. Whereas the glucocorticoid resistance seems clinically evident, we do not know of cases where such patients have gone into shock on the usual replacement doses of glucocorticoids. Nevertheless, because of the overall clinical picture of adrenal insufficiency, we recommend treating the symptoms in these patients by administering increased dosage of glucocorticoids followed by a tapering of the steroid dose as tolerated.

A third situation has been described in patients with AIDS,[76] some of whom have been reported to have frank Addisonian symptoms such as weakness, gastrointestinal upset, and hypotension in the presence of elevated (usually) levels of plasma cortisol. The peripheral blood cells of these patients were found to be resistant to the actions of glucocorticoids to block thymidine uptake.[76] The incidence of this problem is not known, but we urge caution in approaching it. Whereas glucocorticoids can be useful for treating certain problems with AIDS, such as pneumocystis pneumonia,[77] glucocorticoid administration has also been associated with activation of Kaposi's sarcoma.[78] The catabolic and additional actions of glucocorticoids when given in excess may be deleterious for these patients.

Finally, intrinsic tissue resistance to the therapeutic actions of glucocorticoids has developed in some patients treated with glucocorticoids for asthma; these patients have not been studied after discontinuation of the steroid.[64]

The mechanisms for the development of the acquired glucocorticoid resistance are not understood. It appears that the glucocorticoid resistance is induced by prolonged exposure to high levels of glucocorticoids. The development of this apparent glucocorticoid resistance is variable, and it is not observed in all patients. Whether less clinically apparent glucocorticoid-induced resistance is more common is not known. Nevertheless, glucocorticoids can induce a downregulation of glucocorticoid responsiveness.[79] They decrease the rate of transcription of the glucocorticoid receptor gene with consequent decreases in the levels of receptor mRNA and in the production and levels of the receptors.[79] The glucocorticoid receptors were measured in the patients with glucocorticoid-resistant AIDS although there were changes in the affinity of the receptors for the steroid, receptor levels were, if anything, elevated.[76] The extent to which glucocorticoids induce their own responsiveness through postreceptor mechanisms is not known.

Indications for Evaluation of the Axis

When hypofunction of the HPA axis is suspected, the patient should be considered to be adrenally insufficient and followed as such until the diagnosis is excluded.[2–4, 11] In general, patients seen for the first time who do not give a previous history of prolonged exposure to high levels of glucocorticoids, either with therapy or because of spontaneous Cushing's syndrome, should be evaluated immediately unless they are too ill for evaluation, in which case they should be treated and the diagnosis established at a later date. If the patient does give a history of recent exposure to high levels of glucocorticoids for a prolonged period, is not currently taking them except for replacement, or is known to have recently had corrective surgery for spontaneous Cushing's syndrome, it is ordinarily easier to presume that the patient is adrenally insufficient. Therefore, such patients should be treated with replacement glucocorticoids and evaluated later.

Evaluation of adrenal function in patients with AIDS is particularly important, since these patients are commonly stressed because of their illness. It is also difficult to assess these patients clinically, since they commonly have symptoms such as hypotension, hyperkalemia, gastrointestinal upset, anorexia and weakness, without Addison's disease.

The major reason to evaluate for hyperfunction is to determine whether the patient has spontaneous Cushing's syndrome, which should be treated. There have been extensive studies to determine whether the detection of a suppressed HPA axis in patients with various psychiatric illnesses is helpful with the diagnosis of a serious disorder and whether knowing this would be helpful with therapy.* In general, with these cases, the suppression has been measured by dexamethasone-suppression testing using a protocol that differs from that used to detect the cortisol hypersecretion with spontaneous Cushing's syndrome.[6, 33, 34, 37, 50] To date, there has been very little documentation that this is helpful, and the use of such testing in psychiatric patients remains mostly a research procedure. If it ultimately becomes established that the glucocorticoid excess state in these or other conditions is either helpful or harmful, then such evaluation would be warranted. Hopefully, future studies will address this question.

Clinical Evaluation: History and Physical Examination

Although many manifestations of glucocorticoid excess and deficiency are subtle, important clinical information can be gained from the history and physical examination. The manifestations of glucocorticoid excess (Cushing's syndrome), with plethora, rounded faces, truncal obesity, thin extremities, buffalo hump, and easy bruising are known to most clinicians, and they are commonly observed in patients receiving large doses of glucocorticoids in therapy.[2–4, 11, 13] Many of these manifestations, especially plethora, are observed in individuals with pseudo-Cushing's syndrome (e.g., alcoholics).[30] It is stressed that changes in physical appearance are important. An index of this can be obtained by asking the patient to bring in one or several earlier photographs.

The manifestations of glucocorticoid deficiency include weakness, leth-

*References 1–4, 11, 32–37, 45, 46, 48, 49.

argy, anorexia, weight loss, gastrointestinal complaints, and low blood pressure.[2–5, 12] The blood pressure is low in patients with both primary and secondary adrenal insufficiency, and this is because of the lack of the glucocorticoid component of the deficiency, although it may be worsened by the combined mineralocorticoid deficiency that occurs with adrenal destruction in primary Addison's disease.

The distinction between primary and secondary adrenal insufficiency is suggested by two major differences in clinical manifestations.[2–5, 12] First, primary adrenal destruction results in secondary hyperfunction of the pituitary with elevated levels of ACTH and other POMC-derived peptides such as β-lipotropin, whereas patients with secondary adrenal insufficiency are ACTH deficient. Thus, patients with primary but not secondary adrenal insufficiency usually have increased pigmentation, which is due to melanocyte-stimulating hormone (MSH) sequences contained within the POMC-derived peptides. The pigmentation is particularly prominent in areas exposed to the sun, in skin creases, in scars that form during the time of POMC hyperproduction, in mucosal areas such as the lips, gums and buccal mucosae (particularly important areas in blacks), and in sites where there is pressure on the skin. The finding of pigmented and nonpigmented scars on the patients can help determine the date of onset of the increased POMC synthesis. Hyperpigmentation takes weeks to develop and therefore will not be present in patients in whom adrenal insufficiency has only recently developed. Hyperpigmentation does not occur in patients with ACTH deficiency; these patients typically present with pallor.

With primary adrenal insufficiency, there is also associated deficiency of mineralocorticoids, which leads to volume depletion, hypotension, hyponatremia, and hyperkalemia. Patients compensate for the sodium loss and dehydration by eating more salt and drinking more water; however, the hyperkalemia tends to persist unless the mineralocorticoid defect is treated by administering a steroid with mineralocorticoid activity. Patients with secondary adrenal insufficiency and decreased ACTH secretion may present with dilutional hyponatremia, but these patients only rarely present with hyperkalemia.

Clinical Evaluation: Laboratory Tests

Because the clinical manifestations in many cases are either subtle, nonspecific, or attributable to other causes, laboratory evaluation is usually important. However, in cases in which the diagnosis of adrenal insufficiency is strongly suspected and there is hypotension with concern of cardiovascular collapse, treatment should be initiated without waiting for test results. The diagnosis can be made at a later date. However, even in these cases, the physician can usually either obtain baseline cortisol levels or perform ACTH testing before administering therapy.

Basal Measurements

Plasma Cortisol Determination

The release of cortisol in episodic pulses results in rapid fluctuations in the plasma cortisol.[2, 3, 42, 52] Thus, determinations taken within minutes can vary considerably. In normal subjects, there can be low to undetectable plasma cortisol levels several times during the day, especially in the late afternoon and early evening hours, when the releases of cortisol are more infrequent due to the circadian rhythm. For these reasons, little reliance can be placed on a low basal plasma cortisol level in diagnosing adrenal insufficiency.

The finding of a low normal plasma level also does not exclude the diagnosis. With the progression of either primary or secondary adrenal insufficiency, there is a decrease in the number of cortisol releases, and the occasional releases that do occur can result in transient cortisol levels in the normal range. The absolute lower limit for the basal plasma cortisol level that will exclude adrenocortical insufficiency has not been determined. It has been suggested that the finding of a basal plasma cortisol in the 11 μg/dl or greater range "almost excluded ACTH and cortisol insufficiency",[80] and that patients with morning cortisol levels of 7 to 9 μg/dl or greater following pituitary surgery did not have clinical evidence for adrenal insufficiency.[81] However, there are examples in which the stimulated plasma cortisol has been has high as 14 μg/dl, and the patient required glucocorticoid therapy for hypotension[27]; there are also clear examples of adequate responses to severe stress with stimulated plasma cortisol levels in the 18-μg/dL range.[27] Given this information, we have adopted a rather conservative approach and argue that only the finding of a basal level of cortisol that excludes the diagnosis with stimulation testing (see later), i.e., of 20 μg/dl or greater can be taken to exclude the diagnosis, even though most patients with basal plasma cortisol determinations that are below 20 μg/dl do not have adrenal insufficiency. Thus, when the basal plasma cortisol is below 20 μg/dl, further testing is ordinarily warranted.[2, 8–10]

The determination of a basal plasma cortisol for evaluation of adrenocortical insufficiency may be most helpful with patients in acute situations, such as the patient in the intensive care unit and patients with AIDS who are commonly stressed by concomitant illnesses.[24–28, 82, 83] The plasma cortisol levels in these patients should generally be high. Thus, in some cases in which the basal plasma cortisol is repeatedly low (e.g., <5 μg/dl) in a setting of severe stress, the diagnosis of adrenocortical insufficiency can be made if the overall clinical picture is consistent.

The measurement of basal cortisol levels in assessing spontaneous Cushing's syndrome and other glucocorticoid excess states is also of limited usefulness. In general, more extensive tests are needed.[2–4, 11] Nevertheless, the repeated findings of very high plasma cortisol levels in the unstressed patient with suspected spontaneous Cushing's syndrome, for example, levels of 30 μg/dl or greater, is strongly suggestive of the diagnosis.

Conversely, if the plasma cortisol in such patients is repeatedly undetectable, iatrogenic glucocorticoid administration or intake of glucocorticoids in excess through some other means should be considered. However, in most patients with the common form of the spontaneous syndrome, plasma cortisol levels are commonly not elevated, although the plasma cortisol levels tend to be consistently higher during the late afternoon and early evening in these patients than are the levels in normal subjects. This observation has led to the determination of P.M. plasma cortisol levels for evaluating cortisol hypersecretion. However, these are not entirely reliable, since even in normal subjects there can be pulses in the late afternoon and early evening that make usefulness of the circadian changes less reliable.

Urine-Free Cortisol Determinations

The kidney filters the free steroids in plasma and reabsorbs most of it.[2, 3] About 92% of the total cortisol in plasma is bound to plasma proteins, mostly corticosteroid-binding globulin (transcortin or CBG). However, a small percentage of the cortisol is excreted unchanged and under normal circumstances, the 24-hour urinary cortisol excretion is 20 to 100 μg. The 24-hour urine cortisol is an excellent reflection of the relative total cortisol production. This test is usually referred to as the "urine-free cortisol." This was so named, because the test reflected the urinary cortisol that was unconjugated to other substances such as glucuronide and sulfate. The designation "free" ordinarily refers to the unbound material, and since the cortisol in urine is unbound, the designation urine-free cortisol is accurate. Overall, the urinary-free cortisol excretion provides an integrated assessment of the total cortisol production. The test therefore is an excellent one to assess whether there is glucocorticoid hypersecretion, and it has been standardized for this purpose. It might also be a useful test for evaluating adrenal insufficiency when compensatory influences begin to fail, but it has never been standardized for this purpose.[2] Thus, we recommend this test for initial evaluation of spontaneous glucocorticoid hypersecretion.

Elevated urinary-free cortisol values are seen with spontaneous Cushing's syndrome; they are also elevated with any of the conditions that stimulate the HPA axis as described above.[2, 4, 11] Thus, the test is particularly useful for ruling out the diagnosis of glucocorticoid hypersecretion. False negatives in this setting occur only in the rare setting of episodic Cushing's syndrome and with improper urinary collections. When elevated results are obtained, the physician should then determine whether the glucocorticoid hypersecretion is due to one of the causes of spontaneous Cushing's syndrome or one of the other causes of HPA axis stimulation.

Plasma Adrenocorticotropic Hormone Determination

Basal plasma ACTH levels are not generally useful in the primary diagnosis of adrenal excess or deficiency states but are extremely useful in differentiating between primary and secondary adrenal disorders.[2, 4, 11] In normal individuals basal A.M. ACTH levels range from 20 to 100 pg/ml when measured by traditional radioimmunoassay and 10 to 50 pg/ml with more recent immunoradiometric (IRMA) methods.[2–4] Plasma ACTH levels are elevated in primary adrenal insufficiency, usually to the range of 200 to >1,000 pg/ml.[2–4, 11] In contrast in secondary adrenal insufficiency, plasma ACTH levels are low normal or subnormal, i.e., less than 20 pg/ml.[2–4, 11] With spontaneous Cushing's syndrome A.M. plasma ACTH levels are usually 50 to 200 pg/ml in patients with Cushing's disease and are frequently greater than 200 pg/ml to as high as 10,000 pg/ml in the ectopic ACTH syndrome.[2–4, 11] In patients with primary adrenal tumors or hyperplasia, the plasma ACTH levels are generally less than 20 pg/ml.[2–4, 11]

Stimulation of the Hypothalamic-Pituitary-Adrenal Axis

As discussed earlier, if the basal plasma cortisol is lower than 20 μg/dl, provocative tests are generally required for diagnosis. In the outpatient setting where there is a question of adrenal insufficiency, we find it generally more convenient to perform provocative testing as the initial approach, since the basal cortisol will commonly be less than 20 μg/dl.

Three major means for testing are currently available. These include the rapid ACTH test, the metapyrone test, and the insulin-hypoglycemia test. At this writing, CRH is not available for use. However, since it is likely that it ultimately will be available and be used, it is also described. The preferred test of those currently available is the rapid ACTH stimulation test. This test is simple and results in little patient discomfort. The metapyrone and insulin-hypoglycemia tests are more rigorous but have major disadvantages for patient comfort and safety.[2, 3] Several other tests also have been developed, such as the use of vasopression, but these have largely been supplanted by the tests described following.

Rapid Adrenocorticotropic Hormone Testing

This test utilizes cosyntropin (Cortrosyn, tetracosactrin, Synacthen), a synthetic ACTH 1-24 amino acid peptide that has the full biologic activity of ACTH 1-37. The peptide is injected intravenously or intramuscularly in a dose of 250 μg, and plasma cortisol levels are then measured at 30 to 60 minutes.[5, 7, 8, 10, 83, 84] This dose is in excess of the maximally effective dose.[10] In normal subjects the response is maximal by 30 minutes and persists for about 1 hour. Thus, measurement of stimulated cortisol levels can be taken at any time during this period. With primary adrenal insufficiency, the damaged adrenal cannot respond, and with secondary insufficiency, the secondarily atrophic adrenal also cannot respond.

The results have in general been analyzed in terms of either the absolute peak or incremental cortisol levels that result from the stimulation.[5, 7–10, 83, 84] There now appears to be general agreement that the absolute peak level provides the best assessment. In analyzing the data from a number of these studies, we concur with the formulation of May and Carey[8] who concluded that a stimulated plasma cortisol of 20 μg/dl or greater, provides an acceptable exclusion of the diagnosis. In this study, whereas the peak stimulated plasma cortisol level was proportional to the basal, the incremental change was inversely proportional to the basal; changes of less than 7 μg/dl, a value previously used to assess responsiveness, were common with basal cortisol levels in the 21 to 30 μg/dl range.[8] The results of repeated tests in the same patient generally give an excellent correlation[8]; however, there are several situations in which a marginal result for a test will fall into the clearly normal range on repeat.[8] Other recent studies have confirmed these findings and have additionally shown that the test can be performed at any time during the day.[10, 83]

Whereas it appears most unlikely that individuals who achieve a plasma cortisol level of 20 μg/dl or greater in the basal state or with stimulation will not have adrenal insufficiency, it is more difficult to set a lower limit to the test. As mentioned earlier, there are clearly documented cases of hypotension requiring therapy with stimulated cortisol levels in the 14 μg/dl range[27]; thus, values of this magnitude or lower must be considered as insufficient and the patient presumed to have adrenal insufficiency. However, in marginal cases, it is probably preferable to repeat the workup at a later time.

An abnormal response to the ACTH test establishes the diagnosis of primary or secondary adrenal insufficiency, and these two conditions can then be differentiated with the basal ACTH level measurements. Also, a normal response excludes primary adrenal insufficiency.

In a few patients with partial secondary insufficiency, there can be sufficient ACTH secretion so that adrenal atrophy does not occur. These patients can have normal or near normal responses to ACTH stimulation, but abnormal responses to other tests such as insulin hypoglycemia.[7, 15] Secondary adrenal insufficiency should be suspected when there is a rise in the plasma cortisol from low levels, for example, in the 1 to 5 μg/dl range to the 5 to 10 μg/dl range. However, in spite of these concerns, we do not know of cases, using the aforementioned criteria, where the test has given false-negative results, and most of the confusion in the past has been when the fold rise in plasma cortisol level was used, rather than the maximally stimulated level.

There has been some attention placed on establishing more sensitive indices of detecting milder impairment of the HPA axis.[10, 66] For example, lowering the dose of cortrosyn[10] will allow detection of more subtle abnormalities. However, it is not clear how useful such testing is, since the responses are not correlated with the patient's ability to respond to stress. Therefore, we do not recommend these tests at this time.

Metapyrone Testing

Metapyrone blocks adrenal steroid biosynthesis by inhibiting P450c11, the enzyme responsible for the 11β-hydroxylation of 11-deoxycortisol to cortisol, although other steps are inhibited to a lesser extent.[2, 3] In normal subjects, this block results in decreased cortisol production with consequent increases in ACTH production. The elevated ACTH levels stimulate the adrenal to produce large quantities of 11-deoxycortisol (also called compound S or cortexolone), and the response of this hormone is measured.

The usual protocol is to administer metapyrone 2.0 to 3.0 g (30 mg/kg) orally at midnight; plasma cortisol and 11-deoxycortisol levels are measured at 8:00 A.M. the following morning.[2, 4] The normal response is a plasma 11-deoxycortisol of greater than 7 μg/dL. The test is most useful in assessing patients with suspected secondary adrenal insufficiency who have normal or near normal responses to ACTH stimulation. A positive response indicates an intact HPA axis, and there are few false-positive or false-negative responses.

Whereas this is an excellent test, it suffers from the fact that metapyrone administration causes significant gastrointestinal discomfort, and the patient with marginal adrenal insufficiency is exposed to further inhibition of steroid biosynthesis. The test is generally reserved for those few patients with suspected secondary adrenal insufficiency who have normal or borderline responses to the rapid ACTH stimulation test.[2, 4]

Insulin-Hypoglycemia Testing

Insulin-induced hypoglycemia is a stress that stimulates ACTH and cortisol release in normal subjects.[2, 3] Thus, the test is based on administering insulin in sufficient dosage to lower the plasma glucose level to less than 40 mg/dl. Plasma cortisol levels are then measured at 45, 60, and 90 minutes. A normal response is a peak plasma cortisol level of greater than 18 μg/dl. The test is excellent for excluding the diagnosis of pituitary insufficiency, and it allows the concomitant measurement of the growth hormone response. A normal response excludes adrenal insufficiency and predicts a normal adrenal response to stress. In general, the results of the test show excellent agreement with those of the rapid ACTH stimulation test.* Even though the test is safe when performed with proper caution, it remains a cumbersome procedure that is associated with some patient risk and discomfort. We find that this test is rarely required for assessing adrenal insufficiency and mostly utilize it in certain cases to evaluate panhypopituitarism.

Corticotropin-Releasing Hormone Testing

For this test,[1, 29, 31, 88] CRH is administered, and then the plasma cortisol and ACTH levels are measured. A normal test result requires that the pituitary responds with an increase in ACTH release and that the adrenal responds to the ACTH with an increase in cortisol release. Ordinarily, CRH is administered at a dose of 1 μg/kg body weight, which is lower than the maximally effective dose which is in the 3 to 10 μg/kg range.[1] Higher doses are associated with a significantly higher incidence of adverse side effects, particularly, transient shortness of breath, tachycardia, and decreased blood pressure.[1] The plasma cortisol and ACTH are measured before and at one or two 15-minute intervals after the injection. The stimulation in normal subjects tends to be maximal in about 15 minutes, and the plateau tends to be constant for about 1 hour. Various protocols have been examined, but overall it appears that a cortisol at the 15 to 60-minute

*References 2–5, 7, 9, 11–17, 40, 85–89.

time point provides an acceptable endpoint. These are around 22.5 +/− 5.2 μg/dl.[1]

A lack of a cortisol response provides strong evidence for primary or secondary adrenal insufficiency.[1] These two conditions can then be differentiated with the use of the ACTH level. This will be low to undetectable with secondary adrenal insufficiency due to pituitary or hypothalamic dysfunction, whereas it will be high with primary adrenal insufficiency (aforementioned).

The CRH test can be useful in differentiating hypothalamic from pituitary causes of secondary adrenal insufficiency.[1] Patients with primary pituitary insufficiency, either isolated ACTH deficiency or panhypopituitarism, have depressed ACTH responses to CRH, whereas patients with hypothalamic CRH deficiency have prolonged and exaggerated responses.

In general, a normal response excludes the diagnosis of either primary or secondary adrenal insufficiency. This is virtually always true with primary deficiency, but there is some concern that patients with partial pituitary dysfunction and secondary deficiency may maintain normal responsiveness.

The CRH test is also useful for distinguishing pituitary from ectopic causes of ACTH hypersecretion, although as is the case with dexamethasone suppression testing, there is a some overlap between the two groups.[1, 88, 90]

More recently, there has been increased focus on the use of CRH testing for differentiating Cushing's from pseudo-Cushing's syndromes.[1, 29, 31, 88] The standard CRH test tends to show a blunted ACTH response to CRH with depression and alcoholism, but an enhanced response with Cushing's disease.[1, 30, 88] By contrast, the cortisol response to CRH in depression tends to be normal.[1] In a recently proposed modification,[31] the CRH test is performed 2 hours after the last dose of 0.5 mg of dexamethasone has been administered, every 6 hours for 8 doses (low-dose dexamethasone suppression). The logic for this is that the pituitary is more responsive to the dexamethasone with pseudo-Cushing's syndrome than with Cushing's disease, and that the stimulation of cortisol by CRH in the latter group would show even greater differences than in the nonsuppressed state. The results show a clear distinction between the two groups.[31]

Suppression Testing

Suppression tests are utilized to assess hyperfunction of the HPA axis. These have been developed to diagnose the presence of spontaneous Cushing's syndrome and to determine the specific etiology when it is present. The dominant test used to document the presence of glucocorticoid excess, along with measurements of the urine cortisol, is the dexamethasone suppression test. This test is abnormal in states of excessive HPA-axis activity.

There are both low-dose and high-dose dexamethasone suppression tests.[2–4, 11] The low-dose test is used to detect abnormal glucocorticoid hypersecretion. The high-dose test is used to determine whether the hypersecretion is caused by a pituitary or extrapituitary cause of the disorder. The high-dose test is not described, but in general, a higher dose of dexamethasone (8 mg in an overnight dose, or 2 mg 4 times daily for 2 days) is given. In the presence of documented abnormal glucocorticoid hypersecretion, suppression by about 50% of the plasma cortisol levels is suggestive of Cushing's disease of pituitary origin, whereas a lack of suppression suggests either an adrenal tumor or ectopic ACTH hypersecretion.[2–4, 11]

Low-Dose Dexamethasone Testing

The low-dose dexamethasone test is based on the premise that the normal HPA axis is readily suppressed by even a physiologic dose of a glucocorticoid, whereas with abnormal activation of the axis or components of it, small doses of glucocorticoids do not have such a suppressive influence.[2–4, 11] Various protocols have been studied, and the dose, time of administration, and frequency of administration of the glucocorticoid have been varied. Based on these, two protocols have come into general use. One is the overnight dexamethasone suppression test that we prefer, and the other is a 2-day dexamethasone suppression test.

Overnight, Low-Dose Dexamethasone Suppression Test.—A 1-mg dose of dexamethasone is administered at 11:00 P.M. and the plasma cortisol level is measured at 8:00 A.M. In normal subjects, this protocol will reduce the 8:00 A.M. plasma cortisol level to less than 5 μg/dl, whereas this will not occur with abnormal activation of the axis.[2–4, 11] In general, the finding of a plasma cortisol level of greater than 10 μg/dL is regarded as abnormal, and values in the 5- to 10-μg/dL range are considered as indeterminate with further testing recommended, if the clinical situation so dictates.

Two-Day, Low-Dose Dexamethasone Suppression Test.—For this test, 0.5 mg of dexamethasone is administered every 6 hours for 2 days, and 24-hour urinary cortisol levels are measured during the second day and a palsma cortisol is measured at 8:00 A.M. after the last dose. A normal response is considered to be a plasma cortisol level of less than 5 μg/dL and a urine cortisol level of less than 20 μg/24 hours.[2–4, 11]

Interpretation of Dexamethasone Suppression Testing Results.— As stated earlier, these tests are reasonably accurate in detecting the presence of HPA axis overactivity. A normal response to either of these tests excludes Cushing's syndrome with 98% diagnostic accuracy.[2–4, 11] False-negative results occur rarely in patients with episodic Cushing's syndrome and in patients with abnormally slow metabolism of dexamethasone.[4, 11] "False-positive" results are more common because of activation of the HPA axis by the causes described earlier, other than those causing spontaneous Cushing's syndrome and can also be observed with obesity.

A normal response to the overnight test excludes the diagnosis of Cushing's syndrome with the rare exceptions mentioned above. In patients with equivocal responses in the positive range, the two-day test will provide more convincing distinctions in most cases.[2–4, 11]

Naloxone Blockade

Naloxone is being considered as a potential means to distinguish between Cushing's disease and CNS causes of ACTH hypersecretion.[85, 91] The opioid antagonist, naloxone, probably acting through the opiod delta receptors, can increase the release of ACTH, a finding that has been interpreted to suggest that CRH secretion is under tonic opioid inhibition.[1] Utilizing the postulate that the ACTH hypersecretion in pseudo-Cushing's syndrome is caused by CNS-driven CRH release, whereas that from Cushing's disease is not,[91] studies have been initiated to determine whether the ACTH and cortisol response to naloxone can be used to distinguish these two conditions. The final results are not yet available, but a preliminary analysis of the data suggests that this test may show promise.

Diagnosis of Adrenal Insufficiency

A flow diagram for evaluating adrenal insufficiency is shown in Figure 2. In the critical care setting, where there is hypotension or shock and the diagnosis is suspected, the patient should be treated before waiting for the re-

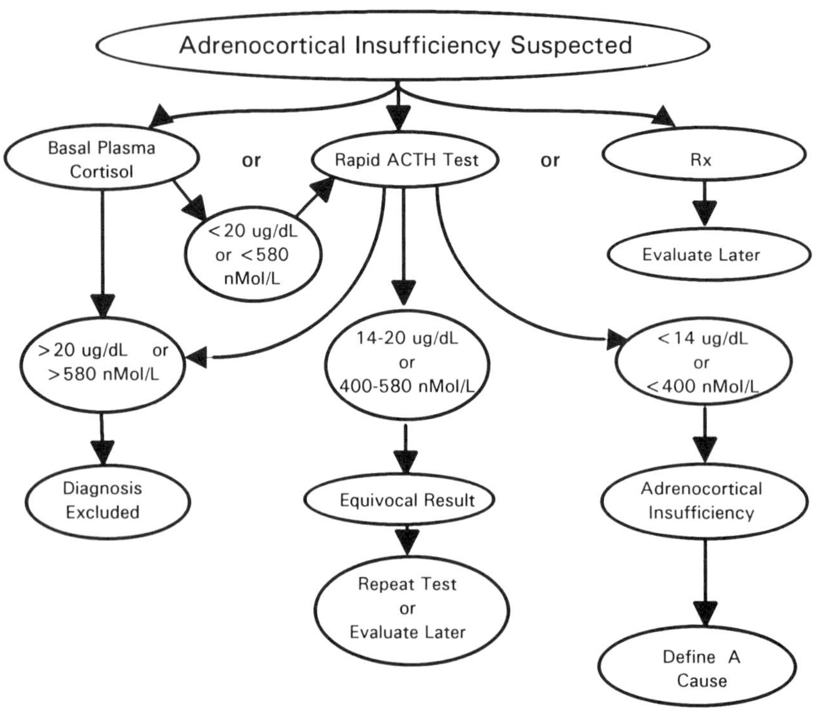

FIG 2.
Scheme for evaluation of adrenocortical insufficiency. ACTH = adrenocorticotropic hormone.

sults of diagnostic tests. Usually, there will be time to obtain either basal or stimulated cortisol samples before therapy is initiated. In any setting, once the diagnosis is suspected, the physician should obtain either a basal plasma cortisol level or perform the rapid ACTH stimulation test. In the outpatient setting, where the patient is not severely ill or stressed, it is more efficient to first perform the rapid ACTH stimulation test, because the basal plasma cortisol level will frequently be low enough to require the stimulation test anyway. However, with severely ill or stressed patients, the stress commonly results in elevated cortisol levels, and a basal cortisol value will suffice. For example, this is commonly the case with patients with AIDS in whom the diagnosis is suspected.

For patients known to have recently been exposed to high levels of glucocorticoids for a prolonged period due to glucocorticoid therapy or spontaneous Cushing's syndrome (but who are no longer receiving glucocorticoids other than for replacement), it is convenient to administer replacement doses of a glucocorticoid (e.g., 5 mg of prednisone daily by mouth at 8:00 A.M.) and monitor the basal A.M. cortisol levels on a monthly basis. This should be done before the patient has taken any steroid that morning, and only if he or she has not taken cortisol for at least 12 hours, or any longer-acting steroids for longer periods. In general, this would imply 24 hours without prednisone or prednisolone and even longer periods for steroids such as dexamethasone. In addition, with certain injected steroids, the glucocorticoid can persist for much longer periods.[13] Once basal plasma cortisol levels have returned to the normal range,[2, 3, 13] then the rapid ACTH test can be performed if necessary.

As discussed earlier, we feel that if the basal cortisol level is 20 μg/dl or greater, the diagnosis of adrenocortical insufficiency is excluded. If it is less than 20 μg/dl, then the rapid ACTH stimulation test is recommended. If the test results in a plasma cortisol level of 20 μg/dl or greater, then the diagnosis is excluded. If the stimulated value is 14 μg/dl or less, adrenocortical insufficiency is likely, and the patient should be followed as such and treated with subsequent evaluations depending on the specific case. If the cortisol level is in the 15- to 20-μg/dl range, then the test should be repeated. Once the diagnosis is made, then primary vs. secondary adrenal insufficiency can be diagnosed by measurement of the plasma ACTH level, which will be high in primary and low with secondary adrenal insufficiency. However, plasma ACTH measurements are rarely necessary to do this after glucocorticoid therapy.

Diagnosis of Glucocorticoid Excess

Figure 3 shows a flow diagram for diagnosing glucocorticoid excess. We recommend first performing the low-dose dexamethasone suppression test. If this test is normal and the clinical suspicion is low, then the diagnosis is excluded, except when there is episodic Cushing's syndrome. If the clinical suspicion is high or if the low-dose dexamethasone suppression test result is abnormal, then a 24-hour urine-free cortisol is obtained. The 24-

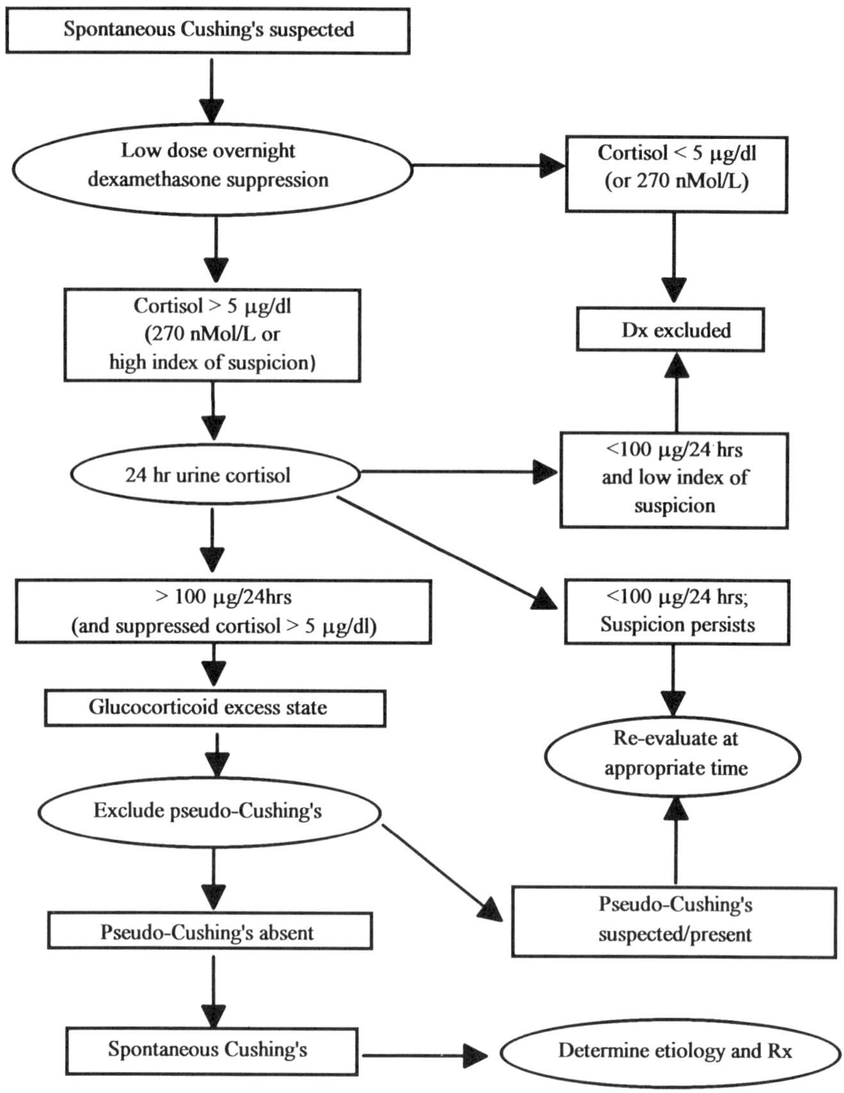

FIG 3.
Scheme for evaluation of spontaneous Cushing's syndrome.

hour urine cortisol level can be normal in the face of an abnormal suppression test in obesity and with the concurrent administration of certain drugs such as barbiturates and anticonvulsants that enhance dexamethasone metabolism. In these states, and in cases where the results are borderline, further workup should be dictated by the degree of clinical suspicion and the overall knowledge of these factors. In many cases a decision to repeat the workup at a later date can be made. If both tests are abnormal, then a glucocorticoid excess state is present. In this case, then the workup involves differentiating the various causes of glucocorticoid excess as described in other sources. The major problem is differentiating spontaneous Cushing's syndrome from pseudo-Cushing's syndrome. As discussed before, promising research is being done to design tests that will help with making this distinction. However, none of these are currently available. Therefore, we ordinarily approach this by utilizing all aspects of the history and physical examination to look for depression, alcoholism, or any of the other causes of pseudo-Cushing's syndrome, and if we think that these are likely, we attempt, if warranted, to reevaluate when these are no longer present. However, it is also recognized, especially given that the incidence of psychiatric problems with spontaneous Cushing's syndrome is so high, that spontaneous Cushing's syndrome may occur in the presence of depression, alcoholism, and other stresses, and that there is no substitute for clinical judgment in these situations.

Perspective

Hyperfunction and hypofunction of the adrenal cortex, which were earlier thought of as rare problems, are now considered as common and major problems. This is due to the emergence of new diseases such as AIDS, the continued use of glucocorticoids in therapy, greater recognition of the presence of adrenocortical insufficiency, and appreciation of the extent of overactivity of the HPA axis in conditions such as stress, alcoholism, and depression.

Our thinking over the years about the function of the axis has expanded greatly, although certain key questions remain unanswered. For example, we still do not know whether the higher levels of glucocorticoids that are produced in stress are helpful or harmful or the optimal dose of glucocorticoid to give the Addisonian patient in stress.

Whereas our ability to diagnose conditions of overactivity and underactivity of the axis has increased greatly, problems remain. We do not have clear criteria for diagnosing adrenal insufficiency, we do not have simple tests to differentiate spontaneous Cushing's syndrome from pseudo-Cushing's syndrome, and commonly, we have difficulty in differentiating the various causes of spontaneous Cushing's syndrome.

Nevertheless, with the combination of clinical judgment and today's sophisticated laboratory tests, it is possible to successfully diagnose and treat these disorders. This brief chapter has attempted to summarize those principles that allow optimization of the information and technology that is currently available.

References

1. Orth DN: Corticotropin-releasing hormone in humans. *Endocr Rev* 1992; 13:164.
2. Baxter JD, Tyrrell JB: The Adrenal Cortex, in Felig P, Baxter JD, Broadus AH,

et al (eds): *Endocrinology and Metabolism,* New York, McGraw Hill, 1986, pp 511–650.

3. Orth DN, Kovacs WJ, DeBold CR: The adrenal cortex, in Wilson JD, Foster DW (eds): *Williams Textbook of Endocrinology,* ed 8. Philadelphia, WB Saunders, 1992, pp 489–620.
4. Tyrrell JB, Aron DC, Forsham PH: Glucocorticoids and the adrenal androgens, in Greenspan FS (ed): *Basic and Clinical Endocrinology,* ed 3. Norwalk, Conn, Appleton and Lange, 1991, pp 323–362.
5. Werbel SS, Ober KP: Acute adrenal insufficiency. *Endocrinol Metabol Clin North Amer* 1993; 22:303.
6. Axelrod L: Glucocorticoid therapy. *Medicine* 1976; 55:39.
7. Lindholm JL, Kehlet H: Re-evaluation of the clinical value of the 30 min ACTH test in assessing the hypothalamic-pituitary-adrenocortical function. *Clin Endocrinol* 1987; 25:53.
8. May ME, Carey RM: Rapid adrenocorticotropic hormone test in practice–Retrospective review. *Am J Med* 1985; 79:679.
9. Nelson JC, Tindall DJ: A comparison of the adrenal responses to hypoglycemia, metyrapone and ACTH. *Am J Med Sci* 1978; 275:165.
10. Dickstein G, Shechner C, Nicholson WE, et al: Adrenocorticotropin stimulation test: Effects of basal cortisol level, time of day, and suggested new sensitive low dose test. *J Clin Endocrinol Metab* 1991; 72:773.
11. Aron DC, Findling JW, Tyrrell JB: Cushing's disease. *Endocr Metab Clin North Amer* 1987; 16:705.
12. Chadosh LA, Daniels GH: Addison's disease. *The Endocrinologist* 1993; 3:166.
13. Tyrrell JB, Baxter JD: Glucocorticoid therapy, in Felig P, Baxter JD, Broadus AE, Frohman LA, et al (eds): *Endocrinology and Metabolism.* New York, McGraw-Hill, 1986, pp 788–817.
14. Baxter JD: The effects of glucocorticoid therapy. *Hospital Practice* 1992; p 111.
15. Stewart PM, Corrie J, Seckl JR, et al: A rational approach for assessing the hypothalamo-pituitary-adrenal axis. *Lancet* 1988; 1:1208.
16. Glascgow BJ, Steinsapir KD, Anders K, et al: Adrenal pathology in the acquired immune deficiency syndrome. *Am J Clin Path* 1985; 84:594.
17. Strauss KW: Endocrine complications of the acquired immune deficiency syndrome. *Arch Intern Med* 1991; 51:1441.
18. Masharani U, Schambelan MS: The endocrine complications of the acquired immunodeficiency syndrome. *Adv Intern Med* 1993; 38:323.
19. Buxi TBS, Vohra RB, Shrishti PB, et al: CT in adrenal enlargement due to tuberculosis; A review of literature with five new cases. *Clin Imaging* 1992; 16:102.
20. McMurray JF, Long D, McClure R, et al: Addison's disease with adrenal enlargement on computed tomographic scanning: Report of two cases of tuberculosis and review of the literature. *Am J Med* 1984; 77:365.
21. Vita JA, Silverberg SJ, Goland RS, et al: Clinical clues to the cause of Addison's disease. *Am J Med* 1985; 78:461.
22. Rao RH, Vagnucci AH: The clinical profile and management of bilateral massive adrenal hemorrhage. *Adv in Endocrinol Metab* 1992; 3:213.
23. Siu SCB, Kitzman DW, Sheedy PF, et al: Adrenal insufficiency from bilateral adrenal hemorrhage. *Mayo Clin Proc* 1990; 65:664.
24. Rothwell PM, Udwadia ZF, Lawler PG: Cortisol response to corticotropin and survival in septic shock. *Lancet* 1991; 1:582.

25. McKee JL, Finlay WE: Cortisol replacement in severely stressed patients. *Lancet* 1983; 1:484.
26. Bagley C: Serum cortisol levels in severely stressed patients. *Lancet* 1982; 1:1414.
27. Jurney TH, Cockrell JL, Lindberg JS, et al: Spectrum of serum cortisol response to ACTH in ICU patients. *Chest* 1987; 92:292.
28. Wade CE, Lindberg JS, Cockrell JL, et al: Upon admission adrenal steroidogenesis is adapted to the degree of illness in intensive care patients. *J Clin Endocrinol Metab* 1988; 67:223.
29. Gold PW, Loriaux DL, Roy A, et al: Responses to corticotropin-releasing hormone in the hypercortisolism of depression and Cushing's disease. *N Engl J Med* 1986; 314:1329.
30. Wand GS, Dobs AS: Alterations in the hypothalamic-pituitary-adrenal axis in actively drinking alcoholics. *J Clin Endocrinol Metab* 1991; 72:1290.
31. Yanovski JA, Cutler GB, Chrousos GP, et al: Corticotropin-releasing hormone stimulation following low-dose dexamethasone administration: A new test to distinguish Cushing's syndrome from pseudo-Cushing's states. *JAMA* 1993; 269:2232.
32. Kling MA, Roy A, Doran AR, et al: Cerebrospinal fluid immunoreactive corticotropin-releasing hormone and adrenocorticotropin-releasing hormone and adrenocorticotropin secretion in Cushing's disease and major depression: Potential clinical implications. *J Clin Endocrinol Metab* 1991; 72:260.
33. Joseph-Vanderpool JR, Rosenthal NE, Chrousos GP, et al: Abnormal pituitary-adrenal responses to corticotropin-releasing hormone in patients with seasonal affective disorder: Clinical and pathophysiological implications. *J Clin Endocrinol Metab* 1991; 72:1382.
34. Holsboer F, Muller OA, Doerr HG, et al: ACTH and multisteroid responses to corticotropin-releasing factor in depressive illness: Relationship to multisteroid responses after ACTH stimulation and dexamethasone suppression. *Psychneuroendocrinology* 1984; 9:147.
35. Carroll BJ, Curtis GC, Davies BM, et al: Urinary free cortisol excretion in depression. *Psychological Med* 1976; 6:43.
36. Roy-Byrne PP, Uhde TW, Post RM, et al: The corticotropin-releasing hormone stimulation test in patients with panic disorder. *Am J Psychiatry* 1986; 143:896.
37. Sachar EJ, Hellman L, Roffwarg H, et al: Disrupted 24-hour patterns of cortisol secretion in psychotic depression. *Arch Gen Psychiatry* 1973; 28:19.
38. Antoni FA: Hypothalamic control of adrenocorticotropin secretion: Advances since the discovery of 41-residue corticotropin-releasing factor. *Endocrinol Rev* 1986; 7:351.
39. Ok Y, Nicholson WE, Orth DN: Role of protein kinase-C in the adrenocorticotropin secretory response to arginine vasopressin (AVP) and the synergistic response to AVP and corticotropin-releasing factor by perfused rat anterior pituitary cells. *Endocrinology* 1990; 127:350.
40. Wittert GA, Stewart GA, Graves MP, et al: Plasma corticotropin releasing factor and vasopressin responses to exercise in normal man. *Clin Endocrinol (Oxf)* 1991; 35:311.
41. Kerrogan JR, Veldhuis JD, Leyo SA, et al: Estimation of daily cortisol production and clearance rates in normal pubertal males by deconvolution analysis. *J Clin Endocrinol Metab* 1993; 76:1505.
42. Katz FH, Romfh P, Smith JA: Diurnal variation of plasma aldosterone, cortisol and renin activity in supine man. *J Clin Endocrinol Metab* 1977; 45:35.

43. Esteban NV, Loughlin T, Yergey AL, et al: Daily cortisol production rate in man determined by stable isotope dilution/mass spectrometry. *J Clin Endocrinol Metab* 1991; 72:39.
44. Udelsman R, Ramp J, Gallucci WT, et al: Adaptation during surgical stress: A re-evaluation of the role of glucocorticoids. *J Clin Invest* 1986; 77:1377.
45. Gwirtsman HE, Kaye WH, George DT, et al: Central and peripheral ACTH and cortisol levels in anorexia nervosa and bulimia. *Arch Gen Psych* 1989; 46:61.
46. Kling MA, Rubinow DR, Doran AR, et al: Cerebrospinal fluid immunoreactive somatostatin concentrations in patients with Cushing's disease and major depression: Relationship to indices of corticotropin-releasing hormone and cortisol secretion. *Neuroendocrinology* 1993; 57:79.
47. Nemeroff CB, Widerlov E, Bissette G, et al: Elevated concentrations of CSF corticotropin-releasing factor-like immunoreactivity in depressed patients. *Science* 1984; 236:1342.
48. Geracioti TD, Orth DN, Ekhator NN, et al: Serial cerebrospinal fluid corticotropin-releasing hormone concentrations in healthy and depressed humans. *J Clin Endocrinol Metab* 1992; 74:1325.
49. Roy A, Pickar D, Doran A, et al: The corticotropin-releasing hormone stimulation test in chronic schizophrenia. *Am J Psych* 1986; 143:1393.
50. Adinoff B, Martin PR, Bone GHA, et al: Hypothalamic-pituitary-adrenal axis functioning and cerebrospinal fluid corticotropin releasing hormone and corticotropin levels in alcoholics after recent and long-term abstinence. *Arch Gen Psych* 1990; 47:325.
51. Mampalam TJ, Tyrrell JB, Wilson CW: Transsphenoidal microsurgery for Cushing's disease. *Ann Intern Med* 1988; 109:487.
52. Boyer RM, Witkin M, Carruth A, et al: Circadian cortisol rhythms in Cushing's disease. *J Clin Endocrinol Metab* 1979; 48:760.
53. Fitzgerald PA, Aron DC, Findling JW, et al: Cushing's disease: Transient secondary adrenal insufficiency after selective removal of pituitary microadenomas; Evidence for a pituitary origin. *J Clin Endocrinol Metab* 1982; 54:413.
54. Perry RR, Nieman LK, Cutler GB, et al: Primary adrenal causes of Cushing's syndrome: Diagnosis and surgical management. *Ann Surg* 1989; 210:59.
55. Donovan DS, Dluhy RG: AIDS and its effect on the adrenal gland. *Endocrinologist* 1991; 1:227.
56. Pulakhandam U, Dincosy HP: Cytomegaloviral adrenalitis and adrenal insufficiency in AIDS. *Am J Clin Pathol* 1990; 93:651.
57. Tapper ML, Rotterdam HZ, Lerner CW, et al: Adrenal necrosis in the acquired immune deficiency syndrome. *Ann Intern Med* 1984; 100:239.
58. Pang S, Wallace MA, Hofman L, et al: Worldwide experience in newborn screening for classical congenital adrenal hyperplasia due to 21-hydroxylase deficiency. *Pediatrics* 1988; 81:866.
59. Graber AL, Ney RL, Nicholson WE, et al: Natural history of pituitary-adrenal recovery following long-term suppression with corticosteroids. *J Clin Endocrinol Metab* 1965; 25:11.
60. Young CA, Williams JR, MadFarlane IA: Unrecognized Cushing's syndrome and adrenal suppression due to topical clobetasol proprionate. *Br J Clin Practice* 1991; 45:61.
61. Schlaghecke R, Kornely E, Santen RT, et al: The effects of long-term glucocorticoid therapy on pituitary-adrenal responses to exogenous corticotropin-releasing hormone. *N Engl J Med* 1992; 326:226.
62. Doherty GM, Nieman LK, Cutler GB, et al: Time to recovery of the hypotha-

lamic-pituitary-adrenal axis after curative resection of adrenal tumors in patients with Cushing's syndrome. *Surgery* 1990; 108:1085.
63. Bertagna C, Orth DN: Clinical and laboratory findings and results of therapy in fifty-eight patients with adrenocortical tumors admitted to a single medical center (1951 to 1978). *Am J Med* 1981; 71:855.
64. Hill MR, Szefler SJ, Ball BD, et al: Monitoring glucocorticoid therapy: A pharmacokinetic approach. *Clin Pharmacol Ther* 1990; 48:390.
65. Christy NP: Pituitary-adrenal function during corticosteroid therapy (editorial). *New Engl J Med* 1992; 326:266.
66. Streck WF, Lockwood DH: Pituitary adrenal recovery following short term suppression with corticosteroids. *Am J Med* 1989; 66:910.
67. Livanou T, Ferriman D, James VHT: Recovery of hypothalamico-pituitary-adrenal function after corticosteroid therapy. *Lancet* 1967; 2:856.
68. Stacpoole PW, Interlandi JW, Nicholson WE, et al: Isolated ACTH deficiency: A heterogenous disorder. *Medicine* 1982; 61:13.
69. Sauter NP, Toni R, McLaughlin CD, et al: Isolated adrenocorticotropin deficiency associated with an autoantibody to a corticotroph antigen that is not adrenocorticotropin or other proopiomelanocortin-derived peptides. *J Clin Endocrinol Metab* 1990; 70:1391.
70. Jensen MD, Handwerber BS, Scheithauer BW, et al: Lymphocytic hypophysitis with isolated corticotropin deficiency. *Ann Intern Med* 1986; 105:200.
71. Malchoff CD, Javier CJ, Malchoff DM, et al: Primary cortisol resistance presenting as isosexual precocity. *J Clin Endocrinol Metab* 1990; 70:503.
72. Chrousos GP, Vingerhoeds ACM, Loriaux DL, et al: Primary cortisol resistance in man: A glucocorticoid receptor-mediated disease. *J Clin Endocrinol Metab* 1983; 56:1243.
73. Nawata H, Sekya K, Higuchi K, et al: Decreased deoxyribonucleic acid binding of glucocorticoid-receptor complex in cultured skin fibroblasts from a patient with glucocorticoid resistance syndrome. *J Clin Endocrinol Metab* 1987; 65:219.
74. Bronnegard M, Werner S, Gustaffson JA: Primary cortisol resistance associated with a thermolabile glucocorticoid receptor in a patient with fatigue as the only symptom. *J Clin Invest* 1986; 78:1270.
75. Lamberts SWJ, Polderman D, Zweens M, et al: Familial cortisol resistance: Differential diagnostic and therapeutic aspects. *J Clin Endocrinol Metab* 1986; 63:1328.
76. Noribiato G, Bevilacqua M, Vago T, et al: Cortisol resistance in acquired immunodeficiency syndrome. *J Clin Endocrinol Metab* 1992; 74:608.
77. Sistek CJ, Wordell CJ, Hauptman SP: Adjuvant corticosteroid therapy for Pneumocystis carinii pneumonia in AIDS patients. *Ann Pharmacotherapy* 1992; 26:1127.
78. Real FX, Krown SE, Koziner B: Steroid-related development of Kaposi's sarcoma in a homosexual man with Burkitt's lymphoma. *Am J Med* 1986; 30:119.
79. Burnstein KL, Cidlowski JA: The down side of glucocorticoid receptor regulation. *Mol Cell Endocrinol* 1992; 83:C1.
80. Hagg E, Asplund K, Lithner F: Value of basal cortisol assays in the assessment of pituitary-adrenal insufficiency. *Clin Endocrinol* 1987; 26:221.
81. Watts NB, Tindall GT: Rapid assessment of corticotropin reserve after pituitary surgery. *JAMA* 1988; 259:708.
82. Udesman R, Norton JA, Jelenich SE, et al: Responses of the hypothalamic-pituitary-adrenal and renin-angiotensin axes and the sympathetic system dur-

ing controlled surgical and anesthetic stress. *J Clin Endocrinol Metab* 1987; 64:986.
83. Patel SR, Jeffcoat WJ: The short Synacthen test in acute hospital admissions. *Acta Endocrinol* 1991; 35:259.
84. Hawkins JB, Burch WM: Rapid tests of adrenocortical function: Intravenous versus intramuscular administration of synthetic ACTH. *North Carolina Med J* 1989; 50:306.
85. Orth DN: Personal communication, 1993.
86. Jackson RV, Grice JE, Jackson AJ, et al: Naloxone-induced ACTH release in man is inhibited by clonidine. *Clin Exp Pharmacol Physiol* 1990; 17:179.
87. Lord JAH, Waterfield AA, Hughes J, et al: Endogenous opiod peptides: Multiple agonists and receptors. *Nature* 1991; 267:495.
88. Loriaux DL, Nieman L: Corticotropin-releasing hormone testing in pituitary disease. *Endocrinol and Metab Clin North Amer* 1991; 20:363.
89. Lindholm J, Kehlet H, Blichert-Toft M, et al: Reliability of the 30 minute ACTH test in assessing hypothalamic-pituitary-adrenal function. *J Clin Endocrinol Metab* 1978; 47:272.
90. Chrousos GP, Schulte HM, Oldenfeld EH, et al: The corticotropin-releasing factor stimulation test: An aid in the evaluation of patients with Cushing's syndrome. *New Engl J Med* 1984; 310:622.
91. Gaitan D, Loosen PT, Burns D, et al: Plasma ACTH response to naloxone in major depressive disorder (MDD), chronic alcoholism (ALC), Cushing's disease (CD), and normal subjects (NL). *Proceedings of the 75th Annual Meeting of the Endocrine Society*. Bethesda, Md, 1993, p 238.

Advances in Internal Medicine® Cumulative Index Volumes 35–39

(The numbers in italics indicate the volume.)

B

G

H

M

N

Q

R

S

T

U

V

X

Y

Z